FUNDAMENTALS OF VETERINARY ANATOMY

NIPA GENX ELECTRONIC RESOURCES & SOLUTIONS P. LTD.
New Delhi-110 034

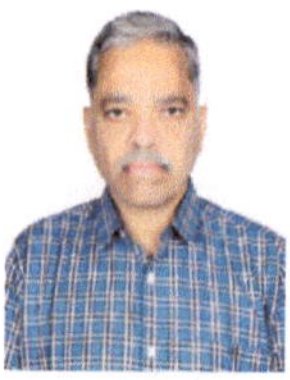

Prof. T.S Chandrasekhara Rao has vast experience of administration for more than 10 years as Dean, Faculty of Veterinary Science SVVU, Tirupati. He served as Director of Research (FAC) for two and half years, Associate Dean College of Veterinary Science, Tirupati for 3 years and Head of the Department of Anatomy, College of Veterinary Science, Tirupati for 12 years. Dr. Rao was Member, Board of Management, KVAFSU, Academic Council, TANUVAS and KVAFSU, Sectoral Committee of Accreditation Board of ICAR, Governing Council, NAVS for two terms, Advisory Body of National Testing Agency, Ministry of HRD, Govt. of India for All India ICAR-UG, PG and JRF/SRF Examination and advisory body of VCI, FAO Fellow at Cornell University, USA, President, Indian Assoc. of Vet. Anatomists for six years and PI of ICAR Ad hoc Research Scheme. He was conferred Bharat Ratna Dr. C. Subramaniam outstanding Teacher award of ICAR and Meritorious Teacher Award of Govt. of A.P. and is Fellow of IAVA,NAVS and IAAVR and authored one text book, two monographs, a chapter in 'ICAR Hand Book of Animal Husbandry" and prepared 12 Laboratory Manuals. He has published 169 research papers, guided 8 research scholars and organized three national Conferences. He was referee for 9 Journals and Member Editorial Board of Indian Buffalo Journal, and Indian journal of Vet. Research. He was Chairman, BSMAC on Basic veterinary sciences for revision of ICAR PG regulations and syllabus 2020 and is also Chairman of the commttee of ICAR for revision of ARS syllabus for basic veterinary sciences (2022). He is on Expert panel for recruitment of Teachers of 16 universities, UPSC and ASRB, Member, Research Council, KVASU and Academic Council, BEST Innovation University and Member, QRT of IVRI.

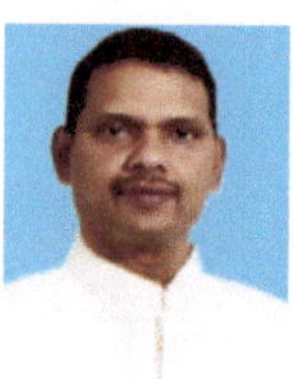

Prof. P. Jagapathi Ramayya is presently working as Technical Officer to Vice-Chancellor of SVVU, Tirupati. He joined in the service as an Assistant Professor on 5-3-1999. His specialization is Developmental anatomy and Histology. He completed his B.V.Sc & AH in 1993 and M.V.Sc during 1997 from ANGRAU and Ph.D during 2007 from GADVASU, Ludhiana. He is recipient of State best teacher award, Fellow Indian Association of Veterinary Anatomists (2016), Dr. A.M Srivastava Award for Best Ph.D thesis, Dr. P.S Lalitha Award (2009) for Best publication in IJVA and Dr. G.Rajeswara Rao Memorial award (2011). He Published 92 research publications in various Journals of National and International repute and he is referee for 8 National and International journals. He guided 5 M.V.Sc and 3 Ph.D students of Veterinary Anatomy. He is Principal Investigator of NAHEP (I.G) project of ICAR, New Delhi. He is author for Text Book entitled "Fundamentals of Developmental Anatomy" Published in 2012. He prepared 6 Lab manuals for U.G and P.G courses and he also Prepared "Virtual Dissection Software of Cow" as an alternative for dissection in Veterinary Anatomy at CVSc, Tirupati.

FUNDAMENTALS OF VETERINARY ANATOMY

T.S. Chandrasekhara Rao
Former Dean, Faculty of
Veterinary Science, SVVU, Tirupati &
Presently Professor and University Head
Department of Veterinary Anatomy
College of Veterinary Science, Tirupati

P. Jagapathi Ramayya
Professor of Veterinary Anatomy &
Technical Officer to Vice-Chancellor
SVVU, Tirupati

Illustrations by
S. Dhilleswara Rao

NIPA GENX ELECTRONIC RESOURCES & SOLUTIONS P. LTD.
New Delhi-110 034

NIPA GENX ELECTRONIC
RESOURCES & SOLUTIONS P. LTD.

101,103, Vikas Surya Plaza, CU Block
L.S.C.Market, Pitam Pura, New Delhi-110 034
Ph : +91 11 27341616, 27341717, 27341718
E-mail:newindiapublishingagency@gmail.com
www: www.nipabooks.com
For customer assistance, please contact
Phone: + 91-11-27 34 17 17 Fax: + 91-11- 27 34 16 16
E-Mail: feedbacks@nipabooks.com

ISBN: 978-93-90175-10-9

Composed and Designed by NIPA.

PREFACE

The text book entitled "Fundamentals of Veterinary Anatomy" has been prepared for the benefit of B.V.Sc &A.H students as per the Veterinary Council of India (MSVE 2016) syllabus. Previously, the Veterinary Anatomy course used to be taught system wise to the BVSc & A.H students in first and second academic years. But in the MSVE 2016 regulations the students have to study the entire Anatomy course in the first professional year only on Regional approach. This prompted us to prepare a book as per the MSVE 2016 syllabus to meet the requirements of the students and Faculty.

The material available in this book has been prepared based on our previous experiences in practical classes and also some information was collected from the standard text books of Veterinary Anatomy and also Madras Veterinary College Lecture Notes prepared by Faculty of Madras Veterinary College, Chennai. In this book every topic is supported by hand drawn diagrams and photographs of original specimens available in the department. To give better pictorial presentation some of the specimens like bones and ligaments of joints are painted and photographed in this book.

Further, the information in this book is made very crisp and optimum and some important points are highlighted, so that students can understand easily, which is highly useful to the students in examination point of view and it creates interest. This text book provides comprehensive knowledge to the undergraduate, postgraduate students, clinicians and faculty in the discipline of Veterinary Anatomy.

The authors highly acknowledge the services of Dr S.Dhilleswara Rao, Assistant professor, Dr T. Sai Urmila and Dr K.Mohana Sujana of this department and P.N.S.S Praneeth for drawing the neat diagrams in this book.

T.S. Chandrasekhara Rao

P.Jagapathi Ramayya

CONTENTS

UNIT 4: THORAX

UNIT 5: ABDOMEN

UNIT 6: PELVIS AND HIND LIMB

LIST OF FIGURES

UNIT 1: General Anatomy

UNIT 2: Fore Limb

UNIT 3: Head and Neck

UNIT 4: Thorax

UNIT 5: Abdomen

UNIT 6: Pelvis and Hind Limb

UNIT 1
GENERAL ANATOMY

1.1 GENERAL OSTEOLOGY

INTRODUCTION

Anatomy is the branch of biological science which deals with the form and structure of organisms. The word "Anatomy" is derived from Greek, means cutting apart (***Ana –separate, tomy-cut***).

The study with unaided eye is **Gross Anatomy / Macroscopic anatomy** while the study of finer details of structure with the aid of a **Microscope is *Histology / Microscopic Anatomy*.**

Gross anatomy is studied in two chief ways:-

1. **Systematic anatomy:** is the study of the structures that make up a discrete body system i.e group of structures work together to perform a unique body function. The divisions are:
   (a) **Osteology** – study of bones of the skeleton
   (b) **Arthrology** - study of the joints
   (c) **Myology** – study of the muscles
   (d) **Splanchnology** – study of visceral organs i.e. digestive, respiratory and urogenital systems.
   (e) **Angiology** – study of circulatory system
   (f) **Neurology** – study of nervous system
   (g) **Aesthesiology** – study of sense organs and common integument.
2. **Topographical anatomy**: is the study in which the different structures are investigated in the order in which they would present themselves in the course of dissection. It is nothing but regional approach.

The application of anatomical facts and their relation to surgery, diagnosis and obstetrical aspects is ***Applied Anatomy.***

Descriptive terms: Certain terms are used in descriptions of the various parts of the body with regard to their position, direction etc.

Ventral or Inferior: The surface directed towards the ground.

Dorsal or Superior: The surface directed away from the ground.

Cranial / Cephalic/ Anterior: refer to the direction towards the head.

Caudal / Posterior: refers to the direction towards the tail.

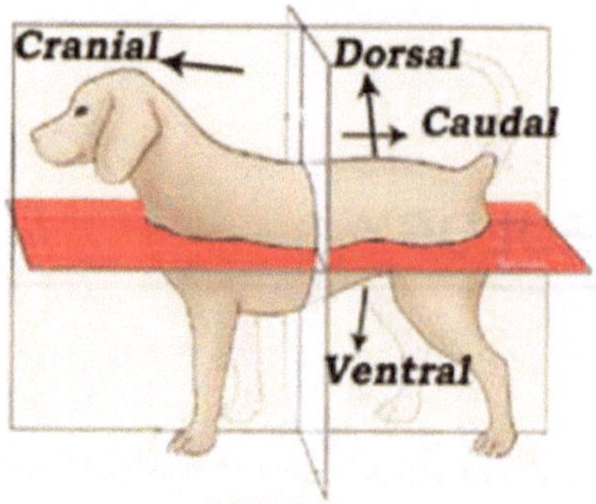

Fig. 1.1: Different Directions

Medial and Lateral: The structre which is **nearer to the median plane** is called ***medial*** and structure **away from the median plane is called *lateral*.**

Superficial and Deep: The relative distances of the structures from the surface of the body are indicated by the terms ***superficial and deep.***

The term **internal and external** express relative distance from the centre of an organ or cavity.

Proximal and Distal express relative distances from the root of the limb and also the direction towards or away from any centre, axis or base (**Fig.1.2**).

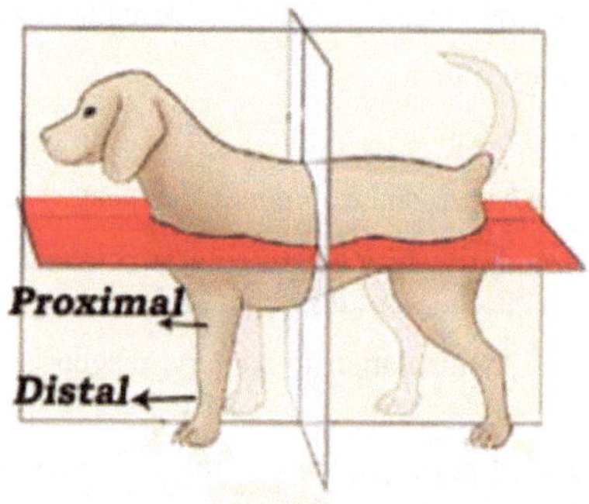

Fig. 1.2: Proximal and Distal

Axial and abaxial are used to denote structures lying towards or away from the central axis of the limb (**Fig.1.3**).

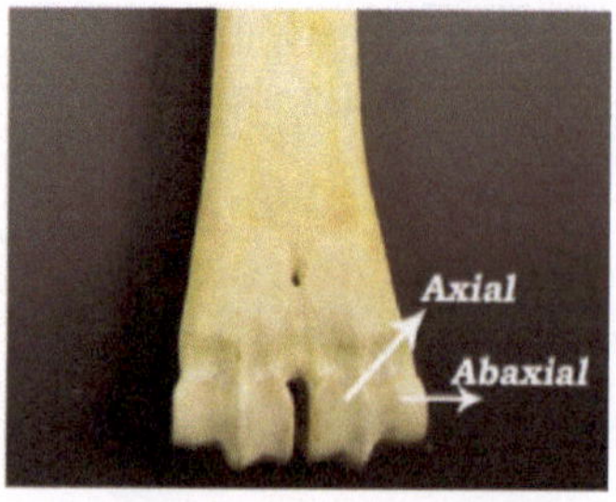

Fig. 1.3: Large Metacarpal

Anatomical Planes: The vertebrate body exhibits three body axes, an **antero posterior or longitudinal axis**, a **dorsoventral or vertical axis** and a **left-right or transverse axis**. Two body axes are necessary to establish an anatomical plane.

1. **The median or sagittal plane**: is established by the **longitudinal and vertical axes** and a cut in this plane is ***called sagittal section*** **(Fig.1.4)**. Planes parallel to sagittal plane but not on the median line are ***called parasagittal planes***.

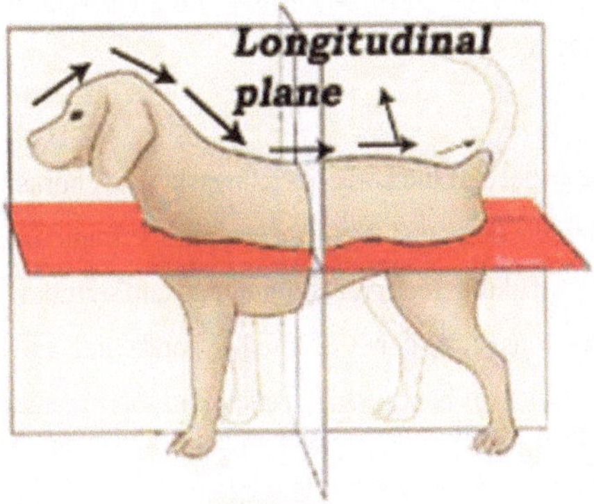

Fig. 1.4: Sagittal Plane

2. **The transverse plane:** is established by the **left-right (transverse) and vertical axes** and a cut in this plane is a ***cross section***.
3. **The frontal or horizontal plane:** is established by the **longitudinal and transverse axes** and a cut in this plane is ***called frontal section*** **(Fig.1.5)**.

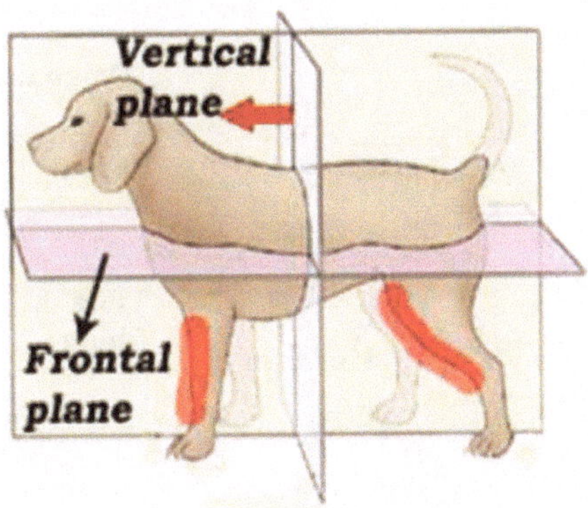

Fig. 1.5: Frontal (Horizontal) Plane

Skeleton is framework of hard structures supporting and protecting the soft tissues of the animals (**Figs.1.6 to 1.10**). The fresh dead bone appears **yellowish white in colour**, while in the living animal it appears **bluish pink. Bones are the hardest structures in the body (excepting the teeth).**

Functions of Bones

1. Support and protect the softer tissues of the body
2. Form the frame work or skeleton of the body.
3. Act as levers to which muscles or their tendons and ligaments are attached and serve as parts of locomotor apparatus.
4. Have bone marrow which is one of the important sources of blood corpuscles.
5. Bones are one of the main sources of calcium.

Classification of Skeleton

1. **Exoskeleton** - found on the surface of the body (eg: claws, hooves, horns).
2. **Endoskeleton** - found within the body and forms the supportive framework. It consists of three parts
   (a) **Axial skeleton** – consists of skull, vertebral column, ribs and sternum (**Fig.1.6**).
   (b) **Appendicular skeleton** - consists of bones of fore (pectoral) limb and hind (pelvic) limb.
   (c) **Splanchnic skeleton** - consists of bones which develop in soft organs. **eg:** ***Os penis*** - in penis of dog; ***Os cordis*** - in heart of adult ox; ***Os phrenic*** - in diaphragm of the camel, ***Os rostri*** - in snout of pigs and ***Os clitoris*** in clitoris of cats.

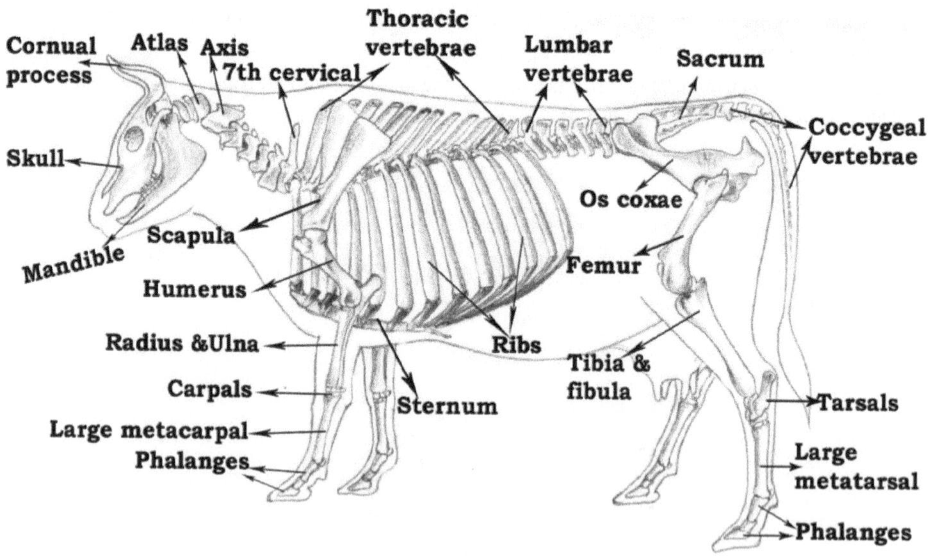

Fig. 1.6: Skeleton of Ox

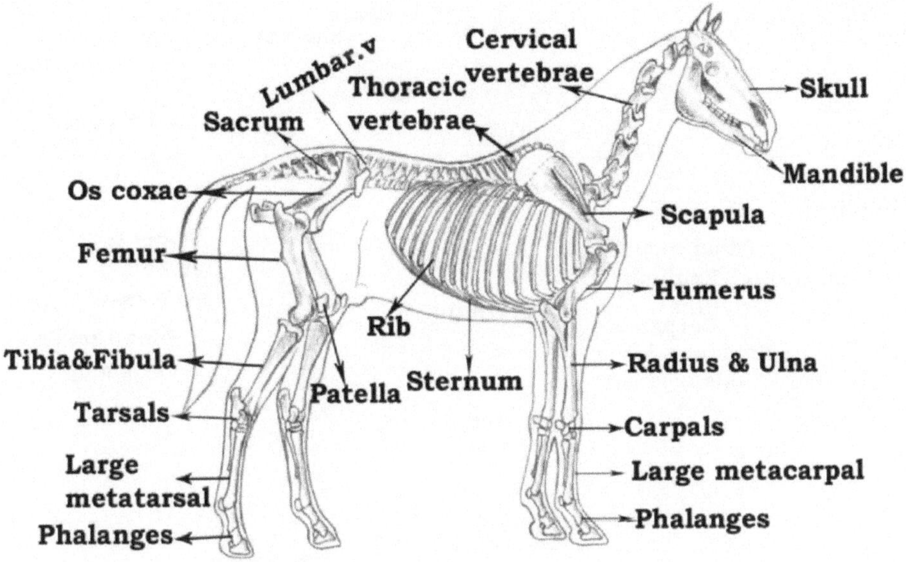

Fig. 1.7: Skeleton of Horse

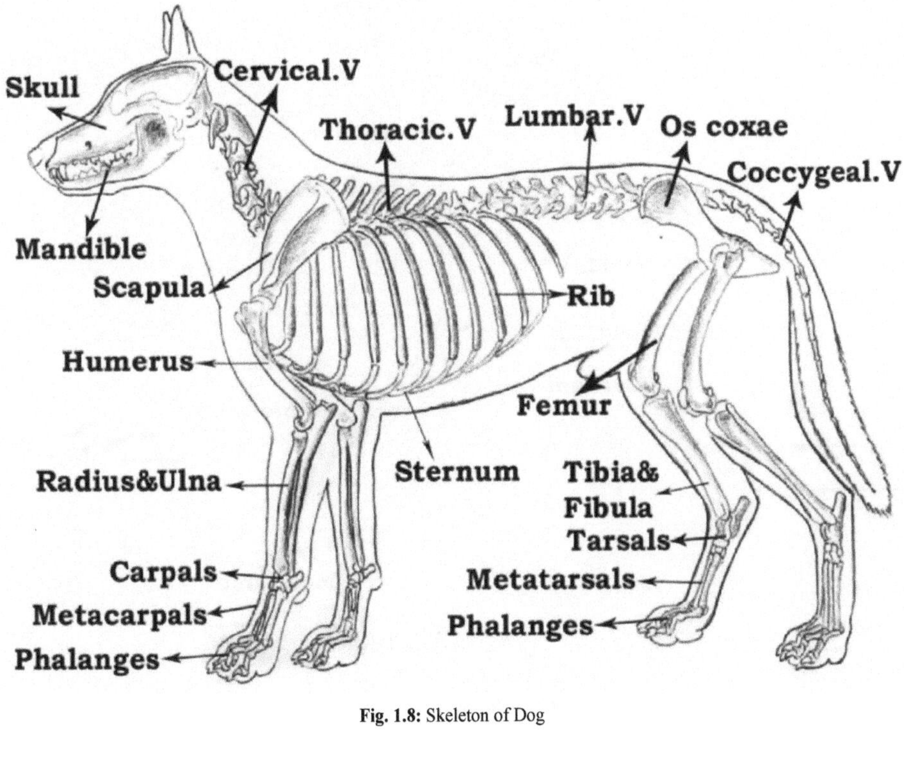

Fig. 1.8: Skeleton of Dog

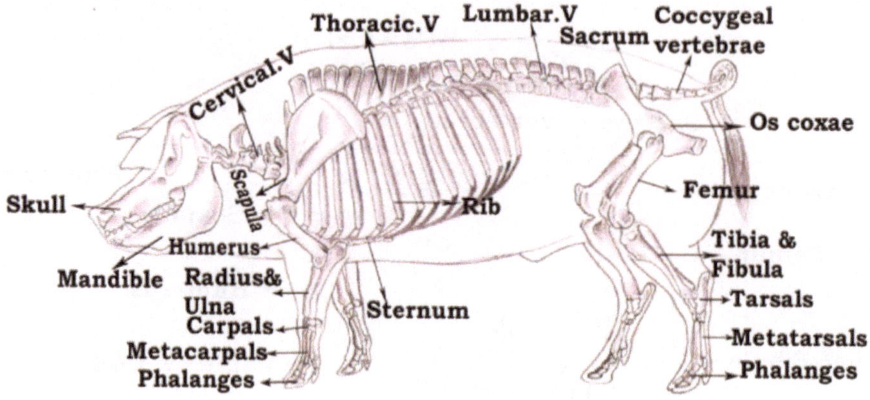

Fig. 1.9: Skeleton of Pig

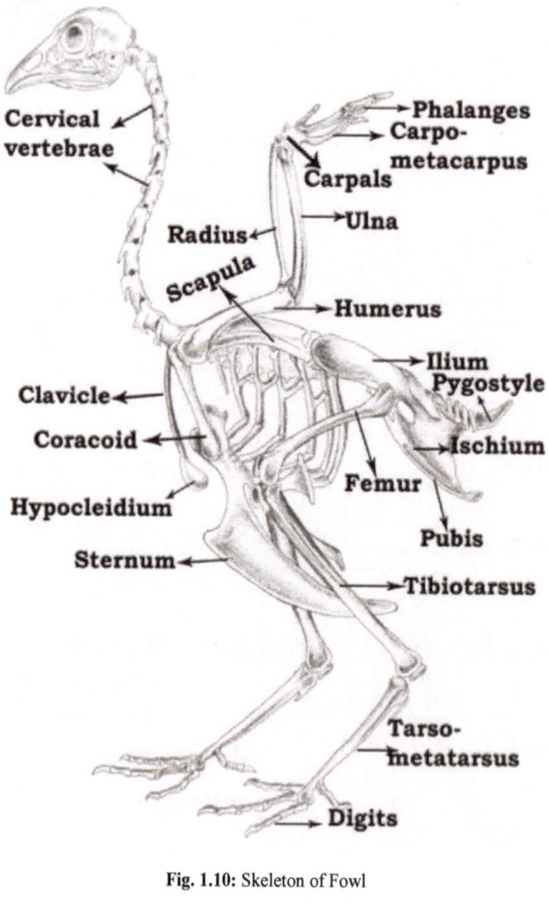

Fig. 1.10: Skeleton of Fowl

Classification of bones

1. Based on structure, bones are classified as **compact and cancellous (spongy) bone**. The **compact bone** is dense, white and forms the outer shell of the bone. Microscopically it shows the ***Haversian systems (osteons).*** The ***cancellous bone*** is made up of delicate plates which intercross with each other forming mesh work with spaces containing marrow in living animal. Haversian systems are absent in this type. ***All the bones except few flat bones of skull contain both the types.***

2. The bones are classified based **on their shape and function** as **long bones, flat bones, short bones and irregular bones.**

   a. **Long bones:** Have a shaft (diaphysis) and two extremities (epiphyses) with well developed medullary cavity in shaft **eg: humerus, femur (Fig.1.11)**. Some long bones do not develop completely and are called **aborted long bones** in which medullary cavity is very small or even absent. **eg: ulna of horse (Fig.1.12).** Some long bones are **elongated** and medullary cavity is completely absent. Such bones are referred to as elongated long bones **eg: ribs (Fig.1.13).**

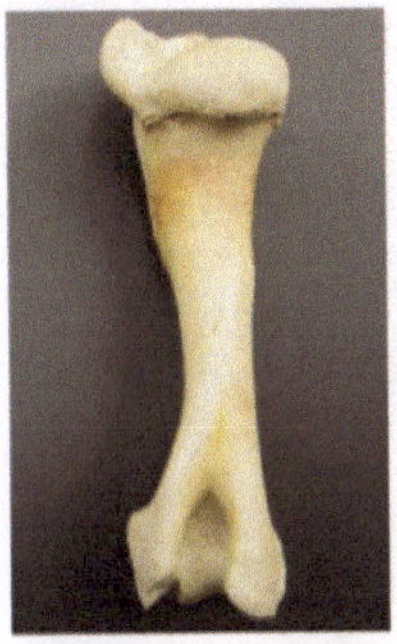

Fig. 1.11: Humerus

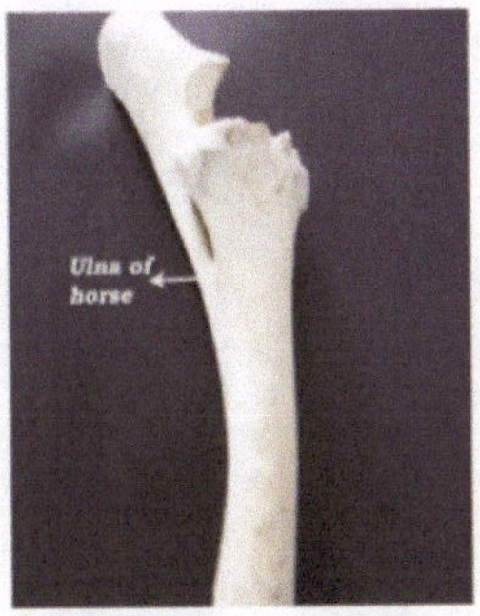

Fig. 1.12: Radius & Ulna

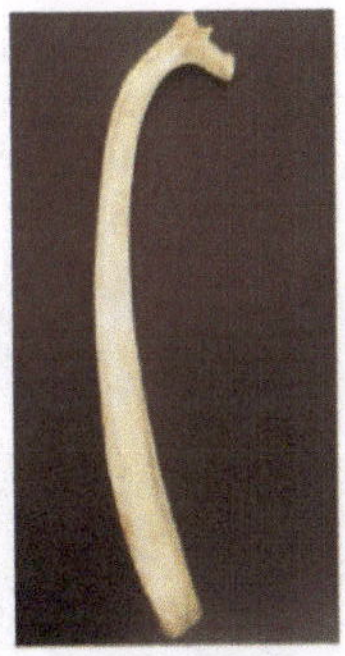

Fig. 1.13: Rib

Epiphyses (extremities) of long bones consists of **an outer compact bone** and **inner cancellous (spongy) bone**, while the the **diaphysis (shaft)** consists of **an outer comapct bone and an inner medullary cavity (Fig.1.14).**

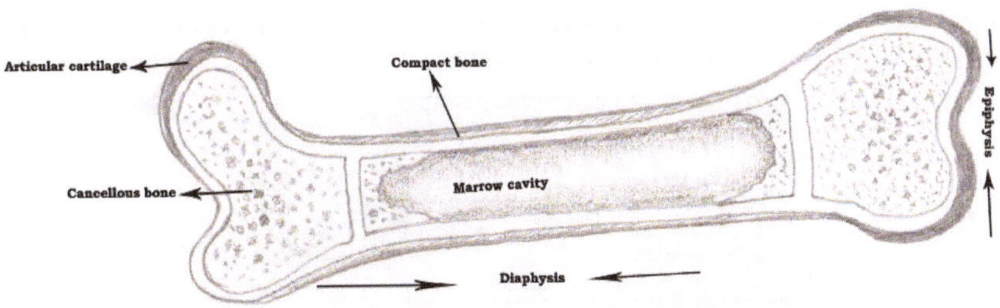

Fig. 1.14: Structure of Long Bone

b. **Flat bones:** These are **plate like and show large surface area for the attachment of muscles** and protection of subjacent structures. There are two layers of compact bone separated by spongy bone (***diploe***) **eg: scapula (Fig.1.15), bones of skull (Fig.1.20).**

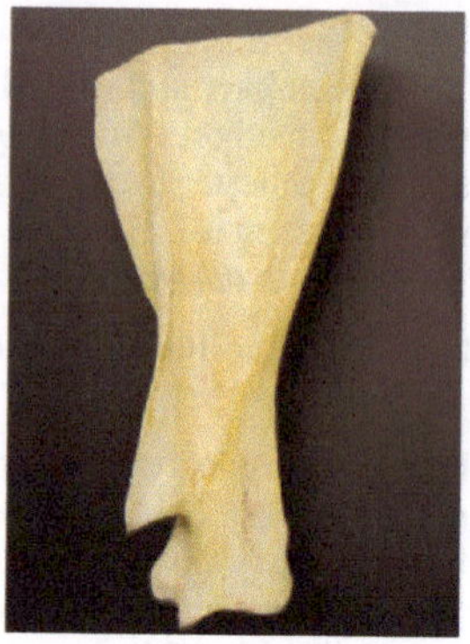

Fig. 1.15: Scapula

c. **Short bones:** Present **similar dimensions of length, breadth and thickness**. Medullary cavity is completely absent in these bones and are mostly made up of spongy bone covered by a thin layer of compact bone. **eg: carpals (Fig.1.16), tarsals. Sesamoid bones** are those short bones which ***do not bear the weight of the body*** but increase the leverage for tendons. **eg: patella, proximal and distal sesamoids (Fig.1.17).**

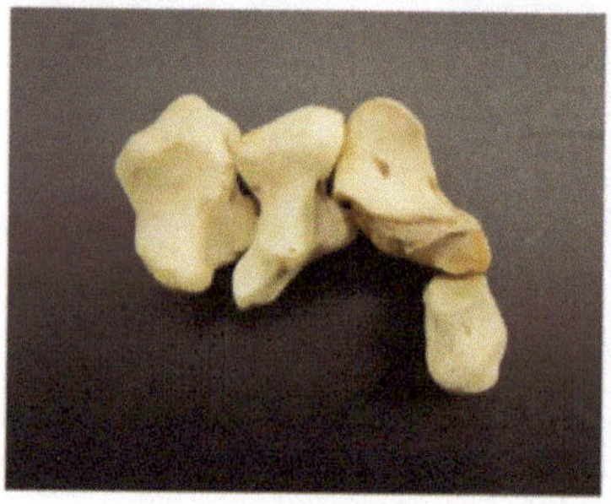

Fig. 1.16: Carpals

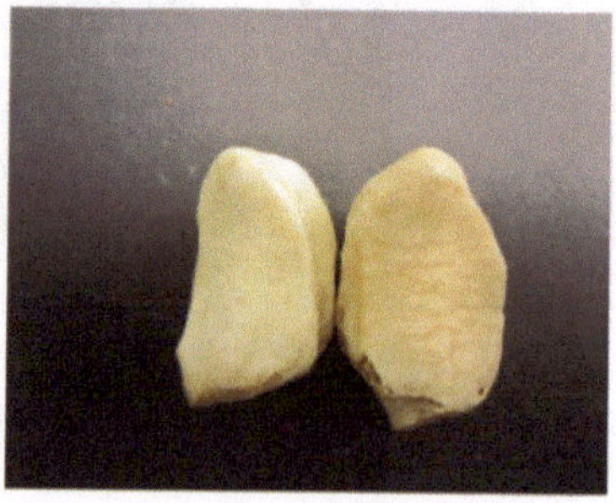

Fig. 1.17: Sesamoids

d. **Irregular bones:** are **irregular in shape because of the presence of processes** and are unpaired bones usually placed on the median line. They resemble short bones in structure. **eg: vertebrae (Fig.1.18).**

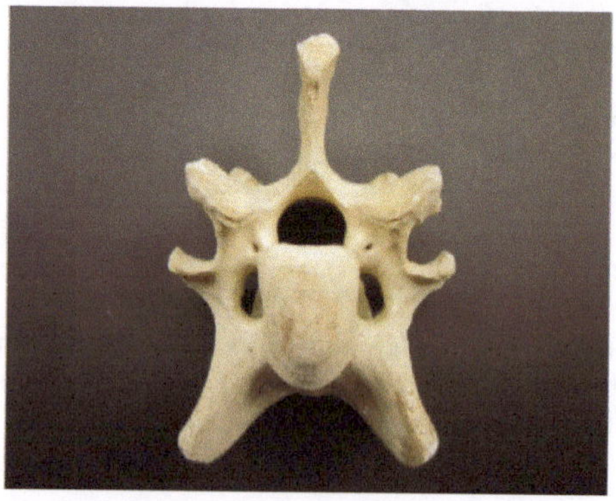

Fig. 1.18: Cervical Vertebra

The short, flat and irregular bones have following appearance on cross section **(Fig.1.19).**

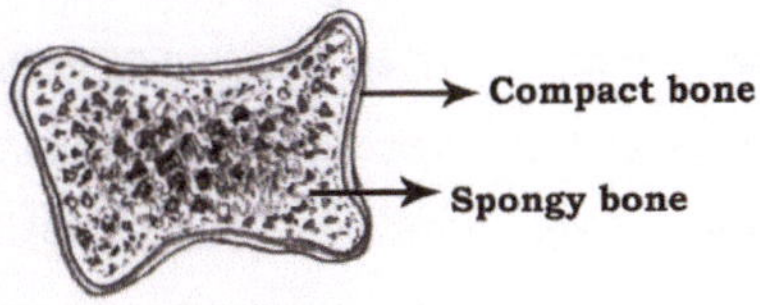

Fig. 1.19: Structure of Short, Flat & Irregular Bones

e. **Pneumatic bones:** Some bones contain air spaces between the two layers of the compact substance instead of spongy bone and marrow and are called **pneumatic bones**. These cavities lined by mucous membrane are termed **sinuses. eg: In mammals**: **frontal (Fig.1.20), maxilla and palatine. In fowl: vertebrae, sternum, humerus (Fig.1.21), femur**. In birds **medullary cavity of long bones** and spaces of spongy bone are partly filled with marrow the remaining part being **occupied by diverticula of air sacs.**

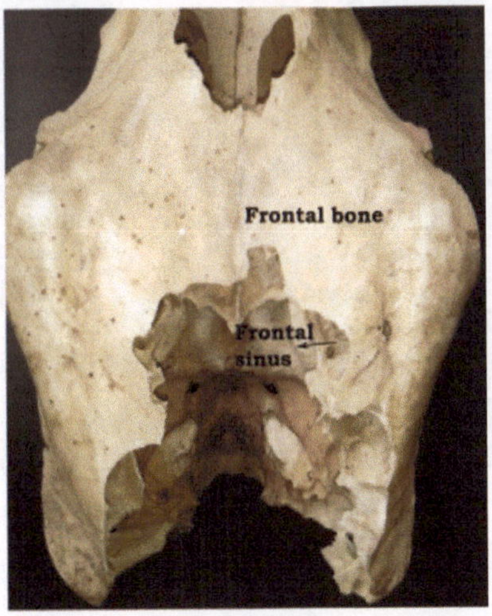

Fig. 1.20: Sinus in Frontal Bone of Skull

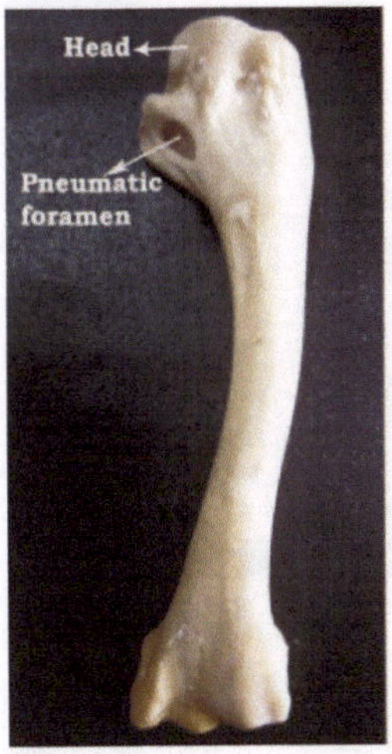

Fig. 1.21: Humerus of Fowl

TERMS USED TO DESIGNATE THE FEATURES OF THE BONES

Facet- is a flat articular surface of a bone.

Process -is a general term for prominence **eg: Acromion process of scapula, (Fig.1.22).**

Tubercle - is a small blunt projection (**eg: Teres tubercle of humerus, Fig.1.24**). If more developed is called tuberosity (**eg. Medial tuberosity of humerus, Fig.1.24**), while a trochanter is the largest of these (**eg. Trochanter major of femur, Fig.1.25**).

Spine - is a pointed projection (**eg. Scapular spine, Fig.1.22).**

Crest - is a sharp ridge (**eg. Tibial crest**).

Head - is a rounded articular area (**eg. Humerus, Fig.1.24**).

Condyle - is cylindrical articular eminence (**eg. Femur, Fig.1.25**).

Epicondyle – is a non-articular projection (**eg**: **Humerus, Fig.1.24**).

Trochlea - is a pulley like articular area (**eg. Femur Fig.1.25**).

Glenoid cavity - is a shallow cup like articular depression (**eg: Scapula, Fig.1.22**).

Cotyloid cavity is a deeper cup like articular depression (**eg: Acetabulum of Os coxae, Fig.1.23**).

Fovea: is a small depression present on a bone (**eg: Fovea capitis present on head of femur)**

Foramen - is a perforation for the transmission of vessels and nerves (**eg: Maxillary foramen**).

Sinus - is an air cavity within a bone or bones lined with mucous membrane which communicates with exterior (**eg: Frontal sinus in frontal bone, Fig.1.20**).

Hiatus - is a depression leading to two or more foramina (eg: ***Maxillary hiatus*** - consisting of ***posterior palatine, sphenopalatine and maxillary foramina***).

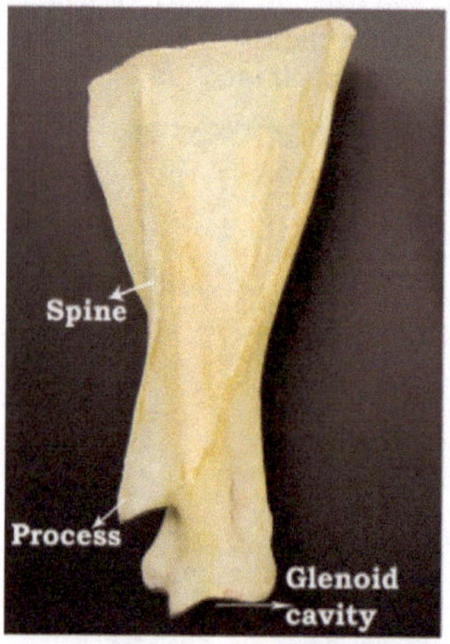

Fig. 1.22: Scapula

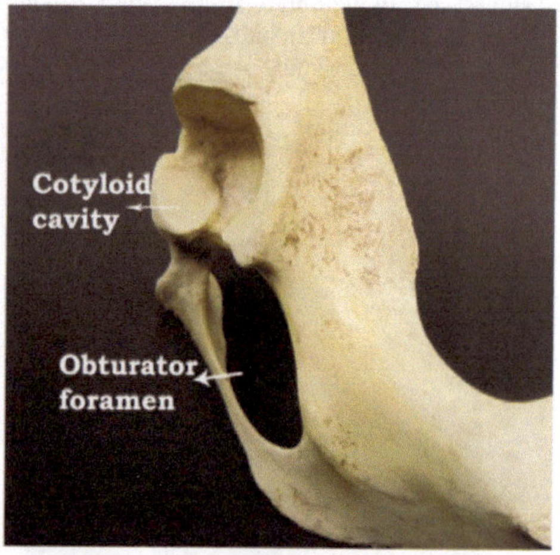

Fig. 1.23: Os Coxae

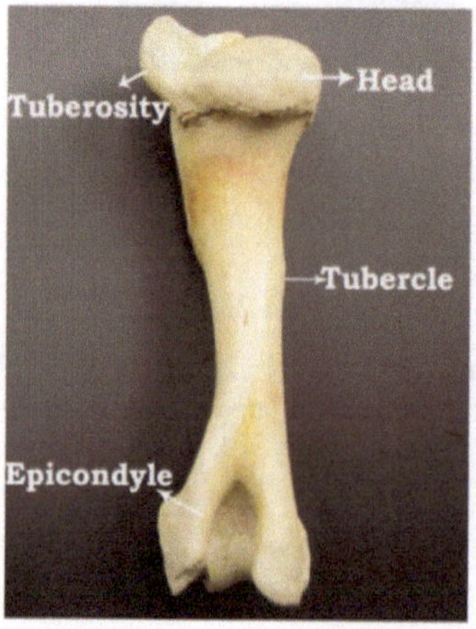

Fig. 1.24: Humerus

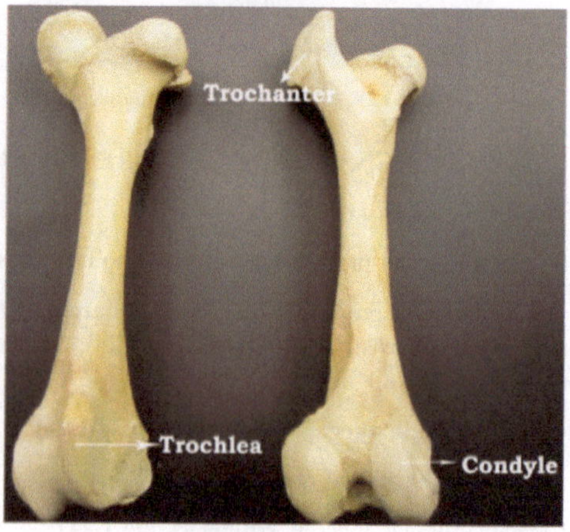

Fig. 1.25: Femur

DIFFERENT REGIONS AND BONES OF PECTORAL LIMB

1. **Pectoral girdle and shoulder region**: Scapula (*shoulder blade*), coracoid and clavicle.
2. **Arm** - Humerus
3. **Forearm** - Radius and Ulna
4. **Manus** consists of

   a. **Carpus** - consisting of small bones arranged in two rows. The number varies with species (**Fig.1.26**).

   b. **Metacarpus** - consists of five bones designated by numbers 1 to 5 but shows considerable modifications in different species (**Fig.1.26, 1.27**).

   c. **Digits** - form the terminal parts of the limbs. The number varies with the species (**Figs.1.26, 1.27**).

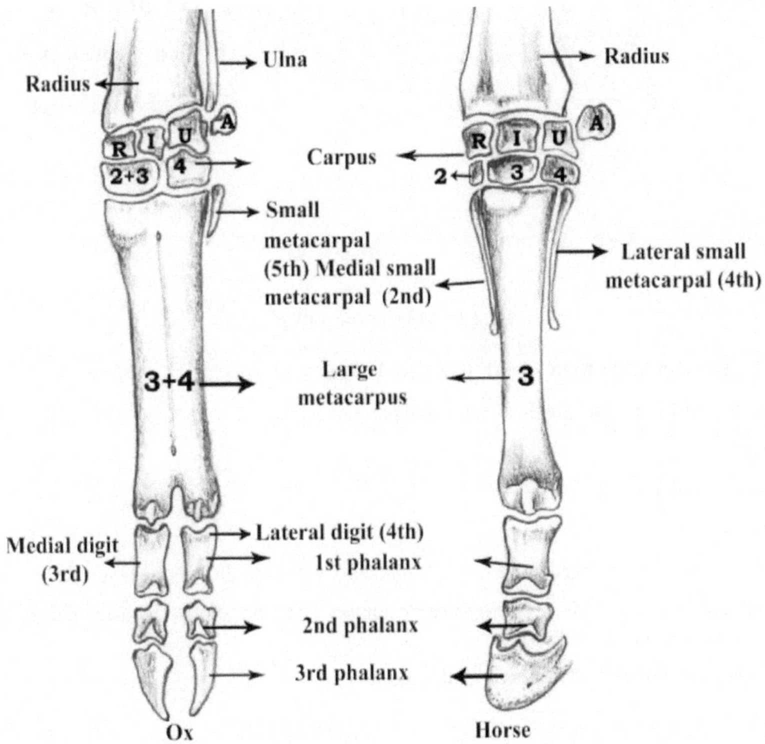

Fig. 1.26: Manus of Ox and Horse

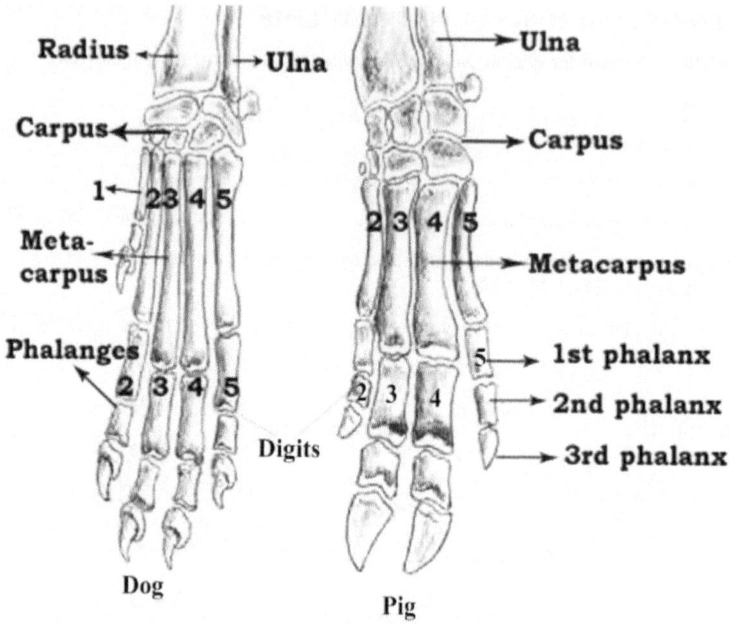

Fig. 1.27: Manus of Dog and Pig

DIFFERENT REGIONS AND BONES OF PELVIC LIMB

1. **Pelvic girdle and hip region**: Ilium, ischium and pubis.
2. **Thigh**: Femur
3. **Leg**: Tibia and fibula
4. **Pes**: Consists of
    a. **Tarsus**: small bones arranged in 3 rows. The number varies with the species **(Fig.1.28).**
    b. **Metatarsus**: consists of 5 bones designated by number 1 to 5 but shows considerable modifications in different species **(Fig.1.28, 1.29).**
    c. **Digits**: The number of digits varies with the species.

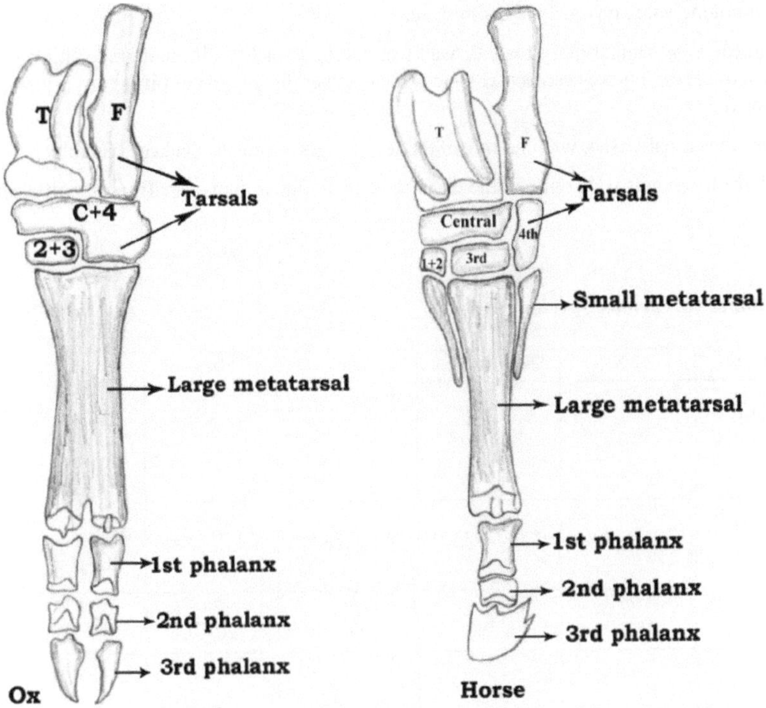

Fig. 1.28: Pes of Ox and Horse

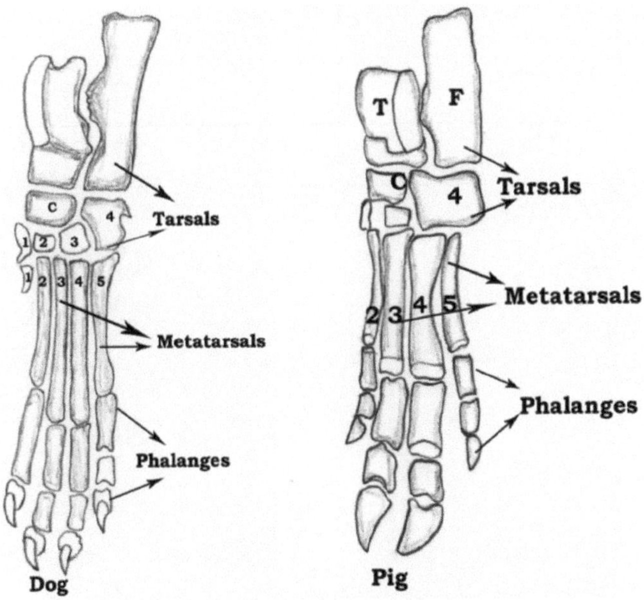

Fig. 1.29: Pes of Dog and Pig

Types of locomotion: Three types of locomotion are.

1. **Digitigrade** is an animal that stands or walks on its digits or toes. In digitigrade animals, more than one segment of the digit makes contact with the ground, either directly (**as in birds**) or via paw-pads (**as in cats and dogs**).
2. **Plantigrades** usually walk with the ***sole*** of the feet (i.e pes) on the ground.**eg: Humans**
3. **Unguligrade** animals walk only on the distal most tips of their digits. **eg: Horses, cattle, sheep, goat and pigs.**

Number of Bones In Various Species

Particulars of bone	OX	Sheep and Goat	Horse	Dog	Pig	Fowl
Skull (including 3 middle ear ossicles, 3 parts of temporal are treated as one)	34	34	34	34	30	38 (including 2 quadrate bones)
Vertebral column	50 ($C_7T_{13}L_6S_5Cy_{19}$)	47 ($C_7T_{13}L_6S_4Cy_{16}$)	54 ($C_7T_{18}L_6S_5Cy_{18}$)	53 ($C_7T_{13}L_7S_3Cy_{23}$)	52-53 (C_7T_{14-15} L_6S_4,Cy_{21})	42 (C_{14},T_7,L-S_{14},CY_7)
Ribs	26 (13x2)	26 (13x2)	36 (18x2)	26 (13x2)	28-30 (14-15x2)	14 (7x2)
Sternum	1	1	1	1	1	1
Thoracic limb	24x2=48	24x2=48	20x2=40	41x2=82	40x2=80	13x2=26
Hind limb (Three parts of os coxae are treated as one)	24x2=48	24x2=48	20x2=40	41x2=82	40x2=80	21x2=42
Other bones	1 (Os cordis)	-	-	1 (Os penis)	1 (Os rostri)	6 (uncinate process)
Total no.of bones in body	208	204	205	279	272-275	169

1.2 GENERAL ARTHROLOGY

An articulation or joint is formed by the union of **two or more bones** or cartilages. Bone is the fundamental part of most joints; in some cases a bone and a cartilage or two cartilages, form a joint. The uniting medium is chiefly fibrous tissue or cartilage or a mixture of these.

Different joints of the animal body (Fig.1.30).

1. Head	1.Sutures between bones of skull 2.Symphyseal joint of mandible 3.Temporomandibular articulation 4.Temporohyoidean articulation 5.Occipito -atlantal articulation
2. Vertebral column	1. Intercentral articulations 2. Interneural articulations 3. Occipito -atlantal articulation 4.Atlanto-axial articulation
3. Thorax	1. Costovertebral articulations (Costocentral and Costotransverse) 2. Costochondral articulations 3. Chondrosternal articulations 4. Sternal articulations
4. Forelimb:	1.Shoulder joint – summit of lateral tuberosity of humerus forms point of shoulder 2. Elbow (cubital) joint – point of elbow is formed by summit of olecranon process. 3. Radio-ulnar articulations. 4.Carpal joint – Radioulnar- carpal, Proximal carpal, Intercarpal, Distal carpal and carpometacarpal articulations 5.Metacarpal articulations 6.Fetlock Joint-metacarpophalangeal joint. 7.Pastern joint: Proximal interphalangeal joint 8.Coffin joint : Distal interphalangeal joint
5. Hind Limb	1.Sacroiliac articulation 2.Hip (coxofemoral) joint 3. Stifle joint a. Femoro patellar articulation b. Femoro tibial articulation 4. Tibiofibular articulations 5. Hock joint 6.Fetlock joint: Metatarso phalangeal joint 7.Pastern joint: Proximal inter phalangeal joint 8.Coffin joint : Distal interphalangeal joint

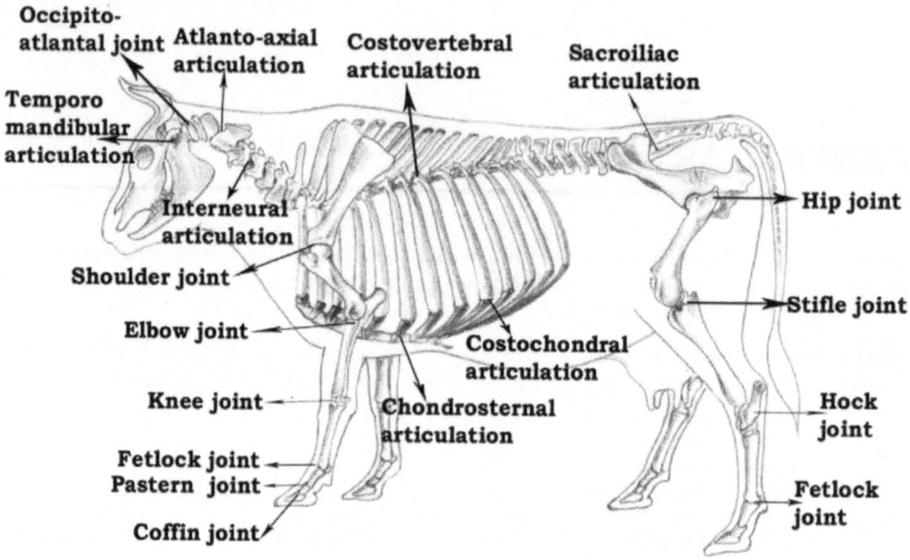

Fig. 1.30: Different Joint Regions of Animal Body

The joints are classified developmentally into three types: (a) ***Fibrous joints***-formerly known as ***synarthrosis*** (b) ***Cartilaginous joints***-formerly known as ***amphiarthrosis*** and (c) ***Synovial joints***-formerly called as ***diarthrosis***.

I. FIBROUS JOINTS: are classified as follows

(1) **Suture:** The term suture is applied to the those joints in the skull in which the adjacent bones are closely united by fibrous tissue – the ***sutural ligament***. The different types of sutures are:

a) ***Sutura serrata***: In this type bones have irregular interlocking margins.

eg: Interfrontal suture (Fig.1.31).

b) ***Sutura squamosa***: In this edges overlap, e.g., **between the squamous part of the temporal and the parietal bone.**

c) ***Sutura plana (harmonia)***: In this edges are plane or slightly roughened. **eg: Internasal suture (Fig.1.31). and suture between horizontal parts of the palatine bones.**

(2) **Syndesmosis:** In these the uniting medium is white fibrous or elastic tissue or a mixture. **eg: union of the shafts of the metacarpal bones.** The original material undergoes ossification with advancing age and the process is then ***known as synostosis.***

(3) **Gomphosis:** This term is sometimes applied to the implantation of the teeth in the alveoli.

(4) **Schindylesis:** One bone is fitted into the groove of another. **e.g. Perpendicular part of ethmoid fitting into vomer.**

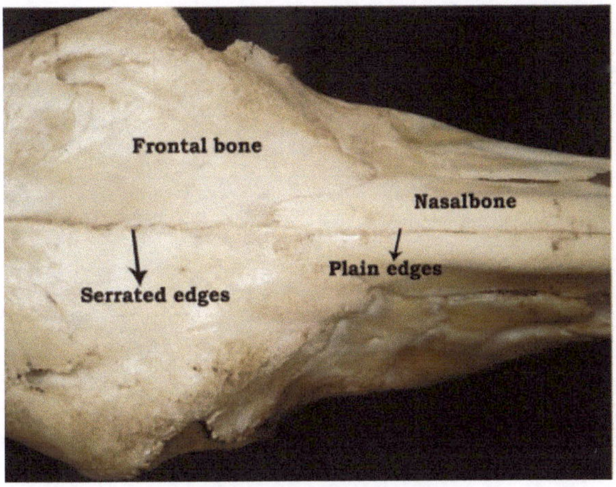

Fig. 1.31: Types of Sutures in the Skull

II. CARTILAGINOUS JOINTS: The bones of cartilaginous joints are united by **fibrocartilage or hyaline cartilage**. Various types of cartilaginous joints are;

1. ***Synchondrosis (hyaline cartilage joints)*:** The opposing bones are connected by **hyaline cartilage.** ***eg: Occipito-sphenoid articulation.***

2. ***Symphysis (Fibro-cartilaginous joints)*:** The uniting medium is **cartilage and fibrous tissue** and the term is restricted to median joints connecting symmetrical parts. ***eg: mandibular symphysis and pelvic symphysis.***

III. SYNOVIAL JOINTS: This group of joints are also ***known as diarthrodial joints***. These are characterized by the presence of a joint cavity with a **synovial membrane** in the joint capsule and by their mobility (**Fig.1.32).** They are often called ***movable or true joints***. The syovial joints are classified into simple and composie joints.

A simple joint is formed by two articular surfaces (***eg: Shoulder joint)***) and **composite joint** (***eg: elbow joint)***) is formed by three or more articular surfaces. The following structures are involved in the formation of synovial joints.

(1) **Articular surface:** The articular surfaces are in most cases smooth. In certain cases the surface is interrupted by non-articular cavities known as ***synovial fossae***.

(2) **Articular cartilage:** The articular cartilages, usually hyaline in type form a covering over the articular surfaces of the bones. The articular cartilages are non-vascular, very smooth and have a bluish tinge in the fresh state. They **diminish the effects of concussion** and **greatly reduce the friction**.

(3) **Articular capsule:** The articular or joint capsule is present around the articulating surfaces. It consists of two layers-an external one, composed of fibrous tissue and an internal one called the ***synovial membrane***. The fibrous layer (***membrane fibrosa***), sometimes termed the ***capsular ligament***, is attached either close to the margins of the articular surfaces or at a variable distance from them (**Fig.1.32).** The synovial membrane secretes a fluid called the ***synovial fluid***, which lubricates the joint; it resembles **white of an egg, but has a yellowish tinge**. It also serves to transport nutrient material to the hyaline articular cartilage. In addition, **it contains albumin, mucin and salts and it is alkaline in nature.**

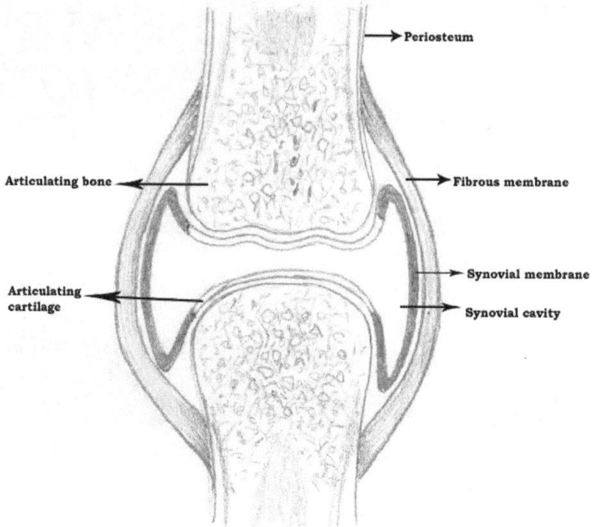

Fig. 1.32: Structure of Synovial Joint

(4) **Ligaments:** Ligaments are strong bands or membranes, usually **composed of white fibrous tissue, which bind the bones together.** They are pliable but practically inelastic. In a few cases, however, e.g., ***the nuchal ligament, they are composed of elastic tissue***, hence, elastic in nature. Those which are situated on the sides of a joint are termed ***collateral ligaments***. Those which connect directly opposed surfaces of bones are termed ***interosseous ligaments***.

(5) **Articular discs and menisci:** These are plates of **fibrocartilage** or **dense fibrous tissue** placed between the articular cartilages. In some joints they divide the joint cavity partially or completely into two compartments. They render articular surfaces **congruent, allow greater range or variety of movements and diminish the concussion *eg: stifle joint and temporomandibular articulation*.**

(6) **Marginal cartilage:** A marginal cartilage is a ring of fibrocartilage which encircles the rim of an articular cavity. It enlarges the cavity and tends to **prevent fracture of the margins eg: Cotyloid ligament present around the acetabulum in hip joint.**

(7) **Vessels and Nerves:** The arteries form anastomoses around the joints and give off branches to the extremities of the bones and to the joint capsule.

MOVEMENTS PERMITTED IN THE SYNOVIAL JOINTS

1. **Flexion** occurs when an angle between two bones is decreased.
2. **Extension** means straightening at a joint which occurs when the angle between the bones is increased.
3. **Abduction** occurs when a part is moved away from the mid sagittal plane of the body or a digit.
4. **Adduction:** occurs when a part is moved towards the mid sagittal plane of the body or the digits.
5. **Circumduction** is a form of motion which occurs when a bone is made to circumscribe a conical space; the base of the cone is described by the distal end of the bone and the apex is the articular cavity.
6. **Rotation:** one segment rotates around the longitudinal axis of the other segment forming the joint.
7. **Pronation and supination** refer to the position and movement of forearm and manus. In supination the volar face of the manus is turned forward / upward and in pronation, it faces backwards / downwards.

DIFFERENT TYPES OF SYNOVIAL JOINTS:

Type of Joint	Articular surfaces	Movement	Examples
1. Arthrodia or gliding joint.	Flat articular surfaces	Gliding	Carpal joint, hock joint and inter neural joints.
2. Ginglymus or hinge joint.	Condyles or convexities with concavities	Extension and flexion	Elbow joint
3. Condyloid or imperfect hinge joint.	Elliptical concavities	Except rotation all movements	Radio-carpal joint
4. Enarthroses or ball and socket joint.	Head with glenoid or cotyloid cavity	Flexion , extension, Circumduction.	Hip joint, shoulder joint.
5. Trochoid or pivot joint.	One segment rotates around the another	Flexion , extension rotation	Atlanto-axial joint
6.Saddle joint	Convexo-cocave and saddle like articular surfaces	Extension, flexion	Interphalangeal articulations of dog

Based on the axes of movement synovial joints are classified as

1. **Uniaxial**: movements in only one plane. **eg: ginglymus, pivot and condyloid joints**
2. **Biaxial**: joints permit movement in two planes at right angles. **eg: saddle, ellipsoidal joints.**
3. **Multiaxial**: The joints permit angular, rotation and circumduction movements. eg: **Ball and socket joint.**

1.3 GENERAL MYOLOGY

Myology deals with the muscles and their structures.

The muscle tissue is classified both morphologically and functionally as ***smooth*** (nonstriated, involuntary), ***cardiac*** (striated, involuntary) and ***skeletal*** (striated, voluntary) ***muscles***.

Smooth muscles: occur principally as masses of spindle shaped cells in the walls of hollow visceral organs and blood vessels as well as in association with the **spleen, inside the eye ball and hair follicles.**

Cardiac muscles: Fibres have cross striations and are arranged in irregular masses, which may be regarded as a **specialized type of striated muscle**. Contractions occur involuntarily.

Skeletal muscles: Consist of bundles of multinucleated fibers. The fibers are cross striated with thick and thin myofilaments. The connective tissue separating muscles from each other and binding them into position are called ***fascia.*** The thicket part of the muscle is the ***belly (venter).*** The presence of an intermediate tendon in some muscles forms two bellies making the muscle ***digastric (eg: Digastricus muscle,* Fig.1.33).**

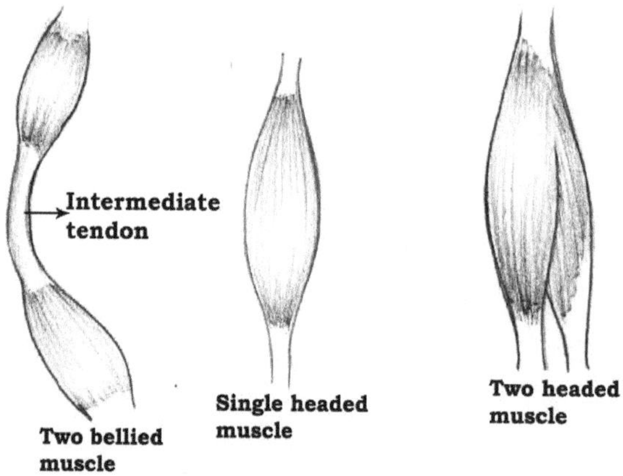

Fig. 1.33: Different Types of Skeletal Muscles

Arrangement of muscle fibers in skeletal muscles: The muscle fibers may have a parallel arrangement, the bundles being perpendicular or oblique or horizontal in respect to the entire muscle. When the parallel fibers attach to the tendon at an angle, the muscle is called ***pennate***. The arrangent may be unipennate, bipennate or multipennate **(Fig.1.34).** The fibers of a ***fusiform (spindle shaped) muscle*** converge upon a tendon at both ends of the muscle.

Unipennate muscle: with two parallel tendon sheets. **eg: Vastus medialis**

Bipennate muscle: two tendon sheets of different directions. **eg: Rectus femoris**

Multipennate muscle: Several tendon sheets of different directions. **eg: Deltoideus**

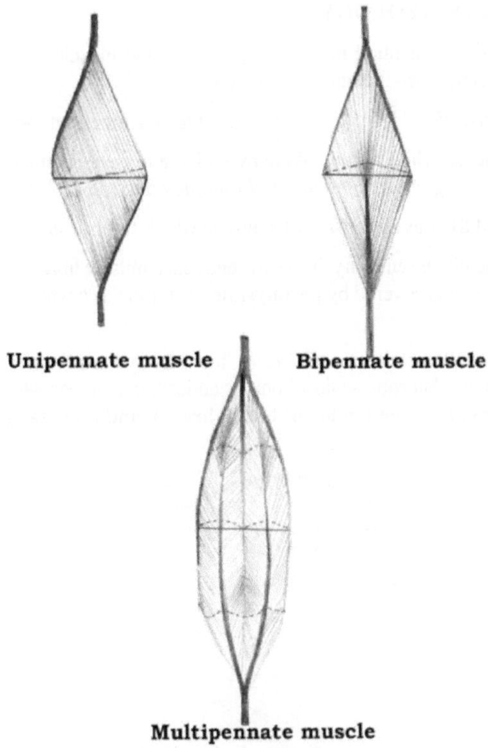

Fig. 1.34: Different Arrangements of Skeletal muscle Fibers

In order to produce skeletal movement the each muscle must traverse at least one joint. Several muscles traverse more than one joint. Certain muscles, by association with the superficial fascia and with firm cutaneous anchorage, move the skin. The muscles which surround natural openings are called as ***sphincters*** **(Fig.1.35).** They are actually arranged in walls of ***tubes or cavities to act as constrictors***.

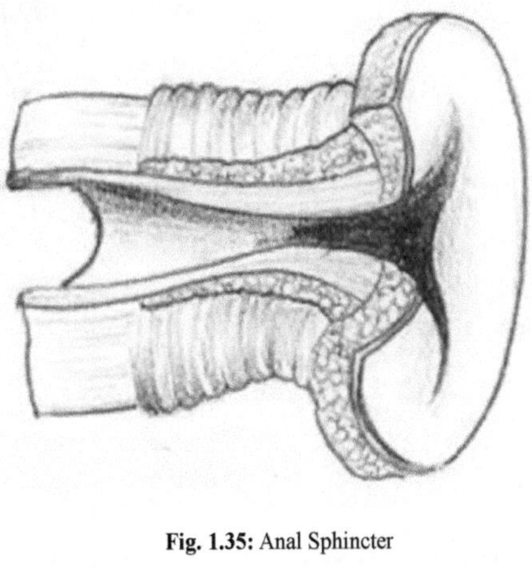

Fig. 1.35: Anal Sphincter

GENERAL TERMS USED IN MYOLOGY

1. ***Origin***: the term "***origin***" is applied to the attachment of the muscle which always or more commonly remains **stationary (fixed)** when the muscle contracts.
2. ***Insertion:*** The term "***insertion***" is applied to the movable attachment of the muscle.
3. ***Tendon***: is a band of dense white fibrous tissue by which a muscle is attached to the bone. **Some muscles have tendon at its origin *eg: Biceps brachii and Complex muscle.***
4. ***Aponeurosis***: is a **broad fibrous expansion** of a muscle which fulfils a similar function as like that of tendon.

A delicate connective tissue sheath, the **endomysium** surrounds each muscle fibre. Several muscle fibres are grouped together to form fasciculus, which is covered by **perimysium**. A muscle as a whole consisted of many fasciculi and is surrounded by **epimysium**.

Synovial bursa: Bursa is thin walled connective tissue sac **lined by synovial membrane and filled with synovial fluid**. These are present where tendon rubs against bone or under ligaments or where the skin moves over a bony prominence. **eg: Synovial bursa between tendon of biceps brachii and bicipital groove of humerus** (**Fig.1.36**).

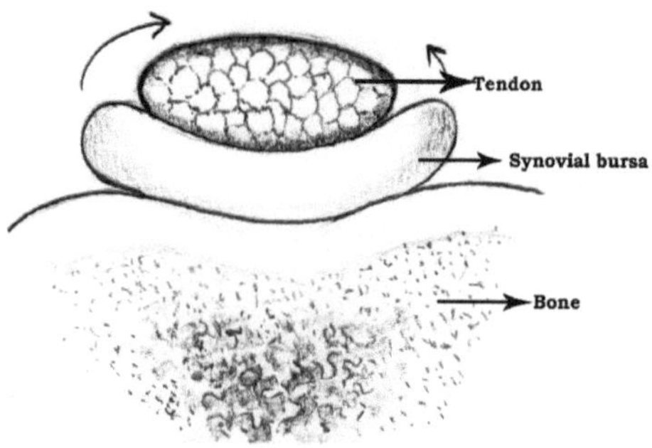

Fig. 1.36: Synovial Bursa

Tendon sheaths (Synovial sheaths): thin walled tube like structures, which envelop the tendon over hard skeletal areas where they are under considerable tension. It is also filled with synovial fluid. **eg: synovial sheath around tendon of flexors and extensors of forearm** (**Fig.1.37**).

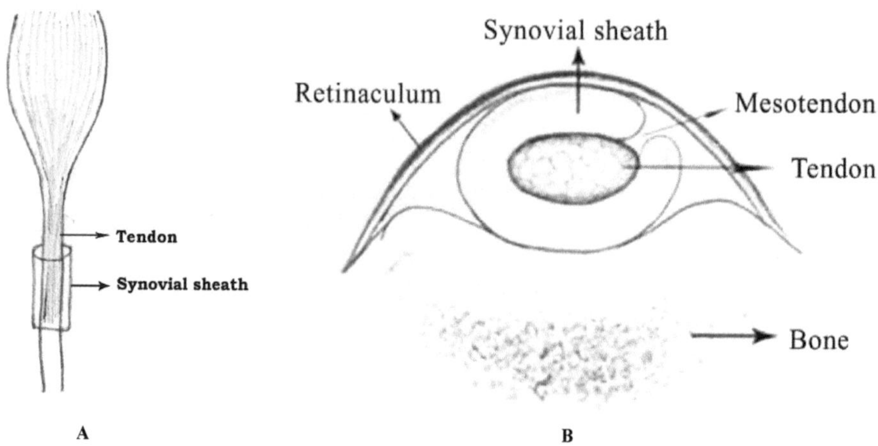

Fig. 1.37: Longitudinal and Cross Section of Synovial Sheath

The Cutaneous Muscle

The cutaneous muscle is a thin muscular layer developed in the superficial fascia. It is intimately adherent to the skin with little attachment to the bones. It is divided in to ***frontal, facial, cervical, omobrachial and abdominal* (cutaneous trunci) parts.**

The frontal part: it is well develoed especially in ruminats. The dorsal part of this muscle is called as ***frontalis*** located between the skin and frontal bone. It is closely adherent to the skin. The muscle fibers are directed from the poll area and the base of the horn ventrally and rostrally toward the superior eyelid, where the fibers spread out in fan like fashion to blend with the orbicularis oculi. Contraction of the muscle fibers will, in part raise the superior eye lid and wrinkles the skin located on the dorsal surface of the forehead (**Fig.1.38**).

The facial part (*m.cutaneous faciei*): consists of a thin and usually incomplete muscular layer, which **extends over the mandibular space and masseter muscle.** A distinct part of it passes cranially to the angle of the mouth and blends with the orbicularis oris, buccinator, zygomaticus and levator nasolabialis. ***This part retracts the angle of the mouth*** (**Fig.1.38**).

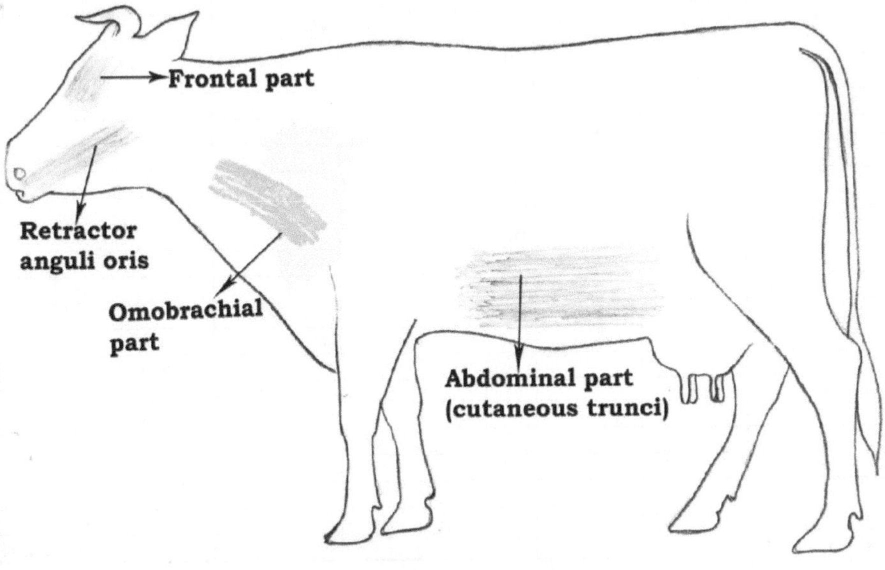

Fig. 1.38: Cutaneous Muscle of Ox

The cervical part (*m.cutaneous colli*): is situated along the **ventral region of the neck.**It arises from the cartilage of the manubrium and a median fibrous raphe.It is thick at its sternal region, but thins out cranially and laterally. On the side of the neck it is attached to the superficial cervical fascia, which acts as its aponeurosis. It is related deeply to the sternocehalicus, brachiocepahlicus (in part) and external jugular vein. Both the ***cutaneous faciei*** (*cutaneous muscle of face*) and ***cutaneous colli*** (*cutaneous muscle of neck*) muscle comprise the ***platysma.***

The omobrachial part (*m.cutaneous omobrachialis*): covers the **lateral aspect of the shoulder and arm.** Its fibres begin at the upper part of the scapular region and extend vertically downwards to the upper part of the forearm. It is **continuous behind with the abdominal part.**

The abdominal part *(m.cutaneous trunci)* of the cutaneous muscle covers a large part of the trunk behind the shoulder and arm (**Fig.1.38**). Its fibers are largely longitudinal and is continuous in **front with the omobrachial part.** A thin tendon from it passes cranially with the pectorals ascends to the lesser tubercle of the humerus and blends with the latissimus dorsi. The two side muscles are **thickest at the ventral part** but as they pass towards the lateral aspects they become thinner and finally towards the spine they become aponeurotic. In the umbilical region, the two muscles are about a hand breadth apart from each other. Cranially, they diverge and partly overlap the deep pectoral muscle. ***The muscle is in general closely adherent to the skin. Its voluntary contraction twitches the skin, thus getting rid of insects or other irritants.***

NAMING OF SKELETAL MUSCLES

The skeletal muscles are named based on their shape, size, origin, position, insertion, action or combination of any two or three of these as mentioned below.

Name	Shape	Size	No.of heads/ bellies	Position	Attachment	Action
Teres	Round					
Deltoideus	Traingular					
Rectus	Straight					
Fusiform	Spindle					
Planus	Sheet like					
Orbicularis	Ring like					
Major		Large				
Longissimus		Longest				
Latissimus		Broadest				
Biceps			Two heads			
Triceps			Three heads			
Quadriceps			Four heads			
Digastricus			Two bellies			
Pectoral				of chest		
Brachii				of arm		
Supraspinatus				above spine		
Infraspinatus				below spine		
Brachiocephalicus					Arm to skull	
Coracobrachialis					coracoid process to arm	
Extensor						Extension
Flexor						Flexion
Adductor						Adduction
Abductor						Abduction
Sphincter						Constriction

***** The above features are used in combination also to name the muscles eg: long digital extensor i.e based on size (long), attachment (digital) and action (extension).***

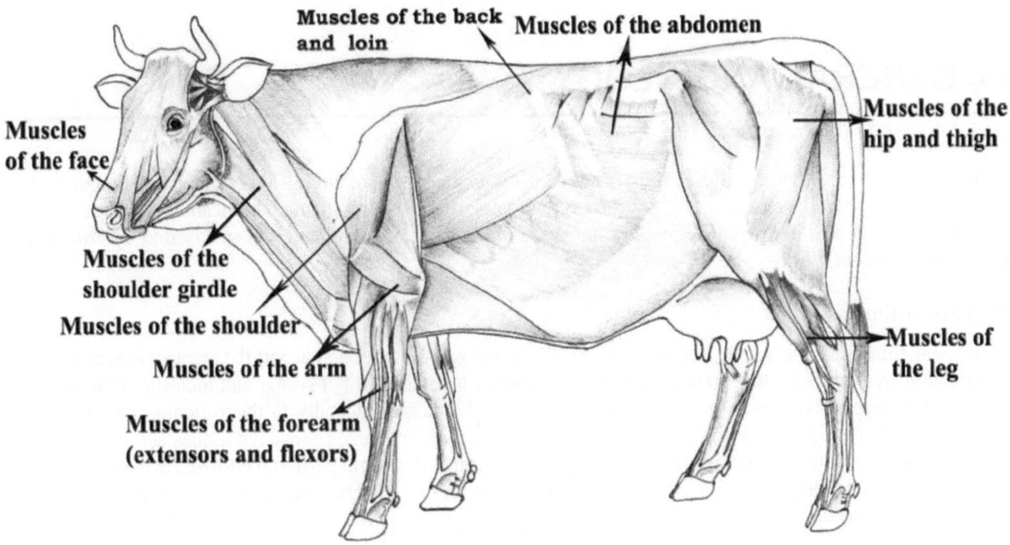

Fig. 1.39: Muscles of the Animal Body

1.4 GENERAL ANGIOLOGY

Angiology is a branch of systematic anatomy which deals with the organs of circulation of blood and lymph. These include the heart, blood vessels (arteries, veins) lymph vessels and lymph glands.The heart is a central hollow muscular organ situated in the middle mediastinal space of the thoracic cavity and it is enclosed in a ***fibro-serous sac, the pericardium.***

The Pericardium

The **pericardium** is a cone shaped fibro-serous sac which encloses the heart and in part the great vessels at its base. It consists of two layers i.e **fibrous and serous.** The **fibrous layer** is thin but strong and inelastic. It is attached above to the great blood vessels at the base of the heart and continues dorsally to the vertebrae and long colli muscle. Its ventral attachment is to the posterior part of the sternum by loose connective tissues and by rhe paired sternopericardial ligaments. The **serous** layer consists of parietal and visceral parts and encloses between the two a potential space containing a thin film of serous fluid the ***liquor percardii***. The visceral part covers the heart and is ***termed the epicardium.***

The Heart

In ox, the heart is relatively small in comparison to that of horse. Its weight varies between **0.4 and 0.5 per cent of the body weight**. Its approximate weight in cows is **2.4 kg and in bulls is 2.6 kg**. It is a cone shaped, hollow muscular organ which occupies the greater part of the middle mediastinal space. The long axis is directed ventrally and backward. The base extends from the ***3rd to the 5th intercostal space***. The **anterior border** is strongly convex and its ventral part is almost parallel with the sternum. The **posterior border** is shorter, nearly vertical, slightly concave and is opposite the fifth intercostal space or anterior border of the sixth rib.

> The **heart field**, clinically important for auscultation and percussion, is an outline of the heart projected on the ***left thoracic wall from the 3rd to the 5th intercostal space in ox***.

The two surfaces are convex and marked by grooves which indicate the division of the heart into four chambers. The grooves are occupied by coronary vessels and fat. The **coronary or transverse groove** indicates the division between the atria and ventricles. The ***longitudinal grooves*** are **left anterior and right posterior** in position. The ***left groove*** begins at the coronary groove behind the origin of the **pulmonary artery** and descends down almost parallel to the posterior border. The ***right groove*** begins at the coronary groove **below the termination of the posterior vena cava** and passes towards the apex but does not reach it. In ox, a shallow **intermediate groove** is also present on left ventricle, which extends from the coronary groove but does not reach the apex.

The interior of the heart is divided by a complete septum into a right and left halves. Each half is subdivided into an **upper atrium and lower ventricle**. The division is indicated externally by grooves.

Location and Shape of Heart in Various Domestic Animals

Species	Location (on left side of thorax)	Shape of the heart
Ox	3rd intercostal space to 5th intercostal space.	Triangular or cone shaped with a wide base.
Sheep and Goat	2nd intercostal space to 5th intercostal space.	Cone shaped with blunt apex in sheep and pointed apex in goat.
Horse	2nd intercostal space to 6th rib.	Cone shaped.
Pig	2nd intercostal space to 5th rib.	Trapezoidal or Valentine shaped
Dog	3rd rib to 6th intercostal space.	Globular or ellipitical in shape
Fowl	Present in cranial part of thoracoabdominal cavity between two lobes of the liver.	Cone shaped with pointed apex

Pulmonary Circulation

The **pulmonary artery** is a large, short vessel which carries venous blood from the right ventricle to the lungs. It curves upward, backwards and medially and divides into ***right and left pulmonary arteries*** behind the aortic arch of the aorta and ventral to the bifurcation of the trachea. A little anterior to the division into branches it is connected to the aorta by the ***ligamentum arteriosum,*** the remnant of the foetal ductus arteriosus. The ***right pulmonary artery is little longer than left.*** The greater size is due to the much larger right lung. It has four secondary branches named according to the lobes of the lung to which they are distributed. The **shorter and smaller left branch** has three secondary branches of which the one to the apical lobe is the smallest.

The **pulmonary veins which carry oxygenated blood are usually 6 to 7 in number** and are devoid of valves. The capillaries arise from the plexus around the alveoli of the lungs and they unite to from large branches accompanying the anterial branches on the ventral face of the bronchioles and finally form the **pulmonary veins which open into the left atrium**.

Systemic Circulation

The aorta is the ***chief vessel*** of the vascular system **(Fig.1.40).** It extends from the left ventricle of the **heart to the level of the fifth lumbar vertebra** where it terminates by dividing into **right and left internal iliac arteries.** The aorta leaves the let ventricle, then reaches the level of the body of the **seventh or eighth** dorsal vertebra runs backwards ***as the thoracic aorta*** between the lungs below the bodies of the dorsal vertebrae. It lies slightly to the left of the median line and reaches the **hiatus aorticus of the diaphragm.** It gradually diminishes in size till about the seventh or eighth dorsal vertebra but **thereafter it rapidly diminishes in calibre.**

Passing through the hiatus aorticus it enters the abdomen ***as the abdominal aorta***, passes backwards below the bodies of the lumbar vertebrae and the psoas minor in contact with the left crus of the diaphragm and the ventral longitudinal ligament. About the **fifth lumbar** vertebra it terminates by **dividing into two internal iliac arteries (Fig.1.40).**

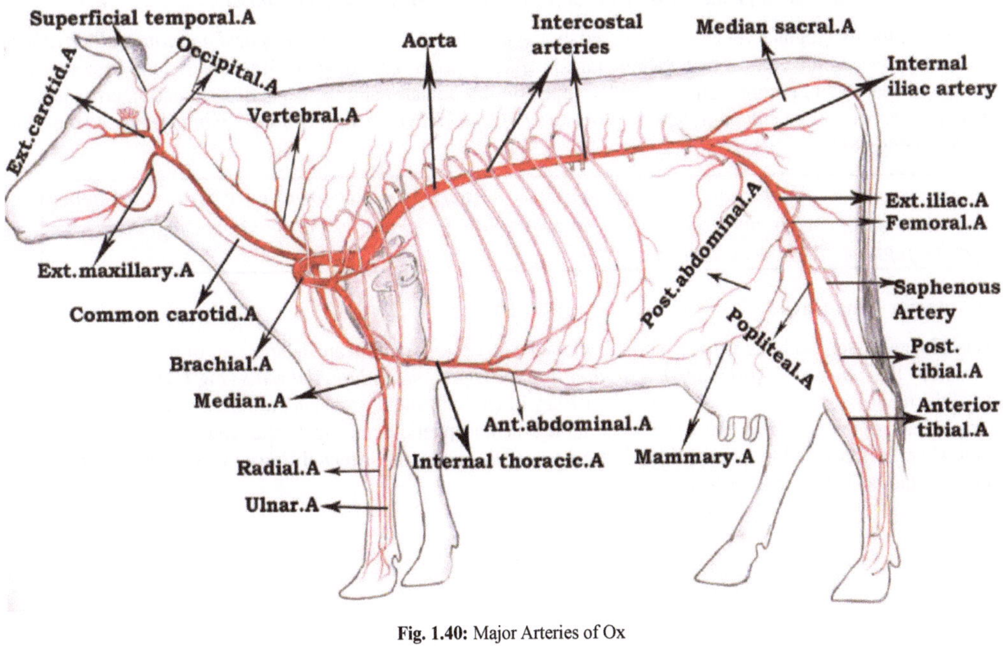

Fig. 1.40: Major Arteries of Ox

Venous System

The veins are distinguished by their **thinner walls**, their frequently collapsed appearance and their capacity, which is invariably greater than that of the associated arteries. They appear blue when filled with clotted blood. Most veins are also distinguished by the presence of valves, which are repeated at intervals along their length. The **valves ensure an unidirectional flow** and prevent reflux of blood when the circulation stagnates. Each **valve consists of two or three semilunar cusps facing each other.**

Most of the veins are the satellites of the arteries and need no special description. Only such of the veins which do not follow arteries (which are not satellite) are dealt here under.

Jugular Veins

There are two jugular veins on each side of the neck **i.e external and internal** and these ***drain the venous blood from the head and neck.***

> The *external jugular vein is used for venipuncture and intravenous injections in ruminants. Its distention and pulsation are signs of heart disease. In addition to the external jugular vein in the neck region, the median caudal or "tail" vein is one of the common locations where blood can be collected from cattle. Fecal contamination has to be avoided when collecting blood from the median caudal vein.*

Internal jugular vein: It is the smaller of the two veins and is formed by the union of ***occipital, thyroid and laryngeal veins***. It passes down the neck in company with the carotid artery, vagus and cervical sympathetic trunk and receives in it course muscular, tracheal and oesophageal radicles and terminates by joining the external jugular to form common jugular vein just in front of the thoracic inlet.

External jugular vein: is **subcutaneous** and occupies jugular furrow except for the first few inches. The vein is covered by skin and fascia and is separated from the common carotid artery, vagosympathetic trunk, recurrent laryngeal nerves and internal jugular vein by the upper border of ***sternomastoideus muscle.***

It is larger of the two jugular veins and is formed by the union of the ***superficial temporal and internal maxillary veins*** on deep face of the vertical ramus of the mandible and parotid salivary gland. It receives along its course the external maxillary vein, parotid veins, auricular veins, muscle radicles and the cephalic vein and internal jugular vein at its termination.The ***common jugular veins and the brachial veins from two sides join to form the anterior vena cava*** **(Fig.1.41).**

> *The sternomandubalris and brachiocephalicus muscles in cattle form the ventral and upper boundaries of the jugular groove. The sternomandibularis muscle is absent in sheep, making the ovine jugular groove less distinct.*

The Anterior Vena Cava

This is a **large vessel** receiving venous blood from the head, neck, fore limb and a large part of the thoracic wall. It is formed by the ***union of the right and left jugular and the right and left brachial veins*** **(Fig.1.41).** It is slightly to right of the median plane. It is a short trunk about 10 to 14 cm long and it passes in the anterior mediastinum below the trachea and right vagus deviating to the right of the brachiocephalic trunk and its branches. It opens into the right atrium where it is covered by pericardium. It receives in its course, the **internal thoracic vein and the thoracic duct** at the thoracic inlet on its superior face.

The Posterior Vena Cava

It is the ***largest venous trunk in the body***. It is formed under the body of the fifth lumbar vertebra by the union of the two common illiac veins (**Fig.1.41**). The **each common illiac vein is formed by the union of the external and internal illiac veins** (*Further course discussed in Unit-4*)

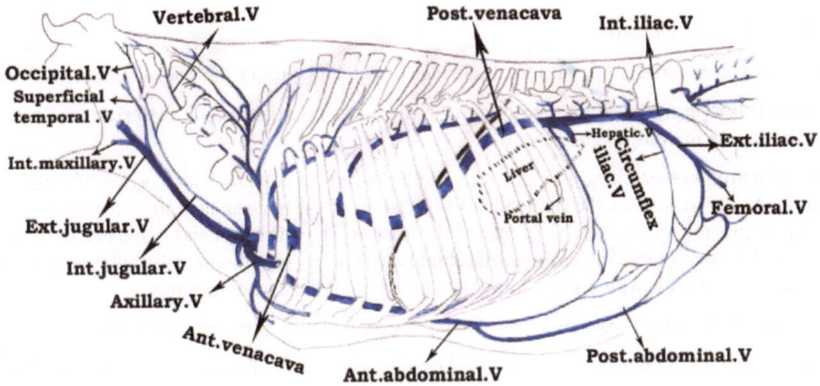

Fig. 1.41: Major Veins of the Ox

Lymphatic System

This system consists of **the lymph nodes and lymph vessels**, containing the lymph. The walls of lymph vessels are very much thinner than those of the veins but are provided with numerous valves. They **give characteristic beaded appearance when they are full.** All the lymph vessels in the body ultimately result by union into two large trunks the **thoracic duct and right lymphatic duct.**

The lymph nodes are intercalated in the course of the lymph vessels. Lymph passes through at least one lymph node before it empties into the venous system. **Lymph vessels which carry lymph to lymph nodes are afferents and those which leave the lymph nodes are efferents.** The haemal lymph nodes are dark red in colour and these have no afferents or efferents but have the blood directly passing through their channels.

Lymph Nodes of Neck and Fore Limb

1. Cervical lymph node: These are placed along the course of the common carotid artery.
2. Costocervical lymph node: It is situated in front of the first rib under the scalenus muscle.
3. Prescapular lymph node: It is situated at the anterior border of the suprasinatus about 10-12 cm above the shoulder joint under the cover of the omotransversarius and brachiocepahlicus muscles.
4. Axillary lymph node: It is placed on the medial face of teres major.

Lymph Nodes of the Head

1. **Atlantal lymph node:** is situated **below the wing of the atlas** under cover of mandiular salivary gland.
2. **Pterygoid**: situated on the upper part of the **lateral face of the pterygoid near the maxillary tuberosity.**
3. **Parotid lymph node**: It is situated superficially on **the lateral face of the posterior portion of the masseter muscle,** partly under the cover of the parotid salivary gland.

4. **Mandibular lymph node**: It is situated on the **lower part of the mandibular salivary gland** below the external maxillary vein and is covered by the tendon of insertion of sternomandibularis muscle.
5. **Suprapharyngeal lymph node**: These are situated close together on the median line of the **dorsal wall of pharynx medial to the great cornu of the hyoid bone.**
6. **Parapharyngeal lymph node:** It is situated on the lateral aspect of the pharynx.

Lymph Nodes of Thoracic Cavity

1. **Intercostal lymph nodes**: These are small glands present in the **upper part of the intercostal spaces.**
2. **Mediastinal lymph nodes**: These are situated in the **anterior, middle and posterior mediastinal spaces along the course of oesophagus.**
3. **Bronchial lymph nodes**: These are right, left, middle and apical brochial lymph nodes. The **right bronchial lymph nodes** are present on the right side of bifurcation of the trachea, near the dorsal border of the right brach of the pulmonary artery on right face of the trachea. The **left bronchial** is situated between the aortic arch and pulmonary artery. The **middle bronchial lymph** nodes are present at the bifurcation of the trachea. The **apical bronchial lymph node** is present at the origin of the apical bronchus.
4. **Pulmonary lymh node**: These are inconstant and found on the cheif bronchi in the lungs.
5. **Diaphargmatic lymh node**: It is a small gland **present close to the foramen vena cavae of diaphragm.**
6. **Sternal lymph nodes**: These are situated **along the course of internal thoracic artery.**

Lymph Nodes of Abdomen, Pelvis and Hind Limb

Abdomen

1. **Gastric lymph nodes**: These are a) **Ruminal** b) **Reticular** c) **Omasal d) abomasal lymphnodes.** These are present along the course of respective blood vessels.
2. **Lumbar lymph nodes**: These are **present in the sublumbar region** along the aorta and posterior vena cava.
3. **Renal lymh nodes**: They are situated along the course of renal vessels.
4. **Coeliac lymph nodes**: They are situated **along the course of coeliac and anterior mesenteric arteries.**
5. **Internal iliac lymph nodes**: They are situated in the angle **between the internal and external iliac arteries.**
6. **External iliac lymph node**: It is situated at the angle of **divergence of the superior and inferior branches of circumflex iliac artery.**
7. **Deep inguinal lymph node**: It is situated between the **external iliac and circumflex iliac arteries.**
8. **Precrural lymph node**: It is situated superficially in **front of the tensor fasciae latae** about a hand's breadth above the patella.
9. **Sacral lymph nodes**: These are medial and lateral glands. The medial lymph nodes are inconstant and present on the **deep face of the sacrosciatic ligament**. The **lateral lymph nodes are present on the lateral face of the sacrosciatic ligament.**
10. **Ischiatic lymph node**: It is a small gland present on the **lateral face of the sacrosciatic ligament at the lesser sciatic foramen** under cover of biceps femoris.
11. **Superficial inguinal lymph node**: It is situated ***above the neck of the scrotum in male*** and above the *posterior border of the mammary gland in female* (**supramammary lymph node**)

The Thoracic Duct

The thoracic duct is the chief collecting trunk of the lymphatic system. It drains lymph from all parts of the body **except the right fore limb, right side of the head, neck and thorax**. It **arises from the cisterna chyli** which is a ***reservoir formed by the union of the lumbar and gastrointestinal trunks***. The ***cistern chyli*** is an **elongated fusiform dilatation situated at the hiatus aorticus** of diaphragm dorsal to the aorta and ventral to the last thoracic and first lumbar vertebrae (**Fig.1.42)**.

The **intestinal trunk** is formed at the ventral face of the posterior vena cava just behind the dorsal border of the liver by the **confluence of the gastric and intestinal trunks**. The **gastric trunk** is on the left of the coeliac artery. The **intestinal trunk** follows on the anterior mesenteric artery. The **lumbar trunk** is formed by the union of the efferents from the iliac lymph glands. It also receives efferents from the lumbar and renal lymph glands.

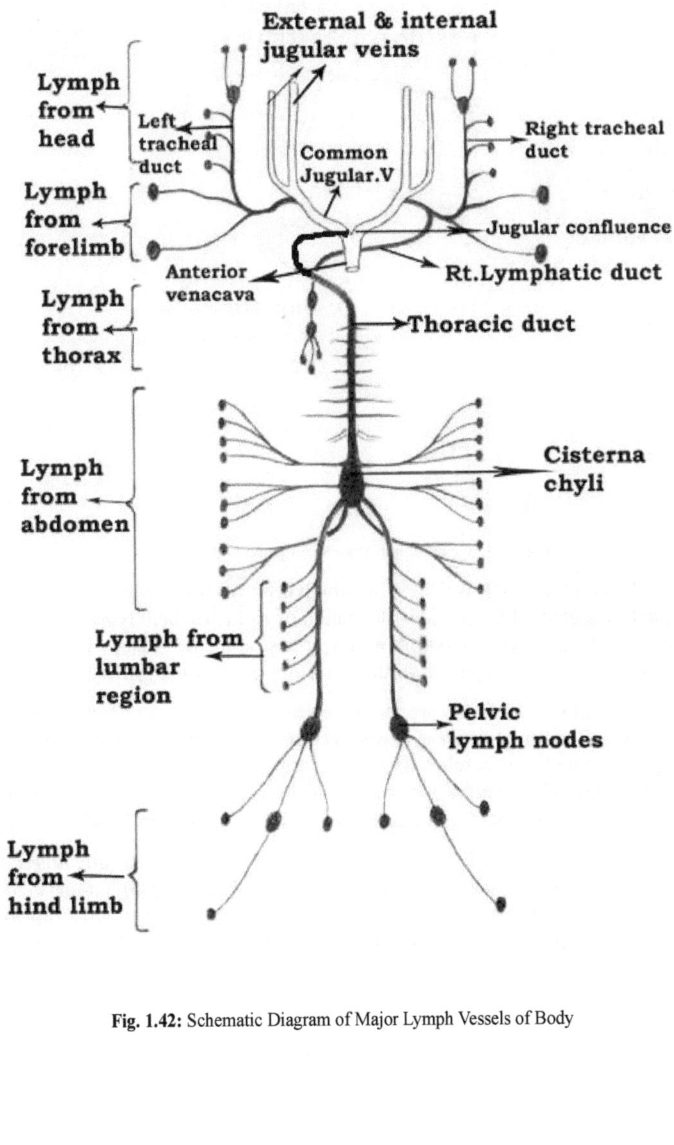

Fig. 1.42: Schematic Diagram of Major Lymph Vessels of Body

The *thoracic duct* arises ***from the cistern chyli*** passes forwards on the right part of the dorsal face of the aorta, covered by pleura and fat. At the **8th or 7th dorsal vertebra**, it inclines ventrally, crosses over the left face of the oesophagus and passes forward on the left face of the trachea to the thoracic inlet. The extra thoracic part is on the deep face of the left scalenus muscle. It curves backwards and inwards under the bicarotid trunk and opens on the dorsal face of the jugular confluence or anterior vena cava. In its course it receives efferents of the intercostal, mediastinal and bronchial lymph glands and at thoracic inlet it receives the efferents from the left posterior cervical lymph node and left tracheal duct.

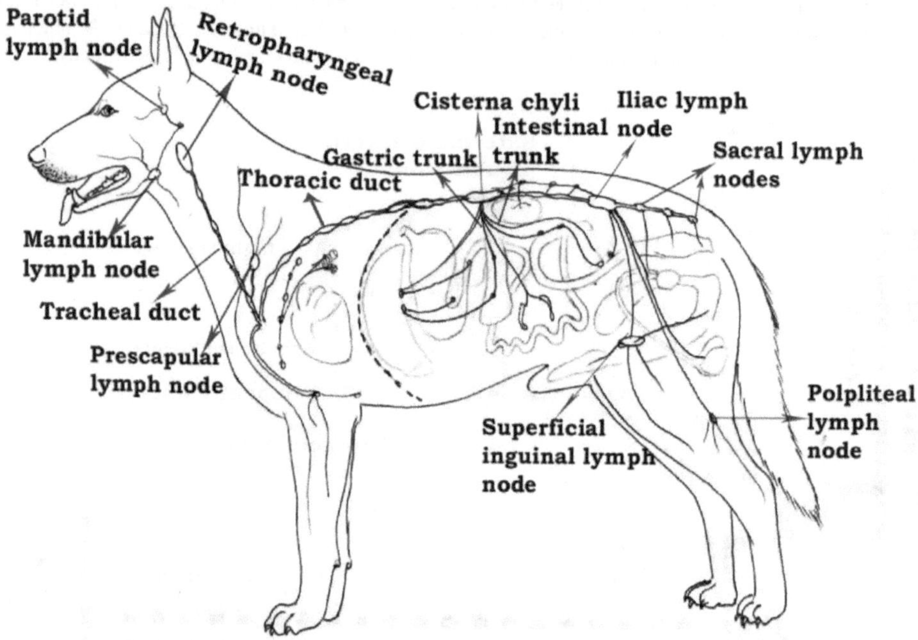

Fig. 1.43: Major Lymph Vessels & Lymph nodes of Dog

Right lymphatic duct: It is a short vessel which **drains the lymph from the right side of the head, neck, right forelimb and right part of thorax**. It is formed by the union of **right tracheal lymph duct** and the **efferents of right posterior cervical and right axillary lymph nodes.** It lies on the deep face of the scalenus muscle above terminal part of the right jugular vein. **It opens into the anterior vena cava (Figs.1.42 and 1.43).**

Tracheal ducts: These are **right and left** and are formed by the confluence of efferent vessels from the **altantal lymph node**. They receive ***efferents of cervical, costocervical and prescapular lymph nodes***. They pass along each side of the trachea and oesophagus in relation to the carotid arteries. The **right duct** joins the efferents of the **posterior cervical and costocervical lymph nodes to form the right lymphatic duct** or it **may join the right common jugular vein**. The **left duct** opens **into the thoracic duct (Figs.1.42 and 1.43).**

Superficial Lymph Nodes: They are useful in diagnosis of diseases like ***theileriosis and tuberculosis*** by palpating enlarged lymphnodes since they are superficially located. These are **1. Parotid lymph node, 2. Mandibular lymph node 3. Prescapular lymph node 4. Prefemoral lymph node 5. Superficial inguinal / supramammary lymph node** (*Figs.1.44 and 1.45*). **5. Popliteal lymph node is** ***superficial in dog*** and it is placed between upper part of **two heads of gastrocnemius** muscle.

The parotid lymph node is located along the rostral edge of the parotid salivary gland. It drains the region of the eye. In the cattle this node is usually inspected in slaughter houses to determine eye cancer.

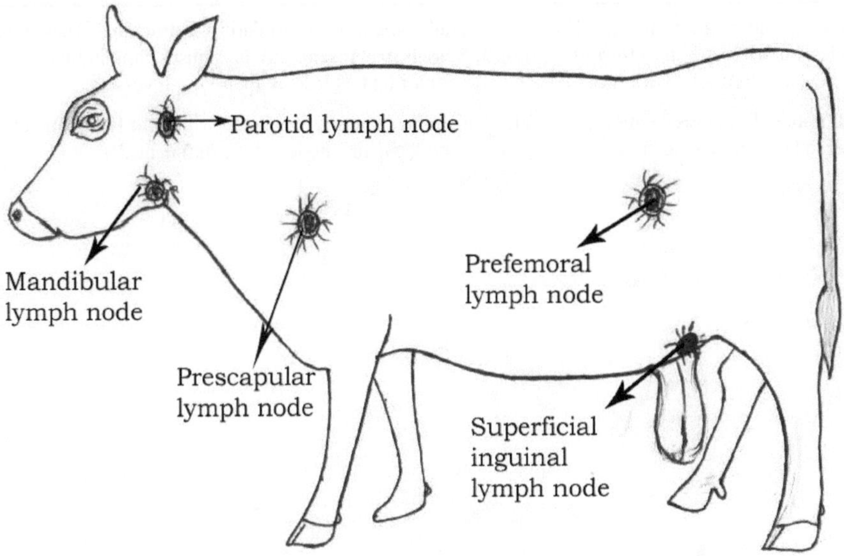

Fig. 1.44: Superficial Lymph Nodes in Male

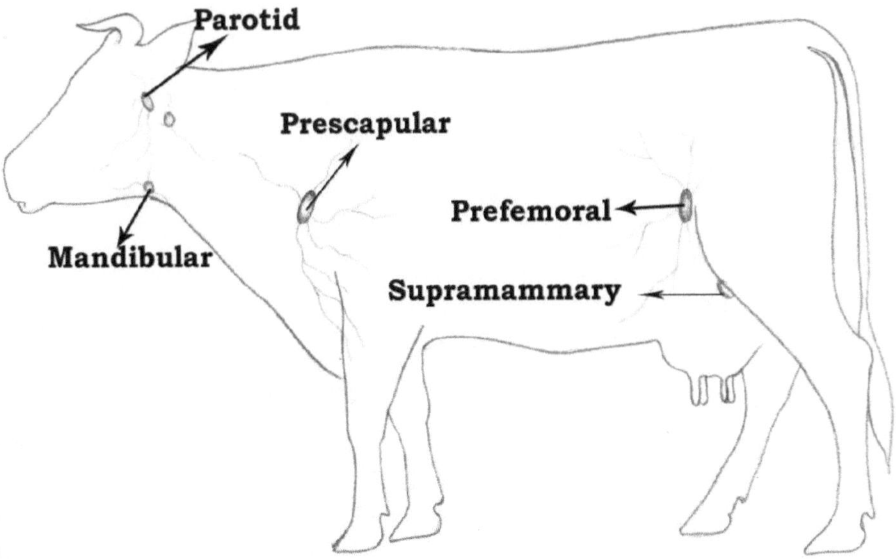

Fig. 1.45: Superficial Lymph Nodes in Female

Superficial inguinal lymph node is also known as ***mammary lymph node*** and drains the lymph from the udder and neighbouring regions (vulva, clitoris and skin of the medial thigh region). The mammary lymph nodes are one on each side of the base of the udder and close to the superficial inguinal ring.

Hemal Nodes: are unique to ruminants. They are generally small, brown to dark red structures. They are similar to lymph nodes, but **afferent and efferent lymphatic vessels are absent** and the sinuses contain blood instead of lymph.They develop during fetal life from lymph node primordia that lose all their lymph vessels.

Hemolymph nodes: In the pig, hemolymph nodes which have sinuses connected with both lymphatic and blood vessels, apper to be intermediate between lymph nodes and the hemal nodes of the ruminants.

1.5 GENERAL NEUROLOGY

Neurology is the study of nervous system. The system is a complex mechanism by which the animal is brought into functional relation with the environment and the functions of the various systems are coordinated.

The nervous system is divided into ***central and peripheral nervous systems.*** The **central nervous system** consists of **brain and spinal cord**, whereas peripheral nervous system is further divided into ***somatic and autonomic nervous systems***.

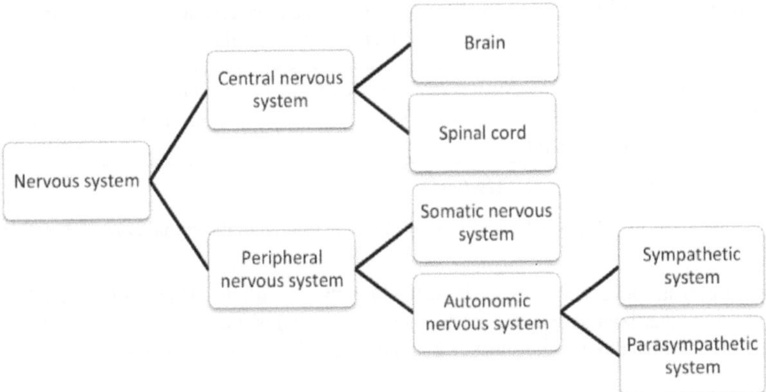

Somatic nervous system: relays impulses from the CNS to skeletal muscles and vice versa.

Autonomic nervous system: Trasmits impulses from CNS to involuntary organs and smooth muscles of the body. The autonomic nervous system is further classified into **sympathetic and parasympathetic nervous systems.**

MENINGES OF THE BRAIN

Dura mater (Dura means ***"Hard"***, mater means ***"Mother")***

It is a **dense tough membrane** of white fibrous tissue. It has cranial and spinal parts which enclose the brain and spinal cord and continuous with each other at the foramen magnum. The **cranial dura mater** is very closely adherent to the internal surface of the cranial bones **eliminating epidural space.** It is composed of two layers, an **outer periosteal layer** which is adherent to the internal face of the cranial bones forming the internal periosteum and an **inner meningeal layer** which is in contact with the next covering. These two layers are separated at certain places to form the venous sinuses lined by endothelium into which veins of brain drain. The internal surface of the dura is also lined by endothelium and is smooth. It forms the outer boundary of the subdural space which contains a small quantity of fluid resembling lymph.The ***subdural space*** is the space between the dura and the arachnoid and contains a thin **film of lymph (Fig. 1.46).**

Folds of Dura mater: They are the falx cerebri, tentorium cerebelli and diaphragm sellae

1. The **falx cerebri** is a ***sickle shaped fold*** of dura mater which is situated in the great longitudinal fissure of the cerebrum.

2. The **tentorium cerebelli** is a ***crescentic fold*** projecting into the great transverse fissure between the cerebral hemispheres and cerebellum.

3. The **diaphragma sellae** is a thick fold of dura mater on the ventral aspect of the brain surrounding the pituitary gland and encloses the cavernous and intercavernous sinuses. It is **perforated above for the** infundibulum centrally and for the ***exit of the emergent artery*** of the retemirabile cerebri and the ***third cranial nerve*** on either side.

The ***spinal dura mater*** is composed only of the **meningeal layer** and forms a very loose tube around the spinal cord. It is separated from the periosteum of the spinal canal by a considerable epidural space which is occupied by connective tissue and fat.

Arachnoid membrane *("Web" like*): It is a very delicate and transparent membrane which is situated between the dura mater and the piamater (**Fig. 1.46**). Its outer face is also lined by endothelium and forms the inner wall of the subdural space. Its internal face is also lined by endothelium and forms outer boundary of the subarachnoid space containing ***cerebrospinal fluid***. The arachnoid membrane furnishes the several strands of connective tissue which join the piameter, thus dividing the subarachnoid space into numerous intercommunicating cavities. The ***spinal arachnoid*** is continuous with that of the cerebral part and it forms a relatively wide tube around the spinal cord so that the latter with the pia mater is surrounded by a considerable quantity of cerebrospinal fluid.

Collection of cerebrospinal fluid can be performed at the occipitoatlantal joint for diagnostic purpose. The joint is punctured between the dorsal arch of the atlas and dorsal aspect of foramen magnum using a long spinal needle.

Pia mater (Pia means ***"Soft,*** mater means ***"Mother"***)

It is a very delicate vascular membrane which closely invests the brain and the spinal cord and sends processes into the brain substance.

The **cerebral pia mater** accurately moulds itself on the brain by dipping it self into all the sulci and fissures. Its external face forms the inner boundary of the subarachnoid space and is lined by endothelium. From its deep face trabeculae are given off which dip into the substance of the brain. The smaller blood vessels ramify in the pia mater forming plexuses.

Folds of pia mater extend into two of the fissures of the brain. One of these is the **telachorioidea of the third ventricle** which enters transverse fissure and forms the roof of the third ventricle. Another fold passes into the space between the cerebellum and medulla and forms the **tela chorioidea of the fourth ventricle**.

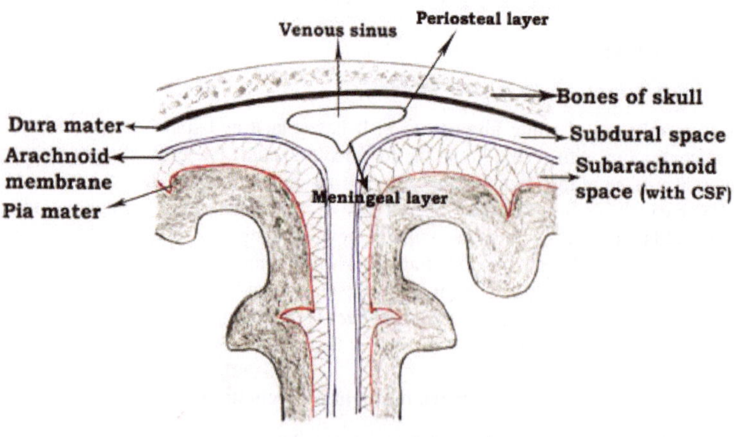

Fig. 1.46: Meninges of Brain

The **spinal pia mater** is thicker and denser. It sends a fold into the ventral median fissure of the spinal cord and also helps to form the dorsal median septum. Along the mid ventral line it forms a thickening the ***linea splendens*** in which the ventral spinal artery passes. On each side it gives of a strong longitudinal band, the ***ligamentum denticulatum*** which lies between the dorsal and ventral roots of the spinal nerves. Its lateral border is serrated and is attached to the dura mater.

PARTS OF THE BRAIN: The mammalian brain consists of 3 parts ***i.e fore brain, mid brain and hind brain.***

Main Division	Sub division	Parts	Cavity
Fore brain (Prosencephalon)	Telencephalon	Cerebral hemispheres Basal nuclei Limbic system	Lateral ventricle
	Diencephalon	Epithlamus Thalmus Hypothalmus	Third ventricle
Mid brain (Mesencephalon)	-	Corpora quadrigemina Cerebral peduncles	Cerebral aqueduct
Hind brain (Rhombencephalon)	Metencephalon	Pons Cerebellum	Rostral part of 4th ventricle
	Myelencephlon	Medulla oblongata	Caudal part of 4th ventricle

The surface of the hemispheres are marked by a number of winding ridges called ***gyri or convolutions*** separated by sulci.

Gray matter: Consists mainly cell bodies and dendrites of neurons. It has a brownish grey color and forms most of the cortex, nuclei of the brain and the ganglia. ***It is placed centrally in spinal cord and peripherally in cerebrum and cerebellum.***

White matter: It is paler tissue of the brain and spinal cord consisting mainly nerve fibers with their myelin sheaths. ***It is placed peripherally in spinal cord and centrally in cerebrum and cerebellum.*** But in brain stem (thalamus, mid brain, pons and medulla oblongata) the white and gray matters are intermingled with each other forming ***reticular formation.***

Ganglion and Nucleus: accumulation of neuronal cell bodies **out side the central nervous system** is called as ***ganglion***, while the term ***nucleus refers*** to accumulation of **neuronal cell bodies within the white matter** and reticular formation of brain stem of central nervous system (**Fig. 1.47**).

Basal ganglia: The basal ganglion is **a group of nuclei (i.e caudate nucleus, putamen and globus pallidum)** located in the basal part of the telencephalon and involved in control of motor functions.

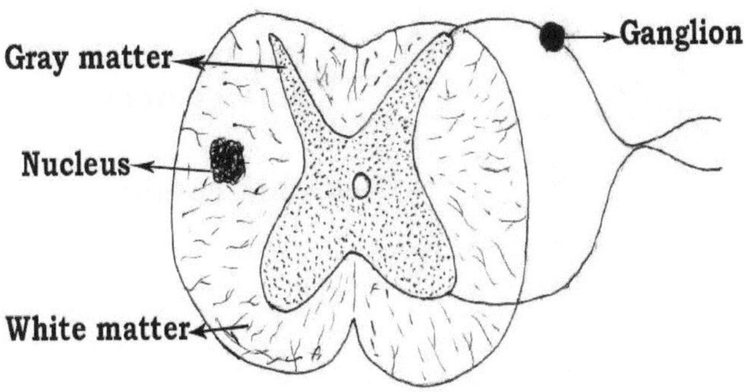

Fig. 1.47: Nucleus and Ganglion

THE SPINAL CORD

The spinal cord is that part of the central nervous system situated in the vertebral canal. It extends from the foraman magnum to about the middle of the sacrum. The spinal cord extends from the medulla oblongata at the foramen magnum and ends at different levels in different species. In ruminants it ends at the level of the **cranial half of the 2nd sacral vertebra**. In ***equines*** it ends caudally at the level of the **caudal half of the 2nd sacral vertebra, In canines it** ends very close to the junction of the **6th and 7th lumbar vertebrae, in pigs it** ends caudally between the cranial edge of the **2nd sacral vertebra and middle of the 3rd sacral vertebra.** In birds spinal cord ends at minute part of the vertebral canal within the **pygostyle.**

The terminal part rapidly narrows to a point called the **conus medullaris**. It is prolonged for a short distance by a slender filament of pia mater called ***filum terminale.*** The **conus medullaris** reaches only the anterior part of the sacral canal and hence the rest of the sacral canal is occupied by the sacral and coccygeal nerves extending backward in the canal for a considerable distance before they pass out of it forming a sort of a bundle in the middle of which is the **conus medullaris and filum terminale**. This arrangement is termed the ***cauda equina*** (**Fig. 1.48**).

The spinal cord is fairly uniform in the greater part of thoracic region but there are two conspicuous enlargements which involve segments with which the nerves of the limbs are connected. The **cervical enlargement begins about the fifth cervical segment** and subsides **at the second thoracic segment corresponding to brachial plexus and the lumbar enlargement** is present at about the **fifth lumbar** vertebra corresponding to **lumbosacral plexus** beyond which the cord ***rapidly narrows to form the conus medullaris*** (**Fig. 1.48**).

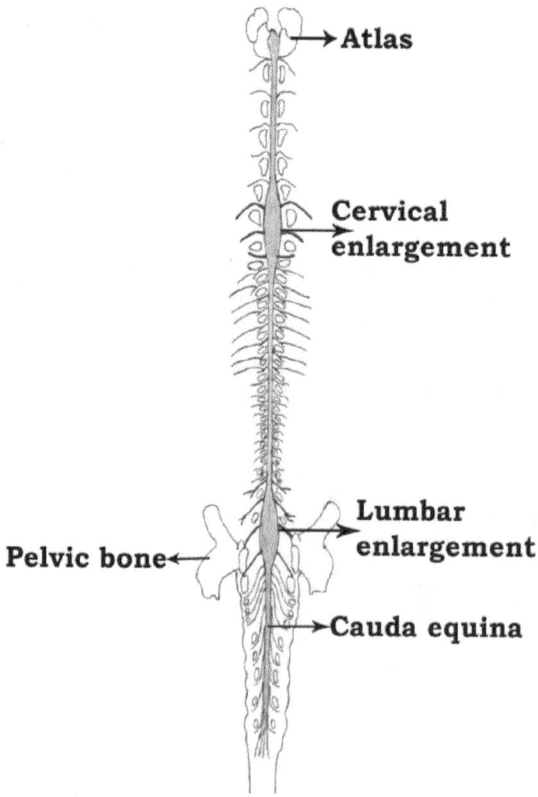

Fig. 1.48: Spinal Cord of Mammals

The surface of the spinal cord is divided into two **equal halves by a dorsal median septum and a ventral median fissure.** The two halves of the cord are connected by commissures of gray and white matter. The **gray commissure** is a transverse band at the base of the **dorsal median septum and is traversed by the central canal of the spinal cord.** The **white commissure** is a bridge of white matter which connects the two ventral columns of white matter **(Fig. 1.49).**

The **gray matter** of the cord as seen in a transverse section resembles roughly the capital letter **'H'** the cross bar being the gray commissure. Each half consists of a **dorsal and a ventral horn.** The **dorsal horn** is elongated, narrow and reaches the surface of the cord at the dorso-lateral fissure at the entrance of the dorsal root fibres of spinal nerves. It contains **sensory neurons.** The apex of the dorsal horn is covered by a mass of translucent nervous tissue, called **substantia gelatinosa** which contains cell bodies in the pain region. The ***lateral horn or intermediate horn* is seen only in the thoracic, lumbar and middle sacral levels.** It contains **autonomic (visceral motor) neurons.** The **ventral horn contains somatic motor neurons** and is rounded, wider and is separated from the surface of the cord by the white matter through which pass the ventral root fibres of spinal nerves **(Fig. 1.49).**

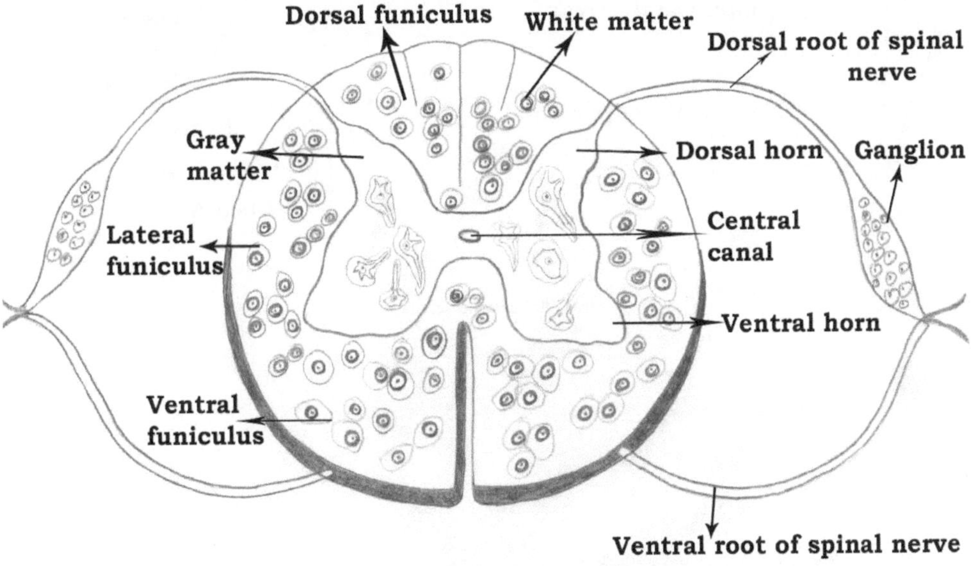

Fig. 1.49: C.S of Spinal Cord

The ***white matter*** consisting chiefly of medullated nerve fibres, is divided into **three pairs of columns or funiculi.** The ***dorsal column*** lies on either side of the dorsal median septum to the dorsolateral groove. The ***lateral column*** is situated between the dorsal and ventral root fibres of spinal nerves and the ***ventral column*** is situated between ventral median fissure and ventral roots of spinal nerves.

SPINAL NERVES: There are **37 pairs of spinal nerves in the ox** (8 cervical, 13 thoracic, 6 lumbar, 5 sacral and 5 coccygeal, **(Fig. 1.50), 42 pairs in horse** (8 cervical, 18 thoracic, 6 lumbar, 5 sacral and 5 coccygeal), **36 pairs in dog** (8 cervical, 13 thoracic, 7 lumbar, 3 sacral and 5 coccygeal) and **36 pairs in fowl** (15 cervical, 7 thoracic and 14 lumbosacral). Each spinal nerve arises from the cord by two roots i.e dorsal sensory and a ventral motor. The dorsal root shows sensory ganglion called ***dorsal root ganglion***. The dorsal root ganglia are **external to the duramater** and are in the **intervertebral foramina** except in the posterior series where they are in the spinal canal. Those of the coccygeal nerves are **intradural.**

Each nerve then divides into dorsal and ventral primary branches of which **former are smaller in size.** These are distributed to the muscles and the skin of the dorsal parts of the body. The **ventral branches** supply in general the muscles and skin of the ventral parts of the body, including the limbs. Each nerve or its ventral branch is connected with adjacent ganglion of the sympathetic system by a communicating branch called the ***ramus communicans***.

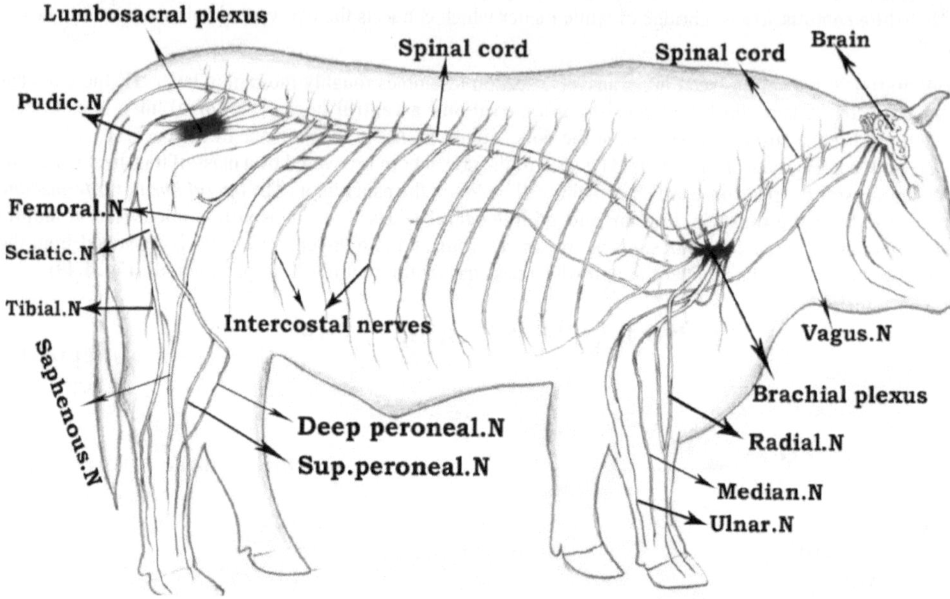

Fig. 1.50: Major Nerves of Ox

1.6 GENERAL SPLANCHNOLOGY

Splanchnology is a branch of Anatomy, which deals with the visceral organs of the digestive, respiratory and urogenital systems. Each of these systems consists fundamentally of a tube lined by mucous membrane, communicating with exterior at one end or both. **In mammals the body cavity is divided into *thoracic, abdominal and pelvic cavities.***

1. Thoracic cavity: is the **second largest** of the three body cavities. It is somewhat like a truncated cone much compressed laterally in its cranial part.

BOUNDARIES OF THORACIC CAVITY (FIG. 1.51)

Dorsally	:	Bodies of thoracic vertebrae, ligaments and muscles connected with them.
Laterally	:	Ribs, costal cartilages and intercostal muscles.
Ventrally	:	Sternum and transversus thoracis muscle
Posteriorly	:	Diaphragm.
Inlet	:	Dorsally body of 1st thoracic vertebra, laterally 1st st pair of ribs, ventrally manubrium sterni.

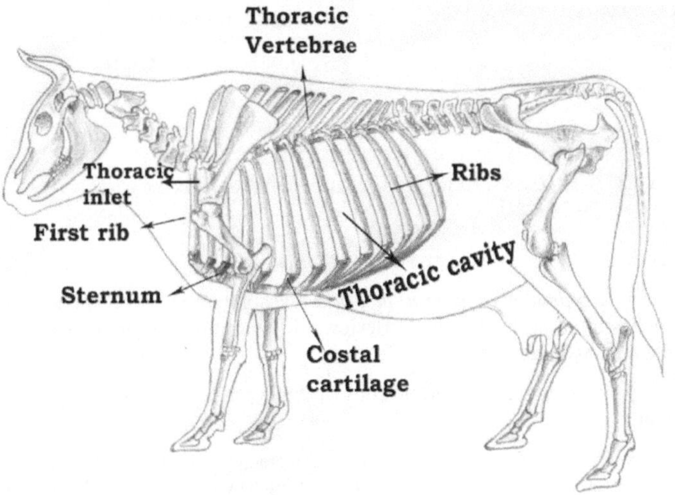

Fig. 1.51: Boundaries of Thoracic Cavity

Pleura: is a serous membrane lining the wall of thorax and organs contained therein. The ***parietal pleura*** lines the walls of thorax and has costal, vertebral, sternal and diaphragmatic parts. The ***endothoracic fascia*** is attached to deep surfaces of ribs, intercostal muscles, sternum and transversus thoracis.

The ***mediastinum*** is a double walled partition formed by **union of vertebral and sternal pleurae,** the former descending down and the latter going up dividing the thoracic cavity into right and left pleural cavities. **It is placed more on the left than on the right (Fig. 1.52).**

Of the **right and left pleural cavities the right is larger**. Each **pleural cavity** is a closed cavity occupied by respective lungs and filled with a small amount of serous fluid. The posterior vena cava and posterior part of right phrenic nerve are also seen in right pleural cavity. A special fold of mediastinal pleura, ***caval fold*** (***plica vena cava***) is seen ***around the posterior vena cava and right phrenic nerve behind the heart.***

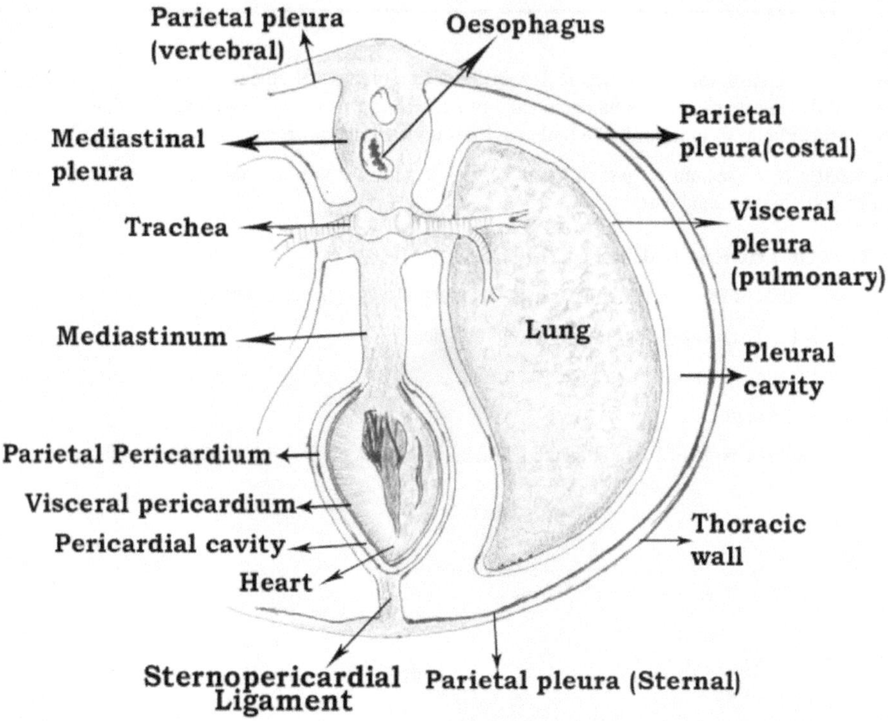

Fig. 1.52: Pleural Reflections

The mediastinal pleura reflects ***as pulmonary (visceral) pleura*** at hilus of lung and covers parietal and mediastinal surfaces of lungs. The **mediastinum** is divided into **anterior, middle and posterior mediastinums by heart, which is located in middle mediastinum.**

Anterior mediastinum: shows trachea, oesophagus and body (thoracic part) of thymus. The thymus lies in ventral part of anterior mediastinum.

Middle mediastinum: shows heart with pericardium, bifurcation of trachea into right and left principal bronchi at the level ***of 5th rib*** and tracheal (apical) bronchus is given off from trachea at the level of ***3rd rib*** to cranial lobe of right lung.

Posterior mediastinum: shows the terminal part of oesophagus, dorsal and ventral trunks of vagus nerves and posterior mediastinal lymph node.

2. ABDOMINAL CAVITY: is the **largest of the body cavities**. It is ovoid in form and compressed laterally. The abdominal cavity contains the greater part of the digestive and urinary organs, part of the internal genital organs, spleen, adrenal glands, certain fetal vestiges, muscles and numerous nerves and vessels.

Boundaries of abdominal cavity (Fig. 1.53)

Dorsally	:	Bodies and transverse processes of lumbar vertebrae, crura of diaphragm, sublumbar muscles.
Laterally	:	Oblique and transverse abdominal muscles, ilia, iliacus muscle, parts of caudal ribs, cartilages of asternal ribs below the attachment of diaphragm.
Ventrally	:	Rectus abdominis muscle, aponeurosis of oblique and transverse muscles and xiphoid cartilage.
Anteriorly	:	Diaphragm
Posteriorly	:	continuous with pelvic cavity at pelvic brim.

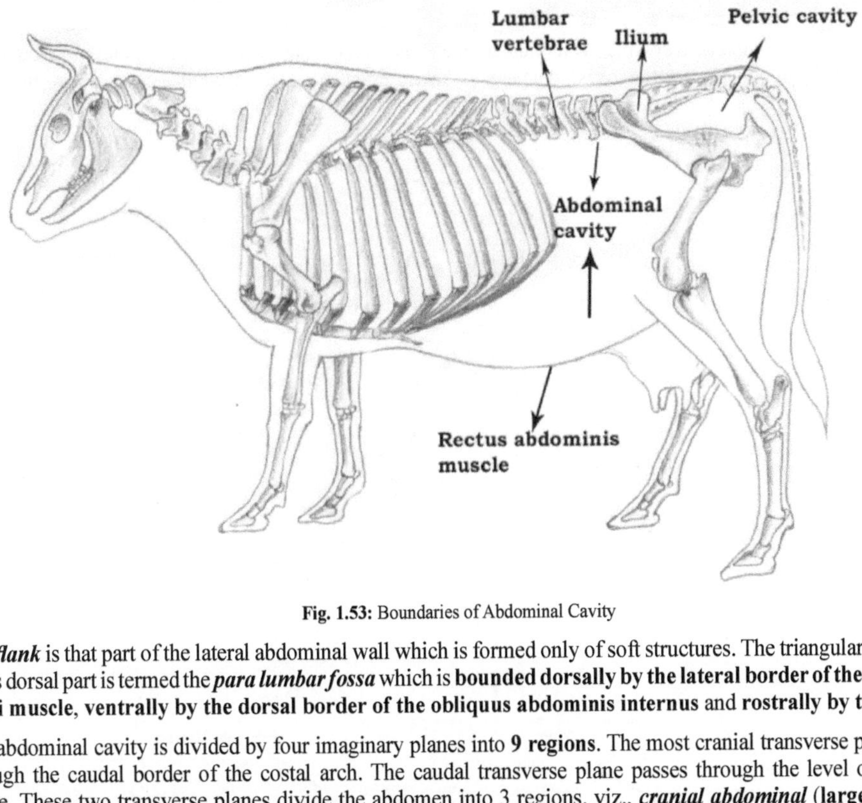

Fig. 1.53: Boundaries of Abdominal Cavity

The ***flank*** is that part of the lateral abdominal wall which is formed only of soft structures. The triangular depression on its dorsal part is termed the ***para lumbar fossa*** which is **bounded dorsally by the lateral border of the logissimus dorsi muscle, ventrally by the dorsal border of the obliquus abdominis internus** and **rostrally by the last rib**.

The abdominal cavity is divided by four imaginary planes into **9 regions**. The most cranial transverse plane passes through the caudal border of the costal arch. The caudal transverse plane passes through the level of the tuber coxae. These two transverse planes divide the abdomen into 3 regions. viz., ***cranial abdominal*** (**largest**), ***middle abdominal and caudal abdominal*** (**smallest**) ***regions*** which are subdivided by longitudinal planes passing through as mentioned below:

Abdominal regions demarcated by transverse planes	Abdominal regions demarcated by sagittal planes		
Cranial abdominal region	Left hypochondriac region	Xiphoid region	Right hypochondriac region
Middle abdominal region	Left lateral abdominal region	Umbilical region	Right lateral abdominal region
Caudal abdominal region	Left inguinal region	Pubic region	Right inguinal region

The walls of the abdominal cavity are pierced by ***five openings***. **Three of them are in diaphragm (*hiatus aorticus, hiatus oesophagus and foramen venacavae*) and two are inguinal canals.** In the **fetus there is an umbilical opening** also.

3. PELVIC CAVITY: is the caudal and smallest of the body cavities. It communicates cranially with the abdominal cavity, the line of demarcation being the terminal line or brim. The pelvic cavity contains the rectum, parts of the internal genital organs, some fetal remnants, muscles, vessels and nerves.

Boundaries of the pelvic cavity (Fig. 1.54 and 1.55)

Dorsally	Sacrum and first three coccygeal vertebrae
Laterally	Parts of ilia, sacrosciatic ligament
Ventrally	Pubis and ischium
Pelvic Inlet	Base of sacrum dorsally, brim of pubis ventrally, Iliopectineal line laterally
Outlet	3rd coccygeal vertebra dorsally, caudal edge of sacrosciatic ligament and semimembranosus muscle laterally and ischial arch ventrally.

Conjugate or ***sacropubic*** diameter which is in median line is measured from the sacral promontory to the anterior end of the pubic symphysis. The transverse diameter is measured at the greatest width i.e just above the psoas tubercle.

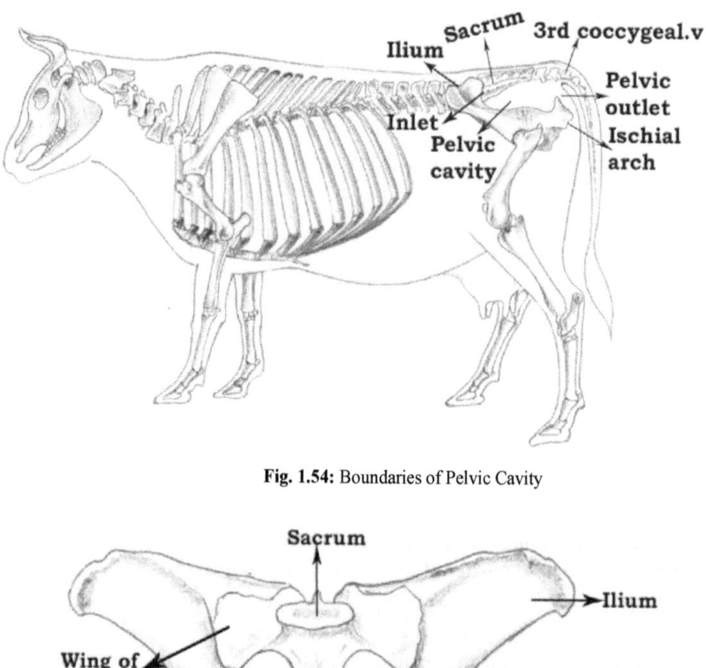

Fig. 1.54: Boundaries of Pelvic Cavity

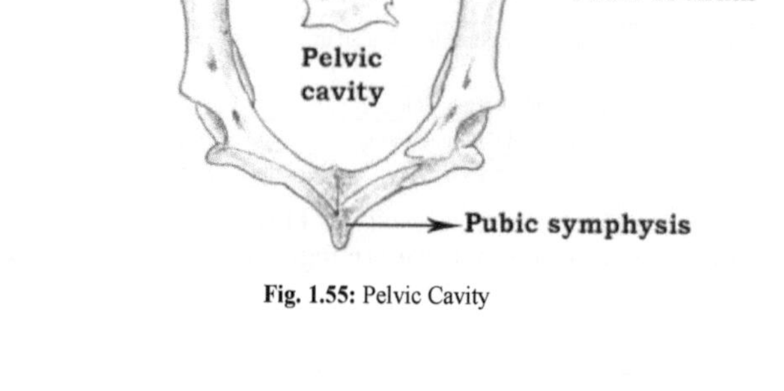

Fig. 1.55: Pelvic Cavity

Digestive System: The digestive system is divided into alimentary canal and accessory structures. The alimentary canal is a muscular tube extending from mouth to anus. It consists of the following consecutive portions. a) Mouth b) Pharynx c) Oesophagus d) Stomach e) Small intestine (Duodenum, Jejunum and Ileum) f) large intestine (caecum, colon, rectum) and g) anus. The accessory digestive structures include teeth, tongue, salivary glands, liver and pancreas.

Respiratory system comprises of nose including nostrils and nasal cavity, nasopharynx, larynx, trachea, bronchi and lungs.

Nose: The nose in domestic animals is incorporated in the face and forms dorsum nasi rostral to the eyes, while in human it projects distinctly from the face. It is supported by cartilages which are variable in form, size and number.

Nasal Cartilages: The free borders of the nasal and incisive bones in mammals provide attachment for the nasal cartilages which support the nostrils.

Urinary system consists of paired kidneys and ureters and unpaired urinary bladder and urethra. The frontal section of the **kidney reveals cortex and medulla**. The **cortex (outer part)** is rich in renal or Malphigian corpuscles which give granular appearance to cortex. The **medulla is the inner part made up of only tubules** and is in the form of renal pyramids.

Male genital system comprises of testicles with their covering (scrotum) and appendages, the ductus deferens, the accessory sex glands, (prostate, seminal vesicles and cowper's glands) urethra and penis with its covering, **the prepuce.**

Female genital system consists of two ovaries and fallopian tubes (oviduct), uterus, vagina, vestibule and vulva. The mammary glands are closely associated functionally with female genital organs.

1.7 General Integument

The skin or the common integument is the protective covering of the body and is continuous at the natural orifices with the mucous membranes of digestive, respiratory and urino genital tracts. It acts as a sense organ concerned in the reception of pain, temperature, touch and pressure sensations. There are various types of nerve endings in the skin some in the epidermis, others in the dermis around roots of hair etc. which serve as the receptors for the above sensations. These include free nerve endings in the epidermis for pain, Merkel's discs, Meissner's corpuscles, peritrichial plexus etc. for touch and tactile sensations., Ruffini's corpuscles for warmth and Krause's corpuscles for cold and Pacinian corpuscles for pressure sensation.

The skin presents fine hairs and numerous sebaceous glands. The skin of the neck form a median ventral fold called the dewlap. In the sheep, cutaneous pouches are present in certain situations i.e. the infraorbital or lacirmal pouch and interdigital pouch. Infraorbital sinus is a cutaneous pouch in sheep rostral to the medial angle of the eye with large odoriferous apocrine and sebaceous glands which produce a fatty secretion. So lacrimal bone shows shallow external lacrimal fossa which underlies the sinus.

APPENDAGES

Hair: The hairs are extremely variable in colour and size in diffeent breeds and individuals. They cover the entire surface of the body and are of two kinds-ordinary and special. The ordinary hair determines the about the lips, nostrils, eyelashes, tragic of external ear, vibrissae of the nostrils or long hairs of the tail forming the brush. Sparse growth of hair and few sweat glands make the buffalo less heat resistant.

The ERGOT is a small piece of horn /horny callosity situated in the tuft of hair at the back of (flexor face) the fetlock joint. It is a vestige of the second and fourth digits (accessory digits) and bear short conical, horny coverings, the structure being the same as the hoof.

The CHESTNUT is a mass of horn on the medial face of the forearm about a hand's breadth above the carpus and on the distal part of the medial face of the tarsus, vestige of the first digit.

1.8 Summary

Axial skeleton - consists of skull, vertebral column, ribs and sternum.

Appendicular skeleton - consists of bones of fore (pectoral) limb and hind (pelvic) limb.

Splanchnic or Visceral skeleton - consists of bones which develop in soft organs.

Os penis :	present in penis of dog.
Os cordis :	present in heart of adult ox.
Os phrenic :	present in diaphragm of the camel.
Os rostri :	present in snout of pigs.

Classification of Bones

1.Long bones:	Have a well developed medullary cavity.	eg: Humerus, femur.
a.Aborted long bones	Medullary cavity is very small or absent	eg: Ulna of horse.
b. Elongated long bones	Medullary cavity is completely absent.	eg: Ribs
2. Flat bones:	Plate like and show large surface area.	eg: Scapula, bones of skull.
3. Short bones:	Present similar dimensions of length, breadth and thickness. Medullary cavity is completely absent.	eg: Carpals, tarsals.
4.Sesamoid bones	Short bones which do not bear the weight of the body but increase the leverage for tendons.	eg: Patella, proximal and distal sesamoids.
5.Irregular bones	Irregular in shape because of the presence of processes and are unpaired.	eg: Vertebrae
6.Pneumatic bones:	Contain air spaces between the two layers of the compact substance instead of spongy bone and marrow.	In mammals: frontal, maxilla, and palatine. In fowl: vertebrae, sternum, humerus, femur.

Falx cerebri is a ***sickle-shaped fold*** of dura mater which is situated in the great longitudinal fissure of the cerebrum.

Tentorium cerebelli. is a ***crescentic fold*** projecting into the great transverse fissure, between the cerebral hemispheres and cerebellum

Diaphragm sellae is a thick fold of dura present on the ventral aspect of the brain which surrounds the pituitary gland.

The spinal dura mater is composed of only the meningeal layer.

The spinal pia mater is thicker and denser. Along the mid ventral line it forms a thickening the linea splendens in which the ventral spinal artery passes.

The subdural space is the space between the dura and the arachnoid and is just a capillary space containing a thin film of lymph.

The lateral horn / intermediate horn is seen only in the thoracic, lumbar and middle sacral levels.

In ox, there are 37 pairs of spinal nerves (8 cervical, 13 thoracic, 6 lumbar, 5 sacral and 5 coccygeal) and 42 pairs in horse (8 cervical, 18 thoracic, 6 lumbar, 5 sacral and 5 coccygeal). 36 pairs in dog (8 cervical, 13 thoracic, 7 lumbar, 3 sacral and 5 coccygeal) and 36 pairs in fowl (15 cervical, 7 thoracic and 14 lumbosacral).

UNIT 2
FORE LIMB

2.1 BONES OF FORE LIMB

SCAPULA

OX: It is a flat, **triangular** bone situated on the **antero-lateral** part of the thorax. It is directed obliquely **downward and forward**. It has two surfaces, three borders and three angles.

The **lateral surface** is traversed by the scapular spine which divides it into the supraspinous and the infraspinous fossae. The **spine** is rough and tuberous in the middle and is prolonged downwards to form the **acromion process (Fig.2.1).** The **medial surface** presents subscapular fossa and its upper part presents anteriorly a triangular rough area and posteriorly a rough line **(Fig.2.2).**

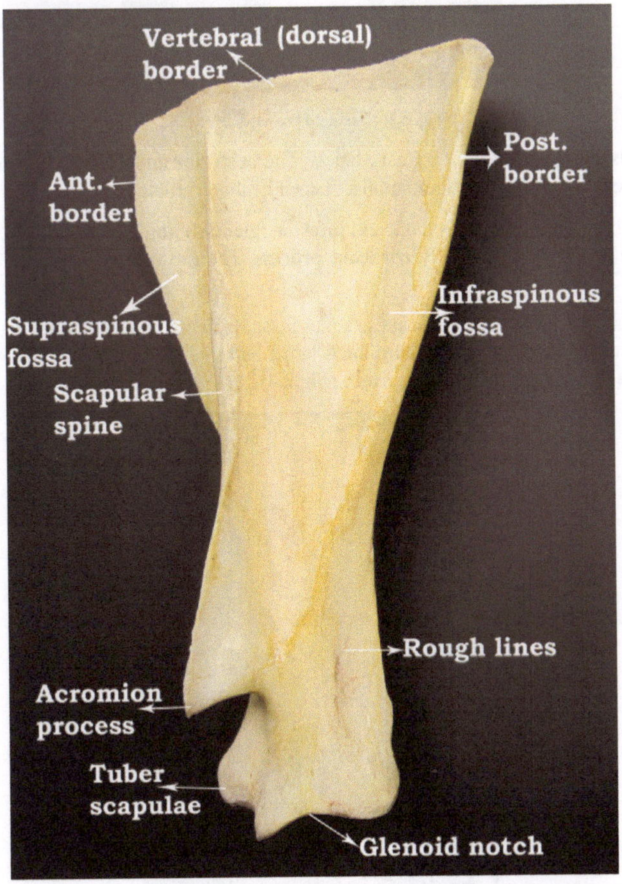

Fig. 2.1: Scapula of Ox -Lateral view

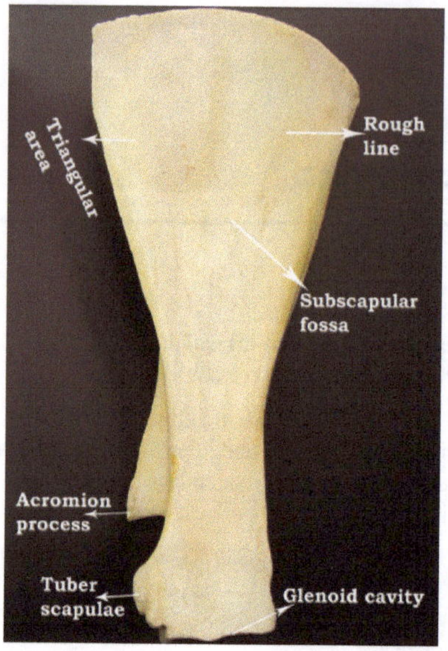

Fig. 2.2: Scapulaof Ox-Medial Veiw

The **anterior border** is convex above and concave below. The **posterior and vertebral borders** are thick and the latter is pitted by impressions into which semicircular shaped hyaline cartilage fits.

The **cervical angle** is thin, **dorsal angle** is thick and **inferior (glenoid) angle** carries the glenoid cavity and tuber scapulae in front. The latter shows medially **coracoid process**. The rim of glenoid cavity shows anterolaterally **glenoid notch**.

Horse: 1.The **acromion process** is absent and subscapular fossa is deeper. 2. The glenoid notch is on anteromedial aspect of rim of glenoid cavity. 3. The **tuber scapulae** is larger and away from the glenoid cavity **(Fig.2.3).** 4. **Two rough triangular areas** are present on medial surface **(Fig.2.4).**

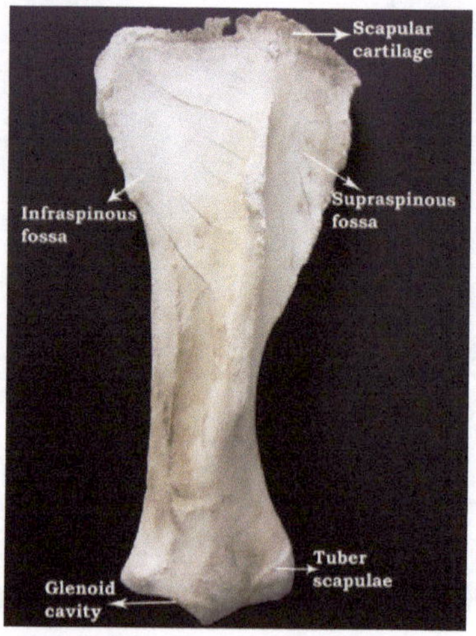

Fig. 2.3: Scapula of Horse- Lateral view

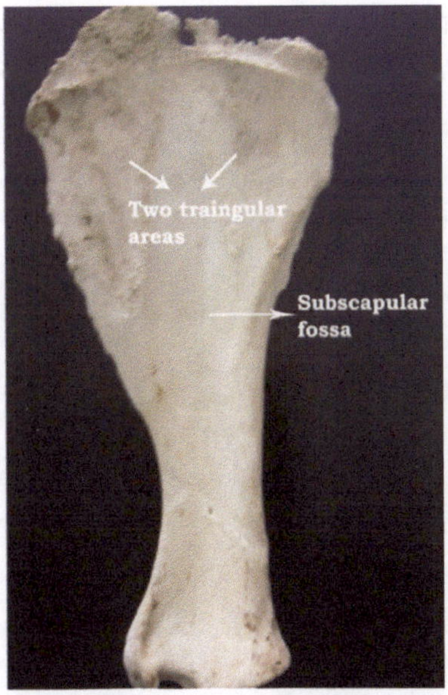

Fig. 2.4: Scapula of Horse -Medial Veiw

Dog: 1.The **scapular spine** is **placed in the middle** dividing lateral surface into equal areas. 2. The **glenoid cavity extends to the inferior face of the tuber scapulae (Fig.2.5).** 3. The **acromion process** overhangs glenoid cavity 4. A **rudimentary coracoid process** is present.

Note: The shoulder girdle in ox and horse is made up of only scapula, while in dog small rudimentary clavicle is also present under brachiocephalicus muscle.

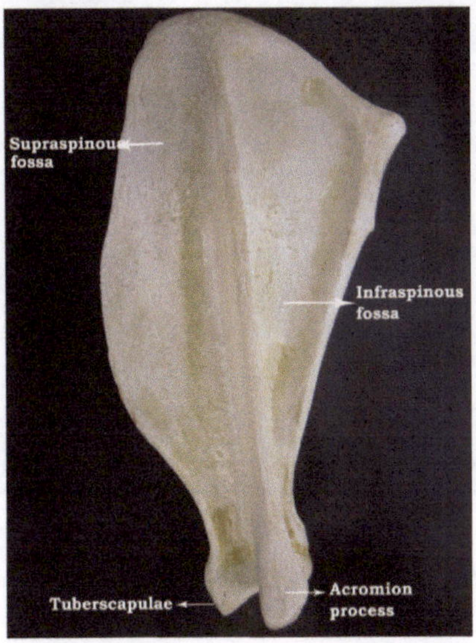

Fig. 2.5: Scapula of Dog -Lateral view

Pig: The scapula is very wide. The spine is triangular and is very wide in its middle which curves caudally over the infraspinous fossa and bears a large tuberosity. Its ventral part bears a small projection (**rudimentary acromion process**).

Fowl: The shoulder girdle shows clavicle, coracoid and the scapula.

Coracoid: is a rod like bone directed backward, downward and inward. The upper extremity presents small articular surface to form the glenoid cavity with scapula. The lower extremity articulates with the sternum **(Fig.2.6).**

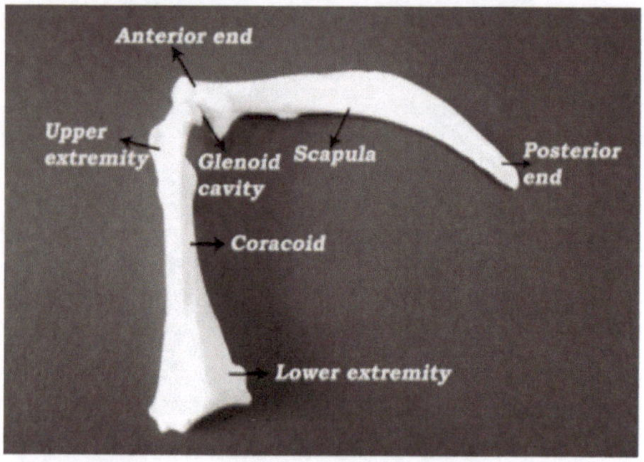

Fig. 2.6: Scapula and Coracoid of Fowl

Clavicle: is a thin bent rod, directed downward and backward. It forms foramen triosseum with scapula and coracoids above. The two side clavicles meet ventrally and form flattened plate called ***hypocleidium*** **(Fig.2.7).**

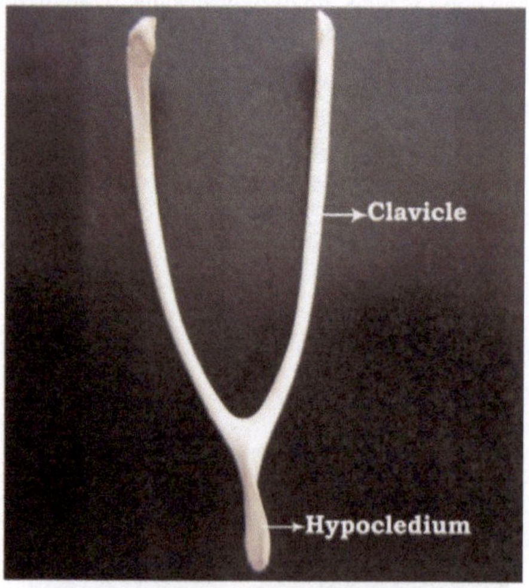

Fig. 2.7: Clavicle of Fowl

Scapula: is a narrow ***sabre shaped*** bone. It lies parallel to the vertebral column and presents a depression laterally which forms the glenoid cavity along with coracoid **(Fig.2.6).** The posterior end lies at the level of the 6th rib.

HUMERUS

Ox: It is a long bone placed obliquely downward and backward between the shoulder joint above and elbow joint below. The shaft has a twisted appearance and shows four surfaces. The anterior surface is triangular. The posterior surface presents nutrient foramen. The medial surface proximal to its middle presents teres tubercle. The lateral surface is in the form of a ***spiral groove***. The crest of humerus separates anterior and lateral faces and extends upward and ends in deltoid tuberosity. The ***deltoid tuberosity*** is continued by a curved line which ends in a tubercle **(Fig.2.8).**

The proximal extremity consists of head, neck, medial and lateral tuberosities. The ***lateral tuberosity*** is large and consists of an anterior summit and a posterior convexity. The former overhangs the bicipital groove. The ***medial tuberosity*** consists of anterior and posterior parts. The intertubular or bicipital groove is present between the anterior divisions of the two tuberosities **(Fig.2.8A).**

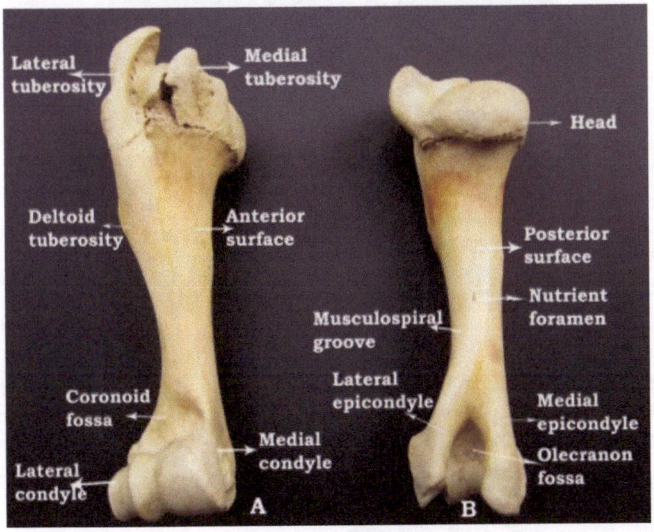

Fig. 2.8: Humerus of Ox (A-Lateral view, B-Posterior view)

The ***distal extremity*** shows medial and lateral condyles, the medial condyle is larger. Above the condyles in front is coronoid fossa, while behind is olecranon fossa bounded by medial and lateral epicondyles **(Fig.2.8B).** The medial condyle is traversed by a sagittal groove which extends into the olecranon fossa and articulates with semilunar notch of ulna **(Fig.2.8A).**

Horse: The **deltoid tuberosity** is more prominent and **bicipital groove** is divided by an intermediate ridge. The **summit of lateral tuberosity** does not arch inward. The coronoid and olecranon fossae are shallower **(Fig.2.9).**

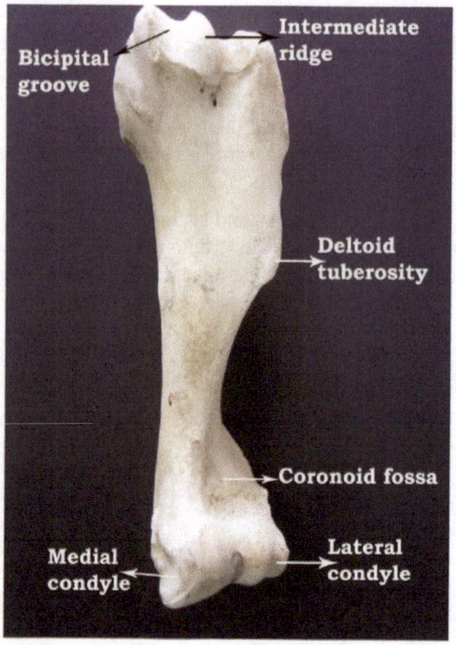

Fig. 2.9: Humerus of Horse

Dog: The shaft is twisted. The musculospiral groove is shallow. The deltoid tuberosity is in the form of a low ridge. The lateral tuberosity is undivided. The ***coronoid and olecranon fossae*** **communicate with each other through the** ***supratrochlear foramen*** **(Fig.2.10).**

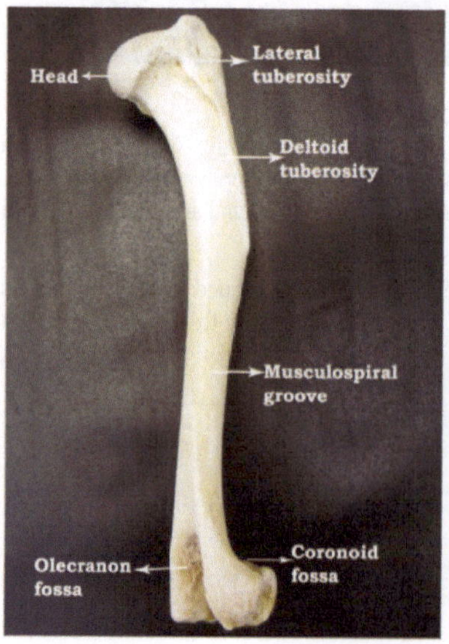

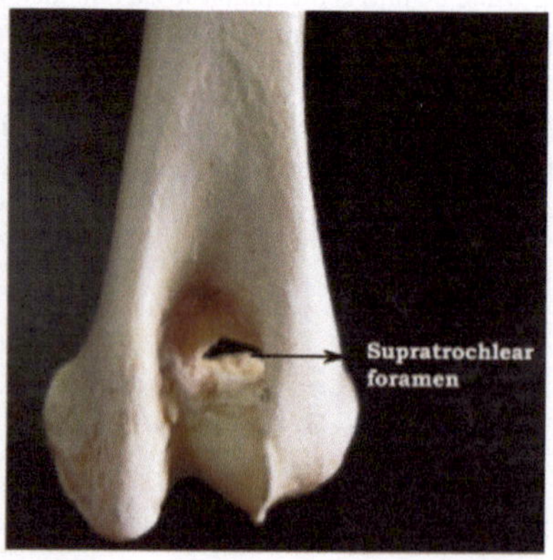

Fig. 2.10: Humerus of Dog

Pig: The humerus has an appearance in profile somewhat like an **italic *f* minus** the cross-bar. The body (shaft) is compressed from side to side. The musculospiral groove is shallow. The deltoid tuberosity is small. The intertuberal (bicipital) groove which is at the front of the medial side; is undivided and almost converted into a canal. The olecranon fossa is very deep.

Fowl: 1.The proximal extremity presents an opening on the medial aspect leading into the air cavity in its shaft. 2. The **head is flattened** 3. **Deltoid tuberosity is in the form of a ridge (Fig.2.11).**

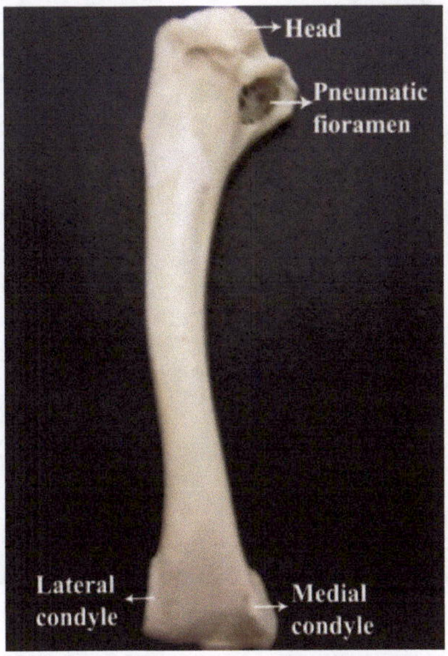

Fig. 2.11: Humerus of Fowl

RADIUS

Ox: The radius is a long bone and the larger of the two bones of the forearm. The shaft has four surfaces: The **dorsal surface** is convex. The **volar surface** is concave and along its lateral border a narrow rough area is present for the ulna **(Fig.2.12).** The **medial face** presents proximally a rough area. The **lateral face** is flattened and limited by the radio-ulnar groove. The proximal extremity presents an articular area which is divided by a sagittal groove into medial and lateral ones. The rim carries anteriorly the **coronoid process** in its middle. Posteriorly just below the rim two facets are present for like facets of ulna. The **dorsomedial aspect** shows an elevated area, ***radial (bicipital) tuberosity*** **(Fig.2.13).** The proximal extremity also shows **lateral and medial tuberosities** of which the lateral tuberosity is more prominent. The **distal extremity** is wider and presents three oblique facets for the **Radial, Intermediate and Ulnar carpals** from within outward **(Fig.2.12).**

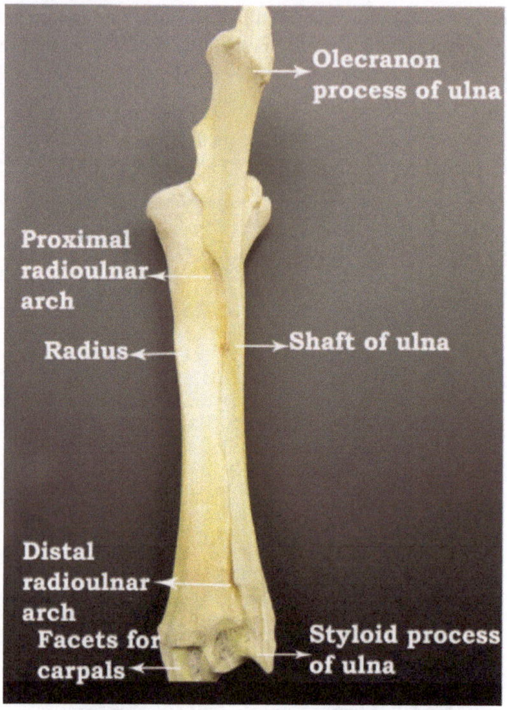

Fig.2.12: Radius and Ulna of Ox- Volar Surface

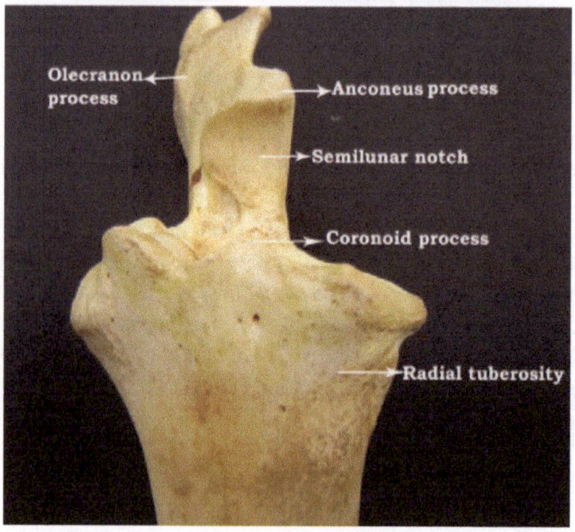

Fig. 2.13: Radius and Ulna of Ox-Dorsal veiw

Horse: The **radial tuberosity** is more prominent **(Figs.2.14&2.15).** The medial border of the volar face presents below the middle a rough elevation for the ***radial (superior) check ligament***. The facets of the distal extremity are ***less oblique***. The lateral facet articulates with **ulnar carpal below** and **accessory carpal behind**.

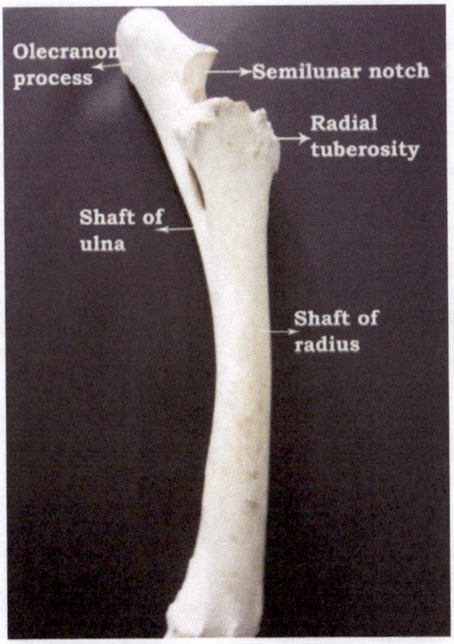

Fig. 2.14: Radius and Ulna of Horse-Lateral View

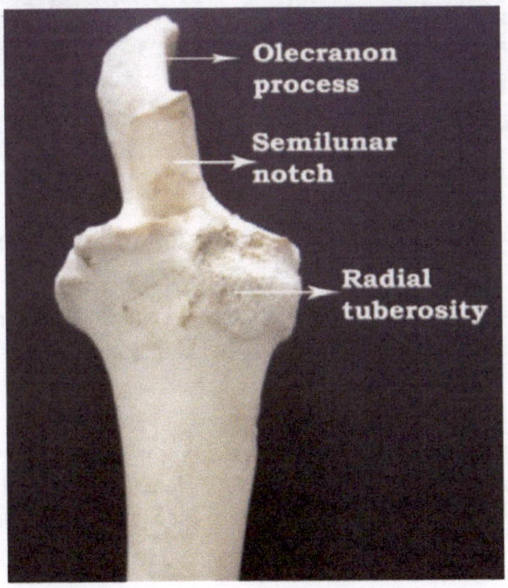

Fig. 2.15: Radius and Ulna of Horse - Anterior view

Dog: The **proximal extremity** is small and bears a concave articular surface. Distal extremity is wide and its **medial border projects downward forming the styloid process of radius** and laterally there is a concave facet for the ulna **(Fig.2.16).**

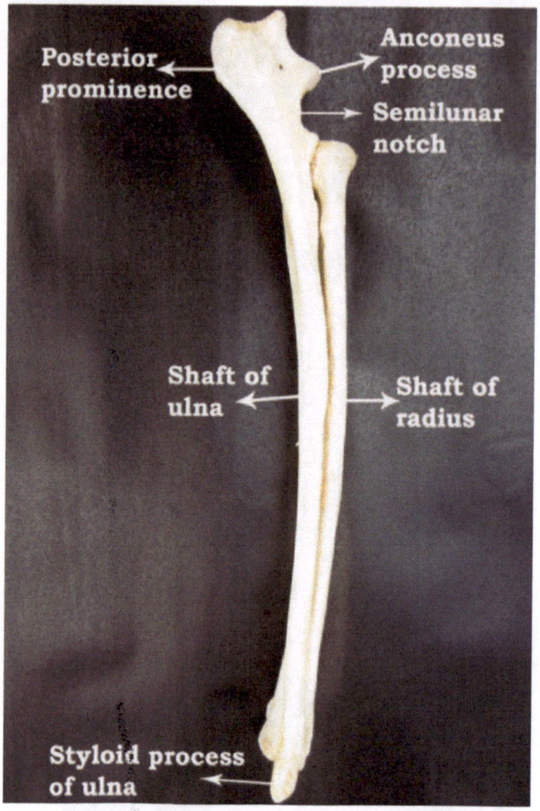

Fig. 2.16: Radius and ulna of Dog-Lateral veiw

Pig: The radius is short and narrow, but thick; the body increases in size distally. The radial tuberosity is represented by a rough area. The distal end or trochlea is relatively large.

Fowl: The **radius is slender**. Its proximal extremity presents concave articular area, while distal extremity is flattened from side to side and articulates with the radial carpal **(Fig.2.20).**

ULNA

Ox: It is a long bone and longer than the radius and located along postero-lateral aspect of the latter. The shaft is three sided hence shows **three surfaces**. The **dorsal face** is rough except at two places where it forms roximal and distal radio ulnar arches. The **medial face** is wide. The **lateral face** presents the radio ulnar groove between it and the radius **(Fig.2.17).**

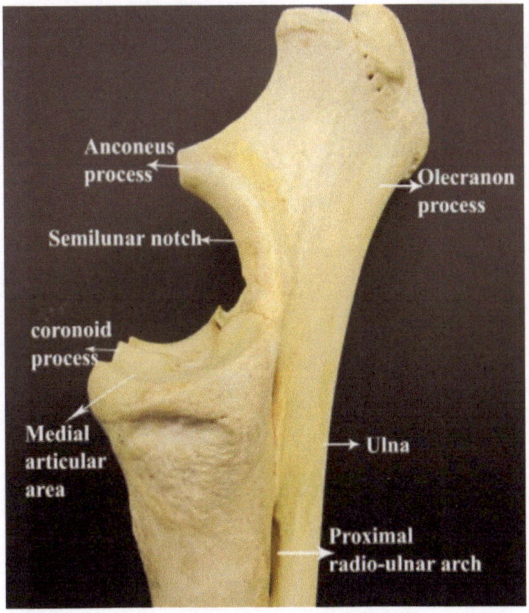

Fig. 2.17: Radius and ulna of Ox

The **proximal extremity** forms the major part of the bone and is made up of the **semilunar notch** and the **olecranon process** the free end of the latter forming the point of elbow **(Fig.2.17).**

The **olecranon process** is quadrilateral in shape and directed upward and backward and its **anterior border** is concave and terminates below as anconeus process. The **posterior border** is thick and concave. The **semilunar notch** is placed below the anconeus process and articulates with distal extremity of the humerus. Below the notch two facets are present for like facets of the posterior aspect of the proximal extremity of the radius **(Fig.2.17).**

The **distal extremity** is fused with the radius and forms the styloid process of ulna and furnishes a part of the facet for the ulnar carpal.

Horse: It is shorter reaching only distal third of the radius. It forms only proximal radio-ulnar arch **(Fig.2.18).**

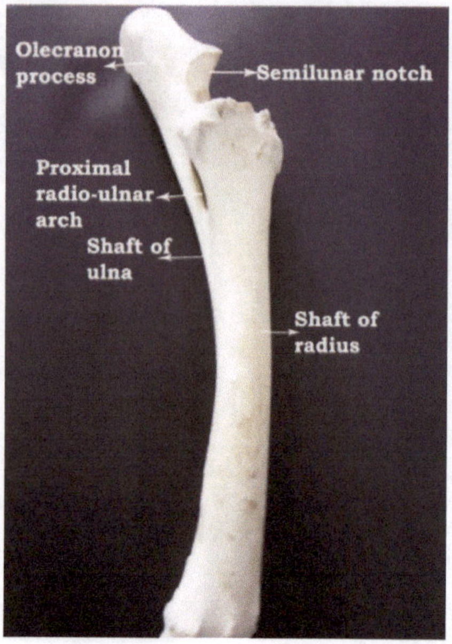

Fig. 2.18: Ulna of Horse- Lateral view

Dog: The ***olecranon process is grooved*** and shows **three prominences** of which the posterior one is large and rounded **(Fig.2.19).** The **styloid process** articulates **dorsomedially with radius** and **below with ulnar and accessory carpals.**

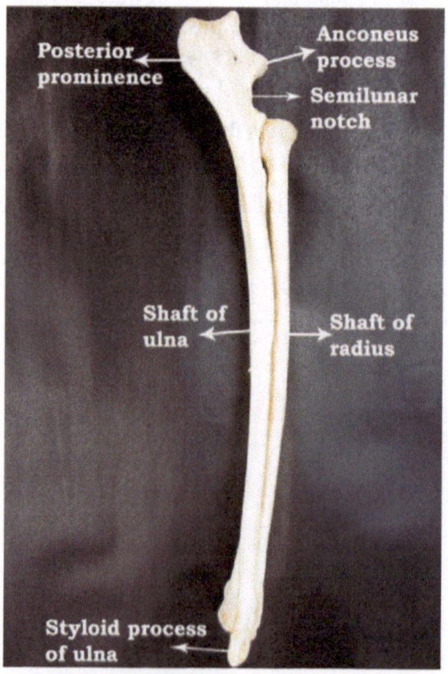

Fig. 2.19: Radius and Ulna of Dog

Pig: The ulna is massive. It is much longer and considerably heavier than the radius; the body is curved.

Fowl: The curved ***ulna is larger, longer and thicker*** than the radius. The proximal extremity has two concave articular areas. The **olecranon process** is short. The ***distal extremity*** presents a trochlea which **articulates with radial and ulnar carpal bones (Fig.2.20).**

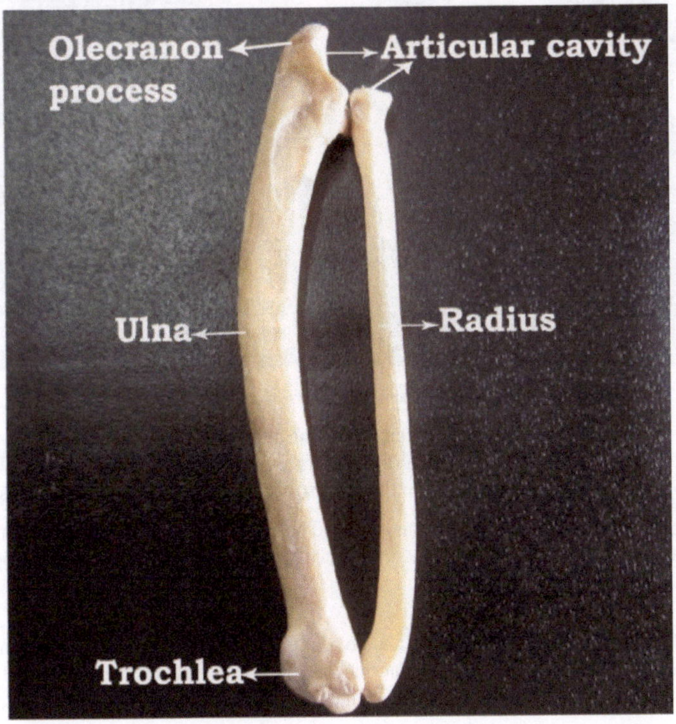

Fig. 2.20: Radius and Ulna of Fowl

CARPALS

Ox: The carpus consists of **six short bones** arranged in two rows, four in the proximal row and two in the distal row.

Proximal row: Radial, Intermediate, Ulnar, Accessory

Distal row: fused 2nd and 3rd, 4th carpal.

Radial carpal: is the ***largest bone of the upper row*** and roughly quadrilateral. Proximal surface is convexo-concave and articulates with radius. The distal face articulates with fused 2nd and 3rd carpal. The lateral surface bears facets for the intermediate carpal. The dorsal, medial and volar faces are continuous and rough **(Fig.2.21).**

Intermediate carpal: is ***wedge shaped***. The apex, which is posterior is prolonged medially. The **proximal face** is convexo-concave and articulates with the radius. The **distal face** is divided by sagittal ridge into two facets the medial one is for the 2nd and 3rd and the lateral one is for 4th carpal. The **medial face** has facets for the radial carpal. The **lateral face** articulates with the ulnar carpal **(Fig.2.21).**

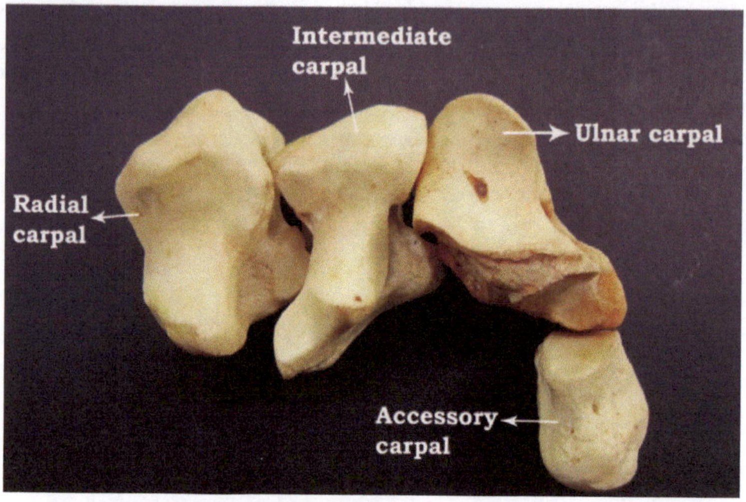

Fig. 2.21: Carpals of Ox (Proximal row)

Ulnar carpal: is ***very irregular***. The **proximal face is oblique** and directed backward and downward. The **distal face** articulates with the fourth carpal. The medial face has facets for the intermediate carpal. The **dorsal face** is convex and rough and posterior face has a facet for the accessory carpal, while **lateral surface** is rough **(Fig.2.21).**

Accessory carpal: is **short, thick and rounded** and situated behind the ulnar carpal. The proximal face is narrow and rough. The distal face is broad and rough. The dorsal face has a facet for the ulnar carpal **(Fig.2.21).**

DISTAL ROW

Fused 2nd and 3rd carpal: is the ***largest carpal***. The proximal face has two facets, the larger medial facet for the Radial carpal and the smaller lateral facet for the Intermediate carpal. The lateral face has facets for the 4th carpal and distal face articulates with the medial facet of proximal extremity of large metacarpal **(Fig.2.22).**

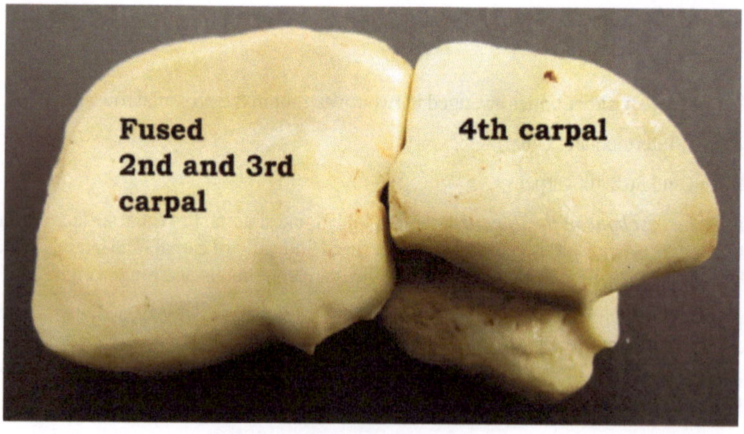

Fig. 2.22: Carpals of Ox (Distal Row)

Fourth carpal: The proximal face has two facets the medial one for the intermediate and the lateral one for ulnar carpal. The distal face articulates with the lateral facet of proximal extremity of large metacarpal. The medial face has facets for the fused 2nd and 3rd carpal. The fused 2nd and 3rd and 4th carpals are quadrilateral **(Fig.2.22).**

Horse: has 7 or 8 bones.

Proximal row: Radial, Intermediate, Ulnar, Accessory

Distal row: 1st carpal (inconstant), second carpal, 3rd carpal, 4th carpal

Radial: is more regularly quadrilateral **(Fig.2.23)**.

Intermediate carpal: The lateral angle of proximal face is more pointed **(Fig.2.23).**

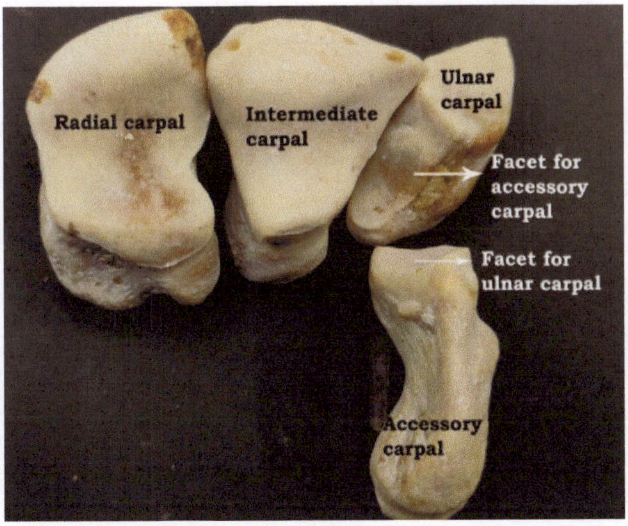

Fig. 2.23: Carpals of Horse (Proximal Row)

Ulnar carpal: proximal face articulates only with the radius.

Accessory carpal: is ***discoid***, its medial face is concave and lateral face is convex and rough. The anterior ***border has two facets, the upper one for radius and lower one for the ulnar carpal*** **(Figs. 2.23. &2.24).**

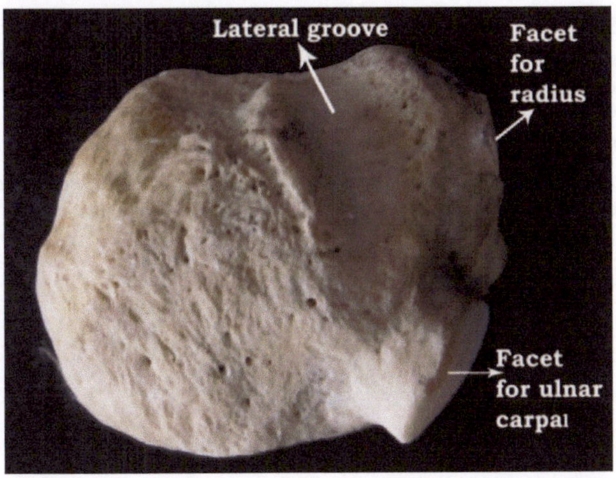

Fig. 2.24: Accessory Carpal of Horse

DISTAL ROW:

2nd carpal: is ***smallest*** bone of the distal row and hemispherical in shape. The proximal face has a convex facet for the radial carpal. The distal face articulates with the medial small and large metacarpals. The lateral face has two facets for the 3rd carpal **(Fig.2.25).**

3rd carpal: is the **largest carpal** in distal row and irregularly triangular. The proximal face articulates with the radial and the intermediate carpals and the distal face with the medial small and large metacarpals **(Fig.2.25).**

4th carpal: The proximal face is convex and articulates with ulnar carpal. The distal face articulates with the large and lateral small metacarpals. The medial face has two facets for the 3rd carpal. The volar face bears a tubercle on its distal part **(Fig.2.25)**..

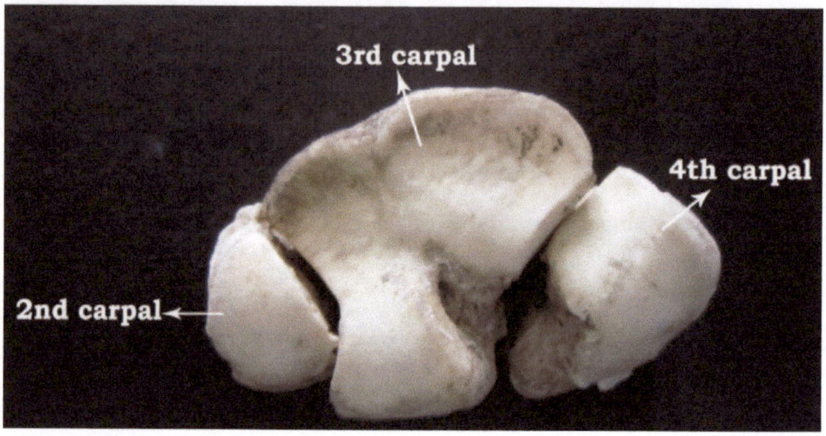

Fig. 2.25: Carpals of Horse (Distal Row)

Dog: Has ***seven bones***, three in the proximal and four in the distal row.

Proximal row: Radio-Intermediate carpal (Fused), Ulnar carpal and Accessory carpal

Distal row: First carpal, Second carpal, 3rd carpal, 4th carpal

The distal row bones articulate with respective metacarpals, while 4th carpal articulates with 5th metacarpal also.

Pig: The carpus comprises **eight bones**, four in each row. The bones of proximal row resemble those of the ox, with the exception of the accessory, which is more like that of the horse but has no lateral groove. In distal row, the **first carpal** is small, elongated from dorsal palmarly and rounded and articulates dorsally with the second carpal.The **fourth is the largest** bone of the row; it articulates with the intermediate and ulnar proximally.

Fowl: There are only two free bones. The ***radial carpal is quadrilateral,*** while the ***ulnar carpal is forked*** **(Fig.2.26).** The bones of the distal row fuse with the metacarpals and form ***carpometacarpus***.

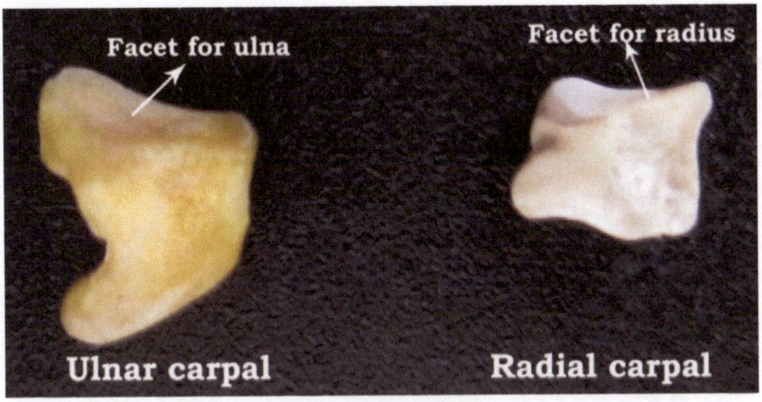

Fig. 2.26: Carpals of Fowl

METACARPUS (*Cannon bone*)

Ox: The metacarpus consists of a large metacarpal (fused 3 and 4th) and rudimentary small (fifth) metacarpal.

The large metacarpal is a long bone. The shaft is semicylindrical and has two surfaces and two borders. The **dorsal surface** is convex and marked by a **vertical vascular groove (Fig.2.27A),** which is traversed by a foramen at either end. The volar face is flat and presents a shallow vertical groove **(Fig.2.27B).** The borders are medial and lateral. The latter at its upper part has the lateral small metacarpal attached to it posteriorly.

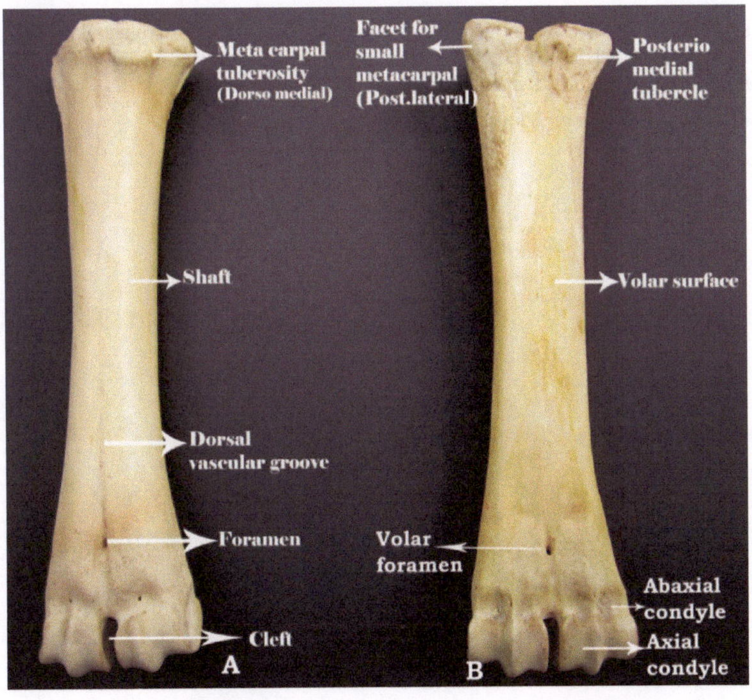

Fig. 2.27: Large Metacarpal of Ox (A-Dorsal and B-Volar surface)

The proximal extremity has two facets separated by a ridge followed by a notch. Of the two facets medial one is larger and is for the fused 2nd and 3rd carpal and lateral one is for the 4th carpal **(Fig.2.28).** At the ***dorsomedial aspect*** the proximal extremity presents ***metacarpal tuberosity*** **(Fig.2.27A)**, while at the **posteromedial** aspect is a **tubercle (Fig.2.27B).**

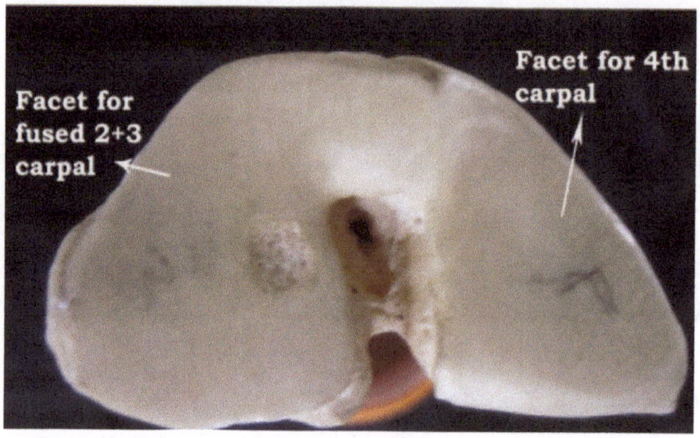

Fig. 2.28: Large Metacarpal of Ox- Proximal view

The **posterolateral** aspect bears a facet for proximal extremity of **small metacarpal**. The distal extremity is divided into two parts by a sagittal cleft. Each part is made up of two (axial and abaxial) condyles separated by a sagittal ridge for articulation with the axial and abaxial articular areas of 1st phalanx. The abaxial condyles are higher and larger and axial condyles are lower and smaller.

The **small metacarpal** is an aborted long bone. This bone is attached to the posterolateral aspect of the proximal extremity of the large metacarpal. The proximal extremity is rounded and bears a small facet on its anterior face for large metacarpal. The distal extremity is pointed **(Fig.2.29).**

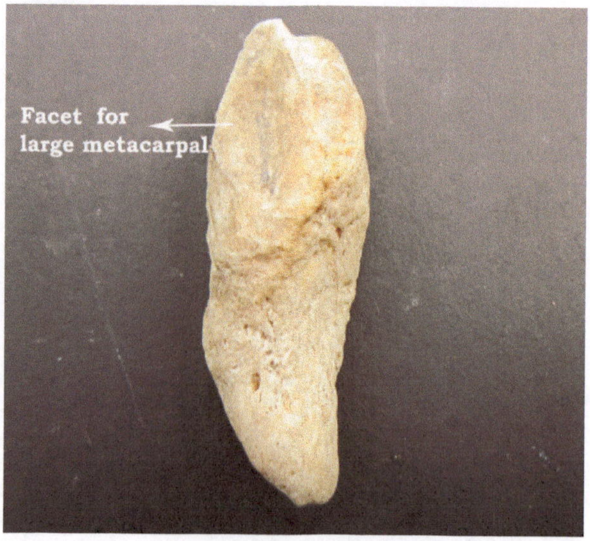

Fig. 2.29: Small Metacarpal of Ox

Horse: The metacarpus consists of one large metacarpal **(3rd)** and two small metacarpals or splints, medial i.e. **(2nd)** and lateral i.e. **(4th)**, **(Fig.2.30).**

Large metacarpal: The vascular grooves on the dorsal and volar faces are absent. The shaft is semicylindrical. The volar face is roughened on either side in its proximal two thirds for the attachment of the splints **(Fig.2.30).** The proximal extremity articulates with the 2nd, 3rd and 4th carpals above and on either side with the proximal extremities of splints. The distal extremity resembles one part of the distal extremity of large metacarpal of the ox **(Fig.2.30).**

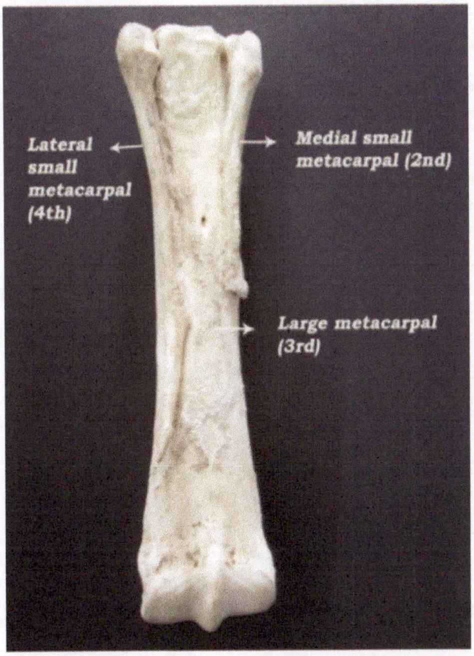

Fig. 2.30: Metacarpus of Horse (Volar aspect)

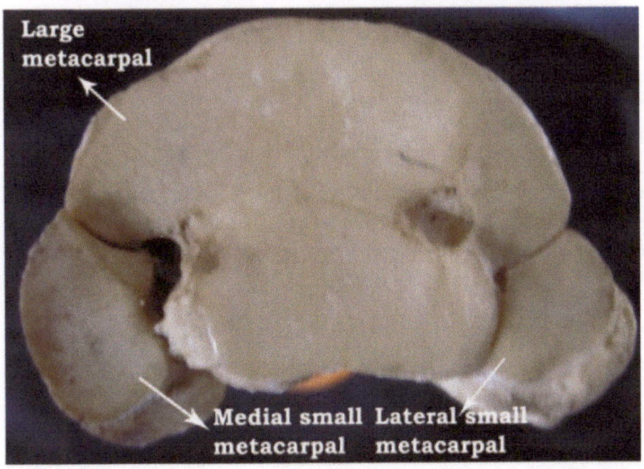

Fig. 2.31: Large and Small Metacarpals of Horse (Proximal view)

Small metacarpals: The shafts of each are three sided. The dorsal face of the proximal extremity bears two facets for the large metacarpal. The medial small metacarpal bears two facets proximally for the 2nd and 3rd carpals, while the lateral small metacarpal presents one facet for the fourth carpal. The distal extremity is in the form of a small nodule **(Figs.2.30&2.31).**

Dog: The metacarpus has five bones. The ***first is shortest***. The ***3rd and 4th are the longest***. The **2nd** is **longer than the 5th**. The proximal ends articulate with each other and the first four with the corresponding carpals above. The 5th also articulates with the 4th carpal above (**Fig.2.32**).

Pig: Four metacarpal bones are present. The first is absent, the third and fourth are large and carry the chief digits (**Fig.2.32**). while the second and fifth are much smaller and bear the "accessory" digits.

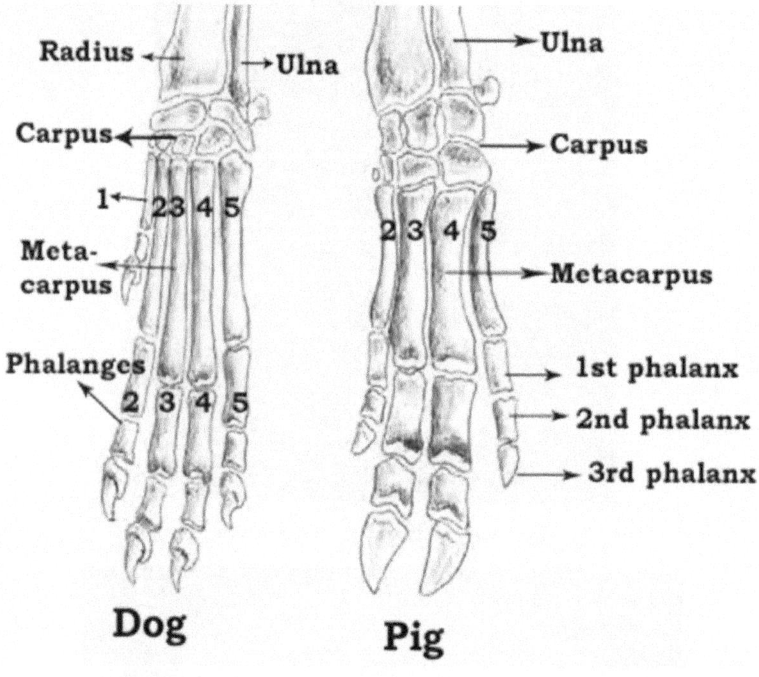

Fig. 2.32: Metacarpals and Digits of Dog and Pig

Fowl: The metacarpus consists of three bony elements which fuse together and with the distal row of carpal bones form a single bone carpometacarpus. The ***first is the most medial*** and is in the form of a nodule. The second and third bones are united at their extremities, leaving a narrow space between their shafts. The **second one is largest (Fig.2.33).**

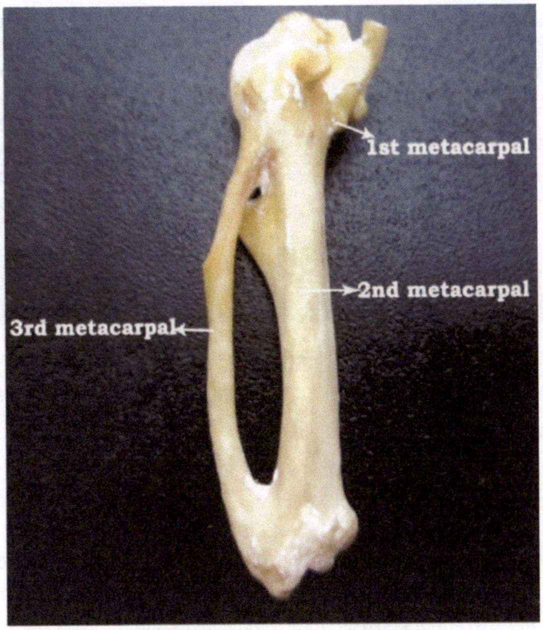

Fig. 2.33: Carpometacarpus of Fowl

Digits and Sesamoids

Proximal sesamoids

Ox: Proximal sesamoids are a pair (axial and abaxial) for each digit, so totally 4 are present in a limb. They are present behind the distal extremity of large metacarpal. Each bone is a three sided pyramid **(Fig.2.34).**

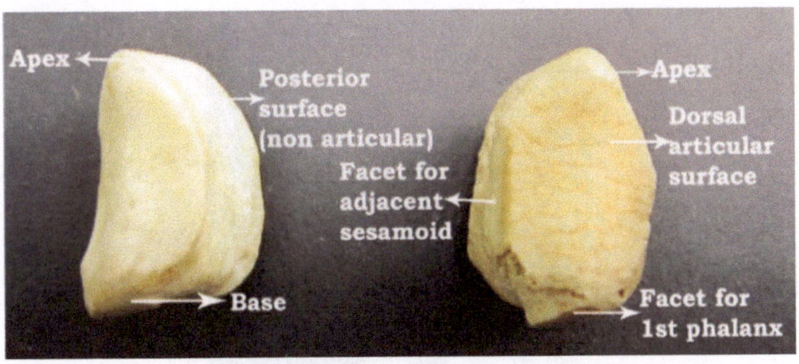

Fig. 2.34: Proximal sesamoids of Ox

The base presents a facet for first phalanx. The dorsal surface articulates with the volar surface of distal extremity of large metacarpal. Each sesamoid presents a facet for articulation with similar facet of its fellow.

Horse: Only one pair of proximal sesamoids in a limb is present and these are ***distinctly pyramidal / triangular*** in shape **(Fig.2.35).** Each articulates only with the large metacarpal but not with either 1st phalanx or with its fellow.

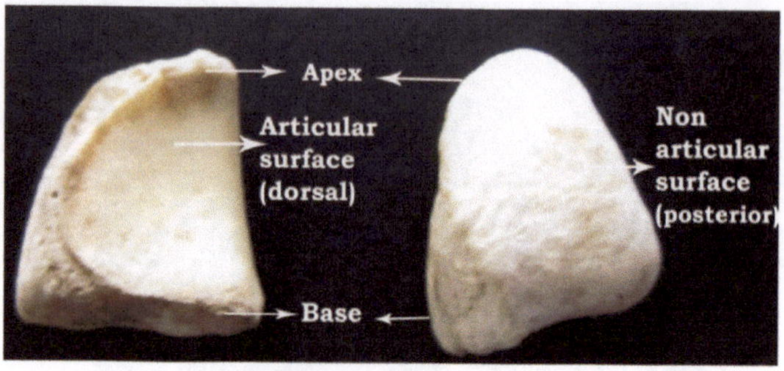

Fig. 2.35: Proximal Sesamoids of Horse

Dog: Nine proximal sesamoids are present, ***one for the first digit and two for each of the other 4 digits.***

Pig: The proximal sesamoids are narrow and ridged palmarly.

Fowl: The sesamoids are absent.

Digits

Ox: Two digits (3rd and 4th) are fully developed and have three phalanges and three sesamoids (2 proximal + 1 distal) each. The 2nd and 5th digits (***dew claws***) are vestigeal and placed behind the fetlock.

Horse: There is only one digit (3rd) and it consists of three phalanges and three sesamoids (2 proximal + 1 distal).

Dog: There are five digits. The **3rd and 4th digits are the longest**. The first digit has two phalanges and one proximal sesamoid and does not come in contact with the ground. The rest have three phalanges and two proximal sesamoids each.

Pig: Each chief digit comprises three phalanges and three sesamoids. The 2nd and 5th digits donot touch the ground.

Fowl: There are three digits. The first and the second digits have two phalanges each. The third digit has one phalanx **(Fig.2.36).**

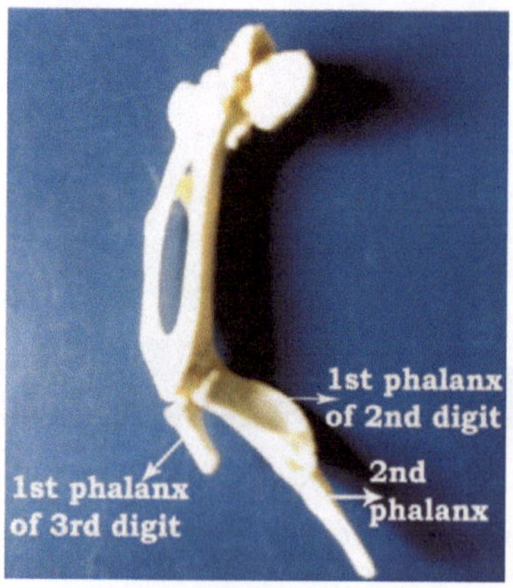

Fig. 2.36: Phalanges of Fowl

Phalanges

First phalanx (*Os suffraginis*):

Ox: is placed between the large metacarpal above and the second phalanx below. It is a long bone. The shaft is four sided **(Fig.2.37).** The proximal extremity is larger than distal and is divided by a sagittal groove into abaxial and axial articular areas which receive the distal extremity of large metacarpal and also shows facets behind for proximal sesamoids. The abaxial articular area is larger and higher, while the axial articular area is smaller and lower. The articular surface of distal extremity is divided by a sagittal groove into two condyles which respond to the proximal extremity of second phalanx

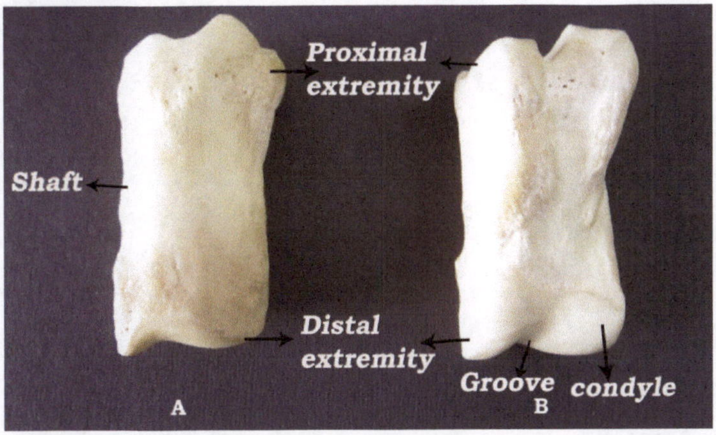

Fig. 2.37: 1st Phalanges of Ox (A-Dorsal and B- Volar view)

Second phalanx (*Os coronae*) is a short bone placed between 1st and 3rd phalanges. The shaft is three sided. The proximal extremity shows two glenoid cavities for 1st phalanx. The distal extremity is smaller and divided by sagittal groove into two condyles which articulate with superior face of 3rd phalanx below and the distal sesamoid behind **(Fig.2.38).**

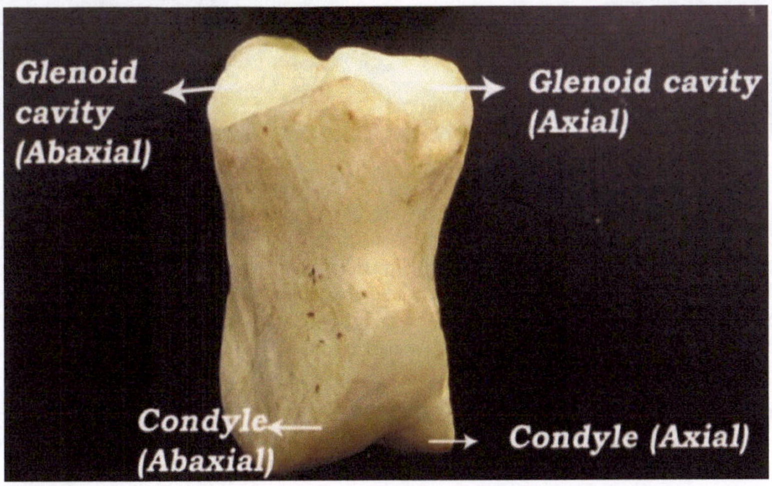

Fig. 2.38: Second Phalanx of Ox (Dorsal view)

Third phalanx (*Os pedis or Coffin bone*) is a short bone consisting of **four surfaces**, **four borders** and an angle. The **superior (articular) surface** presents two articular areas for the distal extremity of the 2nd phalanx and a small facet on volar border for distal sesamoid. The inferior (sole) surface is nearly flat. **The laminar (parietal) surface** is divisible into axial (interdigital) and abaxial surfaces. The slightly concave axial surface is smooth and grooved below and rough and porous above. It presents a large axial foramen near extensor process **(Fig.2.39)**.

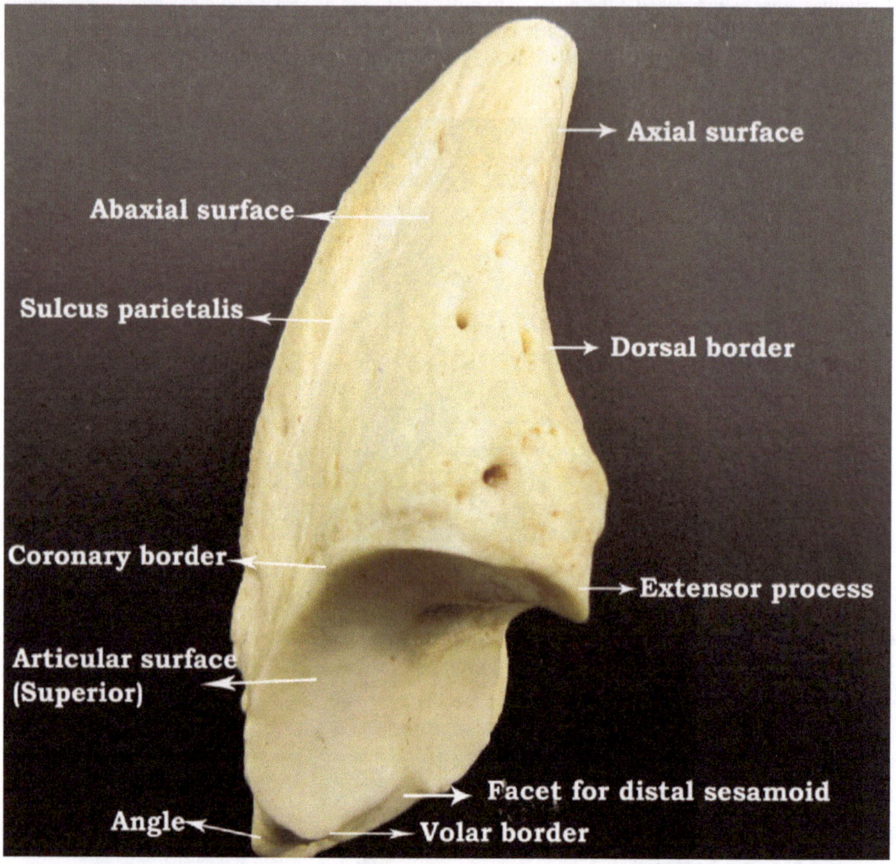

Fig. 2.39: 3rd Phalanx of Ox

The convex **(abaxial) surface** slopes from above downward and becomes steep posteriorly. There is a groove called **sulcus parietalis** on distal part of both axial and abaxial surfaces. The groove on abaxial surface ends caudally at abaxial foramen. **Coronary border** is placed at the junction of laminar and articular surfaces, while rounded **dorsal border** is at the junction of abaxial and axial surfaces and solear border is at the junction of laminar and solear surfaces. At the extreme upper part of the **dorsal border is the** ***extensor process***. The **volar border (ventral)** is thick, while basal (ground / solear) border is distal. The angle is a blunt process at the extreme posterior part of the laminar surface.

Horse: 1st phalanx: The volar face presents ***'V' shaped*** area beginning from the proximal extremity **(Fig.2.40).** The proximal face of proximal extremity is divided by a sagittal groove into two concave areas and no facets are present for proximal sesamoids. The lateral axes bear tubercles **(Fig.2.40).**

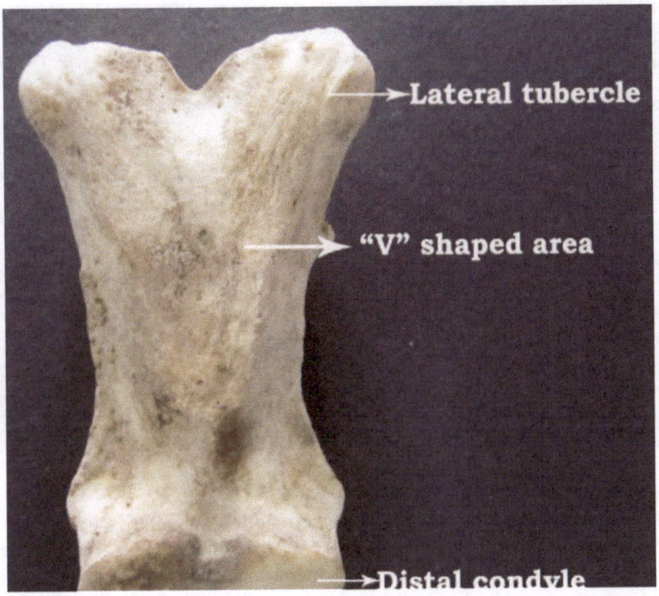

Fig. 2.40: First Phalanx of Horse

2nd phalanx: is short being more wide than long **(Fig.2.41).**

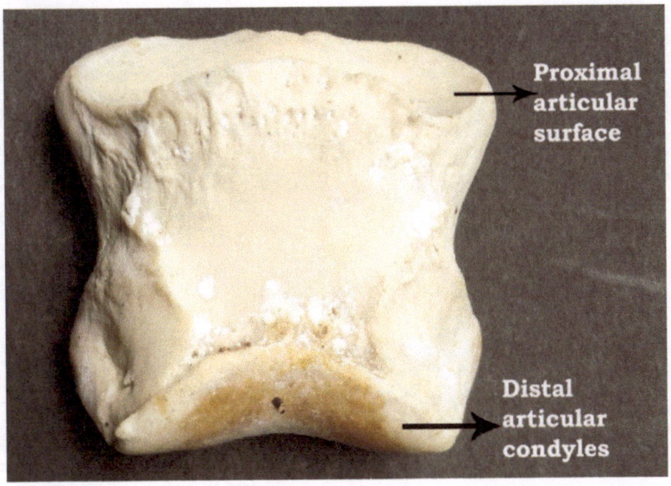

Fig. 2.41: 2nd Phalanx of Horse

3rd phalanx: shows **three surfaces, three borders** and two angles. The **superior face** is adapted to the distal extremity of the 2nd phalanx and distal sesamoid. The **volar fa**ce is divided by the semilunar crest into solear surface and flexor surface **(Fig.2.43).**

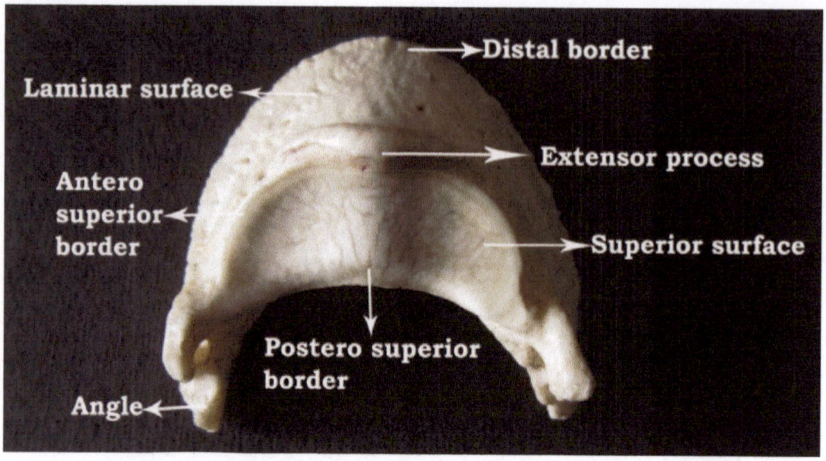

Fig. 2.42: 3rd Phalanx of Horse (Dorsal view)

The **laminar (parietal) surface** slopes from above downwards and becomes steep posteriorly. The surface shows dorsal, medial and lateral parts. The sulcus parietalis is seen both on medial and lateral parts of this surface extending from angles dorsally. The **coronary (anterosuperior) border** bears about its middle the extensor process, while **posterosuperior border** forms posterior limit of the superior surface **(Fig.2.42).** The distal border is irregularly notched with a wider notch in front. The angles or wings project backward and are divided into upper and lower parts by a notch or a foramen **(Fig.2.42).**

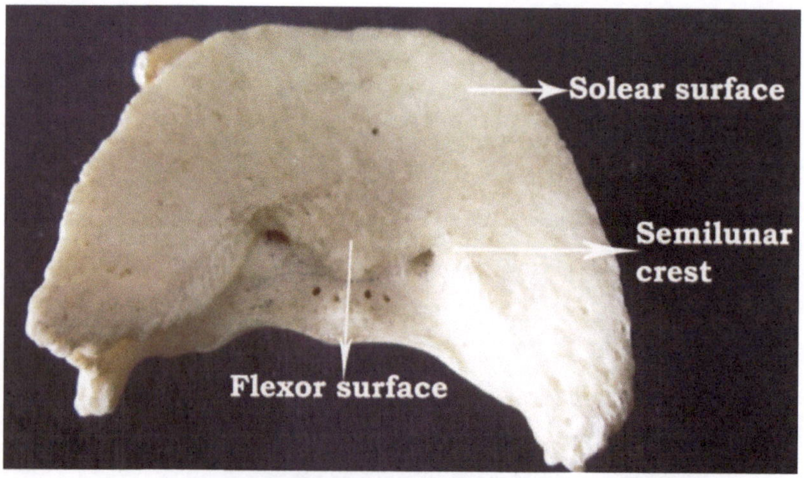

Fig. 2.43: 3rd Phalanx of Horse (Volar view)

Dog: The first phalanges of the chief digit have four sided shafts and the **second phalanges are about 2/3 of the length of the first phalanx (Fig.2.44A).** ***The third phalanges correspond to the shape of the claws.*** The base is encircled by a collar of bone **(Fig.2.44B).** The solear surface bears a flexor tubercle. The ungular process is a curved rod with a blunt pointed free end.

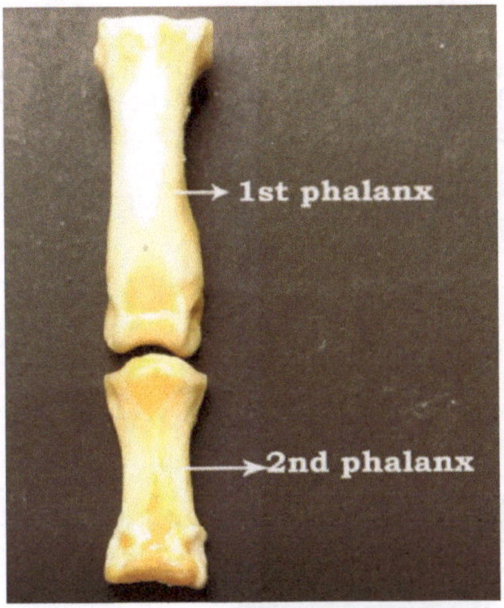

Fig. 2.44A: 1st and 2nd Phalanges of Dog

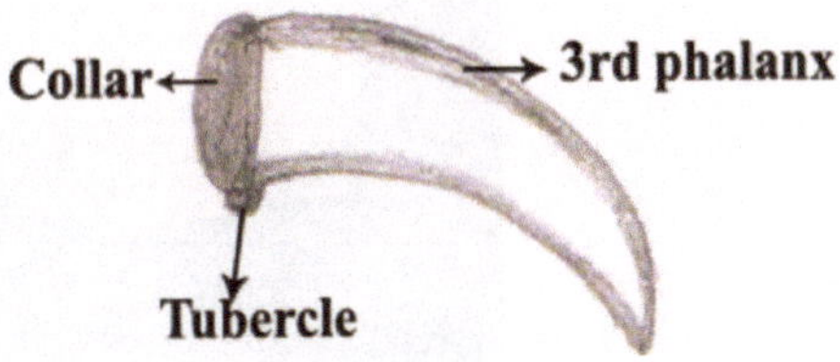

Fig. 2.44B: 3rd Phalanx of Dog (schematic)

Pig: The bones of the chief digits resemble those of the ox in form, but there is no foramen on the axial surface of the extensor process. The phalanges of the accessory digits which donot reach the ground ordinarily, are similar in form but much smaller.

Fowl: The first phalanx can be compared to a ***knife blade*** with a strong back and a sharp edge. The 2nd phalanx is in the form of pointed cone. The phalanx of the third digit is thorn like **(Fig.2.45).**

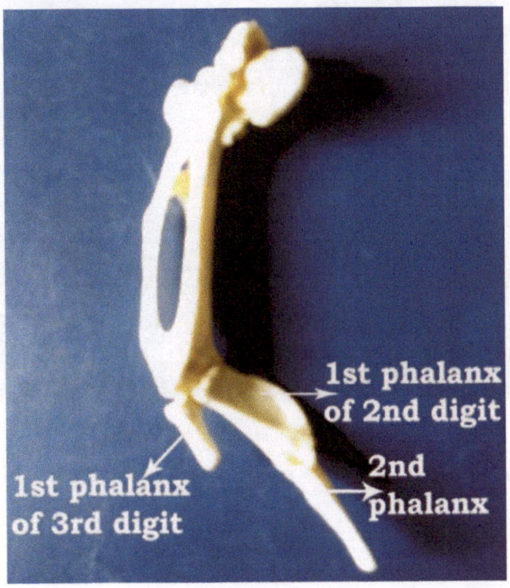

Fig. 2.45: Phalanges of Fowl

Distal Sesamoids

Ox: The distal sesamoid (os navicularis) is placed behind the second interphalangeal articulation. It is **quadrilateral** and presents two surfaces, two borders and two extremities. The anterior (dorsal) face has two facets for the second phalanx. The distal border bears a small facet about its middle for the os pedis **(Fig.2.46).**

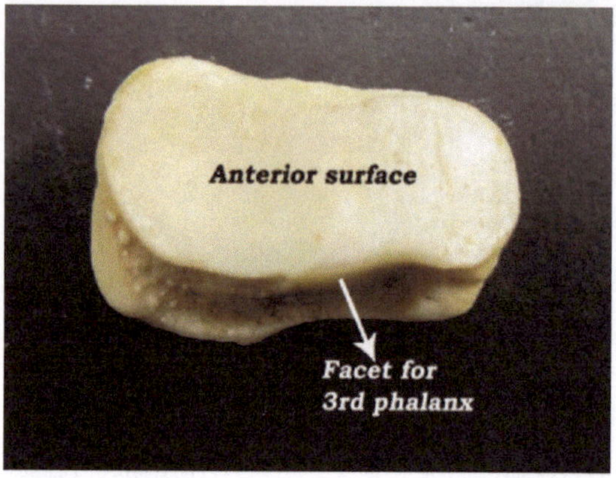

Fig. 2.46: Distal sesamoid of Ox

Horse: The ***distal sesamoid is shuttle shaped*** and longer with narrow extremities **(Fig.2.47).** It is also called as "***navicular bone***" (***analogous to a boat***).

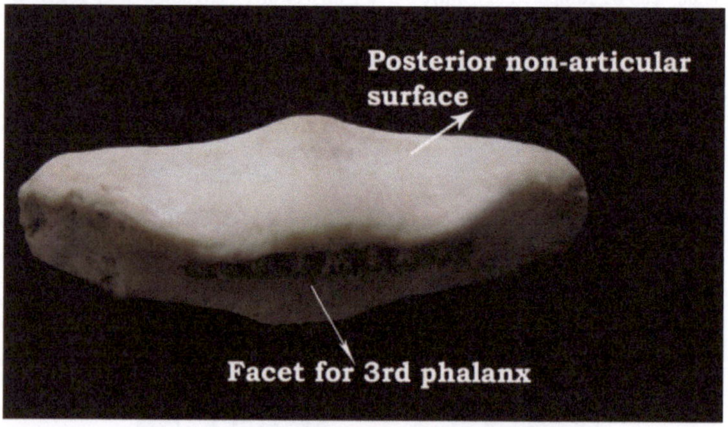

Fig. 2.47: Distal sesamoid of Horse

Dog: The distal sesamoids **are cartilaginous.**

Fowl: absent.

2.2 STUDY OF HOOF

The hoof is the horny box which encloses the distal end of the digit enclosing III Phalanx completely and lower part of II Phalanx and enclosing number of structures sensitive cartilaginous, bony etc.It consists of bony part (2nd and 3rd phalanges) internally, Corium ,modification of dermis of skin in the middle and outermost horny layer ,modification of epidermis of skin. The animals provided with hoofs are called ungulates eg., horse, ox, sheep, goat, camel, pig.

Hoof of the OX : The hoof has only three parts-periople, wall and sole **(Fig. 2.48)**. The frog, lateral cartilages and plantar cushion are absent. It shows three surfaces. The abaxial (outer) surface is convex from side to side and is marked by ridges parallel with the coronary border. Its anterior part is concave from edge to edge. The interdigital (axial) surface is concave and grooved. It touches the opposite one only at its ends. The basal/solar/ ground surface consists of sole and prominent bulb of soft thin horn. The sole is slightly concave and pointed in front and widens behind. The laminar corium shows only primary laminae which are narrower but more numerous. The corium of the bulb is separated from the flexor tendon in natural state by a mass of elastic, fatty tissue analogous with the digital cushion of the horse. There are two hooves in each limb in the ox. The cloven foot takes up the function of diffusing concussion.

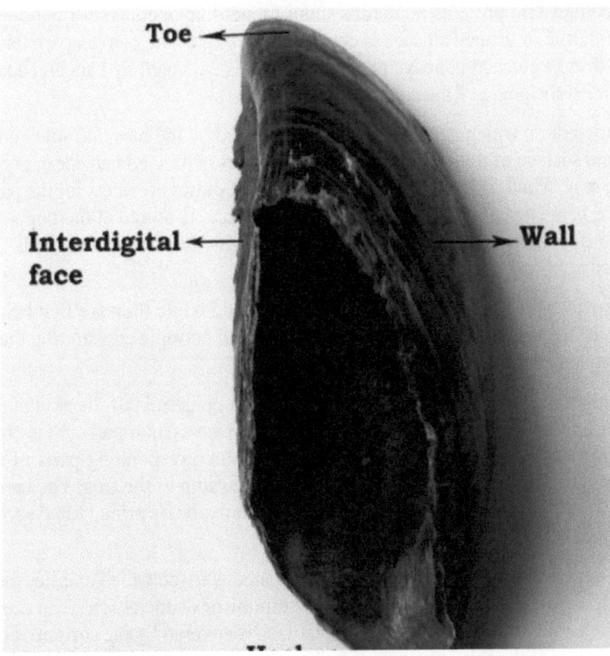

Fig. 2.48: Hoof of Ox

Hoof of the horse : shows three parts wall, sole and frog **(Fig. 2.49 & 2.50)**. The part of the hoof visible when the foot is placed on the ground is the wall which covers the front and sides of the foot and is reflected posteriorly inwards at an acute angle to form the bars. The bars appear on the ground surface of the hoof as convergent ridges which subside in front and are fused with the sole. The frog unites the two bars. There are anterior part (toe), sides-medial and lateral parts (quarters) and the posterior part, angles (heels), two surfaces and two borders of the wall. The external surface is convex from side to side and slopes obliquely from edge to edge. This slope is variable. It is more in the hind limb than in the fore limb. It is steeper at the sides than in front and more on the inside than outside. This surface is crossed by more or less distinct ridges parallel to the coronary border. It is also marked by fine parallel striae which extend from border(edge) to border(edge) indicating the direction of horn tubules of which it is composed.

The internal surface of the wall is concave from side to side and bears about six hundred primary horny laminae extending from the coronary groove to the basal border of the wall and bearing a number of secondary laminae which dove tail with the corresponding laminae of the sensory corium. The proximal /upper coronary border is thin and its outer aspect is covered by a layer of light coloured horn band known as periople at the junction of skin and hoof. It is narrower in front but widens out laterally and completely caps the heels by forming a wide cap or bulb at angle and blends centrally with the frog. The inner aspect of the border is excavated to form two coronary grooves an upper one for the perioplic band and a lower one for the coronary band, designated respectively as the perioplic and coronary grooves. which contain the thick coronary corium in natural state. The groove shows innumerable small funnel like openings occupied by papillae of the coronary corium in natural state. The perioplic groove is narrow at the toe but becomes very wide at the heels while coronary groove is wide in front and becomes narrow posteriorly and blends with the perioplic groove.The basal or ground border comes in contact with the ground and is convex. It is thicker in front and thinner at the sides. Its inner face is united to the periphery of the sole by horn of lighter colour and softer texture which appears on the ground surface of the hoof as the white line.

The crescentic sole constituting greater part of the ground surface of the hoof presents two surfaces and two borders. The internal surface is convex and presents numerous small funnel like openings for papillae of corium of sole in natural state while the external or ground surface is concave and rough. The convex parietal border is joined to the wall by white line. The deeply notched concave posterior border is occupied by bars and apex of the frog.The part between the bars and wall is the angle of the sole.

The frog is a wedge shaped mass which occupies the angle bounded by the bars and sole and extends considerably below these on the ground surface of the foot. It shows four surfaces, a base and an apex. The internal surface bears a central ridge , the frog stay, which is high behind and this surface shows openings for the papillae of corium while external / ground surface bears a central sulcus. The ground surface is united at the upper part with the bars and sole but are free below and prominent at the sides where it unites with the angles of the wall. The apex occupies the central angle of the concave border of the sole and is blunt.

The medial and lateral surfaces join at upper part with bars and sole while they are free below. The base unites at the sides with the angles of the wall where it is covered by expanded periople constituting the bulb of the hoof. The apex occupies the central angle of the concave border of the sole.

The horny hoof is avascular and devoid of nerves. It is a modified epidermis of the skin and receives its nutrition from the corium which is a modified dermis of the skin. The corium is vascular part and is observed between horny hoof and III phalanx and is divisible into five parts which nourish corresponding parts of the hoof i.e. perioplic corium, coronary corium, laminar corium, corium of the sole and corium of the frog. The laminar corium related to internal surface of the wall of hoof and laminar surface of III phalanx, bears primary and secondary laminae which interleave with horny laminae of the wall in natural state.

The digital /plantar cushion is a wedge shaped modified subcutaneous tissue which overlies the corium of the frog in natural state and shows four surfaces, a base and an apex. It diminishes concussion. The deep face is connected to the fibrous sheath of the deep flexor tendon. The superficial face is covered by the corium of the frog. The sides are related to the lateral cartilages of the third phalanx. The base is posterior, subcutaneous and is divided by a central depression into two rounded prominences-bulbs of the cushion. The apex is adherent to the terminal part of deep flexor tendon. It consists of meshwork of white and elastic fibres containing fat.

The lateral cartilages are attached to the angles of the third phalanx. The external face is convex and the internal face is concave. The upper border extends higher up and hence easily palpable. The lower border is thicker and is partly attached to the angle. The posterior end curves towards its fellow.

The hoof is made up of epithelial cells which are more or less keratinsed except at the deepest part-stratum germinativum which by division maintains growth of the hoof. The cells are in part arranged to form horn tubes united by inter tubular horn. The wall consists of three layers : 1. an external layer of periople and stratum tectorium. The periople is made of soft non-pigmented tubular horn which becomes white when the foot is soaked in water. It is continuous with the epidermis of the skin above. The stratum tectorium is a thin layer of horny scales which gives the outer face of the wall below the periople a smooth glossy appearance. 2. The middle layer which forms the bulk of the wall consists of horn tubes which run between the borders and the deep layer of horny laminae composed of non tubular horn. The sole is made up of tubular and non-tubular horn. The frog is composed of softer horn which is not fully keratinized.

The corium furnishes nutrition to the horny hoof. It is composed of the following parts:

1. The perioplic corium is situated in the perioplic groove. It is continuous with the dermis above and is marked off from the coronary corium below and blends with it laterally. It completely blends with the corium of the frog at angles and bears fine papillae which are received into depressions in the horny part and it supplies nutrition to the periople.
2. The coronary corium occupies the coronary groove and furnishes nutrition to the bulk of the wall-middle layer. It has numerous fine papillae. It is wide infront but becomes very narrow posteriorly. It is attached by its deep face to the extensor tendons and cartilages of third phalanx.
3. The laminar corium bears primary and secondary laminae which are inter-leaved with the corresponding horny laminae. It is attached to the laminar face of the os pedis by modified periosteum and supplies nutrition to the horny laminae.
4. The corium of sole nourishes the horny sole. It bears papillae and is continuous with the corium of bars and frog. The deep face is attached to the solar face of the os pedis.
5. The corium of the frog is moulded on the deep face of the frog. Its deep face is blended with the plantar cushion and it nourishes the horny frog.

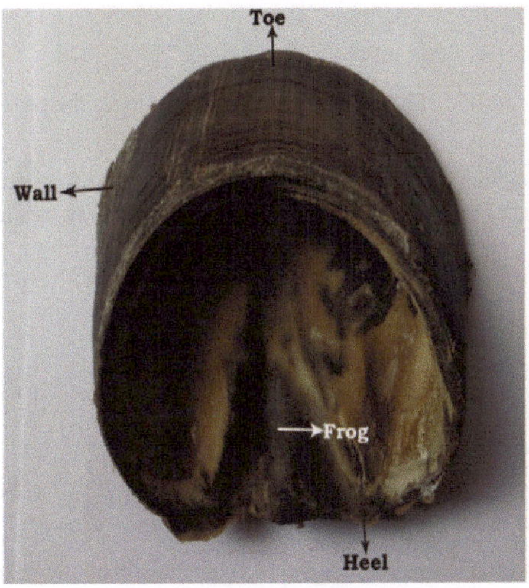

Fig. 2.49: Hoof of Horse-Dorsal view

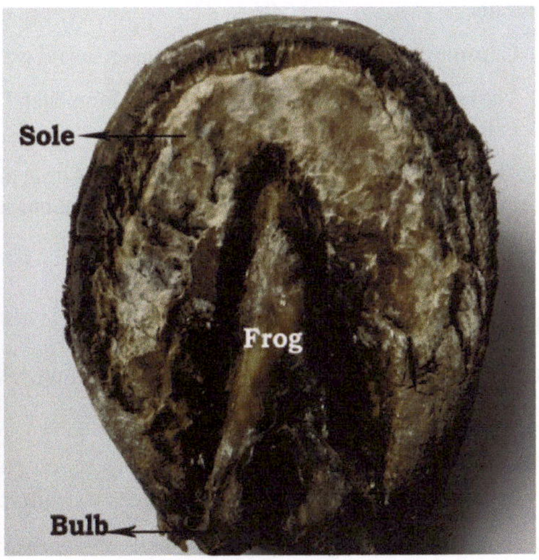

Fig. 2.50: Hoof of Horse- Solear view

2.3 JOINTS OF THE FORE LIMB

Synsarcosis: The attachment of the forelimb with head and trunk by means of muscles like brachiocephalicus, omotransversarius, trapezius, rhomboideus, serratus ventralis, latissimus dorsi, tensor fasciae antibrachii, pectorals (shoulder girdle muscles) is called ***synsarcosis.***

Shoulder Joint

Articular areas: The glenoid cavity of scapula and head of the humerus. The summit of lateral tuberosity of humerus forms point of the shoulder.

Type: Simple, diarthrodial (ball and socket / enarthrosis)

Ligaments: Only capsular ligament is present and has neither collateral nor special ligaments, instead it is supported by strong tendons of muscles of shoulder.

Movements: Chiefly extension and flexion and also circumduction, rotation, adduction and abduction.

Elbow Joint

Articular areas: Condyles of the humerus, articular areas of radius and semilunar notch of ulna. The ***olecranon*** *process forms point of the elbow*.

Type: Composite, diarthrodial (ginglymus).

Ligaments

1. **Capsular ligament** is thick and strong on dorsal aspect and thin on volar aspect.
2. The **lateral collateral ligament** extends from lateral condyle of humerus to lateral tuberosity of the proximal extremity of the radius.
3. The thick **medial collateral ligament** extends from medial condyle of humerus to radius and shows superficial and deep parts, the former attaching to medial border of the radius below the bicipital tuberosity, while the latter attaching to medial tuberosity **(Fig.2.51).**

Movements: Extension and flexion.

Radioulnar articulations:

Articular areas: shafts of radius and ulna mostly along posterolateral aspect of the radius.

Type: simple joint. It is formed at four levels.

The **first radioulnar** articulation is between facets on posterior aspect of radius below the margin of articular cavities and facets on dorsal surface of ulna below semilunar arch. It is diarthrodial in nature.

The **second and fourth** ones are between shafts of radius and ulna above and below proximal and distal interosseous spaces respectively.The **third one** is between the shafts of two bones between proximal and distal interosseous spaces. These are amphiarthroses. The medial and lateral **arciform (transverse)** ligaments covering and connecting shafts of radius and ulna above proximal interosseous space are seen. The three interosseous ligaments uniting the bones at 2nd, 3rd and 4th joints become ossified as the age advances resulting in fusion of bones.

Movements: Inappreciable in all the above joints.
In dog joints between radius and ulna at either end are trochoid.

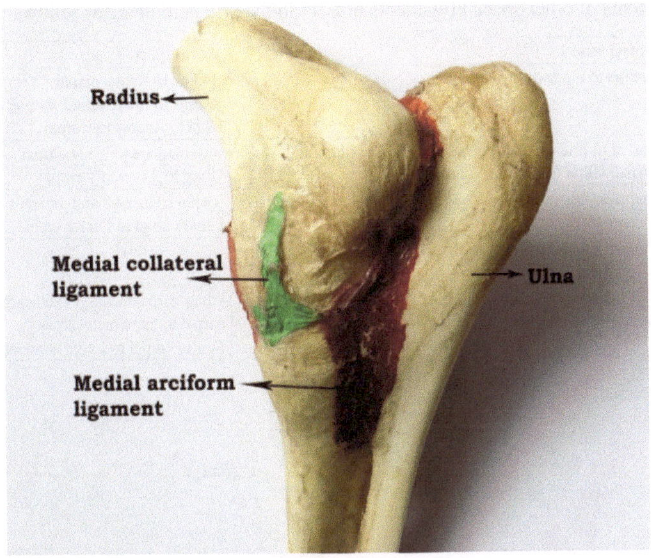

Fig. 2.51: Elbow Joint of Ox

Carpal (Knee) Joint

Articular areas: Distal extremities of Radius and Ulna, articular surfaces of two rows of carpal bones and proximal extremity of large metacarpal **(Fig.2.52).**

Type: composite, diarthrodial. It consists of

a. **Radioulnar carpal joint**: Between distal articular areas of radius and proximal surfaces of Radial, Intermediate and Ulnar carpals and distal articular area of ulna and proximal surface of ulnar carpal. It is an imperfect hinge joint since articular surfaces are oblique and as concavo-convex surfaces of radius and ulna articulate with convexo-concave surfaces of proximal row carpals.

b. **Proximal carpal**: Between Radial and Intermediate, Intermediate and Ulnar, Ulnar and Accessory carpals of proximal row.

c. **Intercarpal**: Between distal surfaces of proximal row carpals (radial, intermediate and ulnar) and proximal surfaces of distal row carpals (2 and 3 fused and fourth).

d. **Distal carpal**: Between 2nd and 3rd fused and 4th carpal of distal row.

e. **Carpometacarpal**: Between distal surfaces of distal row carpals (2nd & 3rd fused and 4th) and proximal extremity of large metacarpal. The joints **b to e** are **arthrodia (gliding)** type.

The joint cavity is subdivided into three compartments corresponding to a, c and e joints. Hence synovial membrane forms three sacs, while fibrous layer is common to all joints. The capsular ligament covering dorsal and volar aspects of the joint are called dorsal capsular (to which extensor tendons are adherent) and volar capsular ligaments. The latter is thick and forms anterior boundary of **carpal sheath / canal,** while **volar annular ligament** (flexor retinaculum) extending across from accessory carpal to medial collateral ligament forms posterior boundary of carpal canal. The medial thick and lateral collateral ligaments extend from distal extremity of radius and ulna respectively to proximal extremity of large metacarpal on respective sides. The interosseous ligaments connect the bones of respective rows and also distal row with large metacarpal.

The details of attachments of other special ligaments present in the articulation are as follows:

	Dorsal aspect	Volar aspect
Radioulnar- carpal	Radius to ulnar carpal (oblique)	Radius to Radial carpal Radius to Intermediate carpal, Radius to Ulnar carpal Ulna to Accessory carpal
Proximal carpal	Radial to Intermediate carpal, intermediate to Ulnar carpal, Ulnar to accessory carpal	Intermediate to Ulnar carpal, Ulnar to Accessory carpal
Inter carpal	Radial to 4th carpal (oblique), ulnar to 4th carpal and also to large metacarpal	Radial to fused 2 and 3 carpal Ulnar carpal to Fourth carpal, Accessory to 4th carpal
Distal carpal	Fused 2 and 3 to 4th carpal	-
Carpo-meta carpal	Fused 2 and 3 carpal to large metacarpal, 4th carpal to large metacarpal	Ulnar carpal to Large metacarpal, Fused 2 and 3 carpal to large metacarpal Fourth carpal to Large metacarpal

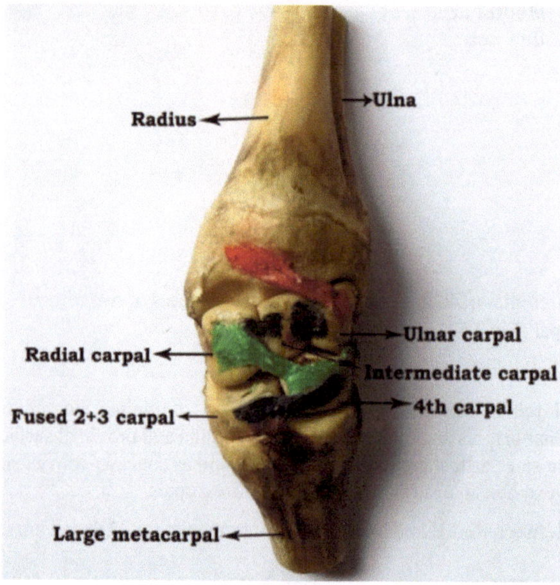

Fig. 2.52: Carpal Joint of Ox

6. Intermetacarpal joints: Between large and small metacarpals. One is between facets on posterolateral aspect of proximal extremity of large metacarpal and facet on proximal extremity of small (lateral) metacarpal (diarthrosis). The other one is amphiarthrosis between shafts of two.

Movements: Limited

Carpal canal: It is formed by ***volar capsular ligament infront*** and ***volar annular ligament behind,*** the latter extends from the posterior border of the accessory carpal to the medial aspect, blending with the medial collateral ligament of the carpus. The canal serves for the passage of ***deep division of superficial digital flexor, deep digital flexor, ulnar artery and median nerve*** **(Fig.2.53).**

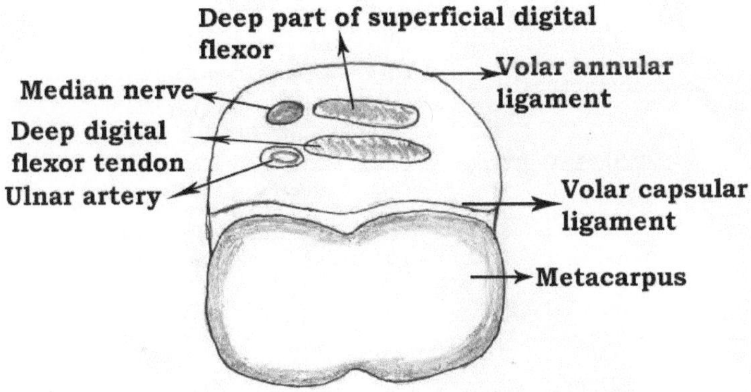

Fig. 2.53: Structures of Carpal Canal (Schematic)

> In horse **superior check ligament** arises from radius below the middle close to medial border and attaches to tendon of superficial digital flexor above the carpus, while **inferior check ligament** is continuation of volar capsular ligament and joins tendon of deep digital flexor.

Fetlock (Metacarpo-Phalangeal) Joint

Articular areas: axial and abaxial condyles of the two parts of distal extremity of large metacarpal above and axial and abaxial articular areas of proximal (1st) phalanx of medial (3rd) and lateral (4th) digits below and axial and abaxial proximal sesamoids behind. The sesamoids articulate with posterior part of proximal extremities of 1st phalanges also by means of their bases.

Type: Composite, diarthrodial (ginglymus).

Ligaments

1. Capsular ligament
2. Axial and abaxial collateral ligaments extending from axial (cleft) and abaxial aspects of each part of distal extremity of large metacarpal to respective aspects of proximal phalanges.
3. The special ligaments are **a.** Proximal or superior sesamoidean ***(suspensory)***ligament, **b.** Lateral sesamoidean ligaments, **c.** Inter sesamoidean and **d.** Inferior sesamoidean ligaments.

The suspensory ligament is actually an interosseous muscle being replaced mostly by fibrous tissue as the age advances. It extends from distal row of carpals and proximal extremity of large metacarpal on volar aspect to proximal sesamoids. It divides **into anterior (muscular) and posterior (fibrous) divisions** in the lower third of large metacarpal.

The **posterior division** divides into two bands which join with those of superficial digital flexor tendon and form two rings (canals) lined by synovial membranes for the passage of two divisions of deep digital flexor tendon **(Fig.2.54).**

The **anterior division** shows six bands **2 axial, 2 abaxial and two middle bands (Fig.2.55).**The axial and abaxial bands attach to respective sesamoids. The slips from abaxial bands also extend to dorsal aspect and attach to tendons of respective (medial and lateral) digital extensors. The **middle bands pass** through axial cleft of metacarpal and reach the dorsal aspect and attach to two divisions of tendon of common digital extensor and also respective (medial and lateral) digital extensor tendons.

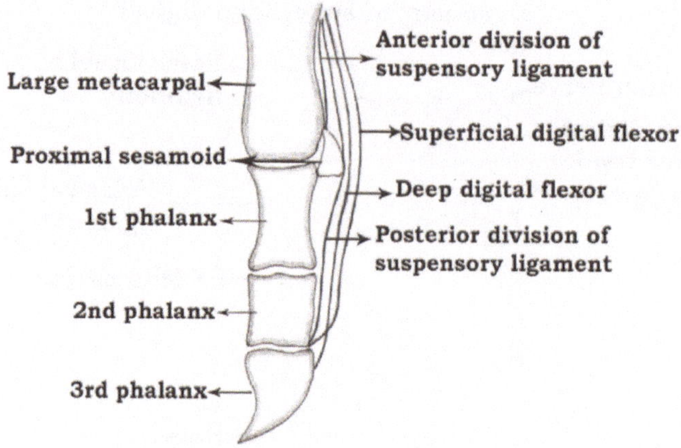

Fig. 2.54: Suspensory Ligament and Digital Flexors-Lateral view

The **three intersesamoidean ligaments** attach the opposite faces of four proximal sesamoids.

The **inferior sesamoidean** ligaments are two straight and two oblique. The two straight ligaments are vertical connecting the bases of the abaxial and axial sesamoids to the proximal extremity first phalanx. The oblique ligaments arising from bases of the sesamoids cross each other and are attached to the first phalanx.

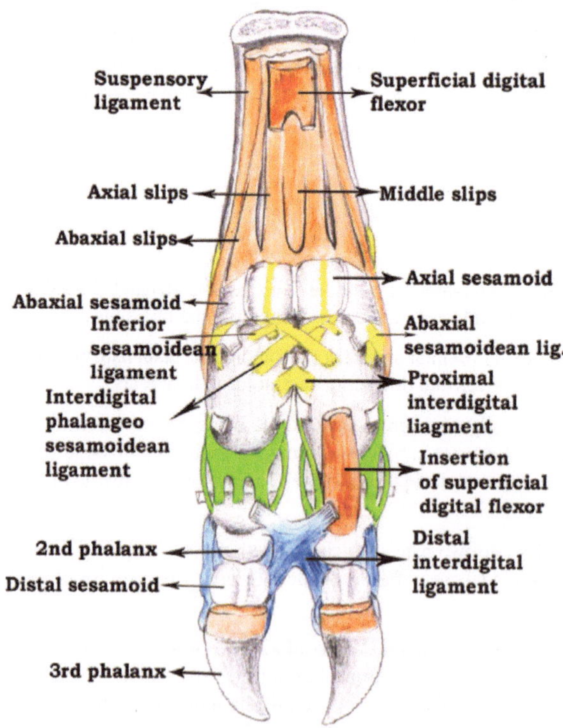

Fig. 2.55: Fetlock Joint-Ox

The **interdigital phalangeo-sesamoidean** ligaments extend from proximal sesamoids of one digit to volar aspect of proximal extremity of opposite first phalanx. The proximal interdigital ligament consisting of intercrossing fibres connect shafts of proximal phalanges of two digits.

Movements: Extension and flexion

> In **horse suspensory ligament** divides into only two (medial and lateral) branches attaching to proximal sesamoids and does not form rings with superficial digital flexor. In **dog the ligament is replaced by interosseous muscles.**

Pastern (Proximal Interphalangeal) Joint

Articular areas: Distal extremity of 1st phalanx above and proximal extremity of 2nd phalanx below.

Type: Simple, diarthrodial (hinge)

Ligaments: Capsular, axial (weak) and abaxial collateral ligaments connecting respective aspects of distal extremity of proximal phalanx and proximal extremity of middle phalanx.

Movements: Extension and flexion.

Coffin (Distal Interphalangeal) Joint

Articular areas: Distal extremity of 2nd phalanx above and proximal articular surface of 3rd phalanx below and distal sesamoid behind.

Type: Composite, diarthrodial (hinge)

Ligaments

1. Capsular ligament
2. **Axial and abaxial collateral ligaments** connecting respective aspects of 2nd and 3rd phalanges.
3. **Distal interdigital** (**cruciate**) ligament extending from abaxial eminence of proximal extremity of 2nd phalanx to distal sesamoid of opposite side and also to axial aspect of 3rd phalanx and distal sesamoid of same digit.
4. **Distal sesamoidean ligament** connects distal sesamoid to volar border of 3rd phalanx.

Movements: Extension and flexion.

2.4 MUSCLES OF THE FORE LIMB

I. Shoulder girdle muscles: These muscles form a group which connect scapula or humerus of the fore limb with the head or trunk. The shoulder girdle muscles are listed below **(Fig.2.56).**

1. **Trapezius**: It is a ***broad triangular*** muscle consisting of cervical and dorsal parts
2. **Rhomboideus**: This muscle is under cover of the trapezius and consists of cervical and dorsal parts.

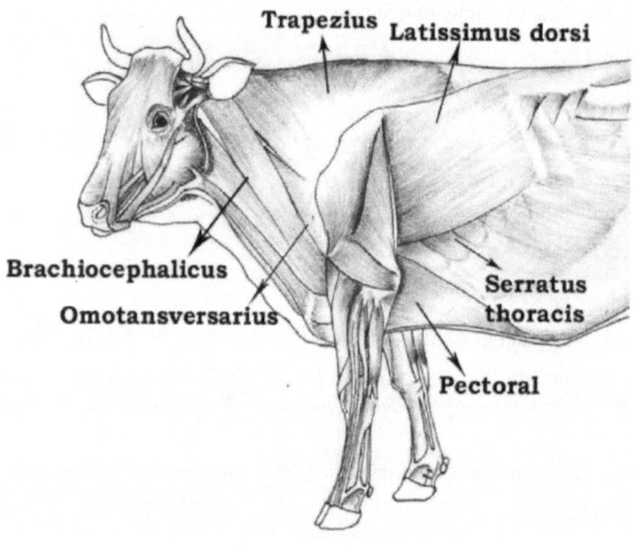

Fig. 2.56: Shoulder girdle Muscles of Ox

3. **Brachiocepahlicus**: This muscle extends from the head, along the neck to the arm, its upper border is in close apposition with the trapezius and the lower border forms the ***upper boundary of the jugular furrow***. It consists of two parts i.e dorsal cleido-occipitalis and ventral cleido-mastoideus.
4. **Omotransversarius**: This muscle is for the most part covered by the preceeding except at the scapular end where it is seen as a broad flat band.
5. **Latissimus dorsi**: It is a very wide muscle extending on the lateral wall of the thorax from the vertebral column to the arm.
6. **Serratus ventralis**: Is a large fan shaped muscle, situated on the lateral surface of the neck and the thorax. It derives its name from the ***serrated ventral edge and shows cervical and thoracic parts.***
7. **Pectorals**: These muscles form a thick mass occupying the space between the lower part of the chest wall and the medial face of the shoulder and arm. They are divisible into two layers superficial and deep. The superficial layer is again divided into anterior and posterior superficial muscles.

MUSCLES OF THE SHOULDER GIRDLE

Name of the muscle	Origin	Insertion	Action
1. Trapezius	Supraspinous ligament, Ligamentum nuchae, Spines of cervical and thoracic vertebrae.	Spine of scapula	To elevate the shoulder and draw the scapula cranially and caudally
2.Omotransversarius	Wing of Atlas and transverse process of axis.	Scapular fascia	To pull scapula upwards and forwards.
3. Rhomboideus	Ligamentum nuchae, Spines of 1st to 7th or 8th thoracic vertebrae	Medial face of scapular cartilage	To draw the shoulder upwards and forwards.
4. Brachiocepahlicus a. Cleido-occipitalis b.Cliedo-mastoideus	 Occipital bone of skull, Ligamentum nuchae, Mastoid process and wing of atlas	Crest of humerus	To draw the limb forwards when the head and neck are fixed. To extend the head and neck when limb is fixed.
5. Latissimus dorsi	Thoraco-lumbar fascia	**The anterior part** in common with the teres major to the teres tubercle of humerus, the **middle part** to the deep face of the long head of triceps and the **posterior part** along with the deep pectoral to the medial tuberosity of humerus.	To flex the shoulder joint
6. Serratus ventralis a. Cervical part (Serratus cervicis)	Transverse process of 3rd cervical to 7th cervical vertebrae and lateral surface of first three ribs.	Medial surface of scapula (anterior triangular area)	To pull the scapula forwards towards the neck.
b. Thoracic part (Serratus thoracis)	Lateral surface of ribs from **4th to 9th**.	Medial surface of scapula (posterior rough line)	To pull the scapula backwards. It acts as a muscle of inspiration.
7.Pectorals: Anterior Superficial pectoral	Ventrolateral aspects of the forepart of the sternum	Anteror edge of humerus along with brachiocephalicus.	To adduct the limb
Posterior Superficial pectoral	Ventrolateral aspects of the forepart of the sternum behind the anterior part.	Fascia of the forearm.	To adduct the limb and to tense the fascia of fore arm.
Deep pectoral	Ventral surface of sternum and tunica flava abdominalis.	Medial tuberosity of humerus	To adduct the limb

MUSCLES OF THE SHOULDER:

These extend from scapula to humerus.

A. Lateral aspect: The following muscles are present on lateral aspect of the shoulder.

1. **Supraspinatus**: This muscle not only fills up the supraspinous fossa but also extends beyond it crossing anterior or cervical border and is in contact with subscapularis.

> ***Subclavius muscle*** is a small round bundle of fleshy fibers arising from the cartilage and ventral end of first rib and inserted to deep surfae of Brachiocephalisus cranial to shoulder joint. ***It is well developed in goats, pigs and horses and absent in dogs.***

2. **Infraspinatus**: This muscle covers most of the infraspinous fossa and extends beyond it posteriorly crossing posterior border.

3. **Deltoideus**: It is a triangular muscle and lies partly on the triceps and partly on the infraspinatus, It consists of two parts, ***acromial and scapular.***

4. **Teres minor**: Present on posterior border of scapula, covered by infraspinatus and scapular part of deltoideus.

Muscles of the Shoulder (Lateral aspect)

Name of the Muscle	Origin	Insertion	Action
1.Supraspinatus	Supraspinous fossa	1. Lateral tendon to summit of lateral tuberosity of humerus. 2. The medial tendon to anterior division of medial tuberosity of humerus.	To extend the shoulder joint
2.Infraspinatus	Infraspinous fossa	a. Superficial tendon to circular rough area below the summit of lateral tuberosituy of humerus b. Deep tendon to convexity of lateral tuberosity of humerus	To abduct the scapula and rotate it outwards and flex the shoulder joint
3.Deltoideus	1.Acromion process of scapula. 2.Posterior border of scapula.	Deltoid tuberosity of humerus	To flex the shoulder and abduct the arm
4. Teres minor	Rough lines in lower part of infraspinous fossa.	Nodule above the deltoid tuberosity of humerus	To flex the shoulder and abduct the arm

B. Medial aspect: The following muscles are present on medial aspect of the shoulder

1. **Subscapularis**: This **shining muscle** occupies the subscrapular fossa and presents ***three fleshy parts.***
2. **Teres major**: This is a flat muscle situated along posterior border of the scapula behind the subscapularis muscle and extends to the teres tubercle of the humerus.
3. **Coracobrachialis**: The muscle lies partly on the medial face of the shoulder joint and the humerus

Name of the Muscle	Origin	Insertion	Action
1.Subscapularis	Subscapular fossa of scapula	Posterior division of medial tuberosity of humerus	To adduct the arm
2.Teres major	Caudal border of scapula	Teres tubercle of humerus	To flex the shoulder and adduct the arm
3.Coracobrachialis	Coracoid process of scapula	Above the teres tubercle and middle third of the anterior surface of humerus	To flex the shoulder and adduct the arm

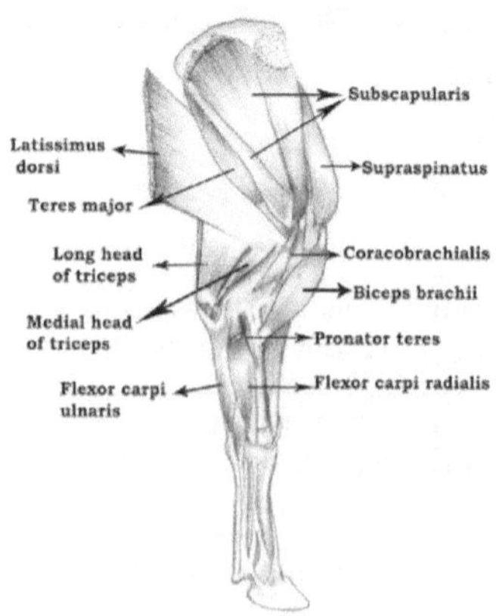

Fig. 2.57: Muscles of the Fore limb-Medial Aspect

III. MUSCLES OF THE ARM

This group consists of muscles grouped around the humerus. Some arise from the scapula and others from the humerus but all are inserted to the forearm **(Fig.2.57).**

1. **Biceps brachii**: It is situated on the anterior face of the humerus. It arises from tuber scapulae (***this muscle is having tendon at its origin***). Under the tendon of origin of biceps brachii there is a large bursa in bicipital groove.
2. **Tensor fascia antibrachii**: This is a **long and narrow band** extending on the medial face of the posterior border of caput longum (long head of triceps).
3. **Triceps brachii**: This is a large muscle which fills up the space between the scapula and olecranon process. ***It is an antigravity muscle.*** It is made up of three heads.
   a. **Long head:** It is the **largest head** and is visible both on the lateral and medial faces
   b. **Lateral head:** It is **quadrilateral** and lies on the lateral surface of the arm below the long head.
   c. **Medial head:** It is the **smallest** and is situated on the medial surface of the humerus below the insertion of coracobranchialis.
4. **Anconeus**: This is a small muscle covering the olecranon fossa.
5. **Brachialis**: This is a curved muscle lodged in the musculo-spiral groove of the humerus.

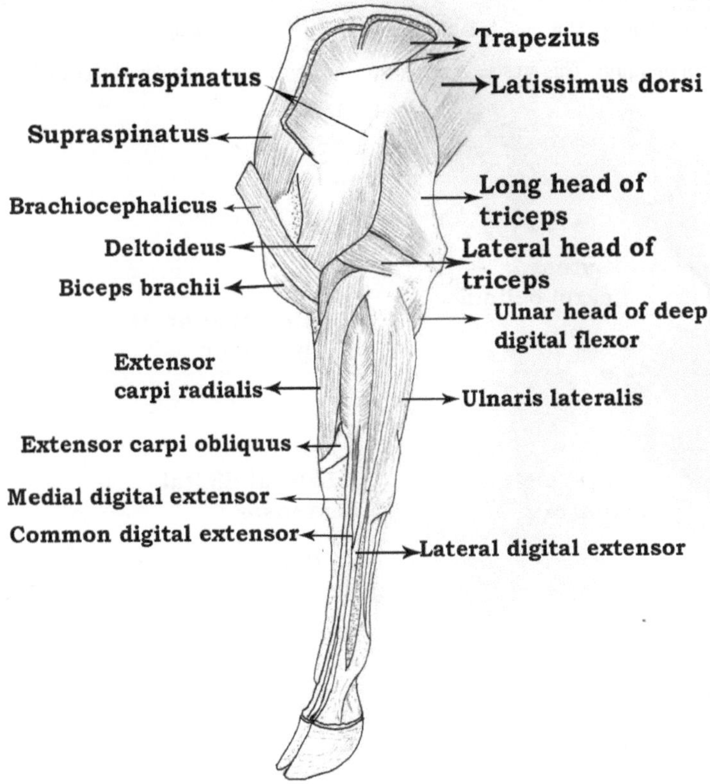

Fig. 2.58: Muscles of the Fore limb-Lateral aspect

Name of the Muscle	Origin	Insertion	Action
1.Biceps brachi	*Tuber scapulae*	*Radial tuberosity*	*Extend the shoulder and flex the elbow*
2. Tensor fascia antibrachii	Latissimus dorsi muscle	Tendon of long head of triceps	To extend the elbow joint
3. Triceps brachii			
a) Long head	Caudal border of scapula	*Olecranon process of ulna*	*To extend the elbow joint and flex the shoulder.*
b) Medial head	Medial surface of shaft of humerus		
c) Lateral head	Lateral surface of shaft of humerus		
4.Anconeus	Margins of olecranon fossa of humerus	Anterior and lateral parts of olecranon process	To extend the elbow joint
5. Brachialis	Musculospiral groove of humerus	Medial surface of radius below the radial tuberosity	*To flex the elbow joint.*

IV. MUSCLES OF THE FOREARM AND MANUS

a) Extensors: These are situated around the ***dorsal and lateral aspects*** of the forearm and extend the carpus and / digits **(Figs.2.58 & 2.59).**

1. **Extensor carpi radialis**: This is the **largest of the extensor** muscle and lies over the dorsal face of radius.
2. **Medial digital extensor**: The muscle is situated lateral to the preceeding.
3. **Common digital extensor**: ***It is the longest extensor of forearm and*** situated lateral to the preceeding. It has two heads of origin i.e lateral epicondyle of the humerus and ulna.
4. **Lateral digital extensor**: This muscle is situated lateral to the preceeding.
5. **Extensor carpi obliquus**: This muscle is situated on the lower part of the dorsal face of the radius and ulna.

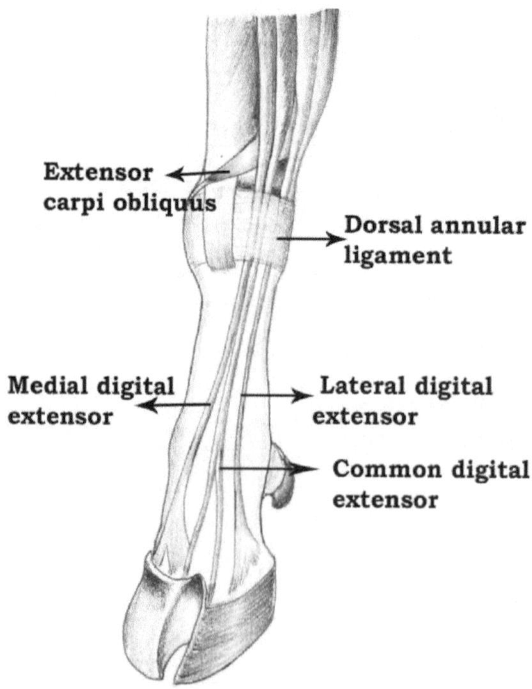

Fig. 2.59: Extensors of Carpus and Digits

1.Extensor carpi radialis (***Largest extensor***)		Metacarpal tuberosity	To extend the carpal joint and flex the elbow.
2. Medial digital extensor		2nd phalanx of medial digit	To extend the carpal joint, fetlock joint and pastern joints of medial digit.
3. Common digital extensor (***Longest Extensor***)	Lateral epicondyle of humerus	Extensor process of 3rd phalanx	To extend the carpal joint, fetlock joint and digital joints (both pastern and coffin) of both the digits.
4. Lateral digital extensor	Lateral collateral ligament of elbow and lateral tuberosity of radius and shaft of radius and ulna.	2nd phalanx of lateral digit.	To extend the carpal joint, fetlock joint and pastern joints of lateral digit.
5. Extensor carpi obliquus	Lateral and dorsal surface of radius and ulna	Postero medial tubercle of Large metacarpal.	To extend the carpus and rotate it outwards.

b) FLEXORS: These muscles are situated around the ***posterior and medial aspect*** of the forearm and flex the carpus and digits. They are arranged in two layers i.e superficial and deep.

SUPERFICIAL LAYER

1. **Pronator teres**: It is small **vestigeal muscle** situated along the medial face of the elbow joint closely blended with the medial collateral ligament of elbow joint.
2. **Flexor carpi radialis**: It is a narrow muscle placed immediately behind the preceeding.
3. **Flexor carpi ulnaris**: It is a wide muscle behind the preceeding and covers the medial surface of the fore arm
4. **Ulnaris lateralis**: It is a large thick muscle situated behind the lateral digital extensor. It is a flexor but arises from **lateral epicondyle** of humerus

DEEP LAYER

5. **Superficial digital flexor**: divides into two parts at the lower third of foearm. i.e **superficial and deep parts.** The superficial part passes over the carpal canal. The deep part passes through the carpal canal in company with the deep digital flexor tendon.
6. **Deep digital flexor**: It is largest of the flexors and is partly under cover of the preceeding and consists of three heads

   a) **Humeral head**-It is the ***largest head,***

   b) **Radial head** – It is the ***smallest & deepest head***

c) Ulnar head- It is most superficial head and placed between ulnaris lateralis and flexor carpi ulnaris.

Name of the Muscle	Origin	Insertion	Action
1. Ulnaris lateralis	Lateral epicondyle of humerus	Accessory carpal bone on its Supero-lateral aspect.	To flex the carpus and extend the elbow
2. Pronator teres	Medial epicondyle of humerus	Medial border of radius.	Inappreciable as it is vestigeal.
3. Flexor carpi radialis	Medial epicondyle of humerus	Posteromedial tubercle of large metacarpal bone	To flex the carpus and extend the elbow.
4. Flexor carpi ulnaris	Humeral head from medial epicondyle of humerus and Ulnar head from olecranon process of ulna.	Accessory carpal bone on its supero-medial aspect.	To flex the carpus and extend the elbow.
5.Superficial digital flexor	Medial epicondyle of humerus	Volar face of 2nd phalanges of both the digits.	To flex the carpal, fetlock and pastern joints and extend the elbow.
6.Deep digital flexor; a) Humeral head	Medial epicondyle of humerus	Volar face of 3rd phalanx of both the digits.	To flex the carpal, fetlock, pastern and coffin joints and extend the elbow.
b) Radial head	Proximal end of shaft of radius near proximal radioulnar arch.		
c) Ulnar head	Olecranon process of ulna		

2.5 BLOOD SUPPLY TO THE FORE LIMB

The brachial artery consists of intrathoracic and extrathoracic parts, the latter supply greater part of fore limb.

EXTRA THORACIC BRANCHES OF BRACHIAL ARTERY

1. **Suprascapular Artery:** It is a small vessel arising from the upper face of the brachial artery about the middle of its extra thoracic course. It ascends and dips in the space between the supraspinatus and subscapularis in company with its satellite vein and suprascapular nerve and divides to **supply the supraspinatus, subscapularis, brachiocephalicus** and the terminal part of the **deep pectoral muscle (Fig.2.60).**
2. **External thoracic artery:** It is a large vessel arising from the ventral face of the brachial artery at about the level of the anterior border of the first rib. It gives number of branches to the **pectoral muscles, axillary lymph gland and skin.**
3. **Subscapular artery:** It is a very ***large vessel as large as the brachial artery***. It arises from its posterior face at the posterior border of the subscapularis muscle. It supplies in its course branches to the **teres major, subscapularis, caput longum, infraspinatus and deltoideus.** Besides these it also gives following branches **(Fig.2.60).**

   (a) The **thoraco-dorsal artery** is given off from the posterior face of the subscapular artery about an inch above its origin. It runs upwards and backwards on the deep face of the ***latissmus dorsi*** and is distributed to it. It also supplies a branch to **the long head of triceps and axillary lymph gland.**

   (b) The **posterior circumflex artery of the humerus** arises from the subscapular artery from its anterior face passes outwards behind the shoulder joint in company with the circumflex nerve and ramifies on the deep face of the **deltoideus.** It supplies branches to **all heads of triceps, brachialis, anconeus, extensor carpi radialis and to the skin.**

   (c) The **circumflex artery of the scapula** arises from the anterior border of the subscapular artery 2" or 3" above the shoulder joint. It divides into medial and lateral branches which supply the **subscapularis and intraspinatus.**

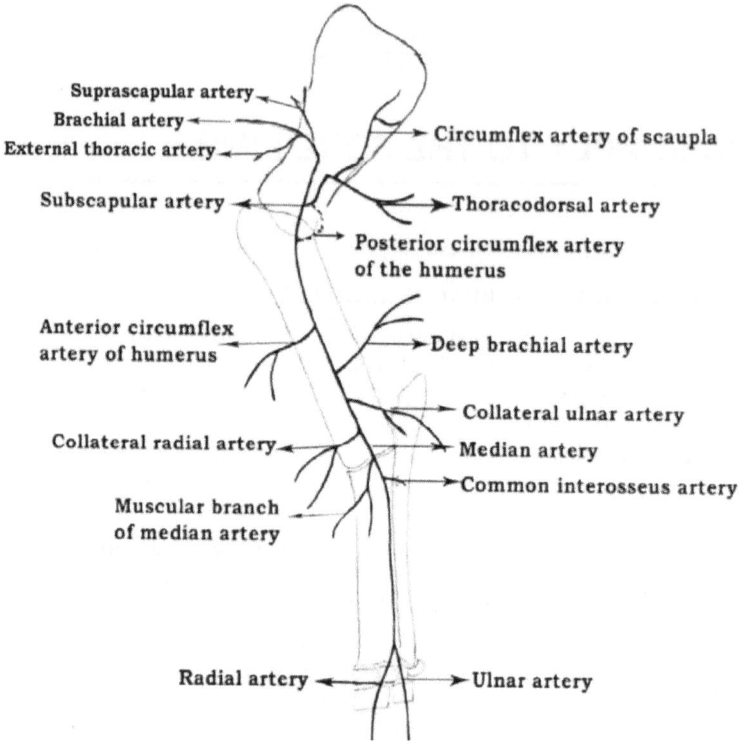

Fig. 2.60: Collateral Branches of Brachial Artery

4. **Anterior circumflex artery of the humerus:** This branch arises from the **anterior face of the brachial artery (Fig.2.60)** at the anterior border of the lower part of teres major, gains the space between the two parts of the **coracobrachialis** in **company with the musculocutaneous nerve** and finally **terminates in the biceps**. It supplies these muscles

5. **Deep brachial artery:** It is a small vessel arising from the posterior face of the brachial artery about the middle of the humerus **(Fig.2.60).** It passes backwards between the long and medial heads of the triceps, supplies these muscles and **tensor fasciae antibrachii.**

6. **Collateral ulnar artery:** This branch arises from the posterior face of the brachial artery and is small **(Fig.2.60).** It divides into ascending branch **supplying long head of triceps, anconeus and descending branch supplying flexor carpi ulnaris and superficial digital flexor of the digit.**

7. **Collateral radial artery:** It is a large vessel arising from the lateral face of the brachial artery. It accompanies musculocutaneous branch of the median nerve under the lower part of of the biceps brachii and **divides into superficial and deep branches (Fig.2.60).** The **superficial branch** runs forwards in company with the cutaneous branch of musculocutaneous branch of median nerve, as a cutaneous vessel. The deep branch gets under the brchialis passes over the capsular liagament of the elbow and passes under extensor carpi radialis. **It supplies all extensor muscles and finally terminates on ulnaris lateralis.**

Median artery: The median artery is the **continuation of the brachial artery** below the level of the medial condyle of the humerus. It passes along the posteromedial face of the radius and divides at variable distance down the forearm into radial and ulnar arteries **(Fig.2.61).**

Collateral branches:

a) A long muscular branch which divides to **supply muscles pronator teres, flexor carpi radialis, flexor carpi ulnaris, superficial and deep flexors of the digit.**

b) **Common interosseous artery:** It is a large branch which **arises from the median artery in** the upper third of the forearm **(Fig.2.61).** It passes outwards through the proximal, interosseous space and continues as the **dorsal interosseous artery**. Before it enters the proximal interosseous space, it gives branches to the humeral and radial heads of the deep flexor of the digit: as it passes through the space, **it supplies the lateral digital extensor and extensor carpi obliquus.**

   The **dorsal interosseous artery** runs down in the groove between the radius and ulna on the lateral face of the forearm under the periosteum. It reaches the level of the distal interosseous space detaches a branch which enters this space, continues its downward course and concurs in the formation of the rete carpi dorsale. The branch detached by it passes through the distal interosseous space gains the volar face of the forearm gives branches to the retecapi volare and is continued down as the lateral deep volar metacarpal artery. This is an extremely fine vessel which passes along the lateral border of the suspensory ligament and by joining the middle deep volar metacarpal and medial deep volar metacarpal arteries forms the deep volar arch above the fetlock, between the large metacarpal bone and the suspensory ligament and is continued as **lateral volar digital artery** on the lateral digit.

Radial artery: The Radial artery is the **smaller** of the **two terminal branches** of the median artery. It descends along the mediovolar border of the radius under the flexor carpi radialis, passes down subcutaneously over the posterior aspect of the carpus under the deep fascia but outside the carpal canal and is continued down as the **medial deep volar metacarpal artery**. The Radial artery gives branches to the formation of the ***rete carpi dorsale and volare*** and another branch which passes between the suspensory ligament and the large metacarpal bone. This branch gives off the **middle deep volar metacarpal artery** and then passes through the foramen at the proximal part of the groove on the large metacarpal bone to anastomose with the **dorsal metacarpal artery**.

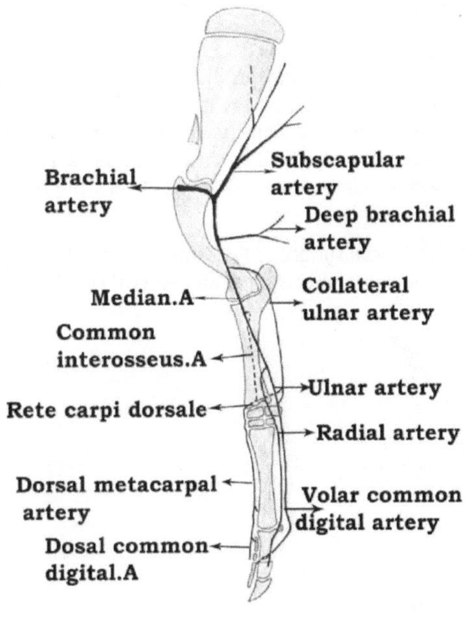

Fig. 2.61: Branches of Median Artery of Ox

The **middle deep volar metacarpal artery** descends down the volar longitudinal groove of the large metacarpal bone and concurs with the branch of medial deep volar metacarpal artery and lateral deep metacarpal artery in the formation of the **deep volar arch above the fetlock between the large metacarpal bone and the suspensory ligament.**

The **medial deep volar metacarpal artery** passes along the medial border of the suspensory ligament gives off fine branches to the tendons and suspensory ligament and skin and at the distal third gives off branch which with the branches of the volar common digital artery forms the superficial volar arch and gives another branch to the deep volar arch. It is continued down as the **medial volar digital artery** on the medial digit.

Ulnar artery: The **ulnar artery is the larger of the two terminal branches of the median artery (Fig.2.61).** It descends under the flexor carpi radialis passes through the carpal canal on the medial face of the tendon of the deep digital flexor and is **continued as the volar common digital artery**. At the lower third, it gives off a branch to form the ***superficial volar arch with medial deep volar metacarpal artery.*** It then enters the interdigital space and divides into two volar proper digital arteries, one for each digit.

Dorsal metacarpal artery: It is very small vessel (often absent) which ***arises from the retecarpi dorsale*** **(Fig.2.61).** It passes down the dorsal metacarpal groove and above the fetlock it is joined by the distal perforating metacarpal artery from the deep volar arch to form the **dorsal common digital artery**. This receives a communicating branch from the volar common digital artery and divides into **two dorsal proper digital arteries (axial digital arteries)** for the two chief digits.

The **axial digital arteries** are directed downward on the axial surface of the digits give branches to the axial part of the dermis/corium and then **enters axial foramina** on the extensor process of third phalanx and within the 3rd phalanx gives number of branches which emerge through the formina in the bone **to supply dermis/corium of hoof.**

Non Satellite Veins of the Fore limb:

Most of the veins are the satellites of the arteries and need no special description. Only such of the veins which do not follow arteries (which are not satellite) are dealt here under.

The Cepahlic Vein

The cepahlic vein is a **subcutaneous vein** on the anteromedial surface of the arm and forearm. It is the ***upward continuation of the medial metacarpal vein.*** This vein passes upward and forward to the tendon of the extensor carpi radialis. Here it enters the groove formed by the **superficial pectoral and brachiocehalicus muscles** and terminates in external jugular vein. In the forearm it is **accompanied by the cutaneous part of the musculocutaneous branch of the median nerve.** The ***medial cubital vein*** is an anastomosis **between the cephalic and median veins** in the region of elbow.

The ***accessory cephalic vein*** lies on the dorsal surface of the carpus and distal part of the radius and is a **tributary of the cephalic vein**. It is formed by the **dorsal metacarpal and several small veins from the carpal joint.**

2.6 NERVE SUPPLY TO THE FORE LIMB

The muscles and integument of the forelimb and some of the muscles of the shoulder girdle and chest wall are supplied by **brachial plexus**. The ***brachial plexus*** is formed by ventral primary braches of ***6th, 7th, 8th cervical and 1st and 2nd thoracic spinal*** nerves. The brachial plexus gives off following branches.

1. **The external thoracic nerve:** This arises from the brachial plexus. Its fibers are derived from ventral branches of 7th and 8th cervical spinal nerves by a common trunk with the ulnar nerve. It gives off a number of branches to the **deep pectoral and cutaneous muscle** and terminates in the skin of the abdominal wall.
2. **The thoraco dorsal nerve:** This nerve supplies **latissimus dorsi muscle**. Its fibres are derived from the **eighth cervical and first thoracic**.
3. **The long thoracic nerve:** The fibres of this nerve are derived from the **seventh and eighth cervicals** and sometimes from the sixth also and it supplies the **serratus ventralis**.
4. **The nerves to pectorals:** These are three or four in number and arise from the anterior part of the plexus and fibers are derived from the ventral branches of **7th and 8th cervical spinal nerves.** Some times the ventral branch of the **first thoracic spinal** nerves is also involved. One of these passes to the deep face of the deep pectoral and another nerve passes to the superficial pectoral and brachiocephalicus.
5. **The suprascapular nerve:** It is the most anterior of all the nerves from the brachial plexus and it is large. It passes forward, downward and outward, gains the space between the supraspinatus and the subscapularis, turns around the lower fourth of the anterior border of scapula and passes under infraspinatus and terminates in teres minor.
6. **The nerves to subscapularis:** They are two or three in number and are derived from the **seventh and eighth cervical spinal nerves**. These nerves are confounded at the origin with the thoracodorsal nerve, suprascapular and circumflex nerves. They supply the three divisions of the subscapularis.
7. **The nerve to teres major:** It is derived from the **seventh and eighth cervical nerves.** It crosses the subscapularis and the teres major and supplies branches to it and also the posterior part of the subscapularis.
8. **The axillary nerve:** It **arises from all the cervicals**. It accompanies the posterior circumflex artery of humerus and reaches the deep face of the deltoideus. It supplies teres major, deltoideus, teres minor and divides into dorsal and ventral branches. The dorsal branch passes under the acromial head of deltoideus and ends in the terminal part of brachiocephalicus. The ventral branch passes under scapular head of deltoideus, over the lateral head of triceps and ***continues down as dorsal or anterior cutaneous nerve of forearm.***
9. **The ulnar nerve:** It derives its fibres from the first thoracic nerve. It arises with the median nerve by a short common trunk. It keeps company with the median nerve till about the middle of the arm, here it detaches a long **cutaneous branch to the skin on the posterior face of the forearm (*posterior cutaneous nerve of fore arm*)**. It gives off branches to the two heads of the **flexor carpi ulnaris, superficial digital flexor and ulnar head of the deep digital flexor.** At the lower one third of the fore arm this nerve lies relatively **superficial between the flexor carpi ulnaris and ulnaris lateralis muscles** and it is the preferable site for ulnar nerve block / neurectomy operation.

The **superficial branch** emerges between the flexor carpi ulnaris and ulnaris lateralis muscles, runs down subcutaneously behind the insertion of the tendon of the flexors, runs superficially over the carpal sheath downward and outward over the metacarpal region and is continued as the **lateral dorsal abaxial digital nerve** on the dorsal and abaxial aspects of the lateral digit.

The **deep branch** descends deeply under the deep fascia behind the carpus over the carpal sheath, supplies branches to the suspensory ligament below the carpus, unites with a branch of the lateral branch of the median nerve and runs subcutaneously as the **lateral volar abaxial digital nerve** on the volar and abaxial aspect of the lateral digit.

10. **Musculocutaenous nerve:** This nerve arises from the anterior part of the brachial plexus behind the suprascapular nerve and derives its fibres chiefly from the seventh and eighth cervical nerves. **It joins the median nerve by a large short branch to form a loop in which the brachial artery passes.** The nerve then runs in the space between the divisions of the **coracobrachialis** in company with the **anterior circumflex vessels**, gives off a branch to this muscle and reaches the **biceps brachii** and terminates in it.

11. **The Median nerve:** derives its fibres from the eighth cervical and the first thoracic nerves. It is united at its origin by a branch from the musculo-cutaneous nerve to form a loop in which the brachial artery is suspended. The median nerve passes below the elbow beneath the pronator teres. It then runs down along the forearm between the radius and flexor carpi radialis muscle. It passes through the carpal sheath descends to the lower third of the metacarpus and divides into **lateral and medial branches (Fig.2.62).**

Branches of median nerve

(a) The **musculocutaneous** branch arises from this nerve about the middle of the humerus from its anterior face passes under cover of the biceps and divides into muscular and cutaneous branches. The muscular branch supplies the **brachialis.** The **cutaneous branch supplies the skin in front and medial aspect of forearm as *medial cutaneous nerve of fore arm.***

(b) Immediately below it gives off muscular branches to **pronator teres, flexor carpi radialis, superficial digital flexor, humeral and radial heads of deep digital flexor.**

The terminal branches are ***medial and lateral*** **(Fig.2.63).** The ***medial branch*** divides into medial and lateral divisions. The medial division of medial branch, after giving small braches to the rudimentary digit is continued down as **medial volar abaxial digital nerve on volar and abaxial aspect of medial digit**. The **lateral division** joins the **medial division** of the lateral branch to form the **volar common digital nerve (Fig.2.63).**

The **lateral branch** also divides similarly into medial and lateral divisions. The medial division forms the ***volar common digital nerve*** with lateral division of medial branch of median nerve and the **lateral division** joins the deep branch of the ulnar nerve to form the **lateral volar abaxial digital nerves** to supply volar and abaxial aspects of lateral digit **(Fig.2.63).**

In buffaloes the median nerve divides into volar common digital and medial volar abaxial digital nerves only, while lateral volar abaxial digital nerve is formed exclusively by the deep branch of ulnar nerve.

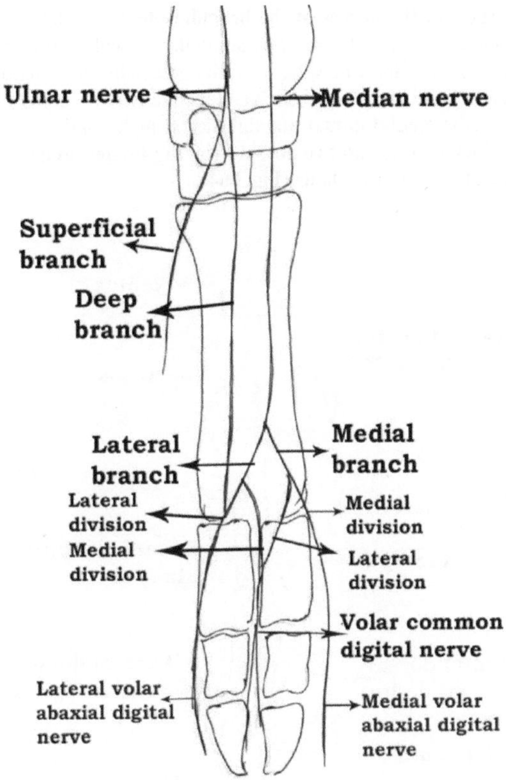

Fig. 2.62: Course of Median Nerve

The **volar common digital nerve** passes into the interdigital space and divides into two volar axial digital nerves to supply volar and axial aspects of both the digits.

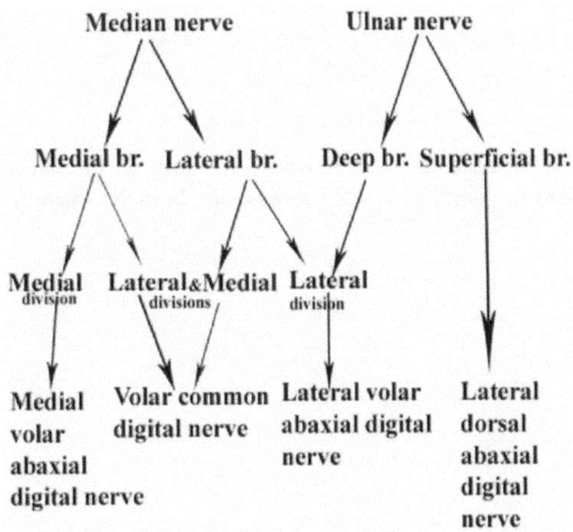

Fig. 2.63: Terminal Branches of Median and Ulnar Nerves

12. Radial nerve: It is the **largest of the nerves of the brachial plexus**. Its fibres are derived from the seventh and eighth cervical and first thoracic nerves. The nerve passes in the musculo spiral groove between the triceps and brachialis, reaches the anterior aspect of the elbow, between the brachialis and extensor carpi radialis. It continues down the anterior face of forearm in relation to cephalic vein, then down the carpus and metacarpus. It detaches at about the middle of metacarpus the **medial dorsal abaxial digital nerve** and continues down the metacarpus as dorsal common digital nerve which divides into **two dorsal axial digital nerves** at the upper part of the interdigital space to supply dorsal and axial aspects of two digits **(Fig.2.64).**

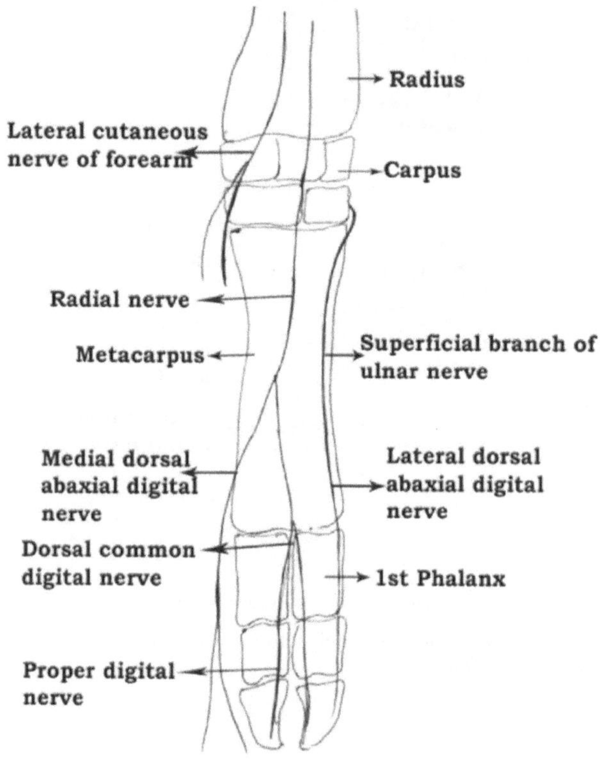

Fig. 2.64: Course of Radial Nerve

It supplies brachialis and anconeus and cutaneous branch to the skin on the lateral part of the forearm **(*lateral cutaneous nerve of fore arm*)** and furnishes a large thick muscular branch to ***supply all the extensors and ulnaris lateralis of forearm.***

2.7 NERVE BLOCKS AND NEURECTOMIES OF FORE LIMB

Nerve blocks: are done for temporary blocking of pathway for passage of impulses by injecting local anaesthetic solution resulting in desensitization and paresis in the region controlled by the nerve to relieve pain.

Neurecetomy: Neurectomy is the division and removal of a piece of nerve.

Indications

i. To relieve pain and to improve usefulness of the animal.

ii. Lameness due to chronic conditions.

iii. Splints, ringbone, navicular disease, laminitis (Horse).

1. Median Nerve block and Neurectomy

Site: Below the medial tuberosity of the radius at the groove between caudal border of the radius and flexor carpi radialis muscle **(Fig.2.65).**

2. Ulnar nerve block and Neurectomy

Site: A few inches above the accessory carpal **(Fig.2.65).**

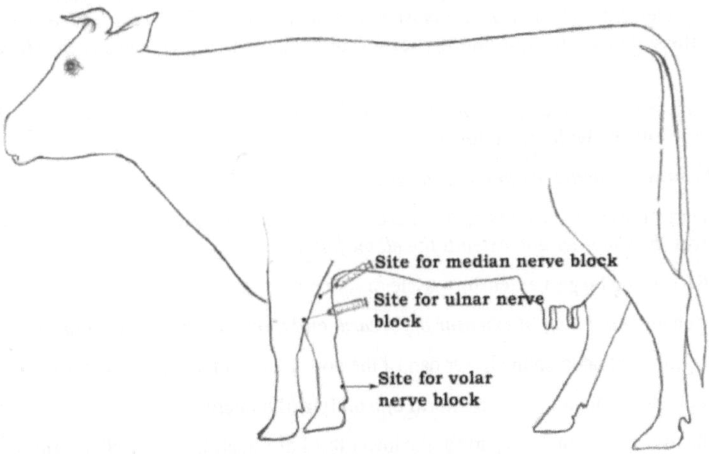

Fig. 2.65: Sites for Nerve Blocks of Fore Limb

3. Volar nerve block and neurectomy

Site

i. **High volar block:** 5 to 7 cm above the fetlock in the depression between suspensory ligament and deep flexor tendon both on medial and lateral aspects.

ii. **Low volar block:** Midway between the fetlock and coronet in between deep digital flexor and superficial digital flexor both for medial and lateral digits.

2.8 SUMMARY

Ox: The carpus consists of **six short bones** arranged in two rows, four in the proximal row and two in the distal row.

The radial carpal is the ***largest bone of the upper row and*** **Fused 2nd and 3rd carpal is largest in the distal row.**

The ***metacarpal tuberosity is present at dorsomedial aspect of large metacarpal.*** **Small metacarpal** is present at the **posterolateral** aspect of large metacarpal.

Horse: In radius the medial border of the volar face presents below the middle a rough elevation for the ***radial check ligament.*** **Accessory carpal** is ***discoid in shape.*** The anterior ***border has two facets, the upper one for radius and lower one for the ulnar carpal.***

Dog: The ***coronoid and olecranon fossae*** communicate with each other through the ***supratrochlear foramen.***

Has seven carpal bones, three in the proximal and four in the distal row. The metacarpus has five bones. The ***first is shortest***. The ***3rd and 4th are the longest***. The **2nd** is **longer than the 5th**.

Nine proximal sesamoids are present, ***one for the first digit and two for each of the other 4 digits.***

Fowl: ***Hypocleidium-*** The two side clavicles meet ventrally and form flattened plate called ***hypocleidium***. There are only two carpal bones. The ***radial carpal is quadrilateral,*** while the ***ulnar carpal is forked***. The metacarpus consists of three bony elements. The ***first is the most medial*** and is in the form of a nodule. The **second one is largest. There are three digits**. The **first and the second digits have two phalanges each**. The **third digit has one phalanx.**

Brachiocephalicus muscle forms the ***upper boundary of the jugular furrow***. It consists of two parts i.e dorsal **cleido-occipitalis and ventral cleido-mastoideus.**

Biceps brachii ***is the muscle having tendon at its origin***.

Triceps brachii is a large muscle which fills up the space between the scapula and olecranon process. It is made up of three heads. ***It flexes the shoulder and extends the elbow joint.***

Extensor carpi radialis is the **largest extensor** muscle of fore arm.

Common digital extensor ***is the longest extensor of forearm and it inserts on extensor process of 3rd phalanx.***

Extensor carpi obliquus is situated on the lower part of the dorsal face of the radius and ulna.

Ulnaris lateralis: is the flexor but arises from **lateral epicondyle** of humerus.

Superficial digital flexor divides into two parts at the lower third of forearm. i.e **superficial and deep parts.**

Deep digital flexor: is ***largest*** of the flexors and consists of three heads

a) **Humeral head-**It is the ***largest head,***

b) **Radial head** – It is the ***smallest & deepest head***

c) **Ulnar head-** It is most superficial head and placed between ulnaris lateralis and flexor carpi ulnaris.

Collateral Branches of Brachial artery

Name of the artery	**Collateral branches**	**Muscles supplied**
1.Suprascapular Artery		Supraspinatus, subscapularis, brachiocephalicus and the terminal part of the deep pectoral muscle.
2.External thoracic artery		Pectoral muscles, axillary lymph gland and skin.
3. Subscapular artery (largest collateral branch)	1. Thoraco-dorsal artery	*Latissmus dorsi*
	2.Posterior circumflex artery of the humerus	All heads of triceps, brachialis, anconeus, extensor carpi radialis and to the skin.
	3.Circumflex artery of the scapula	Subscapularis and Infraspinatus.
4. Anterior circumflex artery of the humerus *(It accompanies the musculo cutaneous nerve)*		Coracobrachialis and biceps brachii.
5. Deep brachial artery:		Long and medial heads of the triceps and tensor fasciae antibranchii.
6. Collateral ulnar artery		Caput longum, anconeus and flexor carpi ulnaris and superficial digital flexor of the digit.
7. Collateral radial artery		All extensor muscles and ulnaris lateralis.

Brachial plexus is formed by ventral primary braches of ***6th, 7th, 8th cervical and 1st and 2nd thoracic spinal*** nerves.

NAME OF THE NERVE	MUSCLES SUPPLIED
1. External thoracic nerve	Deep pectoral and cutaneous muscle.
2. Long thoracic nerve	Serratus ventralis muscle.
3. Thoracodorsal nerve:	Latissimus dorsi muscle.
4. Axillary nerve:	Teres major, deltoideus and teres minor.
5. Ulnar nerve	Flexor carpi ulnaris, Superficial digital flexor and ulnar head of the deep digital flexor.
6. Musculo cutaenous nerve	Coracobrachialis and biceps brachii.
7. Median nerve:	Pronator teres, flexor carpi radialis, superficial digital flexor, humeral and radial heads of the deep digital flexor.
8. Radial nerve *(Largest nerve)*	*Brachialis, Triceps, anconeus* **and** *all the extensors and ulnaris lateralis.*

Cutaneous Nerves of Forearm

Lateral cutaneous nerve	Radial nerve
Anterior cutaneous nerve	Axillary nerve
Medial cutaneous nerve	Median nerve.
Posterior cutaneous nerve	Ulnar nerve

UNIT 3
HEAD AND NECK

3.1 BONES OF THE HEAD AND NECK

Skull: The skull of domestic animals has **two sets of bones** i.e **facial and cranial** bones. The ***facial bones*** are placed in **front** and ***cranial bones*** are placed **caudally.**

Facial bones: The paired facial bones are premaxilla, maxilla, nasal, pterygoid, lacrimal, turbinates, malar and palatine bones. The unpaired facial bones are mandible, hyoid and vomer.

Cranial Bones: The paired cranial bones are parietal, temporal and frontal bones. The unpaired cranial bones are occipital, sphenoid, ethmoid and interparietal bones.

FACIAL BONES

MANDIBLE

Ox: Is largest bone of the face and carries lower teeth. It shows two halves joined by **symphysis mandibulae**. It has a body and two rami. The body shows lingual and mental surfaces and alveolar border. The alveolar border shows **eight alveoli** for lower incisors. Each ramus has horizontal and vertical parts **(Fig.3.1).**

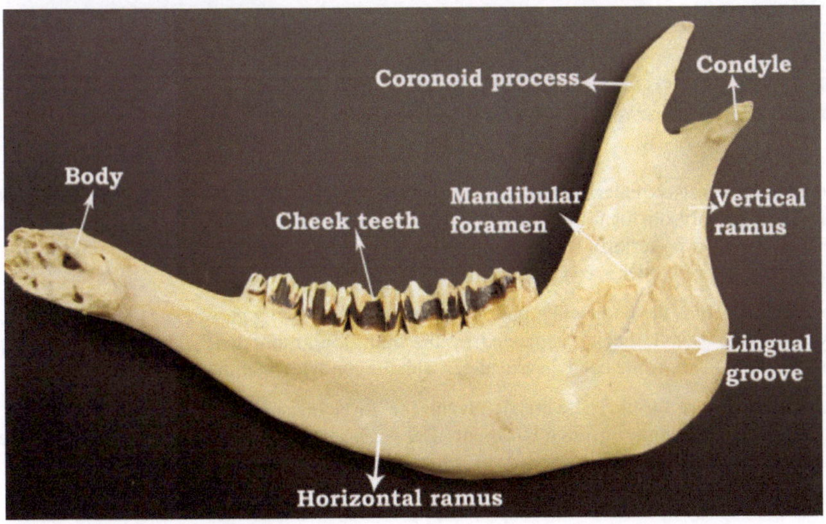

Fig. 3.1: Mandible of Ox-Medial Surface

The diverging rami enclose mandibular space. The **medial surface** of the horizontal part gives attachment to the mylohyoideus muscle. At its junction with the body is a fossa for the geniohyoideus muscles. On the vertical part the rough lines on lower part and mandibular foramen in the middle are present. The lingual groove resulting from contact of lingual nerve leads forwards and downwards from this foramen for lingual nerve **(Fig.3.1).**

The **lateral surface** is smooth and convex in horizontal part and flat in the vertical part. A fossa is present on lateral surface at the junction of horizontal ramus with the body in which **mental foramen,** the external opening of mandibular canal (**inferior dental canal**) is present **(Fig.3.2).** *The manidular canal carries mandibuloalveolar nerve and artery.*

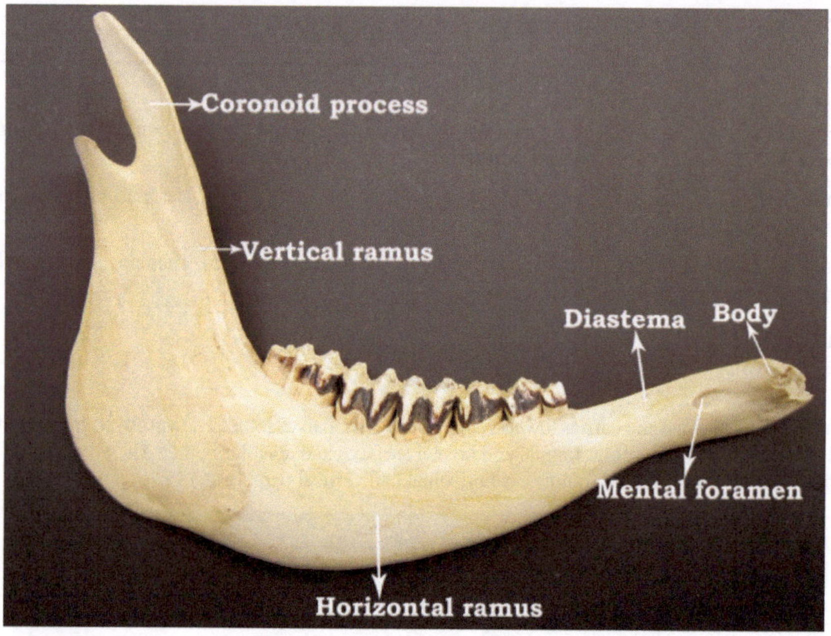

Fig. 3.2: Mandible of Ox- Lateral Surface

The horizontal ramus consists of alveolar and ventral borders. The **alveolar border** shows ***diastema*** (interalveolar space) in front and six alveoli for lower cheek teeth behind. The **ventral border** of horizontal part is convex with a smooth impression posteriorly left by blood vessels. In vertical ramus the anterior border is for muscular attachment, while posterior border is concave and thin.

The anterior extremity joins the body while posterior extremity shows long curved ***coronoid process*** in front and transversely elongated condyle behind separated by the **mandibular notch (Fig.3.2).**The coronoid process is received into temporal fossa, while condyle articulates with the condyle of temporal bone.

Horse: The **two halves are fused**. There are **six alveoli for lower incisors** on body and a little further back two for canines in males. The **lingual groove** is **absent**. The rami are less divergent and **coronoid process is less prominent (Fig.3.3).** There is fovea pterygoidea on anteromedial part of the condyle.

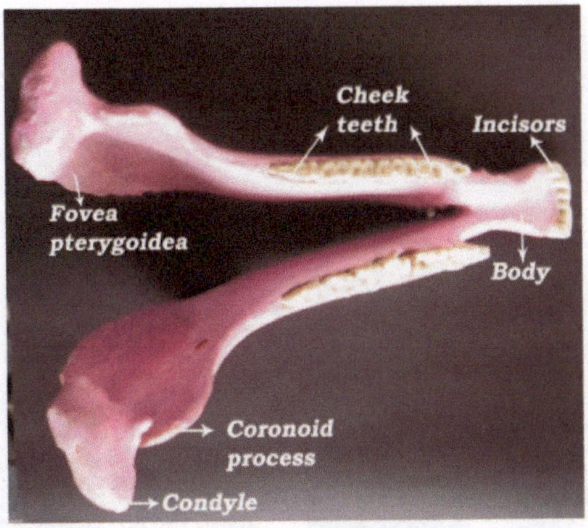

Fig. 3.3: Mandible of Horse

Dog: The two halves do not fuse. The alveolar border of **body shows six alveoli for lower incisors and two for canines.** The **horizontal ramus** shows **seven alveoli** for lower cheek teeth. There are two or three mental foramina on either side. The vertical part is small and shows masseteric fossa laterally and angular process at its posterior border. The condyle is placed very low and the coronoid process is extensive **(Fig.3.4).**

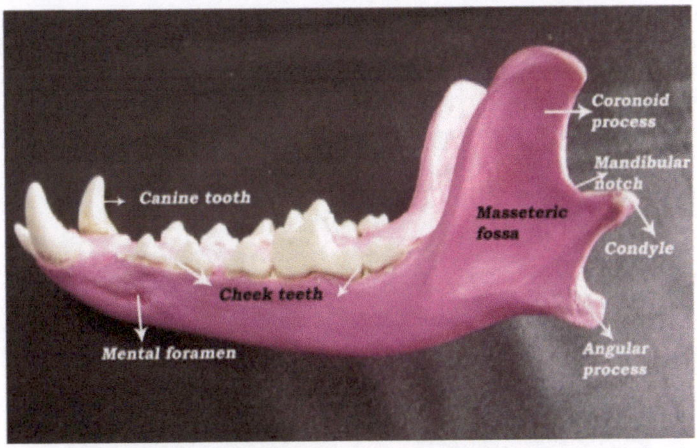

Fig. 3.4: Mandible of Dog

Pig: The bodies are joined at the symphysis and diverge at a greater angle than in the horse or ox. Internally, a pair of **medial mental foramina** are present. On the labial surface there are **lateral mental foramina**. The alveolar border of the incisive part presents ***six alveoli* for incisor teeth *and two alveoli for canine teeth***. The horizontal ramus shows ***seven alveoli for lower cheek teeth***. The **molar part** is very thick and strong.

Fowl: The two halves are fused and posteriorly its articular part joins lower end of **quadrate bone**. Behind this the ventral border is carried upward and backward by a process **(Fig.3.5).**

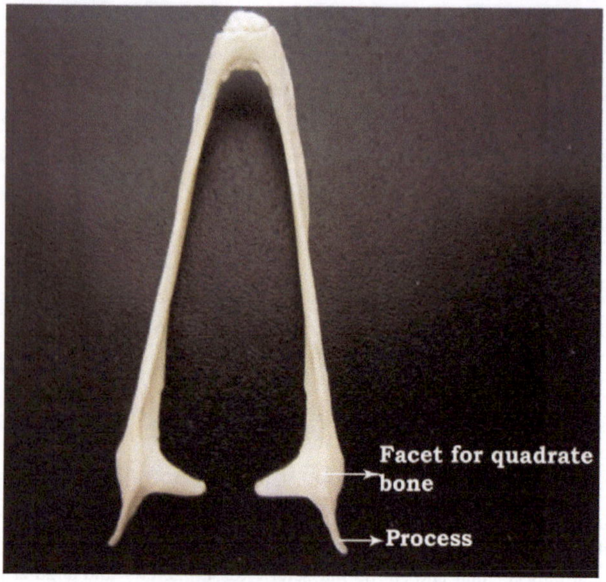

Fig. 3.5: Mandible of Fowl

Quadrate bone of Fowl: It is irregularly four sided bone articulating with temporal above, laterally with the quadratojugal bone, medially with the pterygoid bone and with mandible below. Its anteriomedial angle projects into orbit as a process **(Fig.3.6).** The quadrate bone is the ***homologue of the mammalian incus***. The quadrate bone helps in **extensive opening of mouth**.

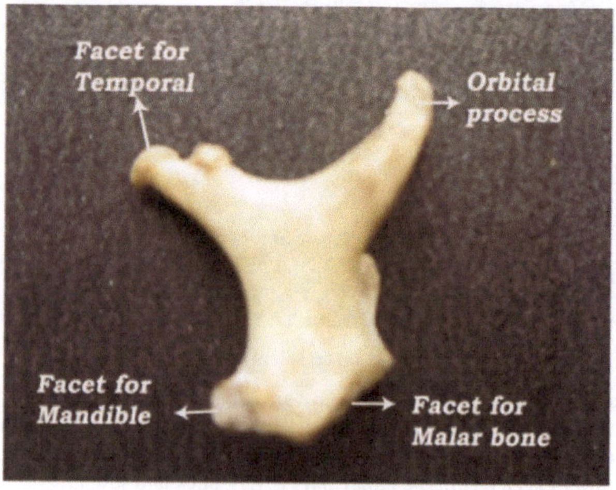

Fig. 3.6: Quadrate Bone-Fowl

HYOID BONE

It shows a **body** (basihyoid) with **lingual process** (glossohyoid) and **four pairs of cornua**. The basihyoid is a short rod placed transversely. The **lingual process** is embedded in the root of tongue. The thyroid cornua are directed upward and backward from the body.

The **keratohyoids** (small cornua) are directed upward and forward and join at their lower ends by concave facet with the cartilage uniting the body and thyroid cornu. Their upper ends join lower ends of the **middle cornua** (**epihyoid**) by cartilage. The **epihyoid** is a small curved rod attached to the small cornua below and great cornu or stylohyoid above **(Fig.3.7).**

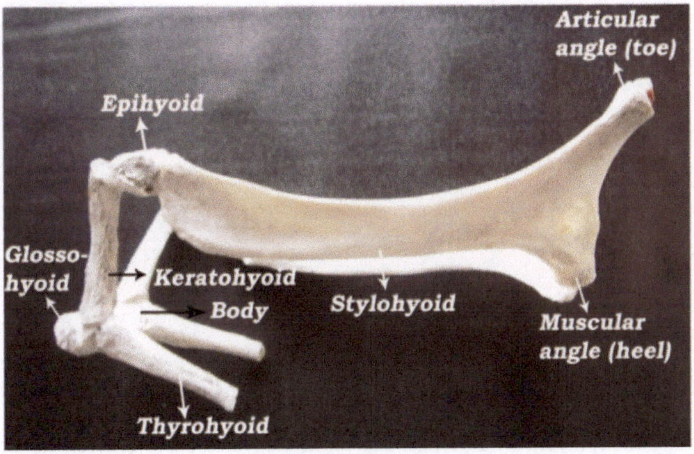

Fig. 3.7: Hyoid of Ox

The **stylohyoid is the largest** part and is directed upward and backward. Its upper end is like a human foot with a **heel (muscular angle)** and **toe (articular angle) (Fig.3.7),** the latter joining hyoid process of temporal bone by cartilage.

Horse: The **glossohyoid is longer and shows pointed free end**. The body and thyrohyoids are fused and along with ***glossohyoid resemble a spur or fork***. The epiphyoid is fused with the stylohyoid **(Fig.3.8).**

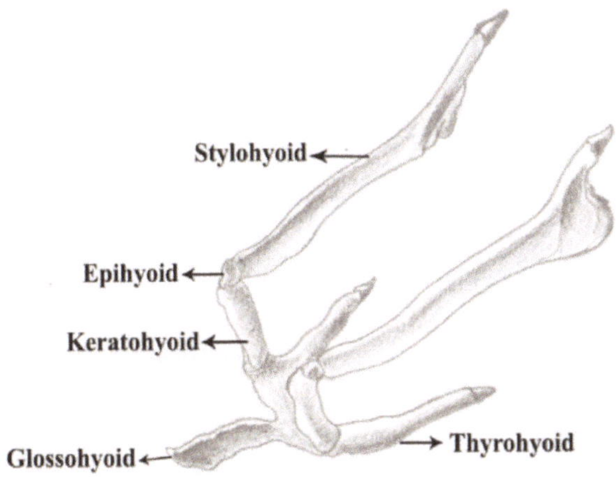

Fig. 3.8: Hyoid of Horse

Dog: The **glossohyoid is absent**. The **epihyoid is longer than stylohyoid**. The latter is twisted **(Fig.3.9).** The thyrohyoids are fused with the body by cartilage.

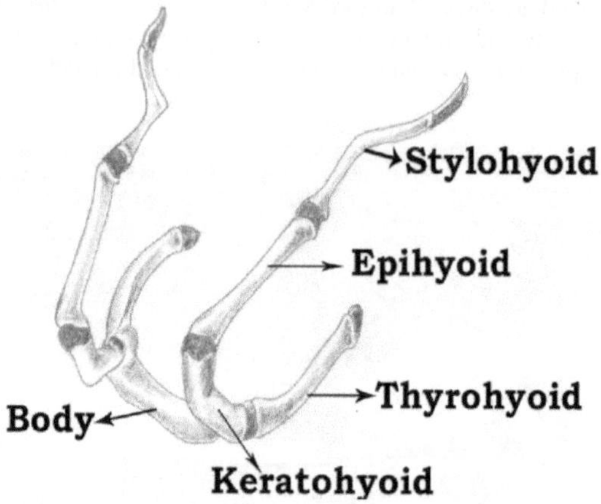

Fig. 3.9: Hyoid of Dog

Pig: The **basi hyoid** is broad rostrocaudally and short transversely. The **lingual process** is very short and pointed. The **thyrohyoids** are wide and curved, concave and grooved dorsally. The **kertaohyoids** are short, wide and flattened dorsoventrally.The **epihyoid** is little longer than the keratohyoids, but is relatively slender. The stylohyoid is very slender rod, slightly enlarged at either end.

Fowl: It shows three median conjoined segments **entoglossal process, basihyal and urohyal** in a sequence and lateral processes at the junction of basihyal and urohyal. Each lateral process shows an **anterior basibranchial** and **posterior ceratobranchial** parts. The latter extends upward and backward **(Fig.3.10).**

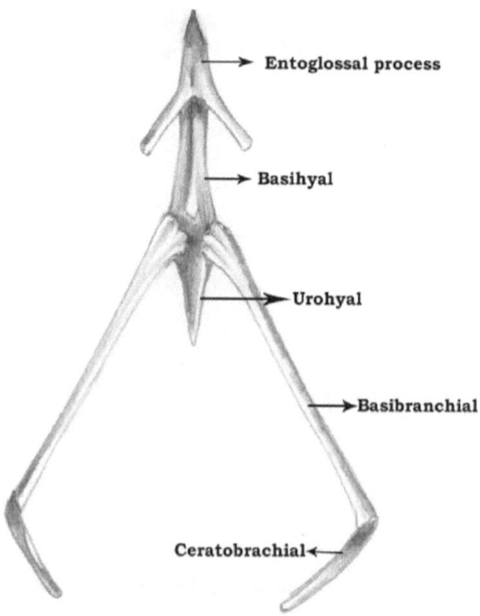

Fig. 3.10: Hyoid of Fowl

VOMER

Ox: is a median bone with two lamina forming a groove to receive septum nasi formed by perpendicular plate of ethmoid and septal cartilage. The lower border rests in a groove formed by palatine processes of maxilla and premaxilla **(Fig.3.11).** The **posterior part of vomer raises from floor of nasal cavity** and expands as two wings to overlap body of presphenoid to form the ***vidian or pterygoid canal***. Because vomer is not attached to the caudal half of the hard palate, posterior nare of one side communicates freely with other **caudal to plane of 2nd cheek tooth**.

> **In buffaloes, the nasal septum** is present throught the floor of the nasal cavity. Hence, the two ***posterior nares are completely separated unlike in ox.***

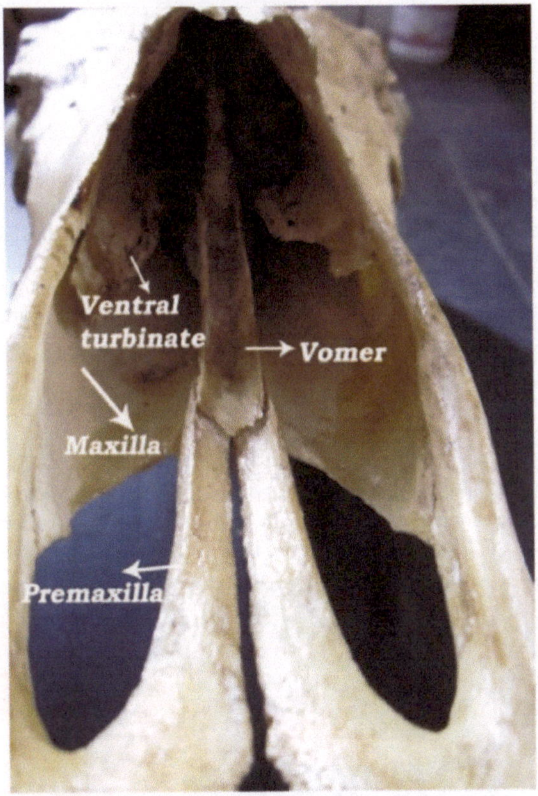

Fig. 3.11: Vomer of Ox

Horse: The posterior part is attached to floor of nasal cavity. ***Hence two posterior nares are completely separated.***

Dog: The posterior part is not in contact with floor of nasal cavity and hence does not separate posterior nares. Near the posterior nares the two laminae curve outward to join incurving lamina of palatine and lamina lateralis of ethmoid to form ***lamina transversalis*** separating olfactory and respiratory compartments **(Fig.3.12).**

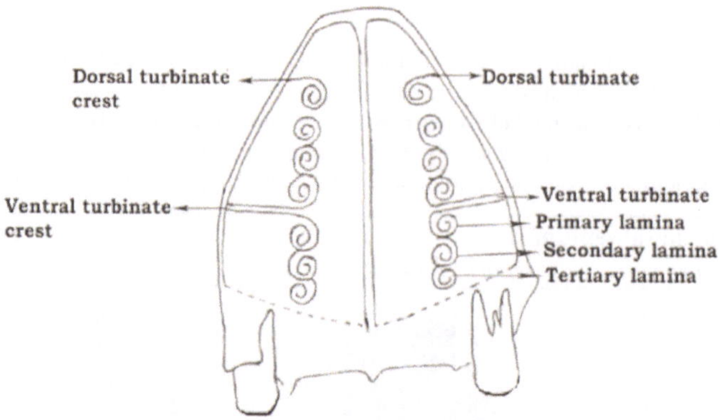

Fig. 3.12: C.S of Nasal Cavity of Dog (schematic)

Pig: It is very long. Its rostral extremity almost reaches the body of the incisive bone and is pointed. Caudally it extends to the level of the presphenoid. It is grooved throught its length to receive the nasal septum. Hence, **the two posterior nares are completely separated.** The extended nasal septum separates the right and left nasopharyngeal meatuses. The caudal half of the vomer articulates with three bones i.e Basal lamina of the ethmoid bone, resulting in a horizontal lamina separating the nasal fundus from the elongate nasopharyngeal meatus ventrally, in its middle third with the perpendicular part of palatine bone ventrolaterally and the caudal third articulates with the expanded part of presphenoid.

Fowl: It is a slender rod extending forward from the sphenoid.

NASAL BONES

Ox: Nasal bone is an elongated curved plate with convex facial surface and concave nasal surface, the latter showing dorsal turbinate crest for dorsal turbinate bone. The posterior extremities of two bones together form projection which is received into the notch formed by anterior ends of frontal bones. The **anterior extremity** shows two processes separated by a notch so that anterior ends of two bones present ***trifid appearance*** **(Fig.3.13).**

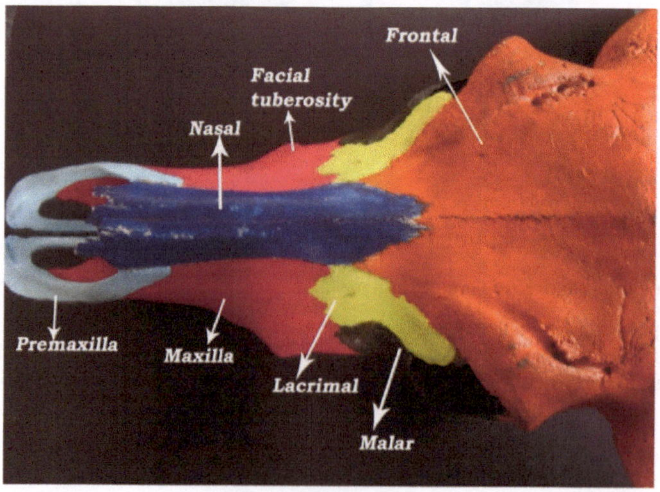

Fig. 3.13: Nasal Bones of Ox

Horse: It is larger and wider. The posterior ends of the two bones together form ***a notch*** into which pointed anterior ends of the two frontals are received. **The anterior end is pointed (Fig.3.14).**

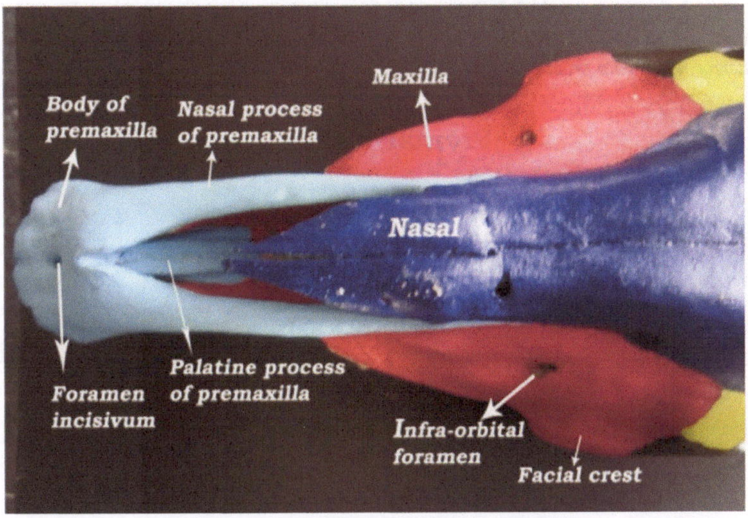

Fig. 3.14: Nasal Bones of Horse

Dog: It is long and wider in front than behind. The anterior ends form a ***semicircular notch and*** posterior ends are like in ox. The **facial surface is concave** in its length and **forms a central groove** with its fellow **(Fig.3.15).** The **medial border projects into the nasal cavity to form the internal nasal crest.**

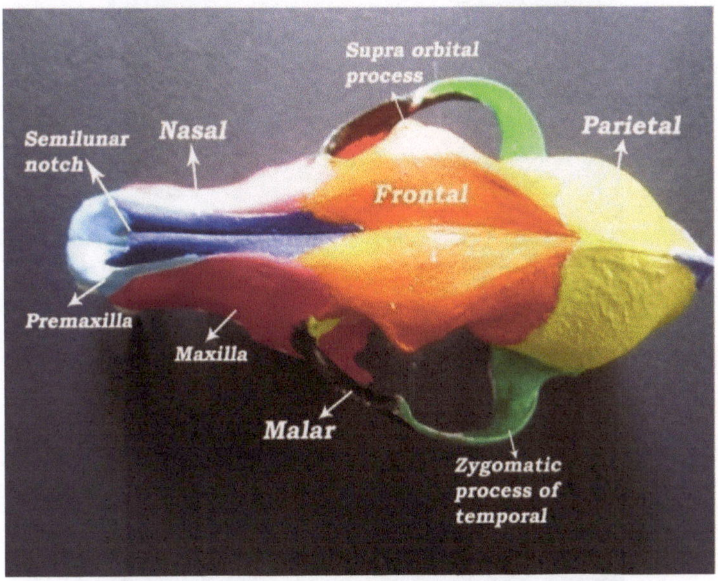

Fig. 3.15: Nasal Bones of Dog

Pig: The rostral one fifth of the bone is free and extends between the laterally curved nasal cartilages. The external surface is flattened, with the exception of the supraorbital sulcus, which crosses the caudolateral surface in an oblique manner.

Fowl: It is a small thin plate showing ***body and frontal, premaxillary and maxillary*** processes. The *processes circumscribe anterior nares with premaxilla and maxilla* **(Fig.3.16 & 3.17).**

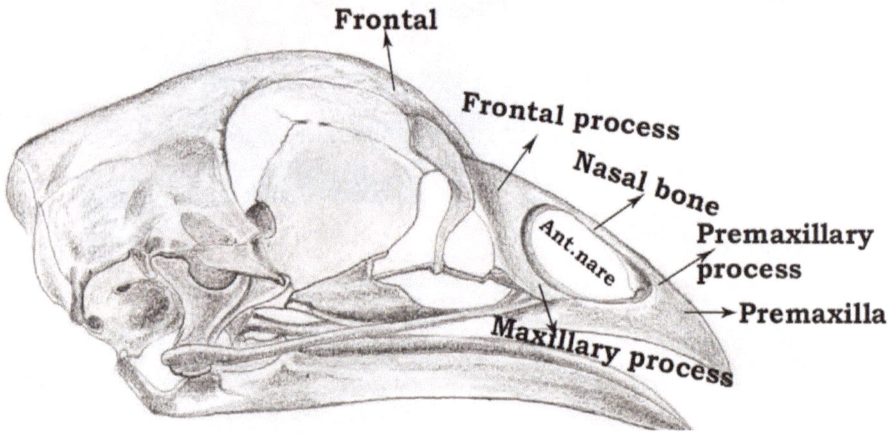

Fig. 3.16: Nasal and Premaxilla of Fowl

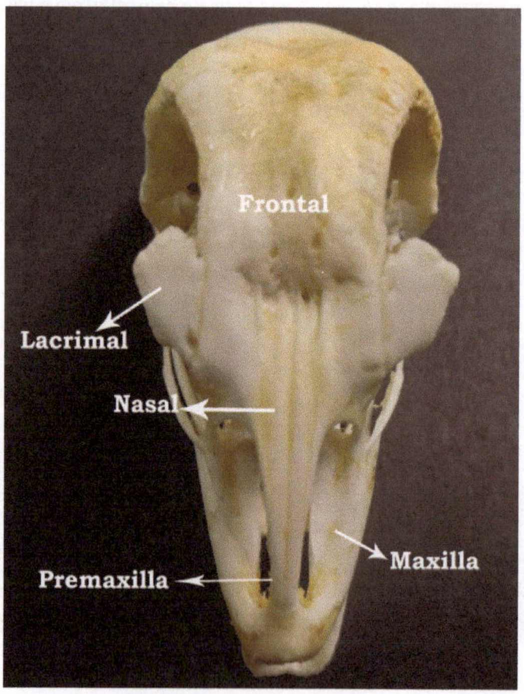

Fig. 3.17: Nasal Bones of Fowl

TURBINATES

Ox: They are delicate scroll like bones two on either side attached to lateral walls of nasal cavity. The **small *dorsal turbinate*** (dorsal nasal concha) is attached to dorsal turbinate crest of nasal bone. The rostral third of the dorsal nasal concha is a thick shelf supported by the basal lamella, which is porous in the ox and of compact bone in the small ruminants. In the caudal two thirds of the concha a spiral lamella is present. It ***coils first ventrally, then laterally and then dorsally***.

The ***larger ventral turbinate*** (***ventral nasal concha***) is divided into rostral and caudal parts. The rostral part consists of a basal lamella and **dorsal and ventral spiral lamellae each of which form subdivided *bullae* (Fig.3.18).** It is attached to ventral turbinate crest of the maxilla by a basal lamina which divides at its inner edge into two plates that are rolled in **opposite directions** to enclose two cavities **(Fig.3.18).**

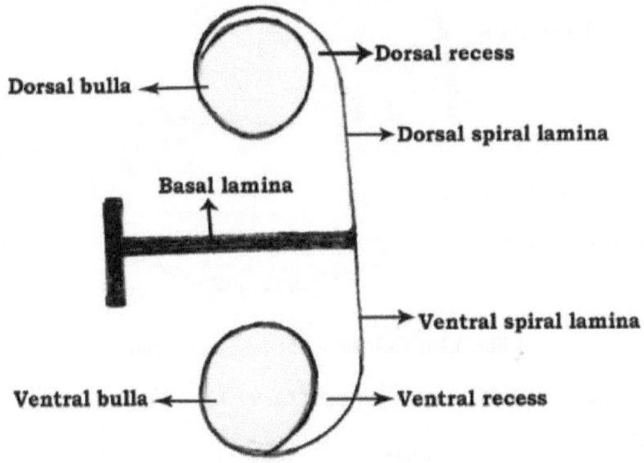

Fig. 3.18: Ventral Turbinate of Ox (schematic)

The medial face of nasal concha is separated from the septum nasi by narrow space called **common nasal meatus.** Between the dorsal turbinate bone and the roof of the nasal cavity is **dorsal meatus.** Between the dorsal and ventral turbinates is **middle meatus.** Between ventral turbinate and floor of the nasal cavity is **ventral meatus (Fig.3.19).**

The ventral meatus is the only one through which a stomach tube can be passed.

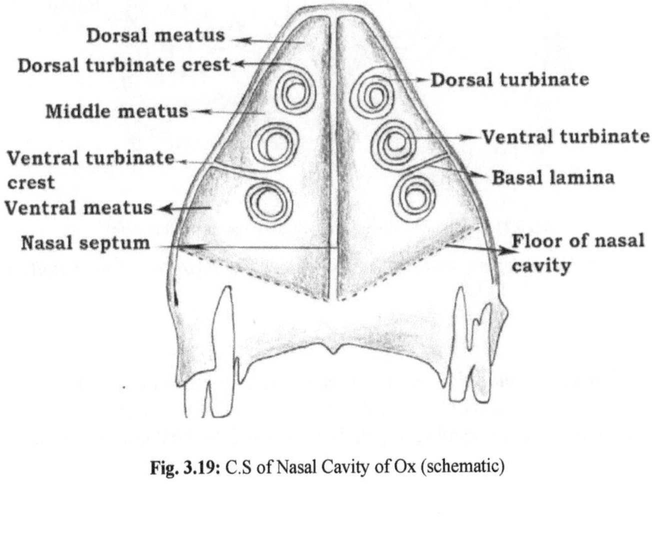

Fig. 3.19: C.S of Nasal Cavity of Ox (schematic)

Horse: The ***dorsal turbinate is larger than ventral one***. Each shows an **anterior coiled part** and **posterior curved portion** which are separated by oblique conchal septa. The coiled parts are rolled towards septum and each other. The basal lamellae of the two conchae project into the nasal cavity from the lateral wall and are continued as spiral lamellae, which coil toward the middle nasal meatus **(Fig.3.20).**

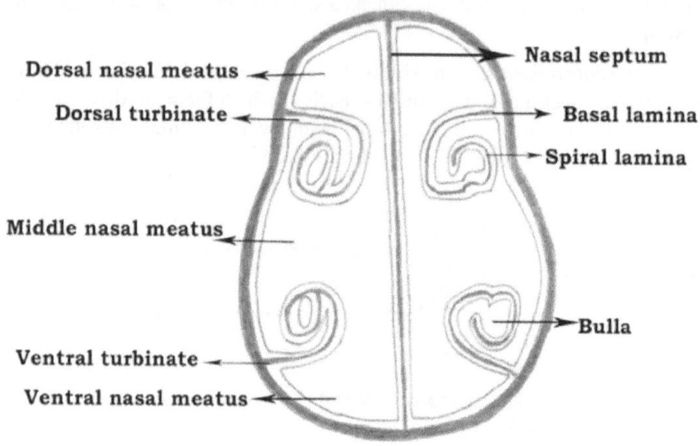

Fig. 3.20: Turbinates of Horse (schematic)

Dog: The larger ventral turbinate is like in ox but shows ***tertiary lamellae*** also **(Fig.3.21).**

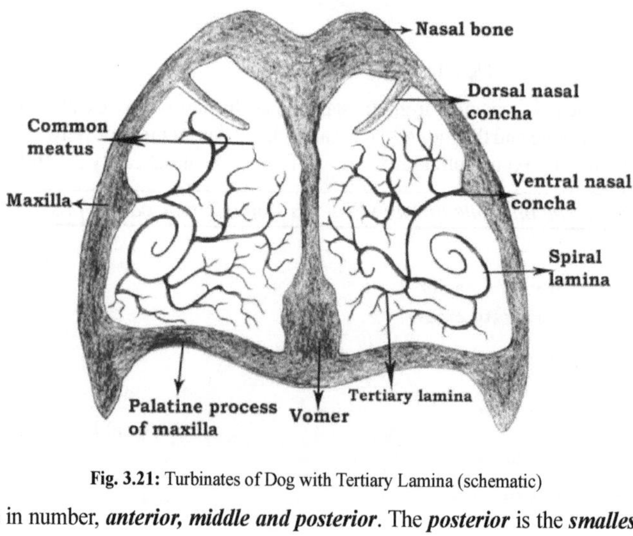

Fig. 3.21: Turbinates of Dog with Tertiary Lamina (schematic)

Fowl: They are three in number, ***anterior, middle and posterior***. The ***posterior*** is the ***smallest*** and the ***middle one is largest***.

PALATINE BONES

Ox: consist of ***horizontal and perpendicular (vertical) parts***, the former forming posterior one-fourth of the bony palate, while the latter forms posterior part of lateral wall of nasal cavity and partly bound posterior nares. The **anterior palatine foramen**, the anterior opening of palatine canal and faint palatine groove are present on horizontal part **(Fig.3.22).** The **vertical part** articulates with **pterygoid medially** and **pterygoid process** of postsphenoid **laterally**. Its upper edge presents a notch which with ethmoid and presphenoid forms ***sphenopalatine foramen.***

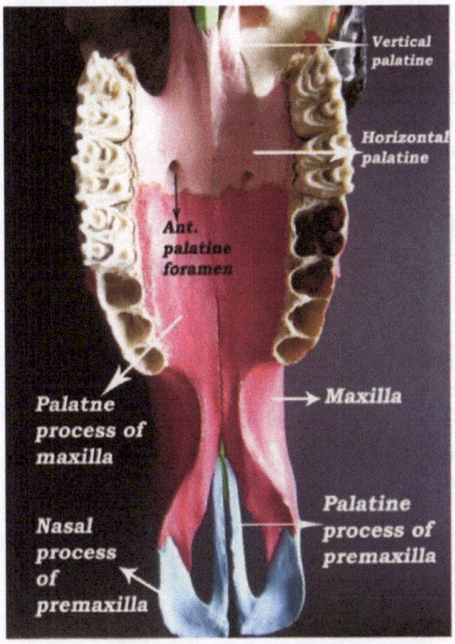

Fig. 3.22: Palatine Bones of Ox

Horse: The **horizontal part is narrow,** while **vertical part is extensive** and **exclusively forms sphenopalatine foramen**. The anterior palatine foramen is formed between the horizontal part and palatine process of maxilla **(Fig.3.23).** The **palatine canal** is formed between the **body of maxilla and vertical part**.

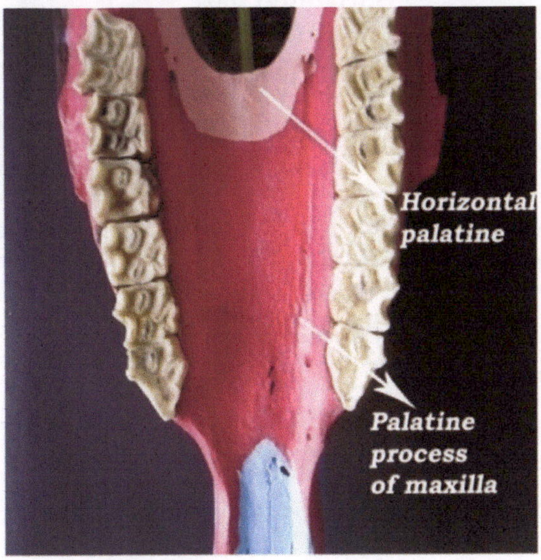

Fig. 3.23: Palatine Bones of Horse

Dogs: Both horizontal and vertical parts are extensive. The lateral surface of vertical part is free and a horizontal plate extends from its nasal surface and meets **incurving lamina from lamina lateralis** and joins **outcurving lamina of vomer** to form ***lamina transversalis dividing caudal part of nasal cavity into upper olfactory and lower respiratory compartments*** **(Fig.3.12).**

Pig: The palatine is **triangular,** with the base caudal and apex rostral. The palatine surface is smooth with the exceptin of an oblique transverse ridge that occurs as the ***palatine crest***. Lateral to the crest **minor palatine foramina** are present, rostral to which the **major palatine foramen** is present. The **nasal surface** is deeply hollowed and has a median nasal crest which extends dorsally and articulates with the vomer.The perpendicular part is slightly concave on its nasal surface.

Fowl: It is narrow in front and wide behind. It forms lateral boundary of posterior opening of the nasal cavity and part of roof of mouth. It meets pterygoid and sphenoid behind and premaxilla and maxilla anteriorly.

PTERYGOID

Ox: Is a thin plate of bone forming lateral wall of posterior nares. Its **lateral face is covered by perpendicular part of palatine and pterygoid process** of postsphenoid. The **extreme upper part** of this face forms **vidian canal** with the **basisphenoid**. The free **lower extremity** forms **hamulus pterygoideus (Fig.3.24).**

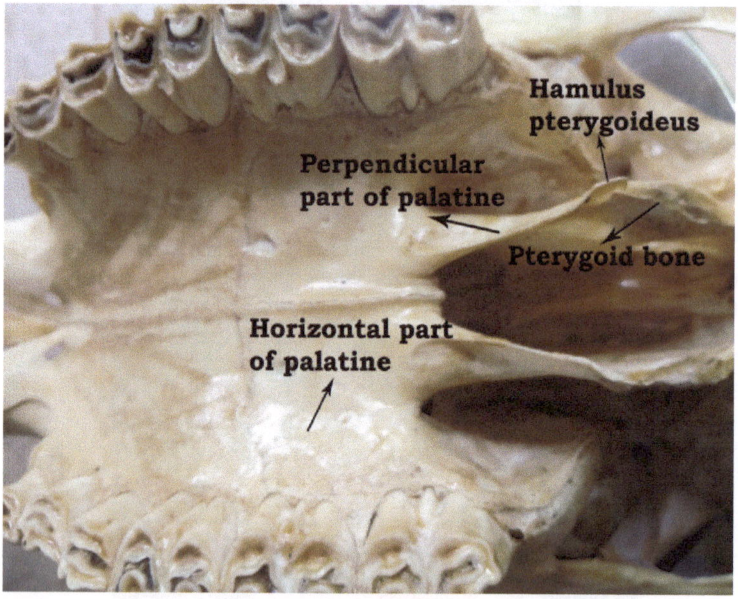

Fig. 3.24: Pterygoid of Ox

Horse: It is shorter and narrower. The lateral face articulates with the vomer also.

Dog: It is wide, short and quadrilateral.

Pig: Each is nearly vertical in direction and is narrow in its middle and wide at each end.

Fowl: It is *rod shaped bone between sphenoid medially and quadrate laterally* **(Fig.3.25).**

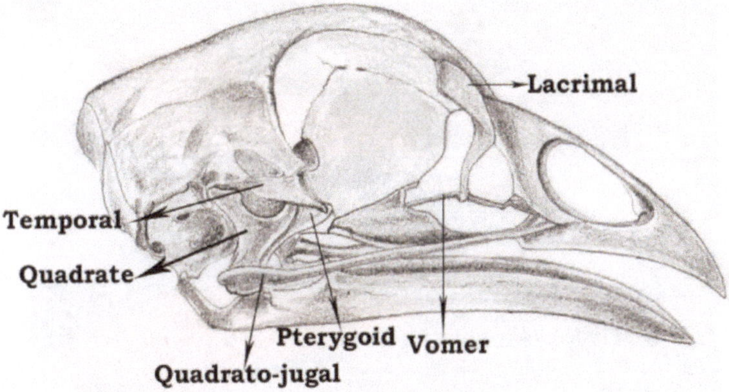

Fig. 3.25: Pterygoid of Fowl

PREMAXILLA

Ox: It forms anterior part of upper jaw and shows a body and nasal and palatine processes. The labial surface of body is convex and oral surface is concave.The body does not show any alveoli since upper incisors are absent. The medial edge forms lateral boundary of the ***incisive fissure along with its counterpart*** **(Fig.3.26).**

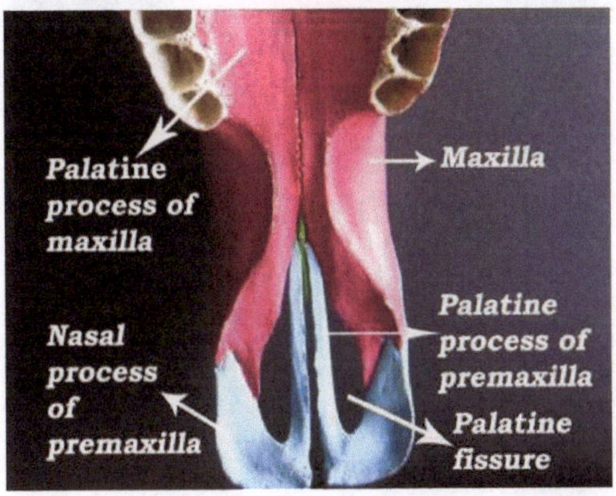

Fig. 3.26: Premaxilla of Ox

The nasal process projects upwards from the body and joins body of maxilla forming lateral wall of the nasal cavity. The ***palatine process*** is smaller and forms anterior part of bony palate.Lateral to **palatine process is a large oval palatine fissure (Fig.3.26).** The lateral boundry of fissure is formed by nasal process.

Horse: The body is thicker and shows ***three alveoli*** for incisors. The medial surface joins opposite one and forms **foramen incisivum (Fig.3.27).** ***Palatine process*** is wide hence **palatine fissure is narrow (Fig.3.28).** The ***nasal process is longer*** and presents at its junction with the maxilla an alveolus for canine tooth.

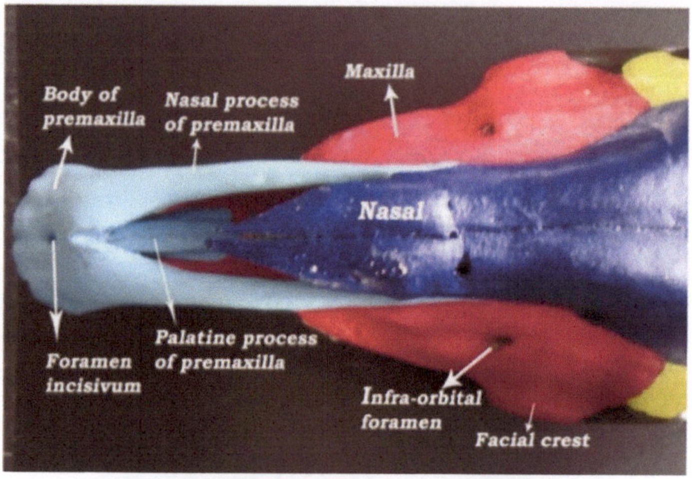

Fig. 3.27: Premaxilla of Horse (Dorsal veiw)

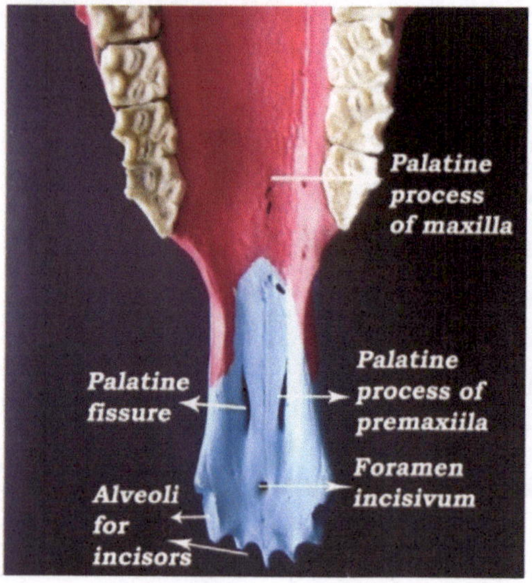

Fig. 3.28: Premaxilla of Horse (Ventral view)

Dog: The body shows three alveoli for incisors and with maxillary bone forms an alveolus for the canine tooth.

Pig: The fusion of the two bones along the midline is incomplete, therefore forming the narrow incisive fissure. The incisive bone concurs in the formation of hard palate and ***bony nasal aperture***.

Fowl: The ***premaxilla forms the skeleton of the upper portion of the beak***. The premaxillae fuse and form anterior boundary of the external opening of the nasal cavity. It presents **three pairs of processes,** ***palatine processes*** which meet the palatine, the ***maxillary processes*** meeting the maxilla and ***nasal processes*** meeting the nasal and frontal bones **(Fig.3.29).**

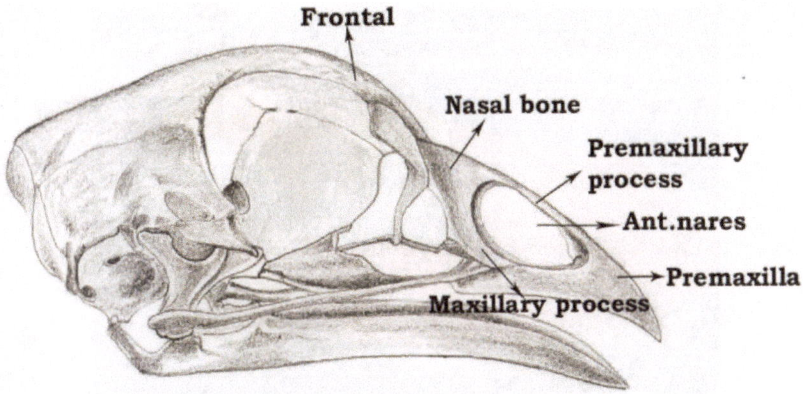

Fig. 3.29: Nasal and Premaxilla of Fowl

MAXILLA

Ox: It is the ***largest*** *bone of the* upper ***jaw***. It shows **body, palatine and zygomatic processes.** The convex external surface of body presents ***infraorbital foramen***, the rostral opening of the infraorbital canal at the level of **the first cheek tooth**, while at the ***level of 3rd or 4th cheek*** tooth is the facial tuberosity extending upward and backward as ***facial crest*** **(Fig.3.30).** The internal face presents ventral turbinate crest for lamina of ventral turbinate below which is lacrimal groove **for nasolacrimal duct.**

The ***dorsal border*** is irregular, while ***ventral (alveolar) border shows six alveoli*** posteriorly for cheek teeth and is free anteriorly **(Fig.3.30).** The **anterior extremity** is pointed. Behind the last alveolus is alveolar tuberosity, while maxillary tuberosity forms posterior extremity of the bone medial to which **maxillary hiatus with sphenopalatine, maxillary and posterior palatine foramina** is present.

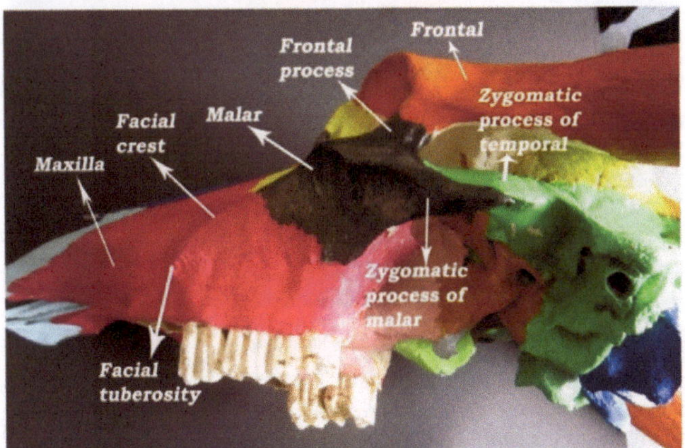

Fig. 3.30: Maxilla of Ox

The **zygomatic process** projects from posterior extremity and is overlapped by the malar. The **palatine process** forms large part of bony palate. Its oral surface shows **palatine groove.**

Horse: The **facial crest is prominent**. The ***infraorbital foramen*** is at the level of ***third cheek tooth*** **(Fig.3.31).**

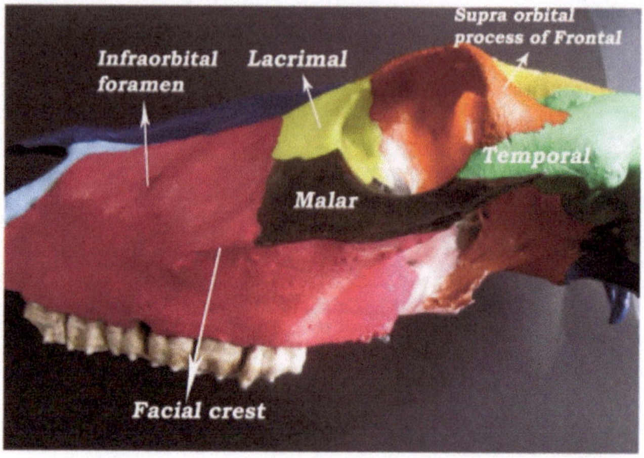

Fig. 3.31: Maxilla of Horse

Dog: The **facial crest is absent**. The infraorbital foramen is as in the horse. The ***maxillary and alveolar tuberosities are absent***. Behind the last alveolus there is a pterygoid process. There are ***six alveoli for upper cheek teeth*** and there is a large alveolus for canine tooth at the junction with the premaxilla **(Fig.3.32).**

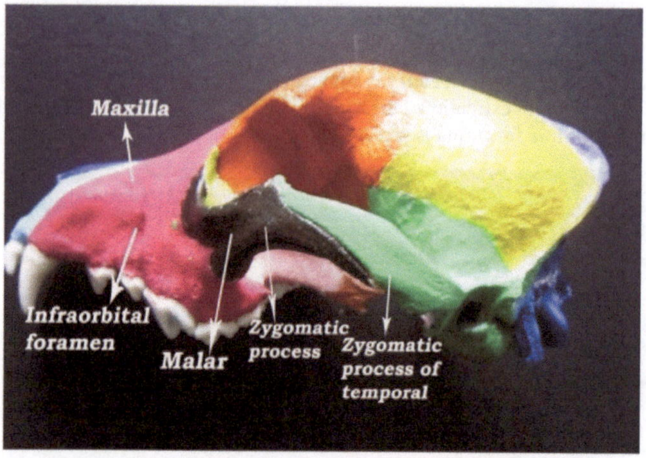

Fig. 3.32: Maxilla of Dog

Pig: The facial surface of the body is smooth and concave. Facial tuberosity is absent. Near the center of the bone is the infraorbital foramen. Dorsal to the zygomatic crest and rostral to the infraorbital foramen the concavity of the facial surface is referred to as the ***canine fossa***. The **zygomatic process** is a short, strong projection from the caudolateral surface of the body. The **frontal process** is greatly reduced and is overlapped by the lacrimal bone and concurs in the formation of nasolacrimal canal.The **palatine process** is very long and forms major portion of the bony palate.

Fowl: It is a slender bone placed on the sides and partly on the floor of the nasal cavity. The ***two palatine processes do not meet but join palatine and vomer posteriorly*** **(Fig.3.33).**

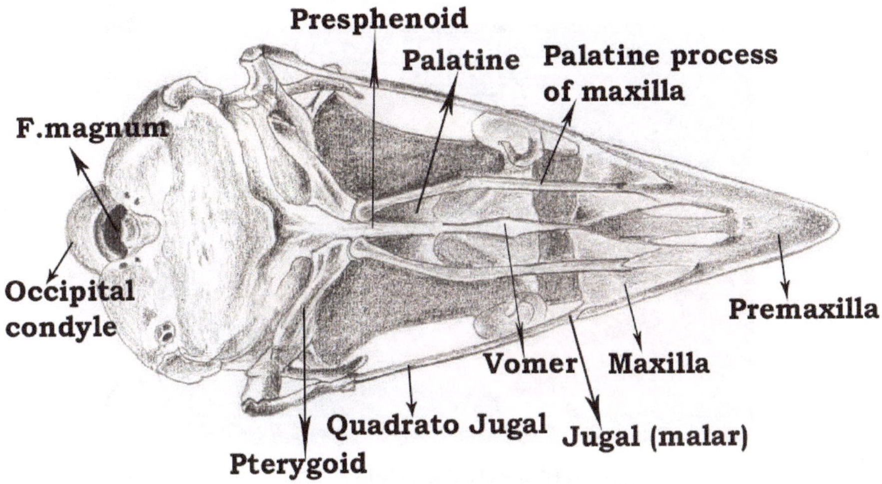

Fig. 3.33: Basal View of Skull of Fowl

LACRIMAL

Ox: It shows facial and orbital parts, the latter forming anterior part and part of medial wall and floor of orbit. The nasal face of facial part shows osseous ***nasolacrimal canal for the passage of nasolacrimal duct***. The ***orbital part bears ventrally thin walled protuberance, lacrimal bulla*** **(Fig.3.34).**

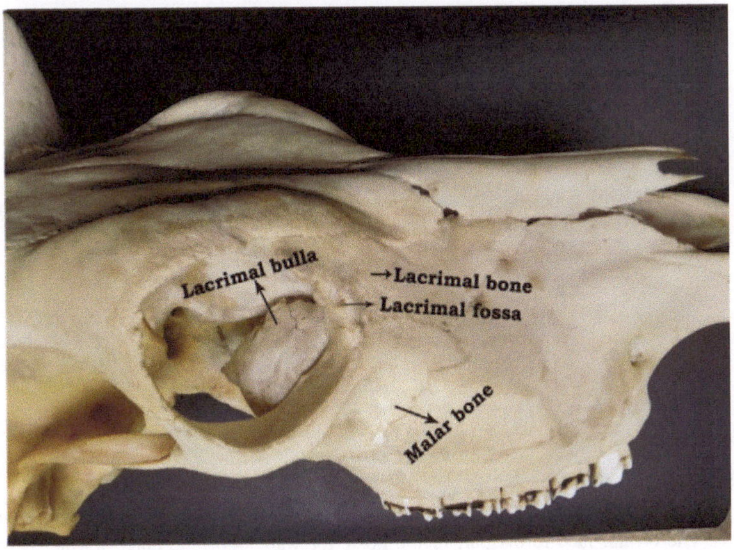

Fig. 3.34: Lacrimal of Ox

Horse: The facial part is less extensive and shows **lacrimal tubercle and the lacrimal bulla is absent (Fig.3.35).**

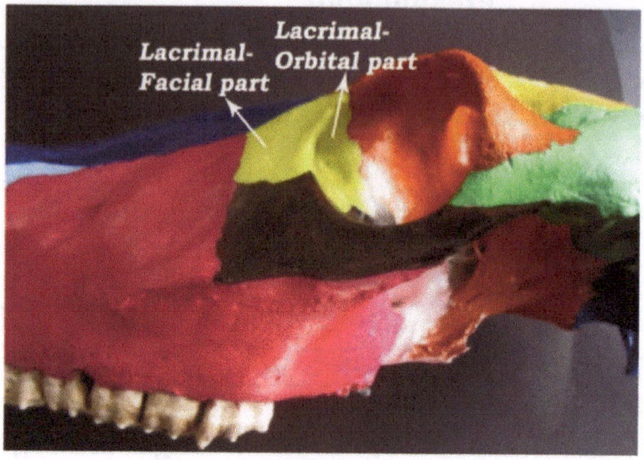

Fig. 3.35: Lacrimal of Horse

Dog: The facial part is very small and does not meet nasal.

Pig: It is irregular in shape. Its orbital face is concave for the presence of the **deep gland of the third eye lid** (***Harderian gland***).

Fowl: It is a **triangular plate of bone at the anterior margin of the orbit**. Its medial edge meets the frontal and the pointed apex projects downward as a long curved process **(Fig.3.36).**

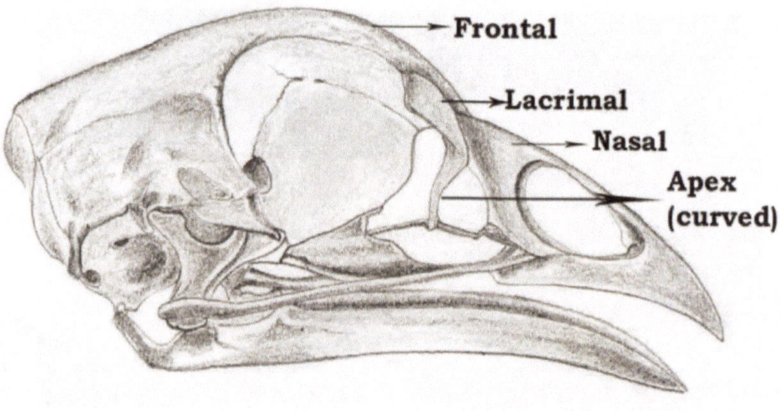

Fig. 3.36: Lacrimal of Fowl

MALAR (Zygomatic bone)

Ox: It is a triangular bone. The external face is marked by **facial crest** which continues over temporal part of zygomatic process. The orbital face forms part of the posterior wall, floor and anterior wall of orbit. The ridge separating two faces forms part of orbital rim.

The ***upper extremity*** shows ***zygomatic (temporal) and frontal processes*** **(Fig.3.37).** The latter joins supraorbital process of frontal to form part of upper margin of orbit while the ***former is overlapped by zygomatic process of squamous temporal to form zygomatic arch*** **(Fig.3.37).**

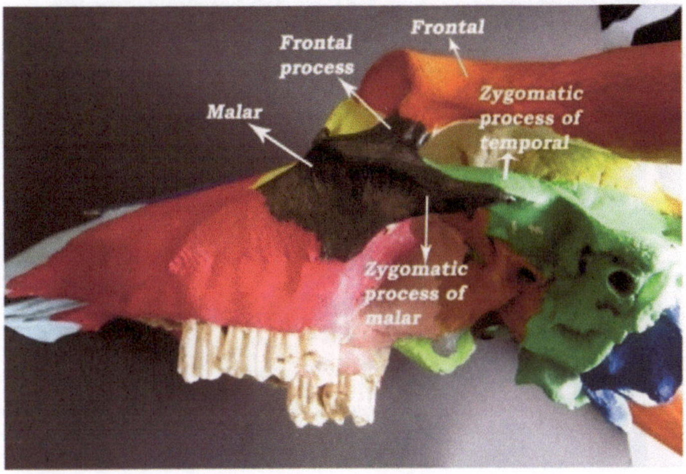

Fig. 3.37: Malar of Ox

Horse: The facial surface is very small. The ***upper extremity is not divided*** and is overlapped by only zygomatic process of sqamous temporal **(Fig.3.38).**

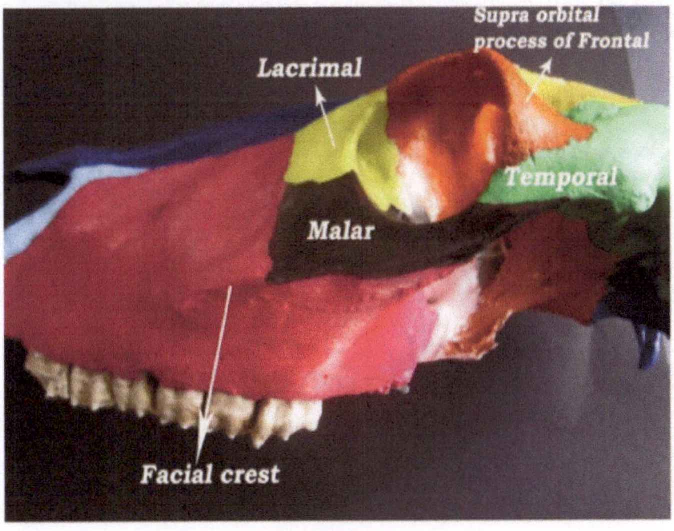

Fig. 3.38: Malar of Horse

Dog: The body shows dorsal ***lacrimal and ventral maxillary processes***. The **zygomatic process forms bulk of *the* bone** and meets zygomatic process of temporal but ***frontal process does not reach supraorbital process*** **(Fig.3.39).**

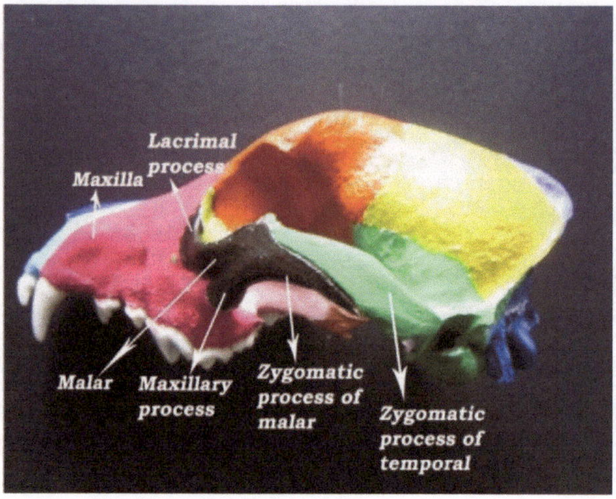

Fig. 3.39: Malar of Dog

Pig: The orbital face is small and deeply grooved. Caudal to the orbital surface a sharp **frontal process** projects dorsally.

Fowl: It is a slender rod of bone extending from **maxilla to quadrate**. The anterior and posterior parts are ***called jugal and quadratojugal*** bones **(Fig.3.40)**.

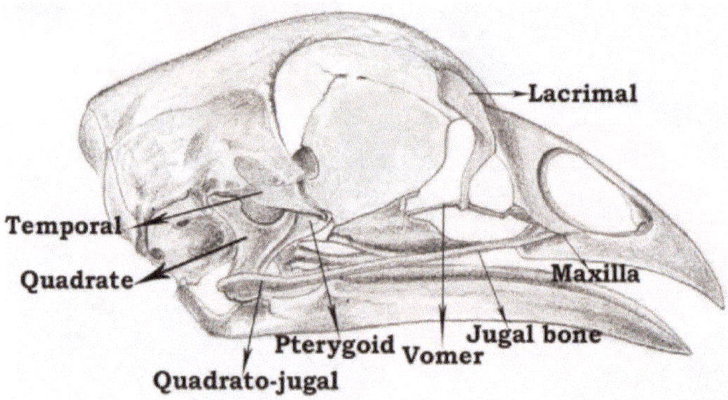

Fig. 3.40: Quadrate and Malar Bones of Fowl

CRANIAL BONES:

FRONTAL

Ox: It is largest of the cranial bones and shows ***body (frontal part), orbital part and temporal part***. The body shows **supraorbital groove and foramen**, the latter is upper opening of supraorbital canal. It presents a central prominence called "***torus frontalis***" at its junction with parietal bone posteriorly and a ***large cornual process or horn core at its posterolateral angle*** **(Fig.3.41)**.

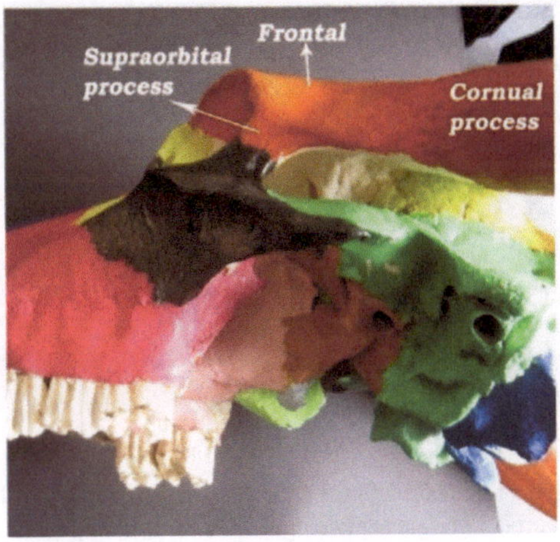

Fig. 3.41: Frontal of Ox

The ***orbital part*** forming **medial wall of orbit** shows orbital opening of supraorbital canal. Close to its posterior edge it forms ***ethmoidal foramen*** with orbital wing of presphenoid. The ***supraorbital process*** forms a part of the rim of orbit and meets frontal process of malar bone **(Fig.3.41).** The **temporal part** forms part of the temporal fossa and joins below with squamous temporal.

Horse: The **supraorbital foramen** perforates root of the supraorbital process. The latter joins zygomatic process of temporal. The **cornual process is absent (Fig.3.42).**

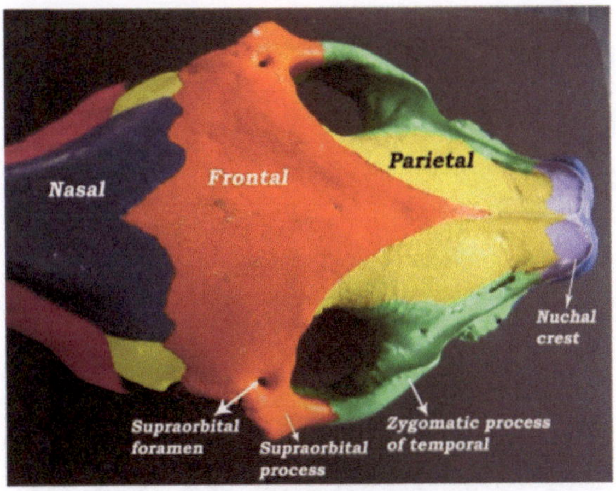

Fig. 3.42: Frontals of Horse

Dog: The body shows a central depression. The **supra orbital foramen is absent** and supraorbital process is short and ***orbital rim is incomplete*** since supraoribtal process joins neither with zygomatic rocess of malar nor zygomatic process of temporal bone **(Fig.3.43).** ***There are two ethmoidal foramina.***

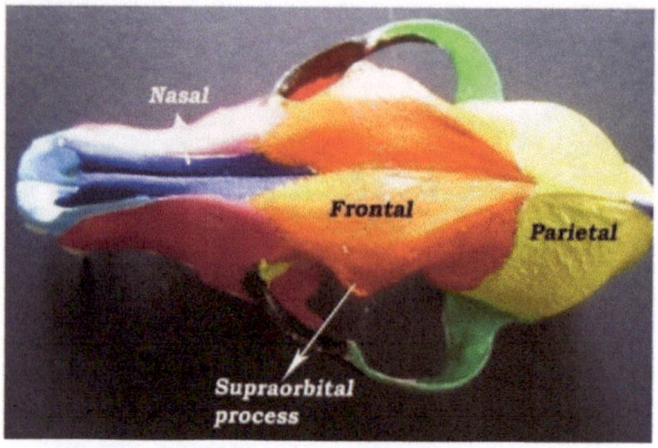

Fig. 3.43: Frontals of Dog

Pig: The squamous part forming the basis of the forehead is thick and excavated by the frontal sinus. Laterally, it is bordered by a semicircular supraorbital margin separating it from the orbital part.

Fowl: It is the largest bone of the cranium. It consists of a body and orbital plate.

OCCIPITAL

Ox: It is situated on the lower part of posterior surface of skull and part of the base of the skull. It shows lateral (exoccipital), squamous (supraoccipital) and basilar (basioccipital) parts (Fig.3.44).

Exoccipital: This consists occipital condyle and paramastoid process on each side between which there is a condyloid fossa with hypoglossal foramen for the passage of hypoglossal (12th cranial) nerve and a condyloid foramen leading to condyloid canal.

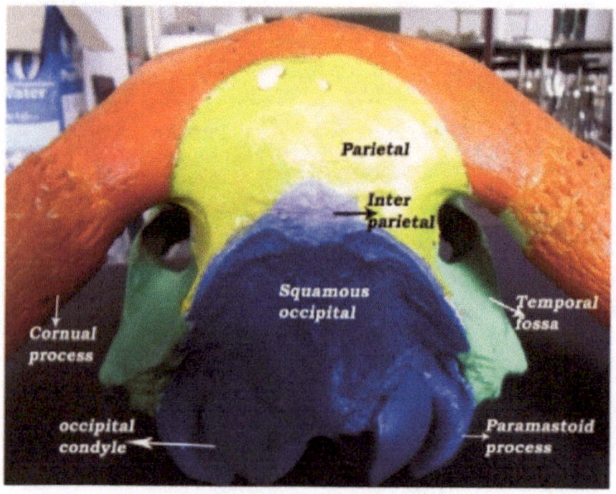

Fig. 3.44: Squamous Occipital of Buffalo

Basioccipital: is a wide thick bar of bone showing two basilar tubercles at its junction with the body of the postsphenoid. It's lateral borders form the medial margins of the foramen lacerum (for passage of IX, X and XI cranial nerves). The exoccipital and basioccipital enclose largest foramen of the skull i.e foramen magnum for continuation of medulla oblongata as spinal cord (Fig.3.44).

Supraoccipital: is a quadrilateral plate of bone between exoccipital, squamous temporal, parietal and interparietal bones. It presents a central external occipital protuberance near its junction with the interparietal for the funicular part of ligamentum nuchae (Fig.3.44). The mastoid foramen is situated on either side at the junction of the supraoccipital with squamous temporal bones. The cranial surface shows internal occipital protuberance below which there is a shallow median fossa for the vermis of the cerebellum.

Horse: Only hypoglossal foramen is present in condyloid fossa. The paramastoid process is narrower and less curved. The basilar part is longer and narrower and the basilar tubercles are smaller. The foramen lacerum is wider (Fig.3.45). The squamous part is crossed by prominent transverse horizontal ridge called nuchal crest (Fig.3.48) and its cranial surface shows a deep central and two shallower lateral depressions.

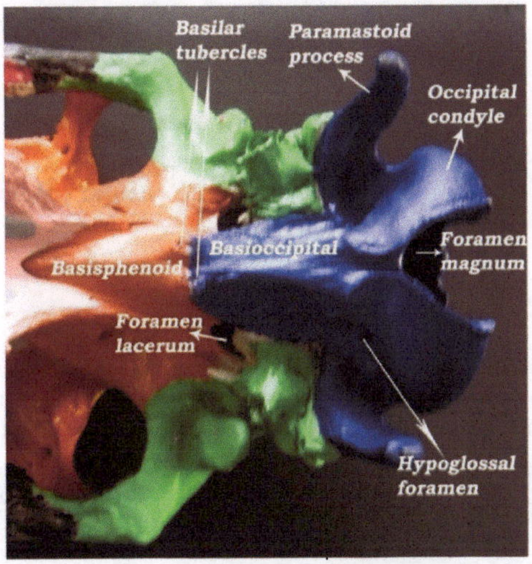

Fig. 3.45: Occipital of Horse

Dog: The **nuchal crest is prominent**, angular and directed backward. The mastoid foramen and condyloid canal are as in ox. The paramastoid process is very short. The wide basilar part joins bulla tympanica on either side and at the junction shows basilar tubercle.

Pig: The basilar part is hexagonal, flattened caudally, narrower and thicker rostrally. The external surface is marked by a narrow, median ridge called the **pharyngeal tubercle**. Ventrally, each lateral part presents a distinct elongated jugular process. Rostromedial to the base of the process, it is marked by a vertical elongate, jugular notch. The squamous part is extensive, flattened and triangular.

Fowl: The occipital condyle is single and placed below the foramen magnum **(Fig.3.46).**

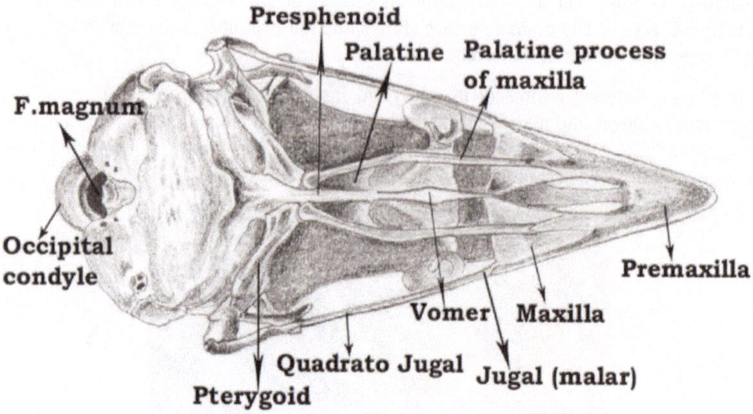

Fig. 3.46: Occipital and Sphenoid of Fowl

PARIETAL

Ox: It is placed on the **posterior and lateral aspects** of the cranium. The **lateral part** forms a part of the **temporal fossa**. The **posterior part** forms posterior wall of the cranium. The junction of two parts is marked by **parietal crest** which is continuous with the temporal crest below and with the frontal crest infront **(Fig.3.47)**.

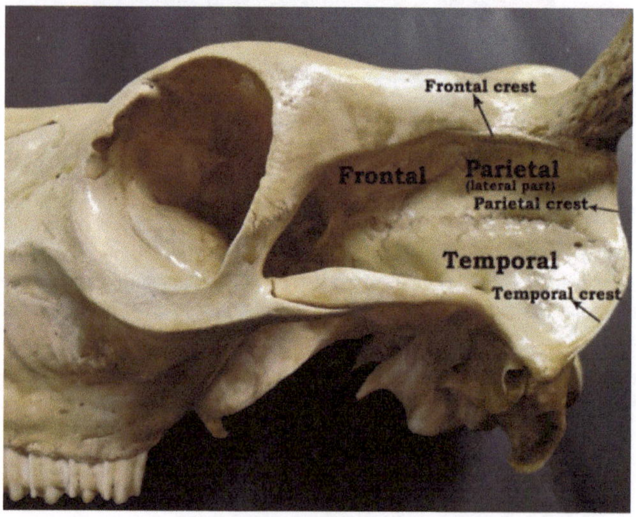

Fig. 3.47: Parietal of Ox

Horse: It is placed on the **superolateral aspect** of the cranium forming its roof. The external surface is marked by **median external parietal** crest above, which bifurcates below to join the frontal crest **(Fig.3.48)**. The posterior border meets the occipital and curves inward and with the temporal forms the parieto-temporal canal.

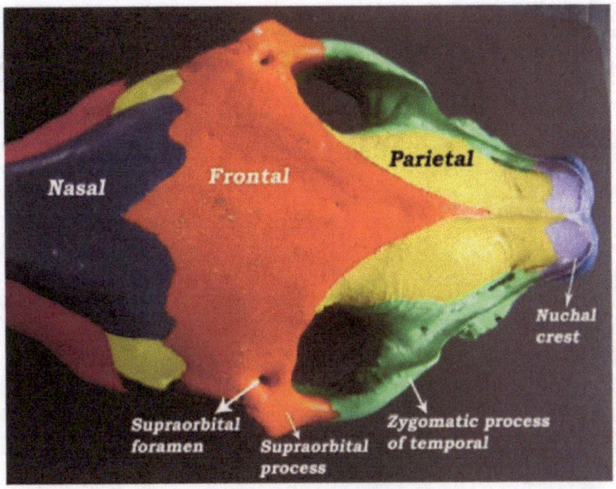

Fig. 3.48: Parietal Bones of Horse

Dog: It is rhomboid in outline and position is like in horse **(Fig.3.49).**

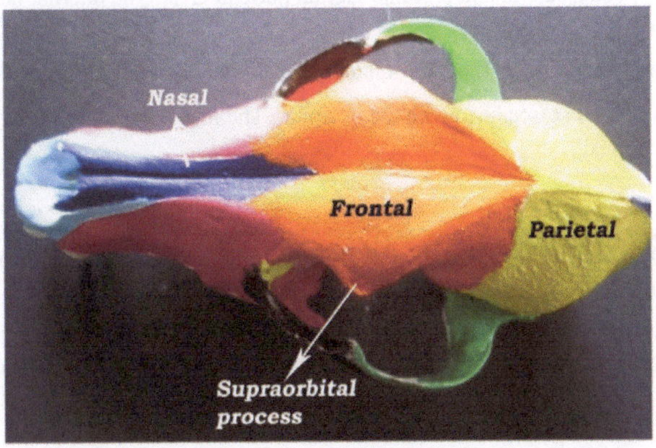

Fig. 3.49: Parietal Bones of Dog

Fowl: It is situated on the posterior part of roof of the cranium.

INTERPARIETAL

Ox: It is a single bone wedged between parietals above and supraoccipital below **(Fig.3.50).**

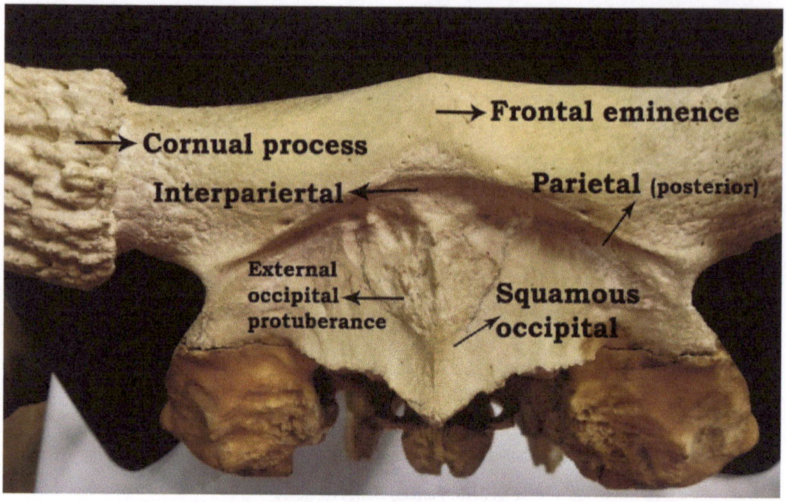

Fig. 3.50: Interparietal Bones of Ox

Horse: The external face is quadrilateral and presents sagittal parietal crest. The internal face presents a three sided process, ***internal occipital protuberance.***

Dog: It bears high posterior part of the parietal crest and large internal occipital protuberance.

Pig: The interparietal bone fuses before birth with the occipital. The internal occipital protuberance is absent.

Fowl: It is absent.

TEMPORAL

Ox: It forms part of the lateral wall of the cranium. It **shows squamous, tympanic and petrous parts**, the latter two parts are related to middle and internal ears respectively.

The ***squamous part*** shows **body and zygomatic process**. The body is divided into two parts by temporal crest, the lateral part forming part of temporal fossa with 2 or 3 foramina and posterior part joining occipital. The **zygomatic process** shows ventrally condyle, glenoid cavity and postglenoid process (behind which there is a postglenoid foramen). The anterior part of zygomatic process meets the zygomatic process of malar.

The ***tympanic part*** shows a curved plate of bone, **external acoustic process enclosing external acoustic meatus**. Above this process there is a mastoid process, while below the external acoustic process, there is a rod of bone called **hyoid process (Fig.3.51).**

The ***stylomastoid foramen*** is placed between **hyoid process and paramastoid process** and **bulla tympanica** whose cavity forms part of the **middle ear cavity (Fig.3.51).** Bulla tympanica, a considerable eminence situated centrally is compressed anteriorly and posteriorly. It is thin walled and encloses cavity which is lower part of the tympanum that is part of the middle ear and it is crossed by irregular bony plates. The muscular or styloid process projects from below bulla. The **petrotympanic fissure** (***Glasserian fissure***) for the passage of ***chorda tympani nerve*** is present lateral to root of this process, while medially there is a groove for **osseous eustachian tube (Fig.3.52).**

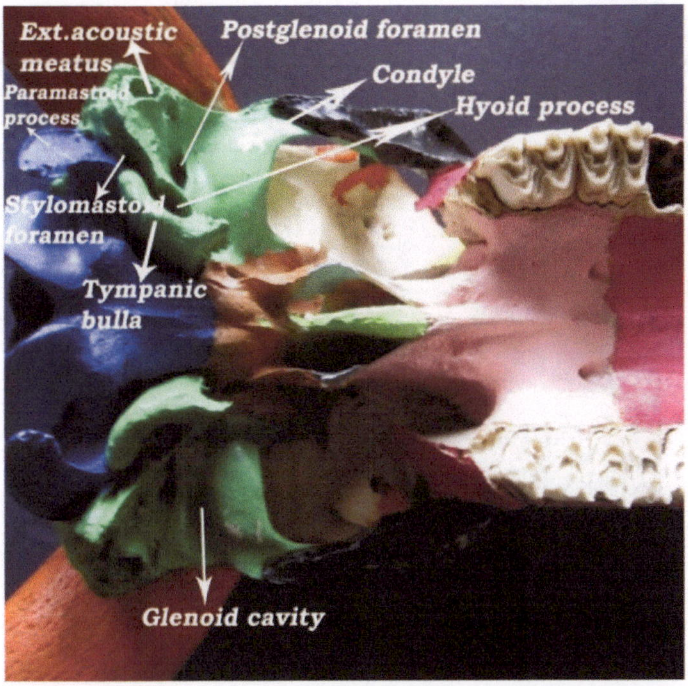

Fig. 3.51: Squamous and Tympanic Parts of Temporal Bone of Ox

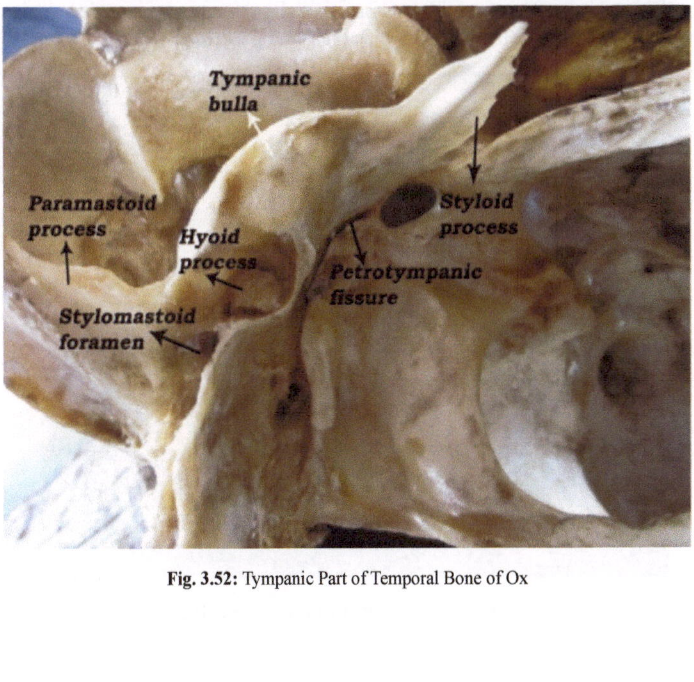

Fig. 3.52: Tympanic Part of Temporal Bone of Ox

The ***petrous part*** houses internal ear. Its smooth medial face presents internal acoustic meatus which is divided by a crest into two fossae **(Fig.3.53).** The superior one is the origin of facial canal (***aqueductus fallopius***) which opens externally at the stylomastoid foramen. It transmits ***facial (7th cranial) nerve***. The inferior fossa presents small foramina for the passage of ***vestibulocochlear (8th cranial) nerve***. Behind the meatus and near the posterior margin of this surface a slit like opening of ***aqueductus vestibulae is present***. Below this is a narrow fissure, the orifice of ***aqueductus cochleae***. The petrosal crest separates anterior face from medial face.

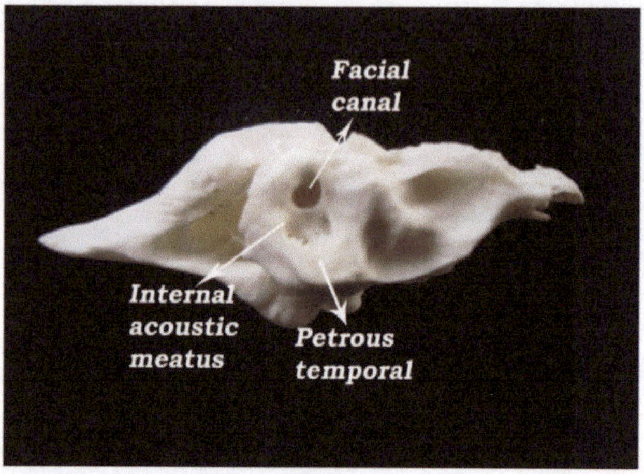

Fig. 3.53: Petrous Temporal Bone of Ox

Horse: The squamous part is larger and shows a posterior triangular process also which joins with occipital above and overlaps mastoid process below. The **zygomatic process** joins both zygomatic process of malar bone and supraorbital process of frontal bone. The **mastoid process** is well developed and tympanic bulla is smaller **(Figs.3.54 & 3.55).** The **stylomastoid foramen** is between hyoid and mastoid processes.

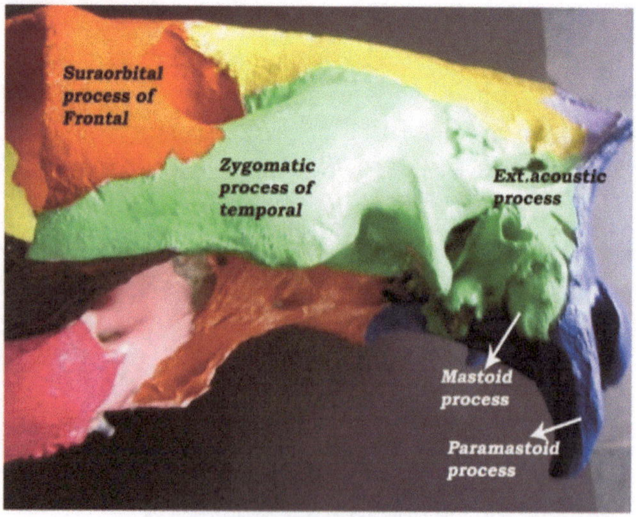

Fig. 3.54: Squamous Part of Temporal bone of Horse

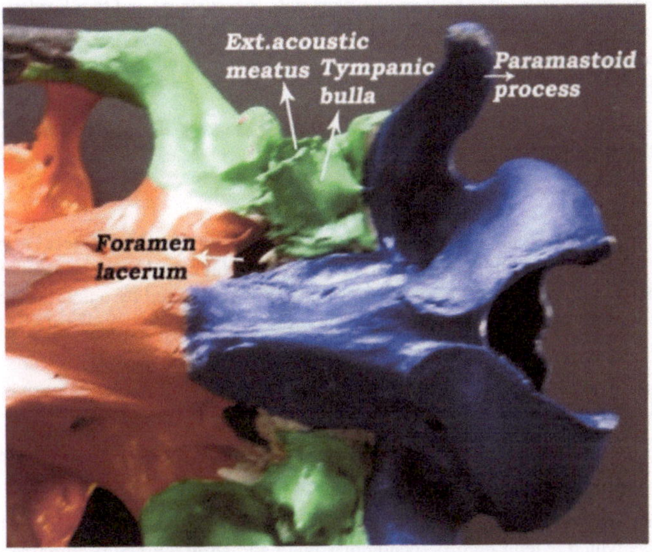

Fig. 3.55: Tympanic Part of Temporal Bone of Horse

Dog: The **zygomatic process** is strongly curved outward and forward and is devoid of condyle, instead a transverse articular groove is present. The **mastoid process** is distinct. The **external acoustic meatus** is very short and wide. The **bulla tympanica** is very large. The **muscular and hyoid processes are rudimentary.** The ***Eustachian opening*** is present lateral to the ***carotid foramen for passage of internal carotid artery*** **(Fig.3.56).** The latter is external opening of carotid canal passing through medial part of bulla tympanica. At the union of **petrous part and basioccipital** is the ***petrobasilar canal***. The petrosal crest is prominent. The medial face of petrous part shows ***floccular fossa*** above the internal acoustic meatus and its anterior angle shows a foramen.

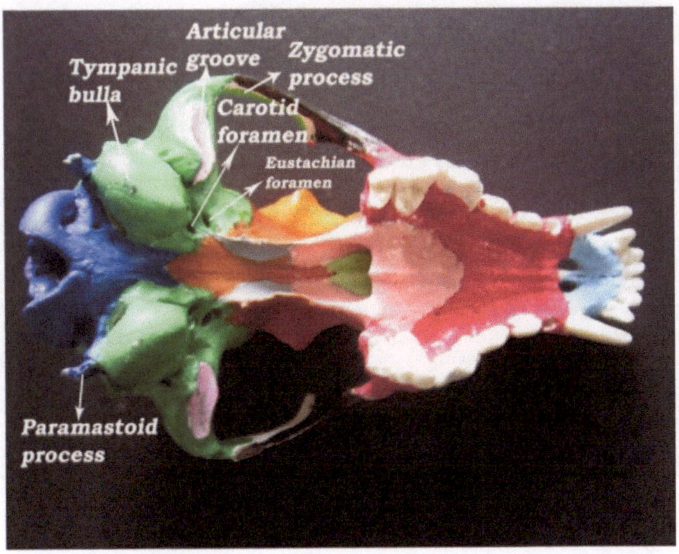

Fig. 3.56: Squamous and Tympanic Parts of Temporal of Dog

Pig: The squamous part is the largest. It is an irregular bone with two surfaces and four borders. The petrous part of the temporal bone is relatively small and irregular in shape. The mastoid process is greatly reduced. The tympanic part is ventral to the petrous part. The tympanic cavity is small and communicates in its ventral wall with the cancellous interior of the bulla.

Fowl: The squamous part shows supraorbital and zygomatic processes, the former fused to that of frontal. It furnishes a facet for the quadrate bone.

ETHMOID

Ox: It is composed of a sieve like **cribriform plate, a perpendicular part and two lateral masses (Fig.3.57).** The cranial surface of cribriform plate is divided by **crista galli (ethmoidal crest) into two deep ethmoidal fossae**. It is considered as intracranial projection of perpendicular plate. It is perforated by numerous small foramina and a large foramen on either side for the passage of **olfactory filaments**. The convex nasal surface shows lateral masses attached to it.

The **perpendicular plate** forms posterior part of septum nasi and its ventral border is received into groove of the vomer. It separates two lateral masses.

Each **lateral mass** has a shape of a half cone and covered by a thin plate of bone, **lamina lateralis** on its lateral face which also forms dorsal margin of sphenopalatine foramen.

Each lateral **mass consists** of delicate scroll like plates of bones termed **ethmoturbinates.** Each mass is made up of **five endoturbinates** which extend upto perpendicular plate and **eighteen ectoturbinates** which do not reach perpendicular plate **(Fig.3.58).**The largest one is dorsal and attached to the nasal bone called **great ethmoturbinate** or **middle (third) turbinate** as it projects between dorsal and ventral turbinates.

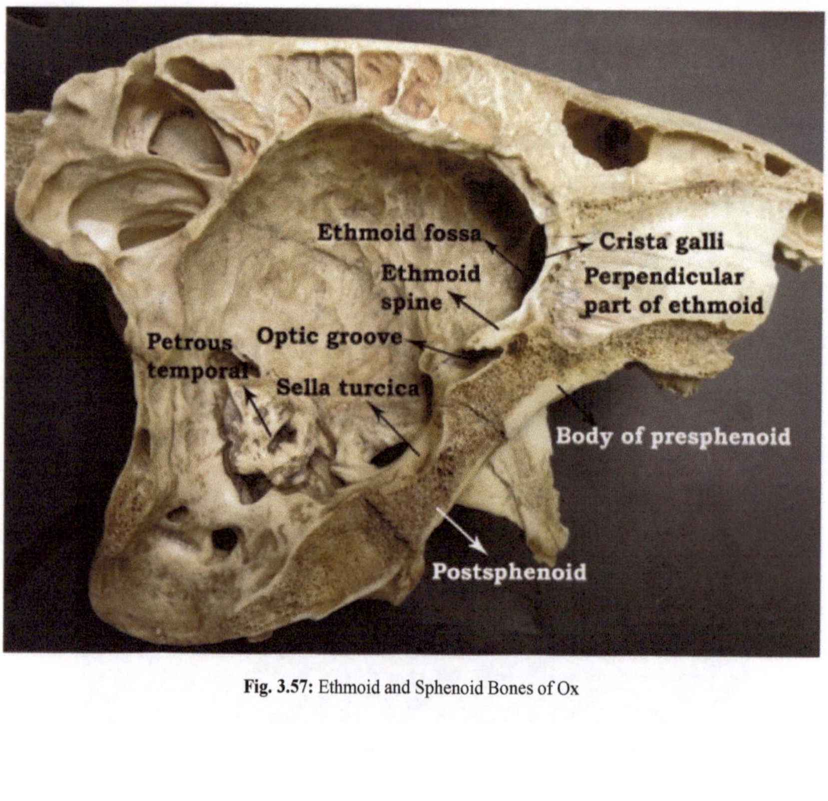

Fig. 3.57: Ethmoid and Sphenoid Bones of Ox

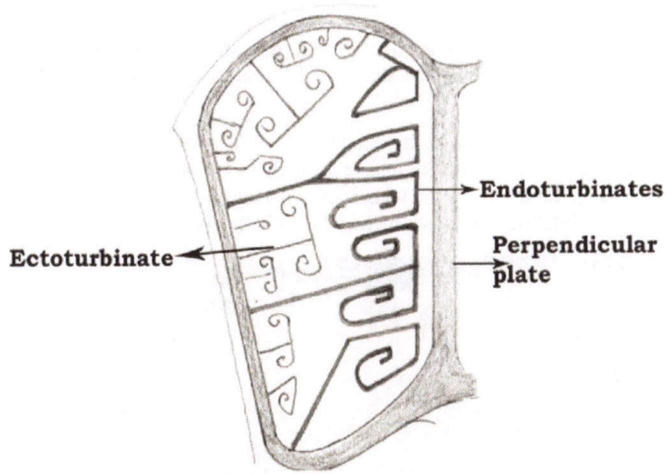

Fig. 3.58: Ecto and Endo Turbinates of Ethmoid of Ox (schematic)

Horse: The lateral masses are made up of **6 endoturbinates and 21 ectoturbinates.**

Dog: Ethmoid is well developed. The cribriform plate **is extensive and olfactory fossae are very deep**. The ***cristagalli*** (***ethmoidal crest***) is ill developed. The perpendicular plate is long. The **lateral masses are well developed** and project into frontal sinus.A shelf like plate extends inward from lower part of lamina lateralis which concurs with similarly **incurved part of *palatine bone* forming *lamina transversalis*** with outcurving plate of **vomer**. There are **four endoturbinates and six ectoturbinates.**

Pig: shows 7 endoturbinates and 13 ectoturbinates.

Fowl: The **lateral masses and cribriform plate are absent**. The **perpendicular plate** forms ***interorbital septum*** with the sphenoid **(Fig.3.59).**

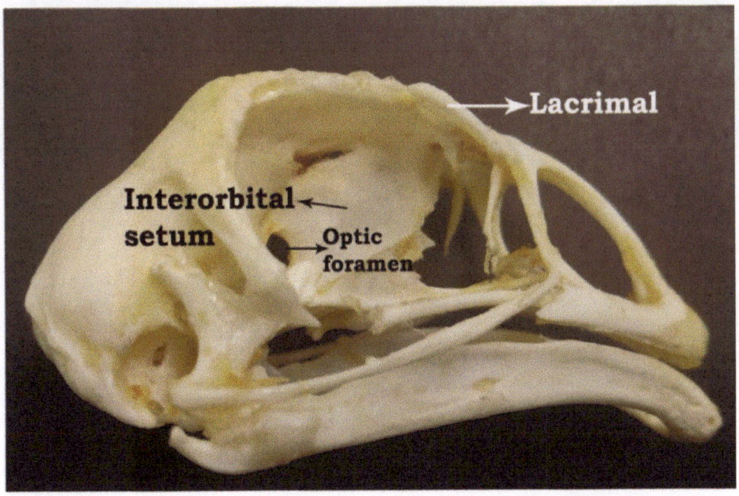

Fig. 3.59: Ethmoid of Fowl

SPHENOID

Ox: It shows two parts, **presphenoid and postphenoid**. The **presphenoid** lying at a higher level shows body and paired orbital wings, while the postsphenoid shows body (basisphenoid) and **paired temporal wings and pterygoid (*subsphenoidal*) processes.**

The body of presphenoid is concealed ventrally by vomer and laterally by pterygoid bones. The internal surface shows ***median ethmoidal spine*** anteriorly which joins crista galli and posteriorly at a lower level is optic groove leading to **optic foramen (Fig.3.60).** The orbital wings curve dorsolaterally from the sides of the body and their lateral faces form part of the orbital wall. They are pierced by optic foramen at the junction with the body.

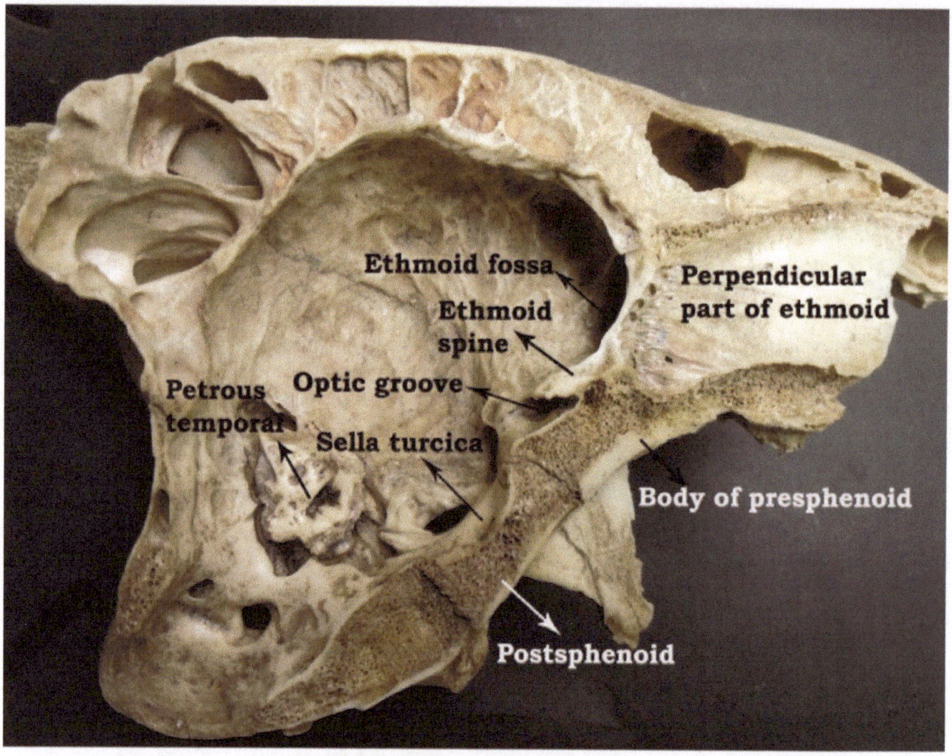

Fig. 3.60: Internal Surface of Pre and Postsphenoids of Ox

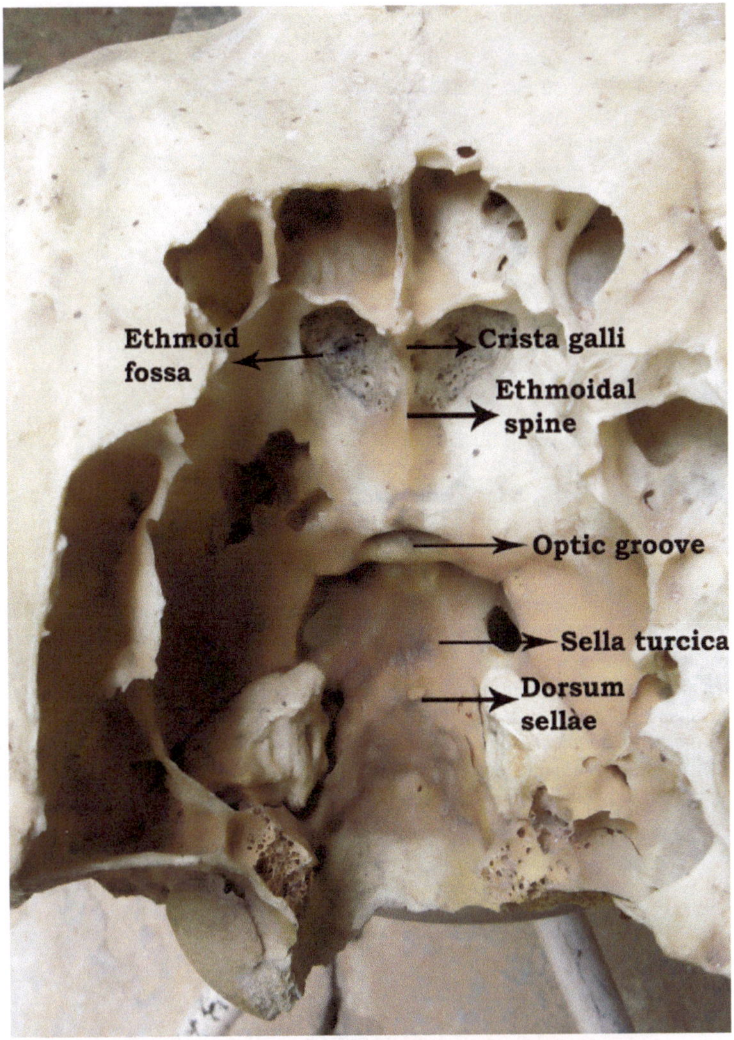

Fig. 3.61: Internal Surface of Pre and Postsphenoids of Ox-Dorsal view

The basisphenoid shows ***sella turcica (pituitary fossa)*** on its internal (cranial) face for lodging of pituitary gland and is marked by a transverse projection at the posterior end (dorsum sellae) which bears posterior clinoid processes on either side **(Fig.3.61).** The **wings are perforated by foramen ovale** (***for the passage of mandibular division of trigeminal nerve***) and their **posterior border** forms **anterior margin of the foramen lacerum** (***for the passage of IX, X, XI cranial nerves***). The **foramen orbitorotundum** (***for the passage of III, IV, VI and maxillary and ophthalmic divisions of trigeminal nerve***) is placed between temporal and orbital wings **(Fig.3.62).** The temporal wings are free anterolaterally forming pterygoid crest. The pterygoid processes are directed downward and forward and their medial surfaces are concealed by pterygoid and join perpendicular part of palatine bones.

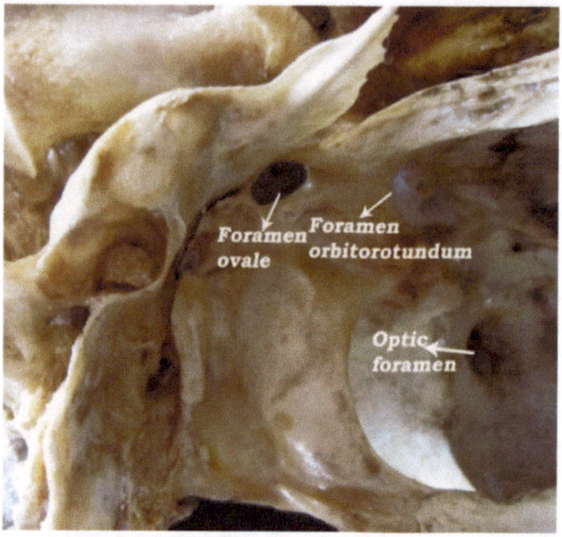

Fig. 3.62: Sphenoid of Ox

Horse: The posterior border of temporal wing forming anterior border of foramen lacerum shows ***carotid, oval and spinous notches*** within outward (***for carotid artery, mandibular nerve and middle meningeal artery*** respectively). The dorsum sellae and posterior clinoid processes are absent. The **foramen orbitorotundum** exists as two separate foramin i.e **foramen orbitale (*for the passage of III, VI and ophthalmic division of trigeminal nerve*) and foramen rotundum** (***for the passage of maxillary division of trigeminal nerve***) separated by a plate of bone. The **trochlear foramen (*for the passage of trochlear nerve*)** is sometimes seen on *the* ***pterygoid crest.*** Caudal to the pterygoid crest a **small alar foramen (alare parvum)** is present **(Fig.3.63).** It is the dorsal opening of a canal which leads from the alar canal and through it the **rostral deep temporal artery emerges.**

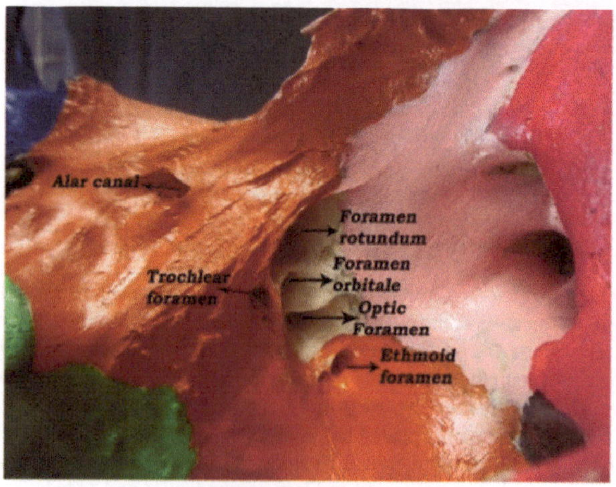

Fig. 3.63: Sphenoid of Horse

Dog: The bodies of pre and postsphenoids are dorsoventrally flattened. The dorsum sellae and posterior clinoid processes are well developed, while anterior clinoid processes project from orbital wings. The **foramen orbitale**

and foramen rotundum exist separately but the ***foramen rotundum*** opens into **alar canal**. The foramen ovale is as in ox. The **temporal wings** are extensive and join with **parietals dorsally** and **carotid notch** with a similar notch on temporal bone forms **carotid foramen (Fig.3.64).**

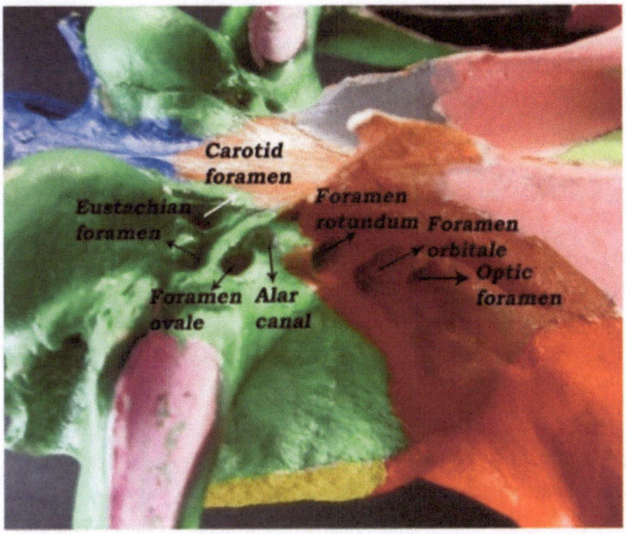

Fig. 3.64: Sphenoid of Dog

Pig: The body of post sphenoid is compressed laterally is somewhat triangular. There is a distinct sella turcica limited caudally by the prominent dorsum sellae. The shallow depression found at this point is termed the ***clivus***. Paired caudal clinoidal processes are also present.

Fowl: It is a triangular in outline **(Fig.3.65).**

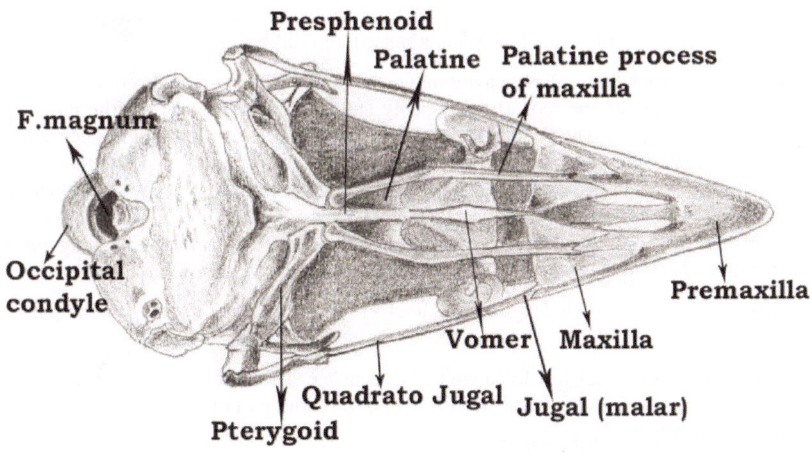

Fig. 3.65: Sphenoid-Fowl

CRANIAL CAVITY

It is an ovoid cavity inclosing the brain with its membranes, associated glands and vessels. Its **roof** is formed by **frontal**. The **lateral wall** is formed by squamous temporal, orbital and temporal parts of frontal, lateral part of parietal and orbital wing of presphenoid.

The **anterior wall** is formed by cribriform plate of ethmoid which separates cranial and nasal cavities. The **posterior wall** is formed by exoccipital and supraoccipital, posterior part of parietal, interparietal and partly by squamous temporal. The **floor** is made up of three parts formed by body and orbital wings of presphenoid, body and temporal wings of postsphenoid and basioccipital respectively. The petrosal crest divides the cavity into cerebral and cerebellar compartments.

In **horse and dog** parietals and interparietals form roof along with frontal and posterior wall is formed exclusively by occipital.

In **fowl** cranial cavity is rounded and wall is thick thus reducing size of the cavity and **roof** is formed by parietals and frontals.

Orbit: It is conical cavity which encloses the eyeball with muscles, vessels and nerves associated with it. The **medial wall** is formed by frontal, lacrimal and orbital wings of presphenoid. The **dorsal wall** is formed by frontal and to some extent by lacrimal. The **ventral wall** is incomplete and is formed by the **malar and to some extent by maxilla**. The **lateral wall** is formed by **supraorbital process of the frontal and frontal process of the malar**. ***In dog lateral wall is incomplete.*** In man orbit is completely surrounded by bone, while in domestic animals bony orbit is deficient caudolaterally. The deficient **caudolateral part of orbital wall is formed by periorbita,** a tough fibrous partially elastic membrane stretching from orbital margin to pterygoid crest.

In **fowl** orbit is oval and very large. The ventral boundary is formed by jugal bone and posterointeriorly it is incomplete.

Pterygopalatine fossa: It is seen ventral to orbit. Its **medial wall** is formed by **perpendicular part of palatine and pterygoid process of postspenoid,** while lateral boundary is formed by maxillary tuberosity. Its deep anterior recess i.e ***maxillary hiatus*** shows maxillary, posterior palatine and sphenopalatine foramina.

NASAL CAVITY

Ox: The nasal cavity is bounded **dorsally** by nasal and to some extent by frontal bones, **ventrally** by palatine processes of premaxilla, maxilla and horizontal part of the palatine, laterally by nasal process of premaxilla, body of maxilla and perpendicular part of palatine bone and turbinate (conchal) bones.

The **turbinate bones** divide each half of nasal cavity into dorsal, middle and ventral meatuses. The **dorsal nasal meatus** is narrow and lies between the roof of nasal cavity and dorsal concha. The **middle nasal meatus** lies between dorsal and ventral conchae. The **ventral nasal meatus** is the largest meatus and lies between the ventral concha and floor of the nasal cavity. The **common nasal meatus** lies between the nasal septum and conchae from roof of nasal cavity to the floor and continuous laterally with the other three meatuses. The **olfactory area is a blind area infront of cribriform plate**, while the **respiratory area** is ventral and leads to posterior nares. The septum nasi does not meet the whole length of the floor of the nasal cavity, hence posterior nares are **not completely divided in ox**, ***whereas in buffalo the two posterior nares are completely separated.***

Horse: The septum nasi meets the whole length of the floor of the nasal cavity and thus **divide posterior nares completely**.

Dog: The nasal cavity is almost completely filled with nasal conchae. The caudal part of the septum nasi fails to meet the floor of the nasal cavity. **Lamina transversalis** divides posterior part of nasal cavity into ***upper olfactory and lower respiratory compartments.***

Pig: Nasal cavity is very long. The septum nasi meets the floor of the nasal cavity throught its length, hence the **two posterior nares are completely separated.**

Fowl: The nasal cavity opens into the mouth and pharynx by narrow slit like opening. The cavity is cone shaped with apex pointing rostrally.

SINUSES OF SKULL

All the sinuses of skull have aperture to nasal cavity. During inflammation aperture may be closed blocking drainage of discharge from the sinus.

Ox: Some of the skull bones show sinuses between two layers of compact bone instead of songy bone. The ***frontal, maxillary, palatine and sphenoidal sinuses are present.*** **The frontal sinus is largest** and is seen in frontal, parietal, interparietal and supraoccipital bones. The two sinuses are separated by a septum and each is divided into smaller spaces by partial septa.The **maxillary sinus** is seen in body of maxilla, lacrimal and malar bones. It communicates with palatine sinus over infraorbital canal. The roots of the last 3 or 4 cheek teeth project into sinus covered by a plate of bone.The **palatine sinus** is seen in palatine process of maxilla and horizontal part of palatine bones. The two sinuses are separated by a septum. The ***smallest sphenoidal sinus is seen in the body of presphenoid and extends into orbital wing***.

Horse: The **maxillary, frontal, sphenopalatine and ethmoidal sinuses are present**. The **maxillary sinus is the largest sinus**. The ventral turbinate and lateral masses of ethmoid are also involved in formation of maxillary sinus. It is divided into anterior and posterior parts by an oblique septum directed inward and upward and both parts are divided into lateral and medial parts by infraorbital canal. The **frontal sinus** is seen in lacrimal, ethmoid and dorsal turbinate also. The **sphenopalatine sinus** is formed in the **body of presphenoid and perpendicular part of palatine bone.** The ethmoidal sinus is the cavity in the largest ethmoturbinate.

Dog: The frontal sinus is confined to frontal bones. The maxillary sinus is small.

Fowl: There are no air sinuses in the skull.

VERTEBRAL COLUMN

Consists of **unpaired irregular** bones. In the adult some vertebrae get fused together with the adjacent ones as single bony mass and are termed **fixed or false vertebrae (eg: Sacrum)**. But other vertebrae remain free throught life and termed **movable or true vertebrae (eg: Axis)**.

The vertebral column is divided for description purpose into five regions - cervical, thoracic, lumbar, sacral and coccygeal regions forming the skeleton of the neck, back, loin, croup and tail respectively.

The number of bones in each region except in coccygeal region is constant in each species so that their number can be expressed as a formula called the vertebral formula. The vertebral formula of domestic animals is given below.

Ox	:	C7	T13	L6	S5	Cy 18-20
Horse	:	C7	T18	L6	S5	Cy 15-21
Dog	:	C7	T13	L7	S3	Cy 20-23
Pig	:	C7	T14-15	L6-7	S4	Cy 20-23
Fowl	:	C-14	T7		LS-14	Cy7

All the bones of the vertebral column which are constructed on the same general plan are termed typical vertebrae. Those that deviate from general plan are atypical vertebrae **eg: atlas, axis**.

A typical vertebra shows **body**, **neural arch**, **paired anterior** and **posterior articular processes**, paired **transverse processes** and **unpaired dorsal and ventral spinous** processes.

1. **Body:** is the fundamental part of the vertebra around which the other parts are grouped. It is in the form of a solid rod. The anterior end is convex and the posterior end is correspondingly concave. The dorsal surface of the body is flat and forms the floor of the vertebral foramen, whereas the ventral surface shows centrally the ventral spinous process for muscular and ligamentous attachment.
2. The **neural arch:** is present on the superior face of the body and it forms vertebral foramen with the body. Each half of the arch is made up of a **vertical pedicle and a horizontal lamina.** The anterior and posterior

edges of the pedicles show notches called **vertebral notches**. These notches form **intervertebral foramina** with the fellow adjacent vertebrae.

3. **Articular processes**: These are four in number two of which are placed on the anterior and two on the posterior edge of the neural arch. They form interneural articulations with preceeding and succeeding vertebrae.
4. **Transverse processes**: They are two in numer for each vertebra. They extend one on either side of the body or lower part of the arch. They vary in size (**well developed in lumbar region**) and shape in the different regions **(Fig. 3.66A).**
5. **Dorsal spinous processes** (**neural spines or superior spines**): They are single, extend from the middle of the dorsal part of the neural arch. They vary in size (**well developed in thoracic region**) and shape in the different regions **(Fig. 3.66A).**
6. **Ventral spinous processes:** These are also single and are situated on the ventral aspect of the bodies of the vertebrae.
7. The **mammillary processes** are situated between the **transverse and anterior articular processes eg. lumbar vertebrae (Fig. 3.66B).**
8. **Accessory processes** are situated between the **transverse and posterior articular processes. eg. lumbar vertebrae of dog (Fig. 3.66B).**

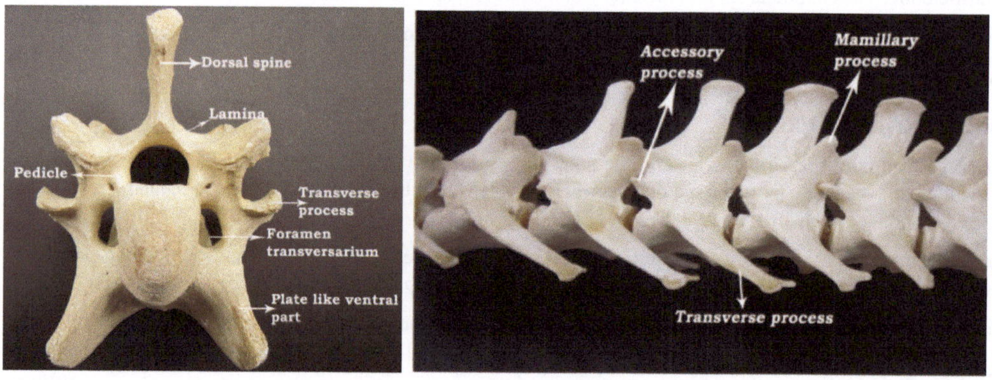

A B

Fig. 3.66: Structure of Typical Vertebra

CERVICAL VERTEBRAE: The first and 2nd cervical vertebrae named as atlas and axis respectively are atypical vertebrae since they deviate from general plan of construction.

ATLAS

Ox: The body and spinous processes are absent. It has the form of a ring from which the wings project laterally **(Fig.3.67).** The **ring consists of two lateral masses** connected by arches. The **lateral masses show articular areas anteriorly for occipital condyles and posteriorly for body of axis (Fig.3.68).**

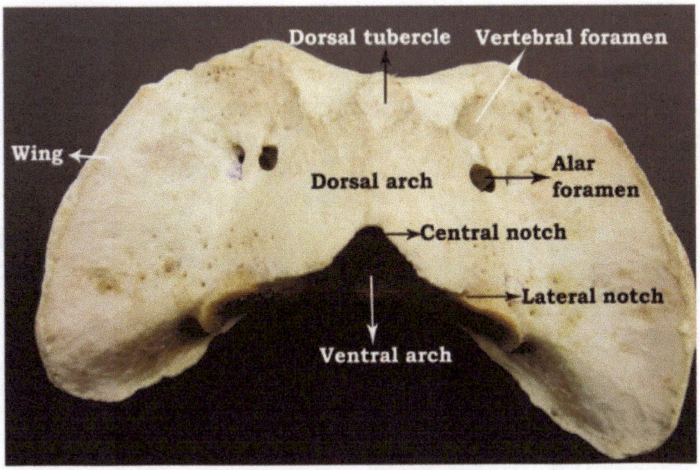

Fig. 3.67: Atlas of Ox- Dorsal View

The **dorsal arch** presents a median **dorsal tuberosity** and its anterior margin is perforated by the **intervertebral foramen** and the posterior border shows a central and two lateral notches **(Fig.3.67).** The **ventral arch** is thicker and less curved and its lower surface presents a tubercle **(Fig.3.68).** The **dorsal surface** of the ventral arch presents a flat articular surface, **fovea dentis** for the dens of the axis in front of which is a transverse rough area for the ligamentum dentis.

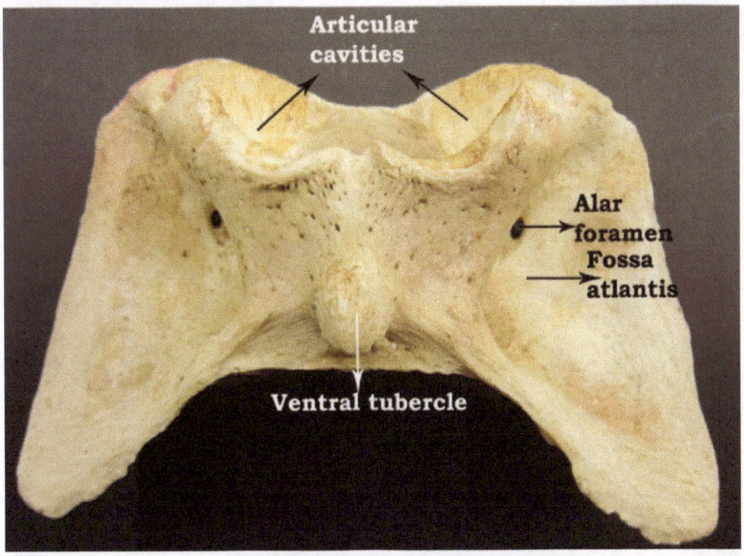

Fig. 3.68: Atlas of Ox-Ventral View

Between the ventral aspect of the wing and lateral mass is a cavity - **fossa atlantis**. At the bottom of the fossa are **two foramina**, the anterior one is called **alar foramen**. The **posterior foramen** pierces the lateral mass and communicates with the vertebral foramen. **(Fig.3.68).**

Horse: The wings slope **downward and outward**. Besides the alar and intervertebral foramina there is a **foramen transversarium** at the posterior part of the wing. The dorsal arch **does not show notches** unlike in the ox. The **posterior articular surfaces are saddle shaped (Fig.3.69).**

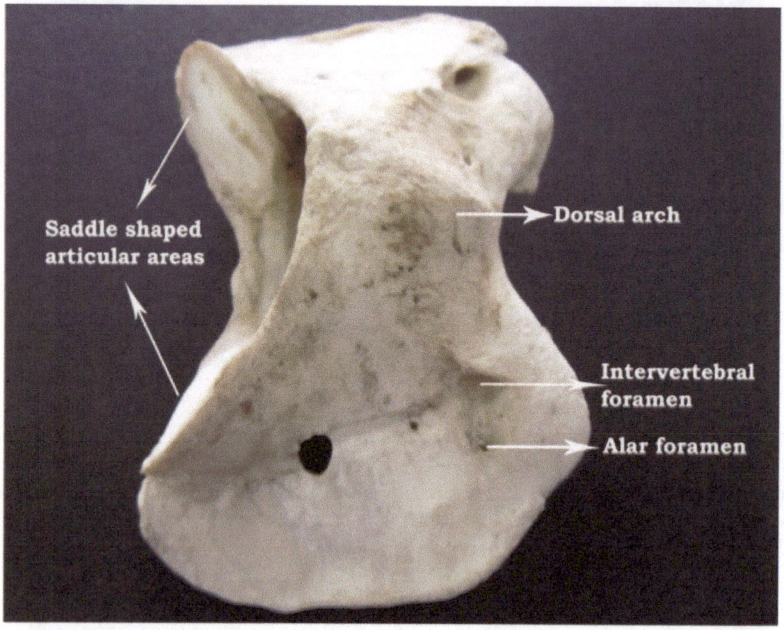

Fig. 3.69: Atlas of Horse- Dorsal View

Dog: The ventral arch is narrower.The dorsal arch is strongly convex and **alar notch** is present instead of alar foramen. **Foramen transversarium is present (Fig.3.70).**

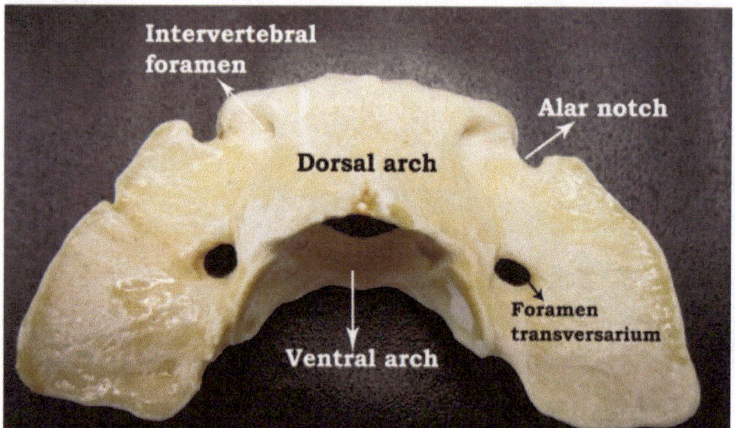

Fig. 3.70: Atlas of Dog- Dorsal View

Pig: The dorsal tubercle of the atlas is large. The ventral tubercle is long, compressed laterally and projects back under the axis. The transverse process (wing) is flattened and bears a caudal tuberosity.

Fowl: It is ring like and the **ventral arch presents concave articular area for single occipital condyle**. Posteriorly there are **three facets** for axis one median on the ventral arch and two on the posterolateral aspects of the dorsal arch **(Fig.3.71).**

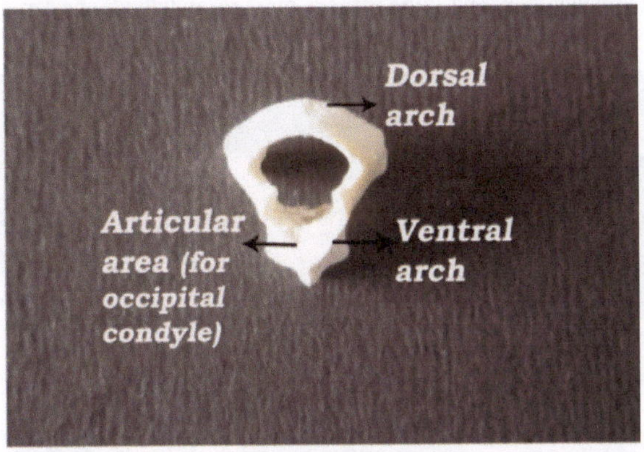

Fig. 3.71: Atlas of Fowl

AXIS

Ox: Axis is the **longest vertebra**. The anterior articular processes are absent. The **odontoid process** is sprout like and its **dorsal surface** is concave and rough for the attachment of odontoid ligament, while its **ventral surface** articulates with dorsal surface of ventral arch of atlas. On each side of the root of this process body presents a flat articular surface which articulates with posterior articular surface of atlas. The **posterior extremity** of the body presents concavity for the anterior convexity of body of 3rd cervical vertebra. The **pedicles present notches posteriorly** but in the place of **anterior ones are large intervertebral foramina (Fig.3.72).**

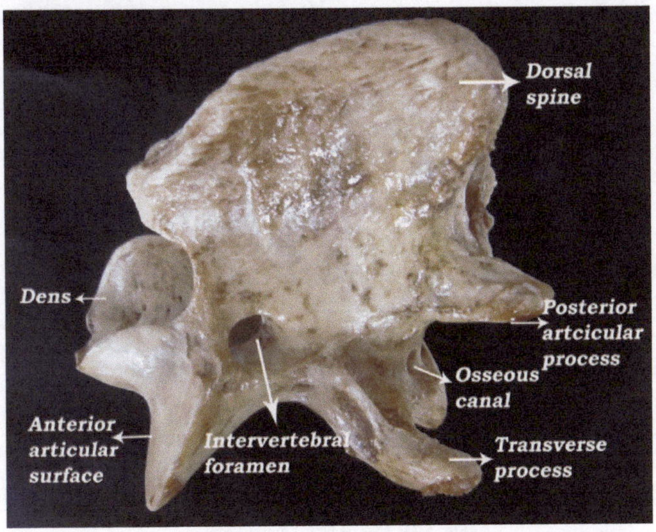

Fig. 3.72: Axis of Ox- Lateral View

The posterior articular processes resemble those of the succeeding vertebrae. The **foramen transversarium** when present is in the form of an **osseous canal** passing through the root of the transverse process. The dorsal spine is very long and its summit is narrow infront and thickens and widens posteriorly. The **ventral spine** is in the form of a ridge **(Fig.3.72).**

Horse: The body is larger. The **dens is longer, narrower and more pointed**. The anterior extremity presents an undulating **saddle shaped** articular area. The **spine is more massive** and divides posteriorly into two ridges which terminate on posterior articular processes **(Fig.3.73).**

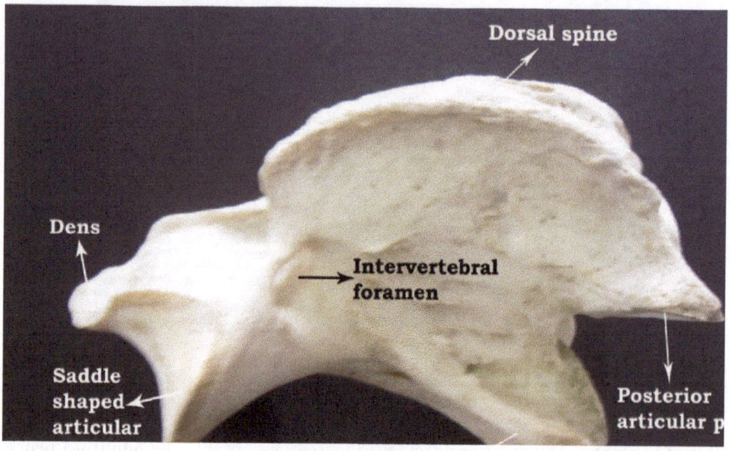

Fig. 3.73: Axis of Horse-Lateral View

Dog: The **dens is rounded and very long**. The **anterior articular areas which flank the dens are very oblique**. The **spine is of great size** and overhangs the dorsal arch of atlas. ***The anterior notches are large and are never converted into foramina*** **(Fig.3.74).**

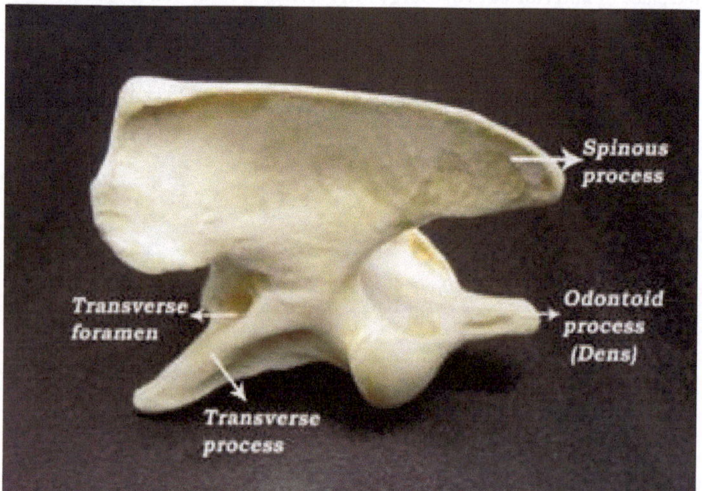

Fig. 3.74: Axis of Dog-Lateral View

Pig: The axis has a large spinous process which is directed dorsally and caudally. The dens is a thick cylindrical rod. The transverse process is very small and the transverse foramen is often incomplete.

Fowl: The anterior articular processes are present and articulate with the facets on the posterior aspect of the dorsal arch of atlas. The **dens articulates with occipital condyle** also in addition to ventral arch of atlas. The **body** presents below the dens a concave articular area for articulation with the ventral arch of atlas. The **dorsal and ventral spines are present, while the transverse process is absent (Fig.3.75).**

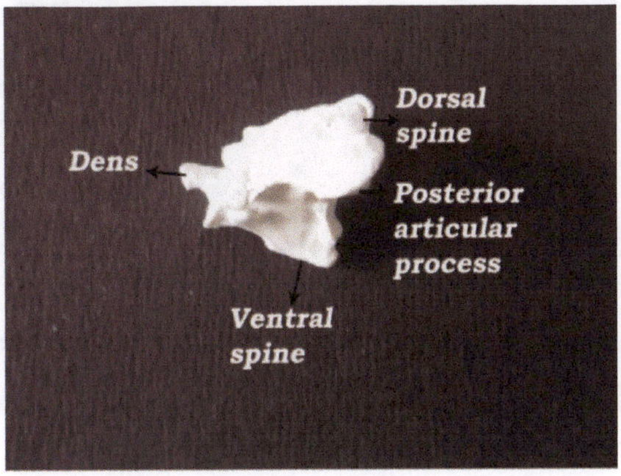

Fig. 3.75: Axis of Fowl

THIRD TO SEVENTH CERVICAL VERTEBRAE

Ox: The bodies of these vertebrae are long and their length decreases from 3rd to 7th. The ventral surface of 3rd to 5th vertebrae presents a median ventral spinous process which is in the form of a sharp ridge becoming less prominent posteriorly and is tuberculate at its posterior end. The marked convexity and concavity in the anterior and posterior ends of the bodies of vertebrae is a characteristic feature of this region.

A **continuous plate** of bone connects **anterior and posterior articular processes** of the same side. The transverse process is divided into dorsal and ventral parts except in 7th. The root of the transverse process is perforated by the foramen transversarium except in the 7th. The spinous process is in the form of a low thick rod which is directed upwards and forwards. The spines gradually increase in height from 3rd to the fifth and that of the **third is often bifid** at the summit.

Special features of 6th cervical vertebra:

The body is shorter and wider. The **lower division of transverse process is plate like.** The **dorsal spine is longer than the 5th,** while the ventral spine is absent **(Fig.3.76).**

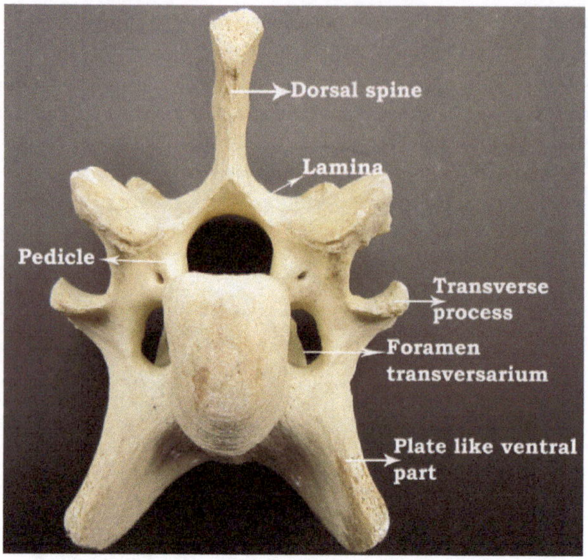

Fig. 3.76: 6th Cervical Vertebra of Ox

Special features of 7th cervical vertebra:

The body is the shortest of all the cervical vertebrae. The **transverse process is** undivided and foramen transversarium is absent. The posterior end of the body presents capitular facets for articulating with the head of the first rib. The **ventral spine is absent**. The **dorsal spine** is very prominent **(Fig.3.77).**

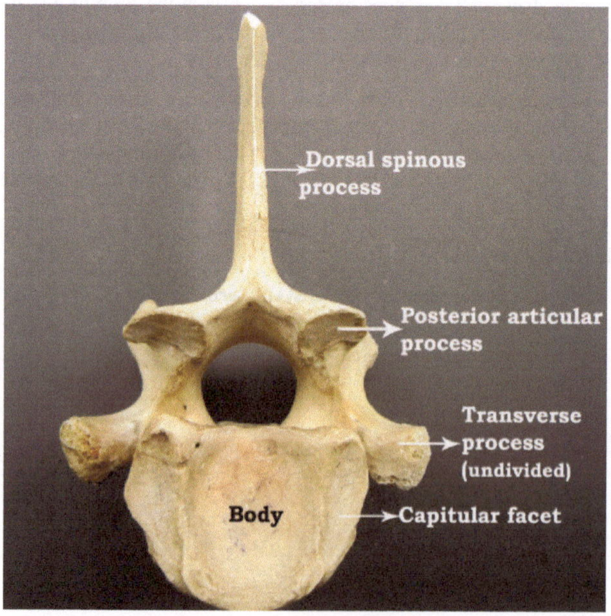

Fig. 3.77: 7th cervical Vertebra of Ox

Horse: 3rd to 5th cervical vertebrae: A continuous plate of bone unites the anterior and posterior articular processes in the fifth, but this plate extends only three-fourth the distance from the posterior articular process in the fourth and only halfway in the 3rd. The spines are less developed and the transverse processes are bifid showing anterior and posterior parts. The articular processes are better developed.

6th cervical vertebra: The **transverse process is trifid.** The third part is plate like and extends below the body **(Fig.3.78).**

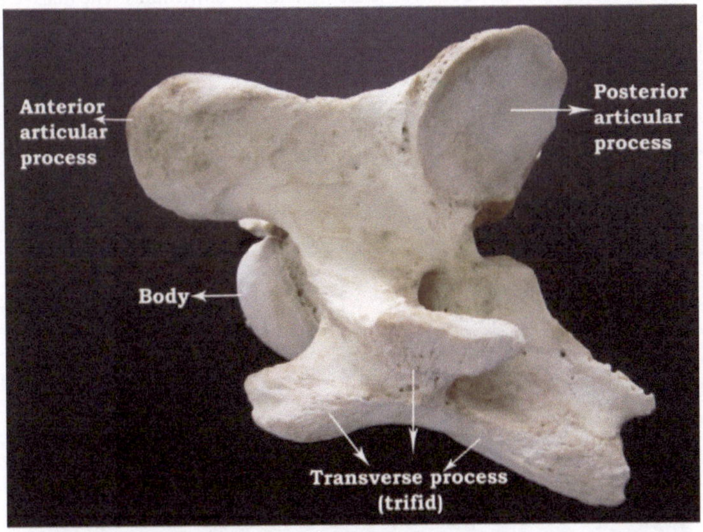

Fig. 3.78: 6th Cervical Vertebra of Horse

7th cervical of vertebra: The dorsal spine is a flattened triangular process and much smaller than that of the ox and the body is larger **(Fig.3.79).**

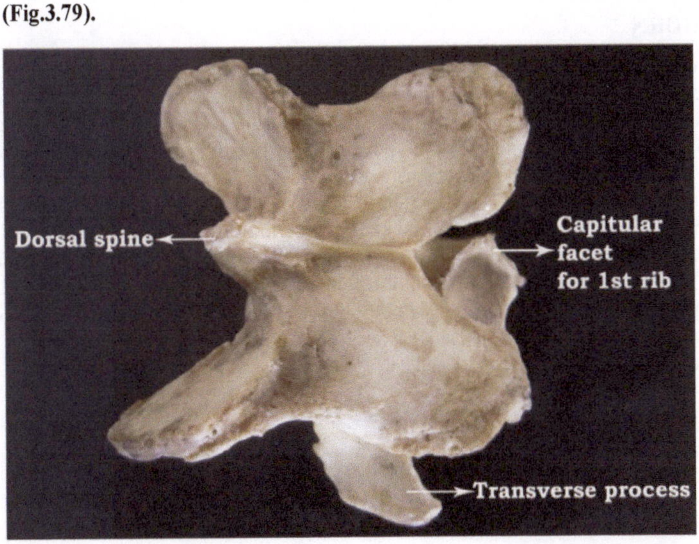

Fig. 3.79: 7th Cervical Vertebra of Horse-(Dorsal view)

Dog: 3rd to 5th cervical vertebrae: Bodies are relatively longer and are compressed dorsoventrally.

6th cervical: The plate like division of the transverse process is extensive and is ridged on its medial face.

7th cervical: The body is short and other features are like in ox.

Fowl: The bodies of the 3rd to 14th cervical vertebrae are rod like. The anterior extremity of the body of each vertebra is concave from side to side and convex from above downwards and the posterior extremity presents the reverse condition i.e. convex from side to side and concave from above downwards. The transverse processes arise from under the anterior articular processes and are prolonged behind by spicules of bone - the **styloid processes.** The latter represent the **cervical ribs (Fig.3.80).** The foramen transversarium is present. No facets for the head of the 1st rib are present on the body of the 14th cervical.

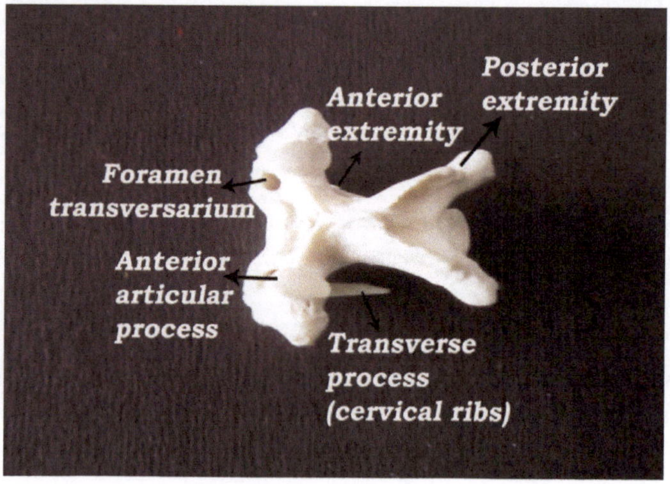

Fig. 3.80: Cervical Vertebra of Fowl

3.2 STUDY OF HORN

Horn : Cornual process of frontal bone (except in polled breeds) in ox enclosed by modified skin in natural state is called Horn. Sensitive and vascular corium covers the bony cornual process followed by external most horny part in natural state. The corium is a modified dermis of the skin while the external most horny part is insensitive and avascular and is a modified epidermis of skin. The horns vary greatly in size, form and curvature and are seen in both males and females. However in males they are generally more strongly developed and broader at base than in females.Horns are unbranched in Bovines The root (base) of the horn is surrounded by a thin layer of soft horn similar to periople of the hoof,which is continuous with the epidermis and is a zone of transitional epidermis called epikeras. Near the root the horn is encircled by variable rings. The corium of the horn is similar to that of the foot. The corium bears papillae and is thick at the root of the horn and thin in the body of the horn. At the apex horn is a solid mass. Horn glands are elongated thickenings of the skin caudomedial to the base of the horn due to increase in size and number of sebaceous glands. In bucks they become swollen and odoriferous during the breeding season. They are smaller in does and castrates. The frontal and parietal bones at the coronal suture exhibit a shallow groove under the position of the glands in Buck.

3.3 JOINTS OF THE HEAD AND NECK

Head: Most of the bones of skull are joined by fibrous tissue (sutures) eg: interfrontal, frontonasal sutures. Sutures get ossified in old age. Certain bones are joined by hyaline cartilage (synchondroses) eg: between basioccipital and basisphenoid. The two halves of mandible are joined by fibrocartilage or connective tissue (symphysis).

1. THE TEMPOROMANDIBULAR JOINT

Articular areas: The condyle and glenoid cavity of squamous temporal and condyle of the mandible with meniscus in between subdividing the joint cavity into upper and lower compartments.

Type: Diarthrodial (hinge and also arthrodia).

Ligaments: Capsular, lateral ligament between zygomatic process and neck of vertical ramus of mandible.

Movements: depression and elevation of the jaws like extension and flexion of hinge joint, to open and close mouth and sliding and gliding (to and fro) movements in mastication.

Note: In fowl presence of quadrate bone facilitates movement of upper jaw also unlike in mammals.

2. HYOIDEAN ARTICULATIONS

- **a)** The temporo hyoidean articulation between articular angle of stylohyoid and hyoid process of tympanic temporal,
- **b)** the inter cornual articulations between stylohyoid and epihyoid, epiphyoid and keratohyoid,
- **c)** basicornual articulation between keratohyoid and basihyoid, **d)** articulation between thyrohyoid and basihyoid and
- **e)** thyrohyoid articulation between thyroid cornu and anterior cornu of thyroid cartilage.

Movements: All are amphiarthroses except basicornual (enarthrosis) and thyrohyoid (syndesmosis) articulations

Vertebral column: The movable vertebrae form common and special articulations. The common vertebral articulations are of two kinds.

a. Intercentral articulations

Articular areas: Bodies of adjacent vertebrae with intervertebral discs in between.

Type: Simple, amphiarthroses. Joint cavities are present in cervical region only.

Intervertebral discs: each of these is made up of fibrocartilage and is interposed between the bodies to which it is intimately attached. These **discs are thinnest in the thoracic, thicker in the cervical and lumbar and thickest in the coccygeal region**.

Ligaments: The **ventral longitudinal ligament** extends from 7th **thoracic vertebra to sacrum** on ventral surface of bodies and intervertebral discs. The **dorsal longitudinal ligament** is present on the floor of vertebral canal on dorsal aspects of bodies and intervertebral discs from axis to sacrum.

Movements: Little

b. Interneural articulations

Articular areas: Facets on anterior and posterior articular processes of neural arches of adjacent vertebrae.

Type: Simple, Diarthrodial (arthrodia in neck & back and trochoid in lumbar region). The movements of vertebral column are dorsal, ventral and lateral flexion and rotation.

Ligaments: Capsular ligament, interspinous ligaments between spines in cervical, thoracic and lumbar regions, ligamentum flava connecting arches of adjacent vertebrae, supraspinous ligament covering spines extending from sacrum to occipital bone.

From 3rd thoracic vertebra onwards towards occipital bone supraspinus ligament becomes elastic in nature and inclines laterally to summits of spines and it is called **ligamentum nuchae** in neck region.

Ligamentum nuchae: consists of dorsal funicular and ventral lamellar portions. The **funicular portion** is paired attaching to external occipital protuberance and **ventral lamellar portion** divides into anterior and posterior parts (**Fig.3.81**).

The **paired anterior** parts extend from funicular portion and attach to spines of **2, 3rd and 4th cervical vertebrae**, while the **unpaired posterior part** extends from spine of 1st dorsal vertebra and attach to spines of **5th, 6th and 7th cervical vertebrae**. It assists extensor muscles of head and neck (**Fig.3.81**).

The nuchal ligament acts as barrier to spread of cervical abscesses between the left and right sides of the neck.

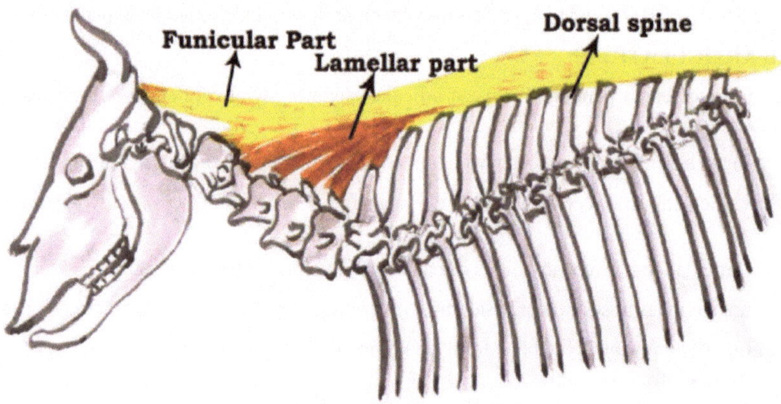

Fig. 3.81: Ligamentum Nuchae of Ox

In horse **lamellar part of ligamentum nuchae does not show anterior and posterior divisions**. In dog interspinous muscles replace interspinous ligaments.

SPECIAL ARTICULATIONS OF VERTEBRAL COLUMN:

1. OCCIPITO-ATLANTAL JOINT

Articular areas: Condyles of exoccipital and glenoid cavities of lateral masses of atlas.

Type: Simple, diarthrodial (ginglymus).

Ligaments

1. Capsular ligament
2. The **dorsal occipito-atlantal ligament** from dorsal margin of foramen magnum to the ring of atlas.
3. **Ventral occipito-atlantal ligament** from ventral margin of foramen magnum to the ring of atlas
4. **Lateral occipito-atlantal ligament** between paramastoid process and anterior margin of wing of atlas.

Movements: Extension and flexion.

2. Atlantoaxial joint

Articular areas: Posterior articular surfaces of lateral masses and dorsal surface of ventral arch of atlas and anterior aspect of body and ventral surface of dens of axis.

Type: Simple, diarthrodial (Trochoid)

Ligaments

1. **Capsular ligament**,
2. **Ventral atlantoaxial ligament** extending from ventral tubercle of atlas to ventral spine of axis,
3. **Dorsal atlantoaxial ligament** extending between posterior border of dorsal arch of atlas and anterior border of neural arch of axis.
4. **Interspinous ligament** between dorsal arch of atlas and spine of axis.
5. **Odontoid ligament** from dorsal surface of dens to rough area on the dorsal surface of ventral arch of atlas.

Movements: Rotation of atlas along with head on axis.

3.4 MUSCLES OF THE HEAD AND NECK

Cutaneous muscle

This is well developed and extensive. It covers whole of the frontal region as frontalis muscle. The part of the muscle extending over the lower jaw and the masseter and buccinator and blending with the orbicularis oris and the angle of the mouth is the retractor anguli oris.

MUSCLES OF THE LIPS AND CHEEKS (Fig.3.82)

1. **Orbicularis oris:** It is the ***sphincter*** around the anterior opening of the mouth but is incomplete in the muzzle. The muscle is present between the skin and mucous membrane of the lips to which it is intimately adherent.
2. **Levator nasolabialis:** The muscle is extensive and continuous above with the frontalis. The muscle divides below into two layers between which the levator labii superioris proprius and the dilator naris lateralis pass through. The deep division is thin and aponeurotic.
3. **Levator labii superioris proprius:** It is a flat narrow muscle extending from the facial tuberosity.
4. **Dilator naris lateralis (Caninus):** It is a narrow band placed between the preceeding and succeeding muscles.
6. **Zygomaticus:** It is a long strap shaped muscle
7. **Incisivus superior:** It consists of an indefinite group of fibres extending from the anterolateral angle of the premaxilla to the deep surface of the upper lip.
8. **Incisivus Inferior:** It is situated in the lower hip
9. **Mentalis:** Lies in the chin ventral to the body of the mandible
10. **Buccinator:** This muscle lies in the lateral wall of the mouth
11. **Depressor labii inferioris:** This muscle lies along the inferior border of the preceeding muscle. It is separable from it only at its anterior part.
12. **Malaris**: It is a broad muscle spreading below the lower eye lid over the buccinator and masseter muscles. It is divided into an **anterior part-levator buccalis** and a **posterior part-** the **depressor palpebrae inferioris**.

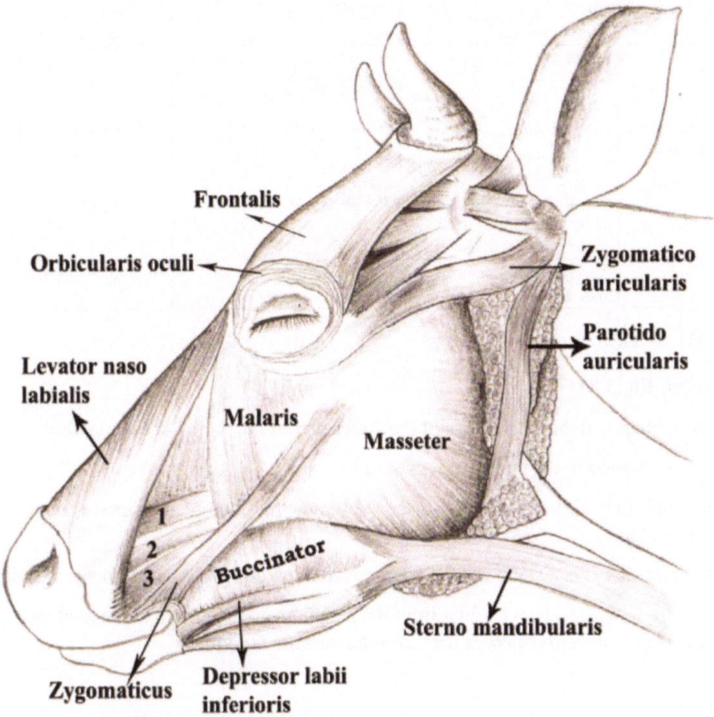

Fig. 3.82: Muscles of the Face

Name of the muscle	Origin	Insertion	Action
Orbicularis oris	Margins of the lips	Upper lip	To close the rima oris and help in suction and mastication
Levator nasolabialis	Rostral part of frontal and nasal bones	Nostrils and upper lip	To dilate the nostril and elevate the upper lip
Dilator naris lateralis (Caninus)	Facial tuberosity	Lateral walls of nostrils	To dilate the nostril
Levator labii superioris proprius	Facial tuberosity	Upper lip	To elevate the upper lip
Depressor labi Superioris	Facial tuberosity	Muzzle and Upper lip	To depress the upper lip
Depressor labi inferioris	Alveolar border of mandible	Lower lip	To depress the lower lip
Buccinator	Alveolar border of mandible	Angle of the mouth	To retract the angle of the mouth and flatten the cheek.
Dilator naris apicalis	Body of premaxilla	Medial wing of nostril	To dilate the nostril
Zygomaticus	Zygomatic process of malar	To the buccinator and orbicularis oris at the angle of the mouth	To retract and raise the angle of the mouth

Name of the muscle	Origin	Insertion	Action
Mentalis	Body of mandible	Skin of chin	To raise the skin to which it is attached
Malaris: a.Levator buccalis (***Ant.part of malaris***)	Facial part of Lacrimal bone	Buccal mucosa ventral to facial tuberosity	To raise the posterior part of cheek
b. Depressor palpebrae inferioris (***Posterior part of malaris)***	Lacrimal bone	Lower eye lid	To depress the lower eye lid
Orbicularis oculi	Skin of eye lids, but some bundles are attached to the palpebral ligament at the medial canthus of eye and to the lacrimal bone.		To close the eye lids
Levator palpebrae superioris	Pterygoid crest opposite the optic foramen.	Upper eye lid	To raise the upper eye lid

MANDIBULAR MUSCLES

(Masticatory muscles, Fig.3.83)

1. **Masseter:** It is situated on the lateral face of the wider part of the ramus of the mandible.
2. **Temporalis:** It is situated in the temporal fossa
3. **Pterygoideus medialis:** This muscle is situated on the medial face of the vertical ramus of the mandible opposite the masseter.
4. **Pterygoideus lateralis:** It is a small muscle situated lateral to the upper part of the preceeding muscle
5. **Digastricus:** It is a long muscle extending from the paramastoid process to the medial face of the horizontal ramus. It presents ***two muscular bellies with an intermediate tendon.***

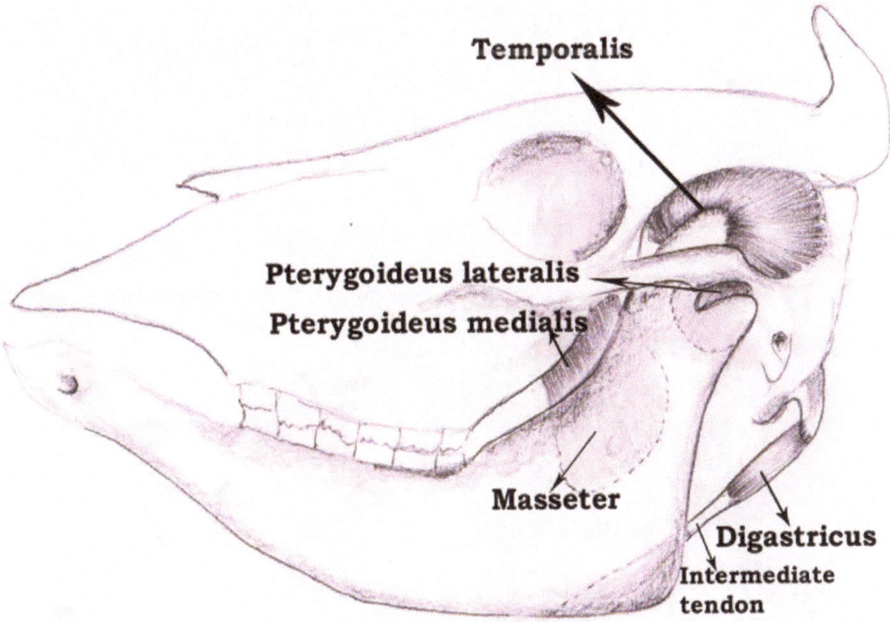

Fig. 3.83: Masticatory Muscles of Ox

Name of the muscle	Origin	Insertion	Action
Masseter	Zygomatic arch, Facial crest and Tuberosity	Posterior border of vertical ramus of mandible	To close the jaws and move the mandible forward and upward
Temporalis	Rough part of temporal fossa	Coronoid process of mandible	To raise the lower jaw
Pterygoideus medialis	Perpendicular part of palatine and pterygoid process of postsphenoid.	Medial surface of the vertical ramus of the mandible behind the mandibular foramen.	To raise the lower jaw and assist in lateral movement of the jaw.
Pterygoideus lateralis	Pterygoid process of post sphenoid	Medial face of neck and condyle of mandible	To move the rami towards the median plane.
Digastricus	Paramastoid process	Medial face of horizontal ramus of mandible near the ventral border.	To depress the lower jaw.

MUSCLES OF THE TONGUE

Tongue consists up of both extrinsic and intrinsic muscles. The origin and insertions of intrinsic muscles are within the tongue.

EXTRINSIC MUSCLES: (Fig.3.84)

1. **Styloglossus:** It is a long muscle present on the ventrolateral face of the tongue
2. **Hyoglossus:** It is a wide flat muscle.
3. **Genioglossus:** It is a wide fan shaped muscle. Its fibres pass up to the body and root of the tongue.

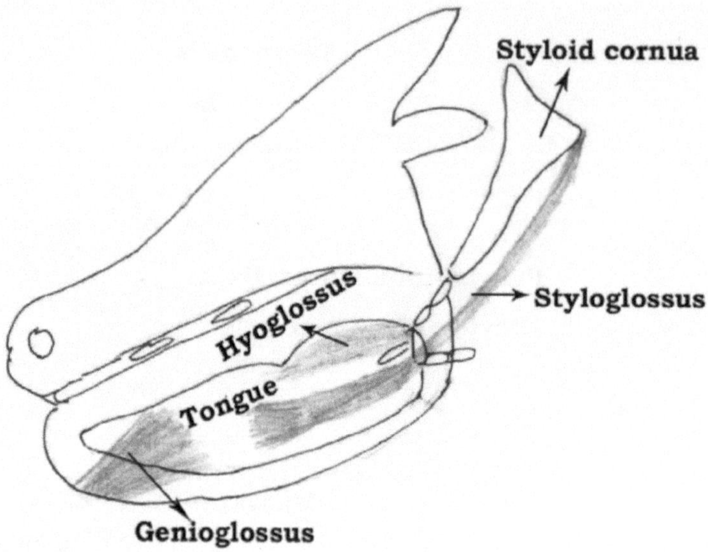

Fig. 3.84: Extrinsic Muscles of the Tongue

Name	Origin	Insertion	Action
Stylo-glossus	Great cornu of hyoid	Tip of the tongue	To retract the tongue and draw it to a side
Hyoglossus	Body of the hyoid	Body and root of the tongue	To retract and depress the tongue
Genio-glossus	Medial face of the ramus of mandible behind the symphysis	Body and root of the tongue	To depress and protract the tongue

MUSCLES OF THE HYOID APPARATUS (Fig.3.85)

1. **Mylohyoideus:** The two muscles form a sling for the tongue.
2. **Stylohyoideus:** Present between muscular angle of great cornu and body of hyoid.
3. **Geniohyoideus:** Present on medial face of the ramus of mandible.
4. **Occipitohyoideus:** Present between paramastoid process and muscular angle of great cornu of hyoid bone.
5. **Keratohyoideus:** Present between posterior part of small cornua of hyoid and thyroid cornu of larynx.
6. **Hyoideus transversus:** A small ***unpaired muscle*** situated between the two small cornua, enclosed by mucous membrane. It raises the root of the tongue.

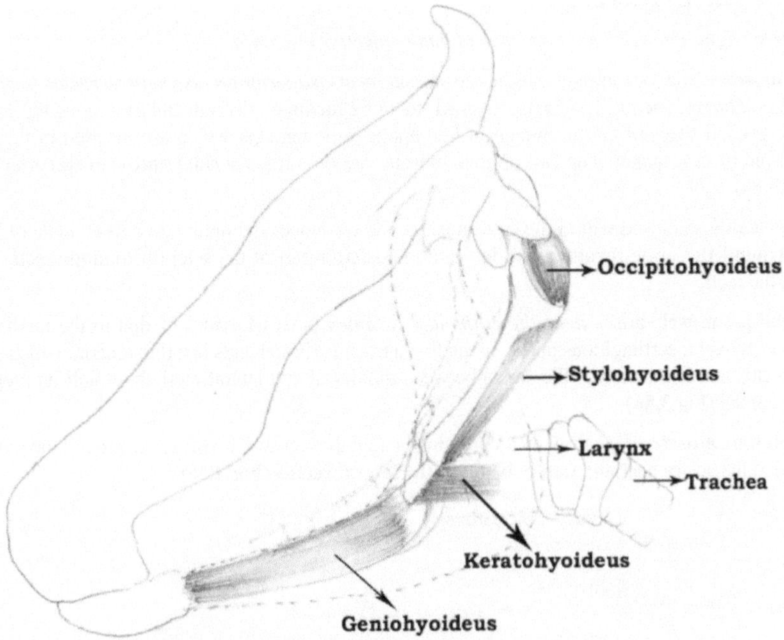

Fig. 3.85: Muscles of the Hyoid

Name	Origin	Insertion	Action
Mylohyoideus	Medial face of the horizontal ramus of mandible below the alveolar border.	Lingual process of Hyoid bone	To raise the tongue and hyoid bone.
Stylohyoideus	Muscular angle of great cornu of hyoid bone	Body of hyoid bone	To draw the tongue and hyoid backwards and upwards
Geniohyoideus	Fossa on the medial face of the horizontal ramus of mandible		To draw the tongue and hyoid forwards
Occipitohyoideus	Paramastoid process	Muscular angle of great cornu of hyoid bone	To draw the great cornu backwards
Keratohyoideus	Posterior border of small cornua of hyoid	Dorsal part of thyroid cornu of larynx	To raise the larynx

MUSCLES OF THE SOFT PALATE

1. **Palatoglossus:** It is a small muscle arising from the lateral border of the soft palate and passing to the tongue.
2. **Tensor palati:** It arises from cartilage of auditory tube and adjacent parts of temporal bone and passes lateral to the levator palati and its tendon gets reflected around the hamulus of the pterygoid bone and spreads in the soft palate. It **tenses the soft palate**.
3. **Levator palati:** It arises from tympanic part of temporal and inserts on soft palate. It **raises the soft palate** towards the root of the pharynx and closes the posterior nares during deglutition.
4. **Palatinus:** It is a small elongated bright red fasciculus lying along with its fellow enclosed in the palatine aponeurosis. It arises from the posterior border of the bony palate and is inserted to the aponeurosis near the free border of the soft palate. **It shortens the soft palate.**

MUSCLES OF THE EYE BALL

There are ***four straight, one rectractor and two oblique muscles*** **(Fig.3.86)**.

The straight muscles: The four straight muscles are ***dorsal rectus (superior rectus), ventral rectus (inferior rectus), medial rectus and lateral rectus***. They **arise around the optic foramen**, diverge and pass along the corresponding aspects of the eyeball forward and terminate in fine aponeurotic tendons which are inserted to the fore part of the sclera in front of the equator. The two oblique muscles are **dorsal (superior) and ventral (inferior) oblique muscles (Fig.3.86)**.

The **retractor oculi** is enclosed within the recti muscles and envelopes the optic nerve. It is made of four bundles which **arise around the optic foramen** and inserted to posterior part of the sclera behind the recti. The bundles alternate with the recti.

The **dorsal oblique muscle** arises ***near the ethmoidal foramen*** passes forward medial to the medial rectus and reflected outwards over a cartilaginous pulley in the fovea trochlearis and ends in a thin tendon; which passes under the superior rectus and is inserted to the sclera between the dorsal and lateral recti about half an inch behind the margin of the cornea **(Fig.3.86)**.

The **ventral oblique muscle** arises from the depression behind the lacrimal fossa curves around the rectus ventralis and is inserted to the sclera near and **partly beneath the lateral rectus (Fig.3.86)**.

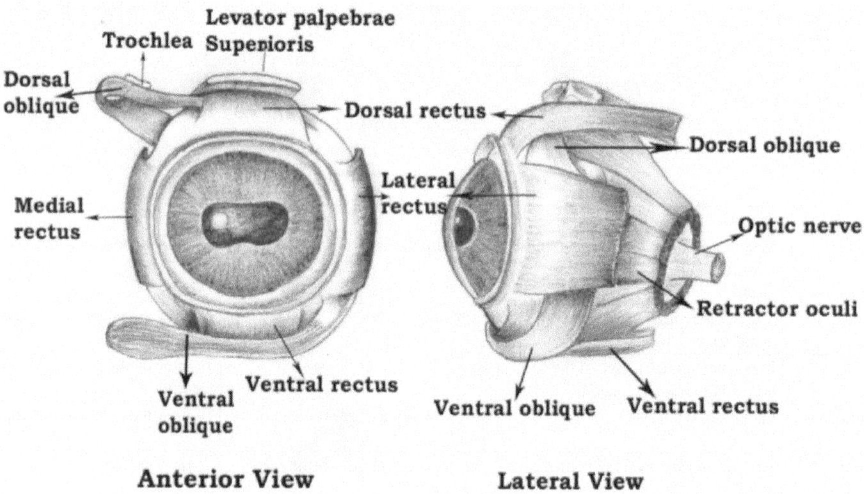

Fig. 3.86: Muscles of the Eye ball

Name	Origin	Insertion	Action
Dorsal rectus	Arise from near optic foramen	Sclera	Rotate the eye ball on trasverse axis
Ventral rectus			Rotate the eye ball on trasverse axis
Medial rectus			Rotate the eye ball on vertical axis
Lateral rectus			Rotate the eye ball on vertical axis
Rectractor oculi	Arises from near optic foramen	Posterior part of sclera behind the rectus musles.	Retract the eye ball
Dorsal oblique	Arises from near ethmoidal foramen	Sclera	Rotate the eye ball on longitudinal axis
Ventral oblique	Arises from depression behind the lacrimal fossa	Sclera *beneath the lateral rectus.*	Rotate the eye ball on longitudinal axis

MUSCLES OF THE PHARYNX (Fig.3.87)

Name	Origin	Insertion	Action
1. Stylopharyngeus	Great cornu of hyoid	Wall of pharynx	Dilator of pharynx
2. Palatopharyngeus	Vertical part of palatine and sphenoid		Shortens the pharynx
3. Pterygopharyngeus	Pterygoid process of sphenoid		Shortens the pharynx
4. Hyopharyngeus	Thyroid cornu of hyoid		Constrictor of pharynx
5. Thyropharyngeus	Lamina of thyroid cartilage		Constrictor of pharynx
6. Cricopharyngeus	Lateral part of cricoid		Constrictor of pharynx

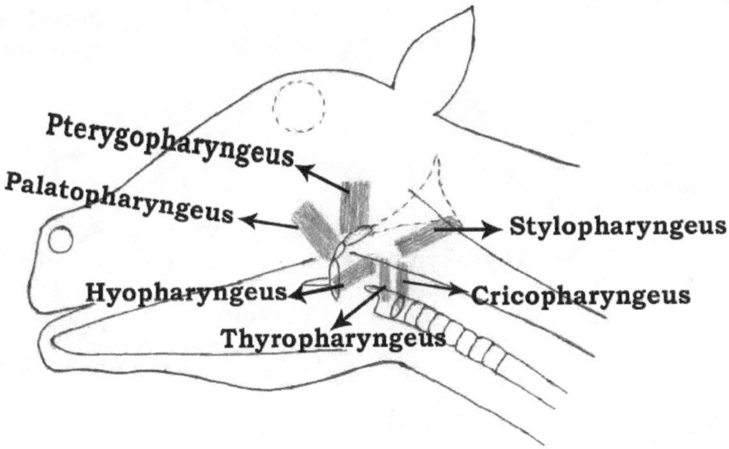

Fig. 3.87: Muscles of the Pharynx

MUSCLES OF LARYNX: consists of both extrinsic and intrinsic muscles.

EXTRINSIC MUSCLES:

1. **Sternothyrohyoideus**: described in neck muscles.
2. **Thyrohyoideus (hyothyroideus)** extends between thyroid cartilage and the body and the thyroid cornu of the hyoid bone.
3. **Hyoepiglotticus** is a small bifid muscle enclosed in the glossoepiglottic fold.

INTRINSIC MUSCLES (Fig.3.88): *Their origin and insertion are within the larynx only.*

1. **Cricothyroideus:** lies on the posterior part of the lateral surface of the larynx.
2. **Cricoarytenoideus dorsalis:** is on the dorsal surface of the cricoid cartilage.
3. **Cricoarytenoideus lateralis:** is on the deep surface of the thyroid cartilage.
4. **Arytenoideus transversus:** is unpaired and lies on the dorsal face of the bodies of the arytenoid cartilages.
5. **Thyroarytenoideus:** It extends from the medial face of lamina of thyroid cartilage to the the arytenoids.

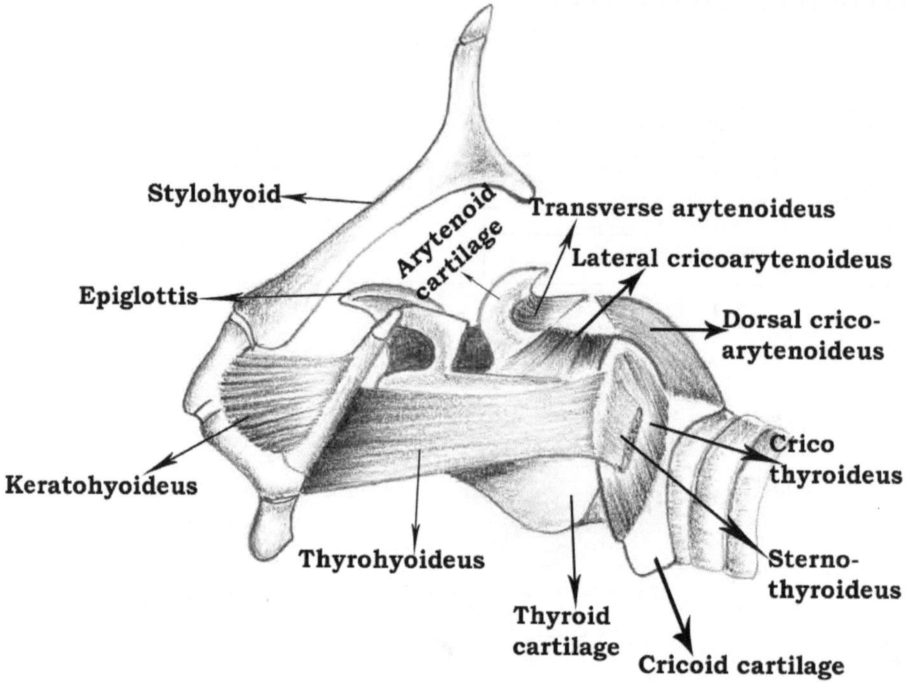

Fig. 3.88: Muscles of the Larynx

Name	Origin	Insertion	Action
Cricothyroideus	Arch of cricoid cartilage	Posterior cornu of thyroid cartilage	Draws the thyroid cartilage and ventral part of cricoid cartilage together and tense the vocal folds.
Cricoarytenoideus dorsalis	Lamina of cricoid	Muscular process of arytenoid cartilage	Dilates the glottis and abducts the vocal process and folds.
Cricoarytenoideus lateralis	Upper part of cricoid	Muscular process of arytenoid cartilage	Closes the glottis by rotating arytenoid cartilage medially and tenses the vocal folds
Areytenoideus transversus (***unpaired muscle***)	Lateral borders of bodies of the arytenoid cartilage		Narrows the glottis
Thyroareytenoideus	Medial face of the lamina of thyroid cartilage	Muscular process of arytenoid cartilage	Closes the glottis and slackens the vocal folds

MUSCLES OF THE EXTERNAL EAR

These are extrinsic and intrinsic. The ***scutiform cartilage is a quadrilateral shaped piece present in front of the base of the ear and acts as a sesamoid.***

EXTRINSIC MUSCLES: (Fig.3.89 & 3.90).

1. **Parotidoauricularis:** it is a thin and wide muscle situated on the parotid salivary gland. It is wide below and narrow above.
2. **Frontoscutularis:** comprises temporal and frontal parts.
3. **Cervicoauricularis:** it extends between neck and base of concha. It shows **superficial, middle and deep parts.**

4. **Parietoauricularis:** is a flat triangular muscle arising from the parietal part of temporal.
5. **Zygomaticoauricularis:** it is made up of two bundles arising from zygomatic arch.
6. **Interscutularis**: It is a very short muscle.

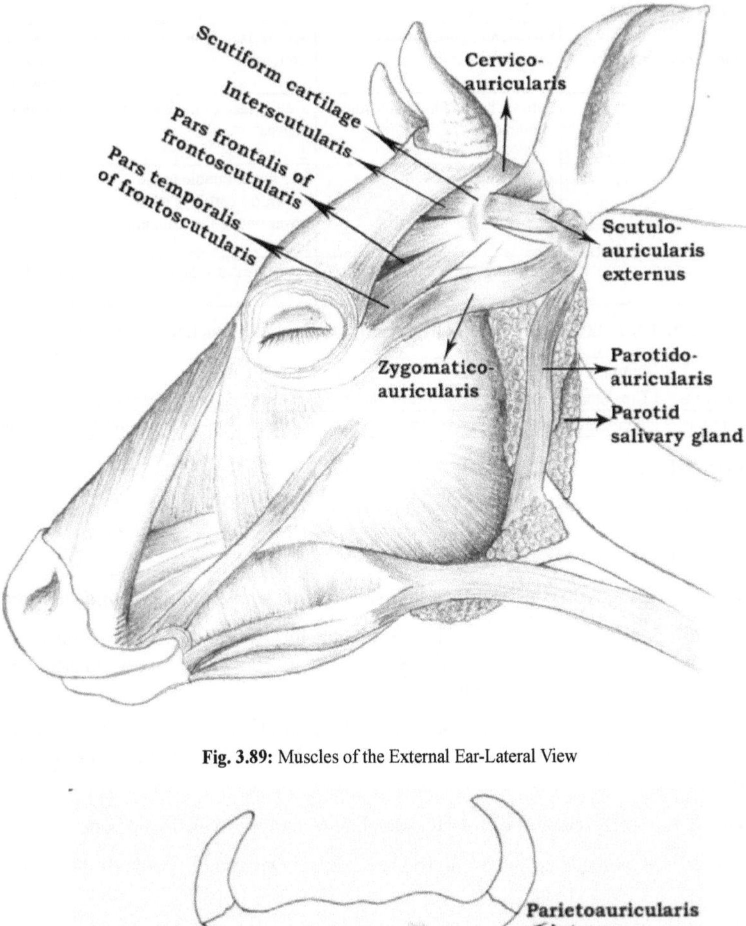

Fig. 3.89: Muscles of the External Ear-Lateral View

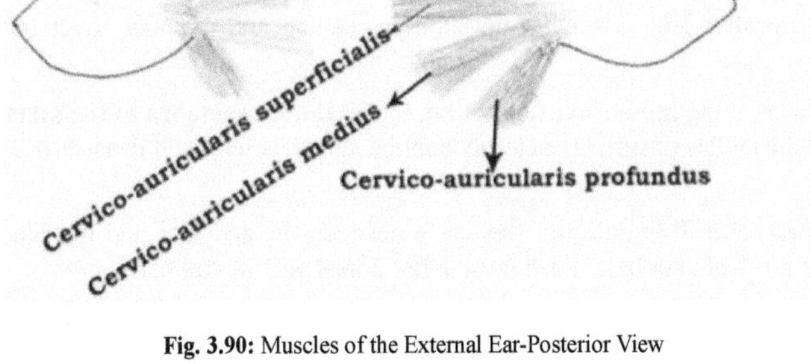

Fig. 3.90: Muscles of the External Ear-Posterior View

Name	Origin	Insertion	Action
1.Parotido-auricularis	Fascia on the lower part of the parotid gland	Conchal cartilage below the angle of junction of its borders.	To incline the ear downwards and backwards.
2.Frontoscutularis *(comprises temporal and frontal parts)*	Zygomatic arch and frontal part of the temporal.	Scutiform cartilage	To adduct the ear
3.Cervico auricularis *(shows superficial, middle and deep parts).*	Ligamentum nuchae and cervical fascia	Medial face of the base of the Concha	To adduct the conchae and direct the opening outwards.
4. Parietoauricularis	Parietal bone behind the frontal eminence	Medial face of the base of the concha	To adduct the ear.
5.Zygomatico-auricularis	Zygomatic process of the squamous temporal	The upper bundle to the scutiform cartilage and the lower one to the front and base of concha.	To prick the ear
6.Interscutularis	Cornual process and frontal crest	Scutiform cartilage	To adduct the ear

INTRINSIC MUSCLES: These are scutuloauricularis externus and scutuloauricularis internus

Name	Origin	Insertion	Action
1.Scutulo-auricularis externus	The outer face of the scutiform cartilage.	Medial part of the base of concha	To prick the ear.
2.Scutulo-auricularis internus	Internal face of the scutiform cartilage.	Anterior aspect of the concha	To prick the ear.

MUSCLES OF THE NECK

The neck muscles are arranged into ventral and dorsolateral groups.

VENTRAL ASPECT MUSCLES OF NECK (Fig.3.91)

1. **Sternocephalicus:** This muscle consists of two divisions i.e ***sterno mandibularis and sternomastoideus.***
    a. **Sterno mandibularis** forms lower boundary of jugular furrow, while sternomastoideus forms internal boundary of jugular furrow separating external jugular vein from common carotid artery and covers the oesophagus, trachea and carotid structures.
2. **Sterno-thyrohyoideus:** It is a long muscle present on the ventral face of trachea. The two side musles are very close at their origin. It divides into two bands at the middle of the neck. **i.e *wider thyroid and narrow hyoid bands.***
3. **Omohyoideus:** It is a small **triangular muscle** extending from neck to the hyoid bone
4. **Scalenus:** This muscle is made up of two divisions i.e dorsal and ventral, between these roots of brachial plexus emerge.
5. **Rectus capitis ventralis major:** This muscle extends from the neck to the basi occipital.
6. **Rectus capitis ventralis minor:** This muscle is placed dorsal and medial to the preceeding.
7. **Rectus capitis lateralis:** This is smaller than the preceeding and is under cover of the obliquus capitis anterior
8. **Longus colli:** This is along muscle extending from the **6th dorsal vertebra to the atlas**. It is situated on the ventral aspect of the bodies of vertebrae closely applied aginst its fellow. It consists of ***thoracic and cervical parts.***
9. **Intertransversales colli:** This occupies the space between the articular and transverse processes on the lateral surface of cervical vertebrae. Each muscle has dorsal and ventral parts.

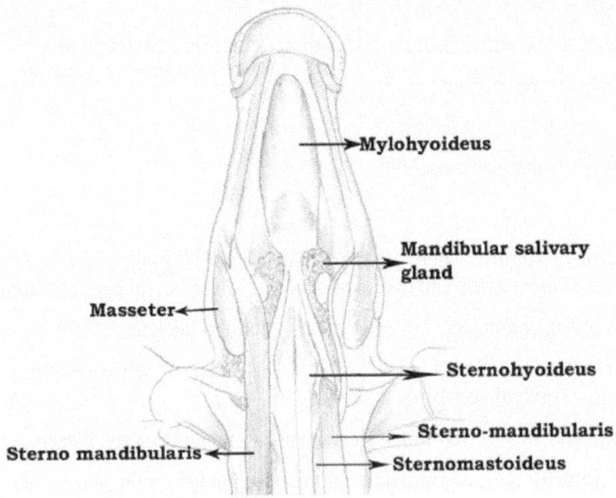

Fig. 3.91: Muscles of Neck-Ventral Aspect

Name of the muscle	Origin	Insertion	Action
1. Sternocephalicus: a. Sterno mandibularis b. Sternomastoideus	Manubrium sterni and 1st costal cartilage	a)Angle of the mandible b) Mastoid process	To flex the head and neck ventrally
2. Sterno-thyrohyoideus	Manubrium sterni	a) Thyroid cartilage of larynx. b) The body and lingual process of hyoid body of the hyoid.	To retract the hyoid bone and tongue
3. Omohyoideus	Transverse processes of 3rd and 4th cervical vertebrae	Body of the hyoid	To retract the hyoid bone and Tongue
4. Scalenus **a) *scalenus dorsalis*** ***b) Scalenus ventalis.***	a) from transverse processes of **4th to 7th cervical** vertebrae b) from transverse processes of **4th to 6th cervical** vertebrae	a)Lateral surface of ***4th rib*** b) Anterior border of ***1st rib.***	To flex the nek or incline it laterally.
5. Rectus capitis ventralis major	Transverse processes of **2nd to 6th** cervical vertebrae	Basilar tubercles	To flex the head or incline it laterally
6. Rectus capitis ventralis minor	Ventral surface of wing of atlas	Basilar tubercles	To flex the occipito-atlantal joint
7. Rectus capitis lateralis	Atlas, lateral to the origin of obliquus capitis anterior.	Paramastoid process	To flex the occipito-atlantal joint
8. Longus colli	Bodies of first six dorsal vertebrae and transverse processes of cervical vertebrae.	Ventral tubercle of atlas.	To flex the neck ventrally
9. Intertransversales colli	Dorsal bundles extend between transverse processes and anterior articular process. Ventral bundles extend between the ventral parts of transverse processes.		To flex the neck laterally

DORSOLATERAL GROUP MUSCLES OF NECK (Fig.3.92).

For description purpose the dorsolateral group muscles of neck are divided in to 4 layers.

First layer: Trapezius, Brachiocepahlicus

Second Layer: Omotransversarius , Rhomboideus and Serratus cervicis

Third Layer: Splenius. it is a triangular muscle

Fourth Layer

1. **Longissimus capitis *et* atlantis**: There are two parallel bundles on the deep face of the splenius. The more medial part is ***longissimus capitis*** and overlapped by the lower lateral part, ***the longissimus atlantis***.
2. **Complexus:** This is a strong muscle covering the ligamentum nuchae
3. **Multifidus cervicis**: This muscle is made up of oblique bundles which are placed over the dorsal surface of arches of the last five cervical vertebrae.
4. **Obliquus capitis posterior**: It is a **quadrilateral muscle** situated chiefly over the wing of atlas and the axis.
5. **Obliquus capitis anterior**: It is a **quadrilateral muscle** situated on the side of the occipitoatlantal joint
6. **Rectus capitis dorsalis major**: It extends from the axis to the occipital along the dorsal median line closely applied to the fellow of the opposite side.
7. **Rectus capitis dorsalis minor**: This muscle lies under the preceeding.

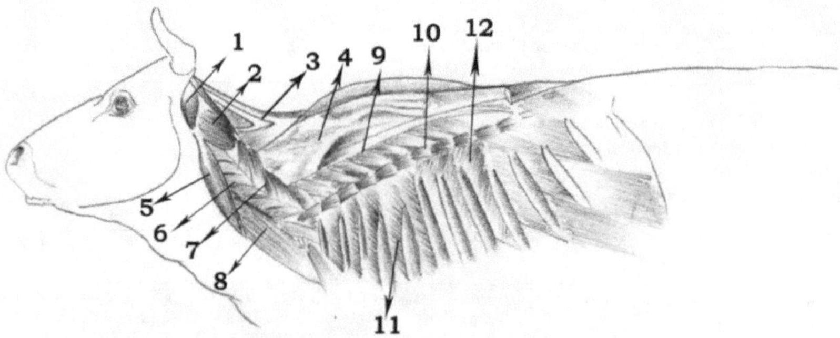

1. Obliquus capitis anterior
2. Obliquus capitis posterior
3. Ligamentum nuchae
4. Complexus
5. Intertransversales longus
6. Intertransversales colli
7. Multifidus cervicis
8. Scalenus ventralis
9. Longissimus dorsi
10. Levatores costarum
11. External intercostal
12. Internal inercostal

Fig. 3.92: Muscles of the Neck and Thorax-Lateral Aspect

Name of the muscle	Origin	Insertion	Action
First layer: 1. Trapezius 2. Brachiocepahlicus	**Described in shoulder girdle muscles** ***Refer shoulder girdle muscles***		***Refer shoulder girdle muscles***
Second Layer: 1. Omotransversarius 2. Rhomboideus 3. Serratus cervicis			
Third Layer: **Splenius**:	Summits of first three or four dorsal spines	Occipital, Transverse processes of first three cervical vertebrae	To elevate the head and neck
Fourth Layer			
1. Longissimus capitis *et* atlantis	Transverse processes of first two dorsal vertebrae	Mastoid process and wing of Atlas	To extend the Head and Neck
2. Complexus	Spines of 3-5th dorsal vertebrae and transverse processes of first 10 dorsal vertebrae	Occipital bone lateral to insertion of ligamentum nuchae	To extend the Head and Neck
3.Multifidus cervicis	Posterior articular processes of last five cervical vertebrae	Spinous and posterior articular processes of preceding vertebrae	To flex the head and neck laterally
4.Obliquus capitis posterior	Spine of axis	Dorsal surface of wing of atlas	To extend the head
5. Obliquus capitis anterior	Cranial border of wing of atlas	Mastoid and paramastoid processes	To extend the head
6.Rectus capitis dorsalis major	*Spine of axis*	*Occipital bone*	To extend the head and neck
7. Rectus capitis dorsalis minor	*Dorsal arch of atlas*	*Occipital bone*	To extend the head

3.5 BLOOD SUPPLY TO THE HEAD AND NECK

The Bicarotid Trunk: The bicarotid trunk continues the brachio-cephalic artery after it detaches the right brachial artery. At the thoracic inlet, it bifurcates into **two common carotid arteries i.e right and left.**

THE COMMON CAROTID ARTERY

Each common carotid artery passes obliquely up the side of the neck diverging from its fellow as it ascends. It is separated from the external jugular vein by the sternomastoideus and omohyoideus muscles. The **common carotid artery terminates at the level of the digastricus by dividing *into occipital, external maxillary and external carotid arteries* (Fig.3.93).**

Carotid sheath contains common carotid artery, vagosympathetic trunk, internal jugular vein (absent in small ruminants) and tracheal duct.

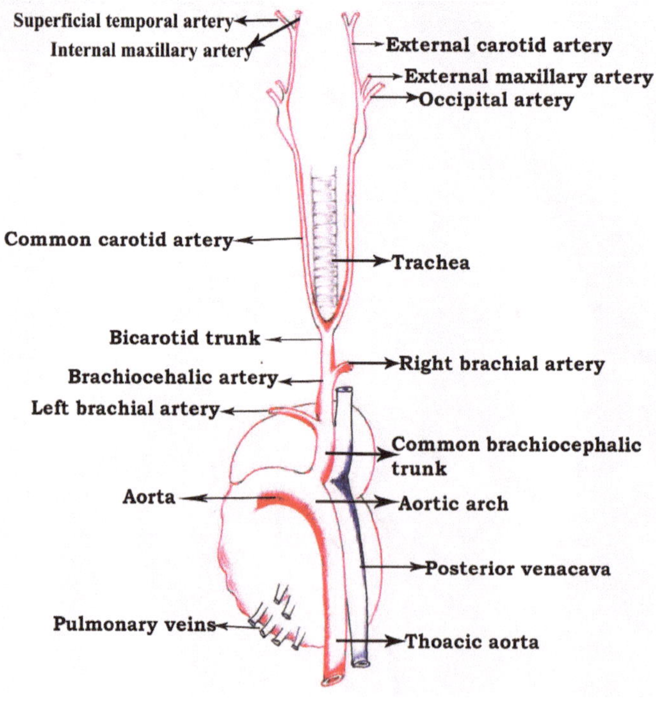

Fig. 3.93: Bicarotid Trunk

Collateral branches: 1.Branches to the trachea and oesophagus.

2. The thyrolaryngeal artery is the largest of the collateral branches. It divides into **thyroid and laryngeal branches.** The **thyroid branch** supplies lateral lobe of the thyroid gland. The **laryngeal branch** divides into ***pharyngeal and laryngeal branches*** of which the former is distributed to the muscles of the pharynx and the latter to the muscles of the larynx.**3.** The **posterior thyroid artery** when present enters the posterior extremity of the lateral lobe of the thyroid gland.**4.** The **inferior parotid artery** to the parotid salivary gland. **5. Muscular branches** to the ventral muscles of neck.

Terminal branches

1. Occipial artery

It is the **smallest of the terminal branches of the common carotid artery.** During its course it gives off **(1) Muscular branches** to the ventral straight muscles of the head. **(2) Branches to the pharynx. (3) Palatine branches to the soft palate. 4.** The ***middle and caudal memingeal arteries*** also arise from the occipital artery pass through the foramen ovale and foramen lacerum respectively and ramify in duramater of the brain.

It is then ***continued as the condyloid artery***. The condyloid artery passes into the cranium through the anterior foramen in the condyloid fossa and joins the vertebral artery in the ***formation of rete mirabile cerebri.***

2. THE EXTERNAL MAXILLARY ARTERY

It arises from the **common carotid artery**, passes downwards and forwards on the lateral wall of the pharynx in company with **the hypoglossal nerve**, reaches the ramus of the mandible and turns round the ventral border of the horizontal ramus rostral to angle of mandible ***in company with the external maxillary vein and the Stenson's duct and the ventral buccal nerve and continues as facial artery after giving inferior labial artery***. Here it is placed subcutaneously and is ***useful for feeling the pulse*** **(Fig.3.94).**

> *The facial artery is used for pulse evaluation in cattle. The artery crosses the ventral border of the mandible infront of the masseter muscle accompanied by the facial vein, ventral buccal branch of facial nerve and stensons's duct of parotid salivary gland. In horses, the facial, masseteric and transverse facial arteries are sites for pulse evaluation.*

Collateral branches

1. **Pharyngeal and palatine branches** to the pharynx and soft palate. **2.** Branches to the parotid salivary gland. **3.** The **lingual artery** is large, runs in company with the glossopharyngeal nerve passes between the hyo and genioglossus muscles in company with the hypoglossal and lingual nerves and reaches the anterior extremity of the tongue. **It supplies branches to the muscles of the tongue and mucous membrane and submaxillary salivary gland. 4.** The **inferior (ventral) labial artery** is a slender vessel which passes in company with the ventral buccal nerve along the inferior border and the deep face of the depressor labii inferioris muscle and it furnishes branches to the muscle **buccinator, cutaneous muscle, skin and the lower lip.**

The **superior (dorsal) labial artery** is continuation of facial artery and supplies branches to **masseter, zygomaticus, malaris and muscles of the upper lip and cheek and terminates in the nostril.**

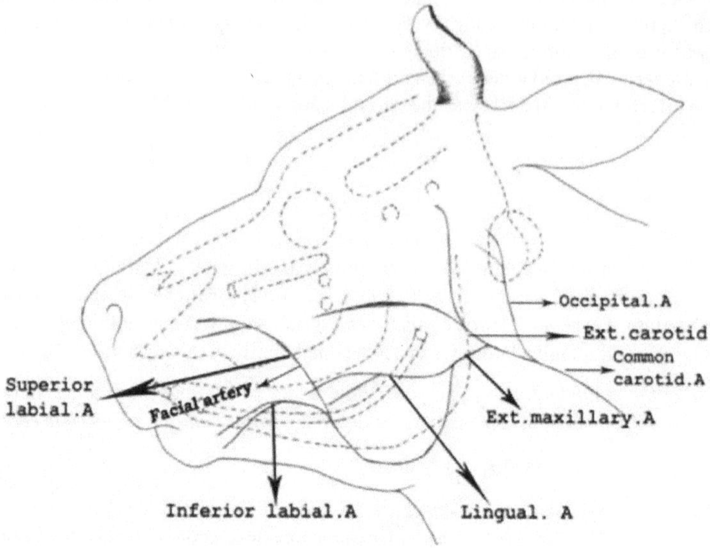

Fig. 3.94: External Maxillary Artery of Ox

3. THE EXTERNAL CAROTID ARTERY

It is the largest of the branches of the common carotid. At the level of the temporo mandibular articulation, it divides into **A.** ***Superficial temporal and B. Internal maxillary arteries.***

Collateral branches:1. Pharyngeal branches to pharynx. 2. Branches to submaxillary salivary gland.3. Branches to parotid salivary gland (***superior parotid artery***).4. Posterior auricular artery which supplies the muscles of the external ear and gives off a stylomastoid branch to the muscles of the middle ear and the tympanic membrane. 5. Muscular branches to temporalis, masseter and medial pterygoideus muscle.

A.THE SUPERFICIAL TEMPORAL ARTERY

It is the **smaller of the two terminal branches** of the external carotid artery. At base of the horn it divides into **anterior and posterior branches** (***cornual artery***) to supply the ***corium of the horn, frontalis and parietoauricularis externus muscles***.

> *Cornual artery, a branch of the superficial temporal artery, should be ligated or clamped at its origin to prevent bleeding in dehorning operations in ruminants.*

Along its course it gives off **1. Anterior auricular artery** to the muscles of the **external ear, temporalis** and skin.

2. Meningeal artery which passes through the temporal canal and **ramifies in duramater. 3. Transverse facial artery** which passes over the masseter in company with the vein and nerve and supplies this muscle. **4. Palpebral** branches to eyelids. **5. Lacrimal branches** to the lacrimal gland. **6. Muscular branches** to *temporalis and frontalis* and cutaneous branches to the skin **(Fig.3.95)**.

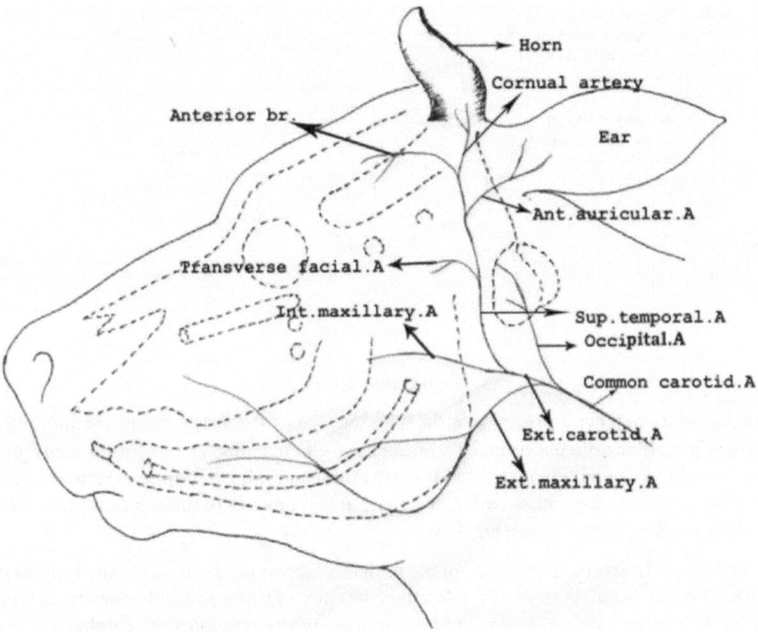

Fig. 3.95: Superficial Temporal Artery of Ox

B.INTERNAL MAXILLARY ARTERY

This is the **larger of the two terminal branches of the external carotid artery**. It passes obliquely forwards and upwards reaches the lower part of the temporal fossa, then turns forwards and runs in ***company with the maxillary nerve*** in the pterygopalatine fossa to the maxillary hiatus. Here it divides into two sets of branches the ***upper set of malar and infraorbital arteries and lower set of greater palatine and sphenoplatine arteries.***

Collateral Branches

1. Branches to the pterygoid muscles (pterygoid arteries).
2. **Parotido-temporal branch** arises from the posterior face of the artery and divides into **parotido-auricular and temporo-meningeal branches**. The former divides into **parotid and auricular branches** of which the former is distributed to the parotid salivary gland and supplies the skin of ear. The **temporo-meningeal** branch enters the **temporal canal and is distributed to the temporalis muscle.** ***This branch is the posterior deep temporal artery.***

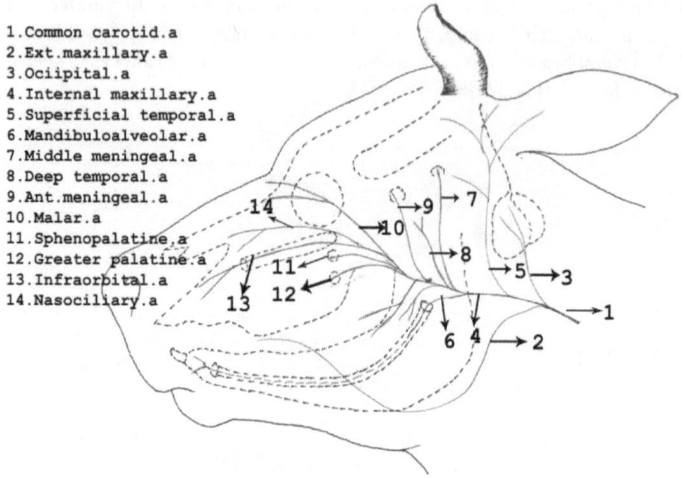

Fig. 3.96: Internal Maxillary Artery of Ox

3. **Mandibuloalveolar artery**: It arises from the anterior face of the artery passes through mandibular canal by enetering through mandibular foramen. During course in mandibular canal it gives alveolar branches to lower cheek teeth. At mental foramen it **divides into labial and inferior dental arteries to supply the lower lip and incisors.** The incisor branch (**inferior dental artery) passes in incisor canal to lower incisors and the alveolar periosteum and bone (Fig.3.96)**.

4. **Caudal rete mirabile artery:** It arises from the posterior face of the artery about the level of the preceeding branch, passes upwards and backwards, **gains the company of the mandibular nerve, enters the cranium through the foramen ovale** and assists in the **formation of the rete mirabile cerebri.**

5. **The anterior deep temporal artery:** It arises from the posterior face, a little above the preceeding, gains the anterior part of the temporal fossa, **enters the deep face of the temporalis muscle** and is distributed to it.

6. **Buccinator artery:** It arises from the anterior face of the artery, passes forwards in company with the buccinator nerve **between the medial pterygoid and the mandible, reaches the maxillary tuberosity**, runs under the masseter and enters the buccinators muscle. It supplies the ***pterygoideus, masseter and buccinators muscles.***

7. **External ophthalmic artery:** ***Eye is supplied by external ophthalmic artery***. The arteries arising from the external ophthalmic artery can be divided into two groups **(Fig.3.97)**.

(A) Arteries supplying eye ball (B) Arteries leaving the orbit to supply adjacent structures

(A) Arteries supplying the eye ball

1. **Short posterior ciliary arteries** penetrate sclera of eye ball near the optic nerve and supply the adjacent choroid in addition to branches to the optic nerve. The latter form the ***central artery of the retina***, the parent vessel for the retinal arteries. **The retinal vessels course dorsally, ventrally, medially and laterally in the form of a cross.**

2. **Long posterior ciliary arteries** pass through the sclera somewhat closer to the equator **(Fig.3.97) and supplyperiphery of the iris.**

3. **The anterior ciliary arteries:** The anterior ciliary arteries penetrate near the limbus (**corneo scleral junction**) and supply the anterior portion of the choroid, the ciliary body and the iris. These arteries anastomose to form

the **greater arterial circle of the iris** from which numerous fine branches pass toward the ciliary body and pupil. Capillaries near the limbus nourish the cornea by diffusion **(Fig.3.97).**

Venous return: The principal venous return is by several ***vorticose veins*** that emerge from the sclera near the equator. Venous blood returning from the retina leaves at the optic disc through small veins satellite to the short posterior ciliary arteries.

B. Arteries that leave the orbit

1. **The *lacrimal artery*** passes forward in the lateral part of the orbital cone and after supplying the **lacrimal gland** ends in lateral part of the eyelids and conjunctiva.
2. **The supraorbital artery** passes dorsally and leaves the orbit through the supraorbital foramen. It ramifies subcutaneously medial to the orbit and givess branches to the **upper eyelid.**
3. **The external ethmoidal artery** has the short intraorbital course. It enters the cranial cavity through the ethmoidal foramen. It passes inward on the cribriform plate and gives off the rostral meningeal artery and nasal branch. The former ramifies in the rostal part of the duramater. The latter passes through the cribri form plate and supplies the **ethmoid labyrinth and adjacent part of the nasal septum.**

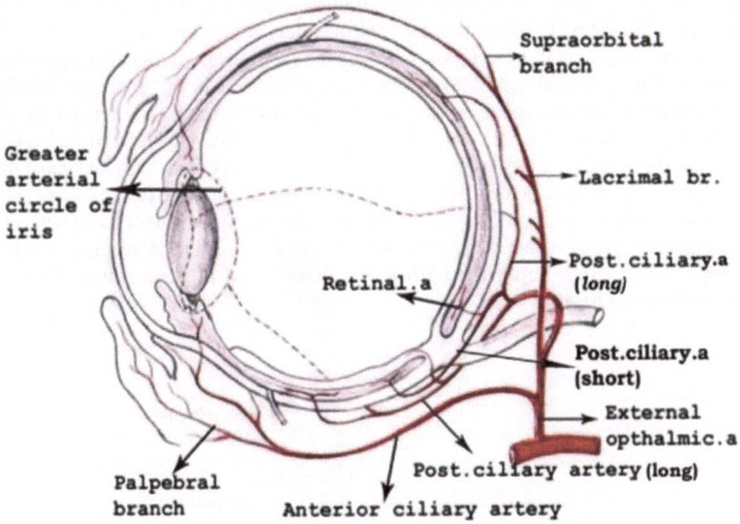

Fig. 3.97: External Opthalmic Artery

Terminal branches of internal maxillary artery

1. **Malar artery**: It is one of the terminal branches of the internal maxillary artery. It runs along the medial wall of the orbit passes along the floor of the orbit. It gives branches to the lower **eyelid and malaris muscle and divides into ascending and descending branches.** The **ascending branch** passes up and **anastomoses with the branch of the superficial temporal artery** and the **descending branch** is the **dorsal nasal artery and supplies the nasal muscles and the nostril.**
2. **Infraorbital artery:** This artery arises in common with the malar artery. It passes downwards and forwards reaches the **maxillary hiatus enters the maxillary foramen, passes in infraorbital canal** and passes out of it through the infraorbital foramen and is ***continued as the lateral nasal artery to supply the*** **nostril.** In the infraorbital canal it gives off branches to the roots of ***the upper cheek teeth.***

3. **Sphenopalatine artery:** This artery arises in ***common with the greater palatine artery,*** crosses the infraorbital artery, ***enters the sphenopalatine foramen in company with the nerve,*** enters the nasal cavity and divides to ***supply the nasal mucous membrane.***

4. **Greater palatine artery:** This is the ***largest of the terminal braches*** of the internal maxillary artery. It enters the palatine canal, comes out of it at the anteriorpalatine foramen, passes forwards in the palatine groove, on the deep face of the hard palate, enters the nasal cavity through the incisive fissure and terminates in the mucous membrane of the anterior part of the nasal cavity. In its course it gives branches to the ***hard palate, nasal branches to the nasal mucous membrane and branches to the dental pad.***

BLOOD SUPPLY TO THE BRAIN

RETE MIRABILE CEREBRI: is a large paired arterial plexus in the hypophyseal fossa. It lies on each side between the pituitary gland and the trigeminal nerve.The right and left plexus communicate posterior to the gland **(Fig.3.98).**

Branches from the internal maxillary artery passing through foramen ovale and orbitorotundum form inside the cranial cavity cranial part of dense arterial anastomotic network, rete mirabile cerebri, while **condyloid artery and vertebral artery contribute to the formation of posterior part.** The internal layer of duramater forms diaphragm sellae dorsal to pituitary gland, while the external layer of duramater is attached to margins of sella turcica. The **larger caudal rete mirabile branch** given from internal maxillary artery opposite the origin of buccal artey / mandibuloalveolar artery / deep temporal artery passes through foramen ovale, while **cranial rete mirabile branches numbering 2-4 arising from internal maxillary artery** opposite the level of origin of external ophthalmic artery pass through foramen orbitorotundum and these two join with opposite ones to form cranial part of rete mirabile cerebri. The condyloid artery, the branch of occipital artery reaching cranial cavity through the hypoglossal foramen and anastomosing with the vertebral artery which reaches the cranial cavity from vertebral canal through foramen magnum and with opposite ones form caudal part of the rete mirabile cerebri. The retia of either side communicate with each other rostral and caudal to the pituitary gland. The rete completely surrounds the hypophysis. Between the two layers of dura mater are cavernous and intercavernous sinuses surrounding pituitary gland in which retemirabile cerebri is located. **So rete mirabile cerebri is bathed in venous blood of these sinuses thereby resulting in cooling of blood reaching the brain.**

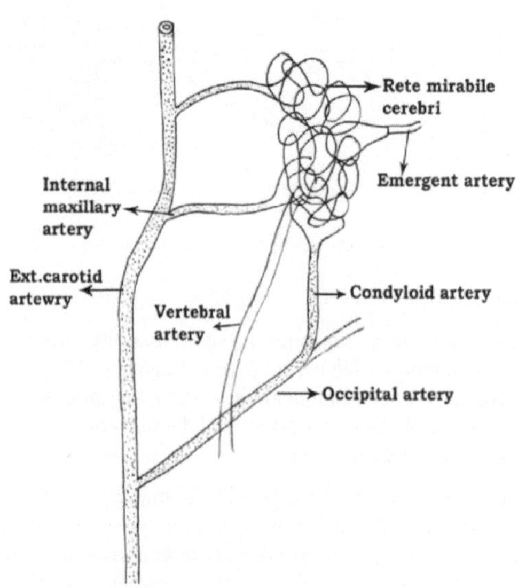

Fig. 3.98: Rete Mirabile Cerebri

CIRCULUS ARTERIOSUS (CIRCLE OF WILLIS)

From the superior face of the rete, on either side a single vessel an **emergent artery arises.** It traverses the cavernous sinus penetrates the diaphragma sellae and divides into two primary branches at the base of the brain. The **anterior primary** branch passes forwards, crosses the optic tract, curves medially and divides into middle and anterior cerebral arteries. ***The middle cerebral artery*** passes laterally gains the ***sylvian fissure*** and divides to supply the **lateral aspect of the cerebral hemisphere**. The **anterior cerebral** artery passes in front of the optic chiasma, gains the great longitudinal fissure and here it is connected to its fellow by a small anastomotic branch, thus completing the ***anterior arc of the circle of Willis***. It divides to supply the medial aspect of the cerebral hemisphere.

The **posterior primary** branch passes backward as the posterior cerebral artery, inclines medially, detaches the **anterior cerebellar artery** to the cerebellum and joins its fellow **to form the basilar artery**, thus completing the ***posterior arc of the circle of Willis***. This artery passes backwards in the central sulcus on the pons and **continues as the ventral spinal artery.** During the course, it detaches the **posterior cerebellar artery**, branches to the pons and medulla and choroid branches to the choroid plexus. The ***ventral spinal artery*** runs along the ventral median fissure of the spinal cord and is *reinforced during its course by branches from vertebral, intercostal, sacral and coccygeal arteries* **(Fig.3.99)**.

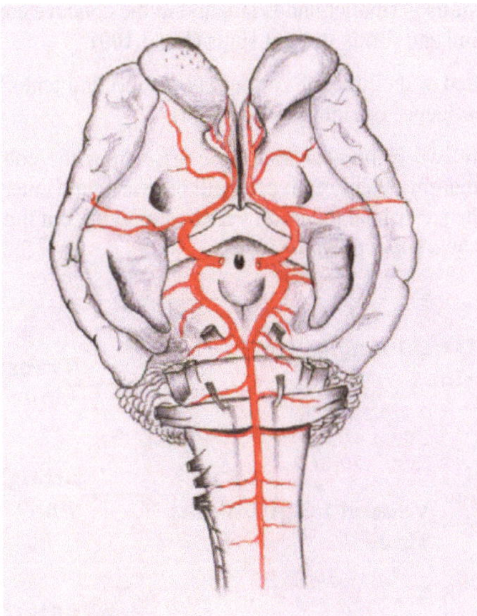

Fig. 3.99: Blood Supply to the Brain (Circle of Willis)

Blood supply to meminges: The ***middle meningeal artery*** **arises from occipital artery** and passes through **foramen ovale** and reaches cranial cavity and ramifies in duramater of the brain, while ***caudal meningeal atery*** **also given from occipital artery** reaches the cranial cavity and meninges through **foramen lacerum**. Another **meningeal branch is given off from the superficial temporal artery** / rostral auricular artery which passes through temporal canal and ramifies in duramater.

VENOUS DRAINAGE FROM THE BRAIN

The venus blood is drained from the brain by small cerebral veins which are *devoid of muscular coat and valves.* **They do not accompany the cerebral arteries**. They lie in the piameter and subarachnoid space. The **ascending cerebral veins** drain the convex and medial faces of the cerebral hemispheres and open into the dorsal longitudinal (some into the transverse) sinus of the duramater. The **descending cerebral veins** drain the ventral part of the convex face of the hemispheres and open into the vena rhinalis posterior. The **basal cerebral veins** form the trunk, the vena rhinalis posterior which joins the dorsal petrosal sinus. The ***deep cerebral veins*** draining the basal ganglia and choroid plexuses join to form the great cerebral vein which passes upwards and backward behind the splenium of corpus callosum and is continued as the straight sinus which joins the dorsal longitudinal sinus. The dorsal cerebellar veins drain into the occipital and dorsal petrosal sinuses. The **ventral cerebellar** veins form the basilar plexus. The veins from pons and medulla join the basilar plexus and the occipital and dorsal petrosal sinuses.

Sinuses of the Dura mater

These sinuses are the venous **spaces between the meningeal and periosteal layers of the dura mater** at places and are lined by endothelium. These receive the cerebral, meningeal and diploic veins form brain, meninges and skull respectively. The sinuses communicate with veins outside the cranium by means of ***emissary veins*** thereby draining venus blood from brain through sinuses to extracranial veins through *emissary veins.*

1. **Dorsal longitudinal (sagittal) sinus** is situated in the convex border of the falx cerebri and receives the ascending cerebral veins. It terminates by joining the straight sinus to form the confluence of sinuses **(Fig.3.100).**
2. **The ventral longitudinal sinus** is smaller and is situated in the concave edge of the falx cerebri. It receives the great cerebral vein behind and forms straight sinus **(Fig.3.100).**
3. **The straight sinus** is situated at the junction of the falx cerebri and tentorium cerebelli. It joins the dorsal longitudinal sinus at the confluence of sinuses **(Fig.3.100).**
4. **The transverse sinuses** are two in number and these arise from the confluence of the sinuses and pass laterally along the convex margin of tentorium cerebelli outwards and enter the temporal canal as the dorsal cerebral vein which joins the superficial temporal vein by emerging out through **postglenoid foramen**. The ***two sinuses are connected by a sinus communicans.***

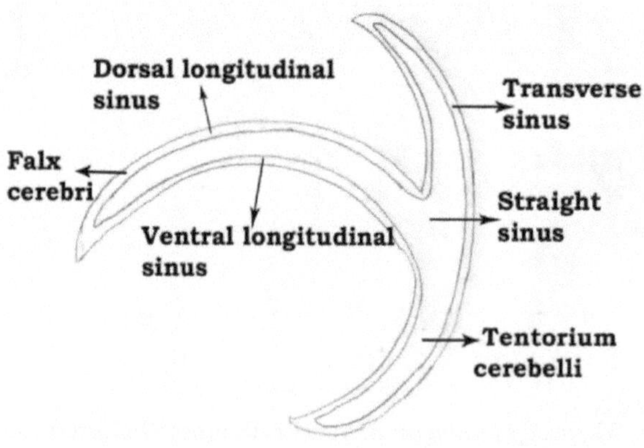

Fig. 3.100: Sinuses of Dura Mater

5. **The dorsal petrosal sinuses** are the direct communication of the venae rhinalis posterior and receive the basal cerebral veins.
6. **The ventral petrosal sinuses** lie along the lateral borders of the basioccipital enclosed in the thick dura closing the foramen lacerum.
7. **The cavernous sinuses** are situated on the internal surface of the temporal wing of the postphenoid on either side of the sella turcica and are connected with each other by an intercavernous sinus behind the pituitary body
8. **The occipital sinuses** are situated in the duramater on either side of the vermis cerebelli.

3.6 NERVE SUPPLY TO THE HEAD AND NECK

BRAIN

The brain consists of 3 parts i.e *fore brain, mid brain and hind brain*.

1. Fore Brain

comprises the median diencephalon and the paired cerebral hemispheres (telencephalon).

Telencephalon: consists of the paired cerebral hemispheres, separated by the **longitudinal fissure**. They are connected across the midline by **commissural fibers** i.e corpus callosum, rostral commissure and the dorsal and ventral commissures of the hippocampus. The surface of the hemisphere shows elevated ridges called ***"gyri"*** separated by grooves called ***"sulci"***. The pattern of the gyri is constant within one species but differs among species. E*ach hemisphere is composed of surface* ***gray matter called cerebral cortex or pallium with*** underlying cerebral white matter. The deep accumulations of **gray matter** are generally referred to as ***basal nuclei*** (**corpus striatum**). The **cortex or pallium** can be divided into **three parts based on** evolutionary history, i.e ***paleopallium, archipallium and neopallium***

1. ***Paleopallium:*** constitutes the ventrl part of the each hemisphere. It is principally **related to the** ***olfaction.*** Its rostral part is provided by an appendage, *the* ***olfactory bulb*** that fits into a recess of the ethmoid bone.
2. ***Archipallium:*** *The next oldest part, forms medial aprt of each hemisphere* extending from the longitudinal fissure into the hemisphere as the ***hippocampus***. It is included in the limbic system, which comprises the cingulated, supracallosal and geniculate gyri, the hippocampal foramation and the dentate gyrus. It is concerned with olfaction.
3. ***Neopallium*** is the the **youngest part**, It is the largest and functionally dominant part of the cerebrum. It is divided from the paleopallium by the rhinal sulcus on the lateral side of the hemisphere and from the archipallium by the splenial sulcus medially.

Fissures and sulci of Brain: The ***great longitudinal fissure*** separates the left and right hemispheres. The ***transverse fissure*** separates the cerebrum from the cerebellum. The ***cruciate sulcus (ansate sulcus)*** runs transversely on the **rostrodorsal aspect of the hemisphere (Fig.3.101).**

Sylvian sulcus is present on **the lateral aspect of cerebral hemisphere (Fig.3.101),** in which ***middle cerebral artery*** ascends. It is a very deep and irregular indentatation with multiple overlapping gyri. The deepest and most prominent sulcus on the dorsolateral side of the hemisphere is the combined rostral, middle and caudal suprasylvian sulci.

The ***coronal sulcus*** is deep and is *directed upward and medially over the frontal pole. The coronal sulcus continues rostrolaterally into the presylvian sulcus, which ends dorsolaterally in the rhinal sulcus* **(Fig.3.101).**

The ***rhinal sulcus*** divides the **cerebral hemisphere from the lateral olfactory stria.**

The ***callosal sulcus*** is on the medial face and separates the corpus collasum from the gyrus fornicates **(Fig.3.102).**

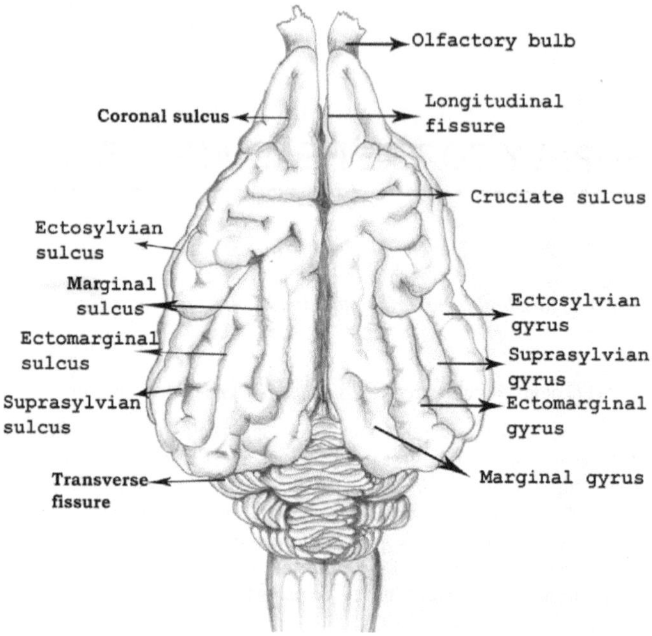

Fig. 3.101: Different Fissures, Sulci and Gyri of Brain (Dorsal view)

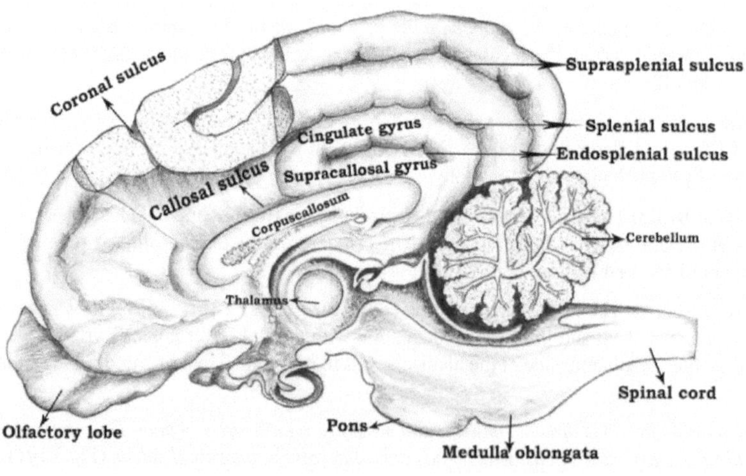

Fig. 3.102: Different Sulci and Gyri of Brain (Medial view)

Different Cortical areas of Telencephalon: The cerebral cortex can be divided into different areas based on their function.

1. **The olfactory area**: is located within the rhinencephalon.
3. **Visual area: is located in lingual gyrus of the *occipital lobe*** between the *anterior and posterior calcarine fissures*.

4. **The auditory area***:* is located predominaltly in the **rostral sylvian gyrus.**
5. ***Motor area:*** is located in the rostral half of the **post cruciate gyrus**.
6. **The gyrus fornicatus:** It contains two gyri (***upper cingulate gyrus and lower supracallosal gyrus)*** and lies on the medial face of the hemisphere between the callosal and callosomarginal fissure **(Fig.3.102).** In this gyrus the area for **taste** is located in its **upper part** (***cingulate gyrus***) and the area for **smell** is located in its **lower part (*supracallosal gyrus*)** which is continous with the hippocampal gyrus.

Different Parts of Telencephalon

For description purpose the neopallium can be divided in to **four regions or lobes**, these are ***frontal, parietal, occipital and temporal lobes.The motor areas*** are mainly located in the frontal lobe which gives origin to the pyramidal motor tract. The ***parietal lobe*** features mainly ***sensory areas, the temporal lobe*** *shows the* ***auditory area and the occipital lobe shows the visual area*** **(Fig.3.103).**

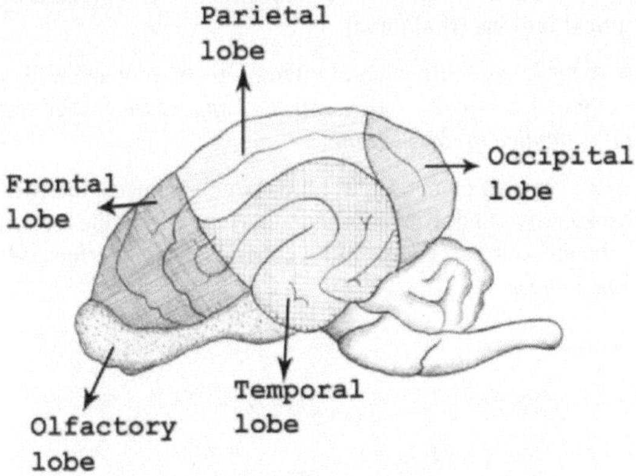

Fig. 3.103: Different Parts of Cerebral Hemisphere

Limbic system: The term limbic system is applied to ***collection of brain structures involved with emotional behaviour***. It consists of **cortical and subcortical components**. The ***cortical part*** comprises *interconnected telencephalic structures namely, cingulate gyri, the piriform lobe and the hippocampus*. The ***subcortical part*** includes components of diencephalon (habenula, thalamus, hypothalamus), mid brain (interpeduncular and tegmental nuclei) and the amygdaloid body **(Fig.3.104).**

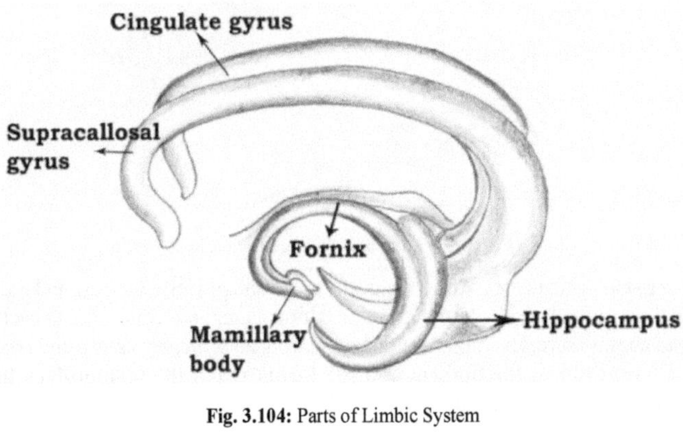

Fig. 3.104: Parts of Limbic System

The ***limbic system*** receives olfactory input from the piriform lobe that initiates mostly visceral motor activities, but also triggers emotional behaviour such as fear, aggression and pleasure. The limbic system has great input on ***thirst, hunger and sexual behaviour*** and is closely related to the reticular formation.

Basal Ganglia (corpus striatum): The basal ganglia consists of masses of gray matter or nuclei, the ***caudate and lenticular nuclei, claustrum and the amygdaloid nucleus*** within the cerebral hemisphere. The ***caudate nucleus*** appears as ***comma*** with a large head bulging into the floor of the lateral ventricle, a body following the caudal bend of the cavity and a tail related to roof of its ventral extension.

The ***lentiform nucleus*** is more lateral and is divided by a fiber intersection into ***medial part, globus pallidum*** and the ***lateral part, putamen***. The **lentiform nucleus** is separated from the **caudate nucleus** by the ***internal capsule*** (capsula interna). Between the putamen and claustrum fibers of the ***external capsule*** pass. A thin band of of white substance separates the claustrum from adjacent cerebral cortex.

The ***amygdaloid nucleus is*** smaller, located near the tail of the caudate nucleus and the ***clastrum*** (**Latin for: close or shut**) is interposed between the lentiform nucleus and neopallium. It is a bilateral structure which **connects to cortical (frontal) and sub cortical regions (thalamus).**

The alternating presence of these nuclei and afferent and efferent fibers, projection fibers and association fibers of white matter in which they are embedded give the region a ***striated appearance*** when sectioned. ***Therefore the term striated body (corpus straitum) is applied to this region.***

Corpus callosum: It is the largest mass of commissural fibres which connects the two cerebral hemispheres. The anterior end the ***genu***, bends backwards and downwards and thins out to from the rostrum which is continuous with the lamina terminalis forming the anterior part of the third ventricle. The ***posterior end is the splenium*** and lies at a higher level than the genu **(Fig.3.105).**

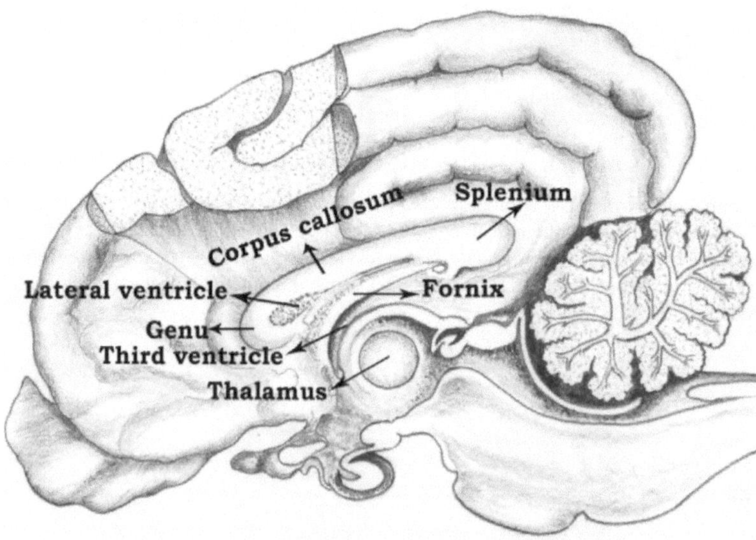

Fig. 3.105: Structure of Corpus Callosum

Hippocampus: This is a **gyrus** which curves from the deep face of the piriform lobe around the thalamus and forms the posterior part of the floor of the lateral ventricle. The two hippocampi are connected to each other at their upper parts by the hippocampal commissure.The hippocampus represents an ***olfactory centre*** and receives fibres from the **piriform lobe** and its **efferent fibres, the fimbria and the fornix reach the mammillary body.** *The fornix is a tract connecting hippocampus with mammillary body*

Types of Nerve Fibers of Brain

1. **Association fibers:** connect parts of the neopallium of the same hemispher **(Fig.3.104).** eg: white fibers of cerebral cortex.
2. **Commissural fibers:** connect the two hemispheres, generally liniking equivalent contralateral parts. ***eg: corpus callosum.***
3. **Projection fibers:** connect cortex with lower parts of the central nervous system ***Eg: internal casule of basal ganglia*** forming croticospinal tract connecting cerebral cortex and spinal cord.

Diencephalon: it comprises three parts: **i.e epithalmus, thalamus and hypothalamus**, which form the roof, walls and floor of the third ventricle, respectively.

Epithalamus: The most dorsal part, comprises the **pineal gland** (***Epiphysis cerebri***), **habenular striae and habenular commissure**. The **pineal gland** is a small, median body projecting dorsally from the brain stem as an evagination of the roof of the third ventricle that is composed only of piamater and ependyma. The **habenular stria** is a fiber bundle that connects the septal area with the **habenular nuclei i.e medial (MHb) and lateral (LHb) habenulae**. The habenular nuclei are interconnected by the **habenular commissure**. ***Habenula is Latin for "little rein"*** acts as a regulator of key CNS neuro transmitters, connecting the forebrain and midbrain within the epithalamus. It is an important pathway in the limbic system. They receive fibers (habenular stria) from the hippocampus and other parts of the telencephalon and send fibers to mesencephalic nuclei.

Thalamus: is the **largest part** of the diencephalon. It forms the lateral walls of the 3rd ventricle **(Fig.3.106).** Its ***dorsal surface faces toward the fornix and floor of the lateral ventricle***. Its ventral surface rests on hypothalamus. Its lateral face is covered by the fibers of internal capsule. The thalamus is composed of *large number of nuclei*. These nuclei have specific functions and collectively form one of the most important relay and integration centres of brain stem. The ***medial geniculate body*** represents the thalamic **relay station of the auditory tract** and acts as a gateway to the centres of perception in cerebral cortex. The ***lateral geniculate body*** is the relay station of the ***optic system. The lateral and medial genicult e bodies constitute the metathalamus.***

Hypothalamus: The term hypothalamus does not refer to any single structure anatomically and includes the wall of the third ventricle below the ***thalamus, optic chiasma, tuber cinereum, infundibulum, mammillary body, subthalamic nuclei*** and posterior perforated substance etc **(Fig.3.106).**

The hypothalamus is functionally important as it contains centres of the sympathetic and parasympathetic systems of auotonomic nervous system regulating visceral activities; **centre for regulation of body temperature, centre for fat, carbohydrates and water metabolism, centre for sleep rhythm etc**. Neurons in the hypothalamus are also concerned in the regulation of secretion of hormones in the pars anterior of pituitary through secretion of chemical mediators or releasing factors into the blood stream (***Hypothalamo-hypophyseal portal circulation***) and in addition, other neurons in the hypothalamus are responsible for secretion of the posterior pituitary hormones which are conveyed by the axons of these neurons (the hypothlamo-hypophyseal tract) to the pars nervosa, where they are released in to the blood stream.

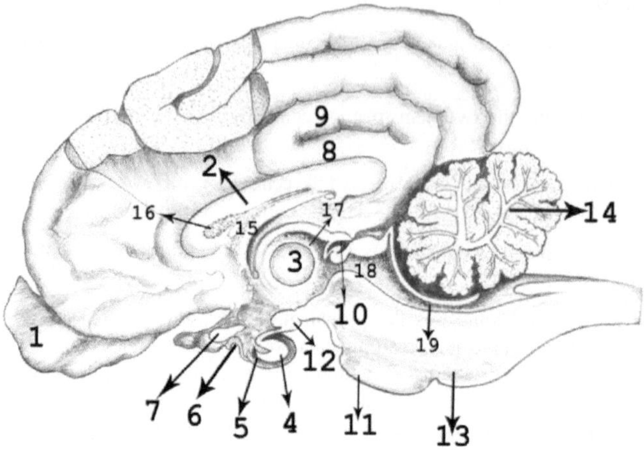

1. Olfactory bulb
2. Corpus callosum
3. Interthalamic adhesion
4. Hypophysis
5. Infundibulum
6. Tuber cinereum
7. Optic chiasma
8. **Supracallosal gyrus**
9. **Cingulate gyrus**
10. Epiphysis
11. Pons
12. Mamillary body
13. Medulla oblongata
14. Cerebellum
15. Fornix
16. Lateral ventricle
17. Third ventricle
18. Cerebral aqueduct
19. Fourth Ventricle

Fig. 3.106: Sagittal Section of Brain

Hypophysis: is a dark and solid body. It is located within a recess of the floor of the cranial cavity, sella turcica. It is hollowed by a recess of the third ventricle by the infundibulum. It is coverd by a fold of duramater.

2. Mid Brain (Mesencephalon)

The mid brain consists **of tectum, tegmentum and cerebral peduncles** in dorsoventral sequence.

Tectum: lies dorsal to the cerebral aqueduct. It has four rounded swellings. The paired caudal swellings, called **caudal colliculi** are widely spaced and are joined by a commissure. They are connected with the ipsilateral **medial geniculate body** (a swelling of thalamus) through a distinct ridge called ***inferior brachium***. The paired **rostral colliculi** are placed higher and closer together and are joined to the **lateral geniculate bodies** by indistinct brachia called ***superior brachium*** **(Fig.3.107)**.

Function: The **rostral colliculi** have visual pathways. They receive visual impulses from the optic tract through the **superior brachium**. Its efferent fibres form the **Tectospinal tract**. ***The posterior colliculi*** are concerned with **auditory pathways**.

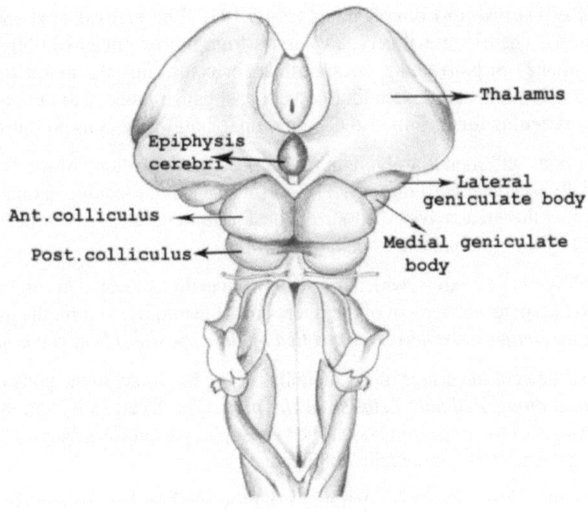

Fig. 3.107: Structure of Mid Brain

Tegmentum: comprises the core of the midbrain and is directly continuous with the corresponding stratum of the metencephalon. Much of it is formed by reticular formation. The principal nuclei are the mesencephalic nuclei of the trigeminal nerves (V), **the trochlear nuclei** (IV) and the **parasympathetic oculomotor nuclei** (III) and the **red nuclei (named from their pronounced vascularity).** The **substantia nigra** is a prominent lamina that can be identified in transverse sections by its darker color which is due to accumulation of pigment within constituent neurons **(Fig.3.108).**

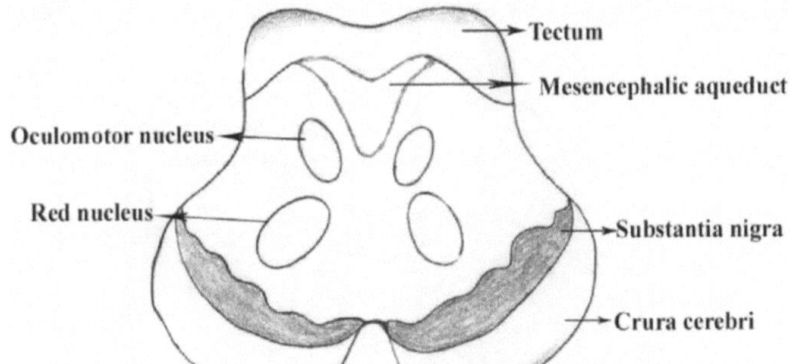

Fig. 3.108: Parts of Mid Brain

Crura cerebri: are visible on the ventral surface of the brain caudal to the optic tract at the base of the brain. They are bound **laterally by the piriform lobes** and **caudally by the pons.** They comprise fiber tracts that are in passage between the telecephalon and caudal brain stem. The **crura cerebri** flank the interpeduncular fossa that contains the **mamillary body, infundibulum of hypohysis and pituitary gland.** The **oculomotor nerves (III)** emerge from the **ventromedial aspect** of the cerebral peduncles. The **trochlear nerves** arise from the **midbrain dorsally**, just caudal to the tectum.

3. Hind Brain (Rhombencephalon)

Comprises the pons, medulla oblongata and cerebellum.

Pons: The pons consists of ventral and dorsal parts (Fig.3.106). The ventral part shows transverse pontine fibers that bulge out ventrally. The trigeminal nerve (V) arises from **motor nucleus in lateral aspect** of the pons. Several other nuclei are situated in pons and are responsible for controlling the motor functions of the body. It has also a large number of ascending and descending nerve tracts, which proceed to the cerebellum as the **middle cerebellar peduncle.** The **reticular formation** also occupies up to half of the pons on transverse section.

Medulla oblongata: The pons and medulla oblongata form successive portions of the brain stem. The medulla oblongata continues caudally as spinal cord directly. The dorsal surface of medulla oblongata is largely concealed by the cerebellum and forms the greater part of floor of the fourth ventricle. Its ventral surface is marked by a median fissure and flanked by longitudinal ridges called ***pyramids***.

Each pyaramid consists of myelinated axons, which originate from neurons located in cerebral cortex and extend to the medulla oblongata and the spinal cord. Most of the fibers cross the midline to form the pyramidal decussation at the spinomedullary junction. ***Hence, muscles are controlled by the opposite side of the brain.***

A transverse ridge crossing the ventral surface of the medulla oblongata caudal to the pons is called ***trapezoid body (corpus trapezoideum), that ontogenetically belongs to the pons.*** The facial (VII) and Vestibulocochlear (VIII) nerves arise from lateral aspect of the trapezoid body. The Glossopharyngeal (IX), Vagus (X) and Spinal accessory (XI) nerves arise from lateral aspect of the medulla oblongata.

Cerebellum: The cerebellum or lesser brain is separated from the cerebral hemispheres by the ***transverse fissure* (Fig.3.109)**. It overlies the pons and greater part of the medulla oblongata and the fourth ventricle **(Fig.3.106)**. The primary fissure subdivides the body of the cerebellum into **rostral and caudal lobes**. The ***rostral lobe*** is subdivided into the narrow ***small lingula***, which is the most rostral part of the vermis. The **larger central lobe** is subdivided into two parts and finally the ***culmen***, which in turn is subdivided into two parts. The lobules of the rostral lobe are designated ***vinculum lingulae, ala lobuli cetralis and lobulus quadrangularis***

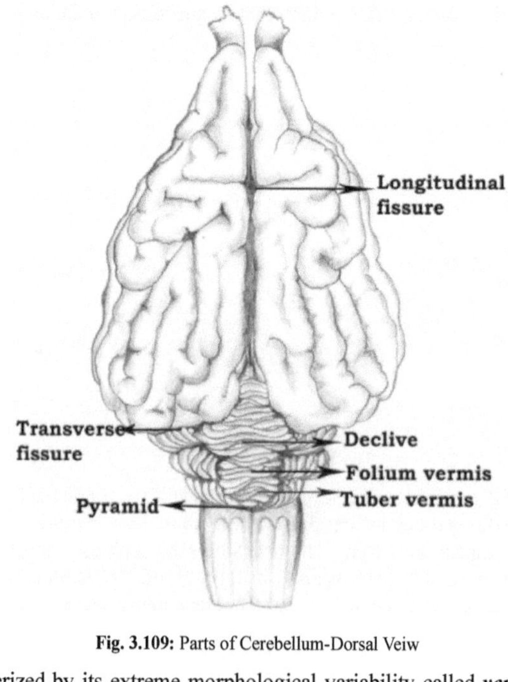

Fig. 3.109: Parts of Cerebellum-Dorsal Veiw

The caudal lobe is characterized by its extreme morphological variability called ***vermis*** (***due to resemblance to earth worm***). The ***vermis is subdivided into*** the ***declive, the folium*** and the ***tuber vermis*** from rostral to caudal. The

pyramid and uvula are the most caudal lobes of the vermis which are related to the dorsal and ventral paraflocculi in the hemispheres **(Fig.3.110)**.

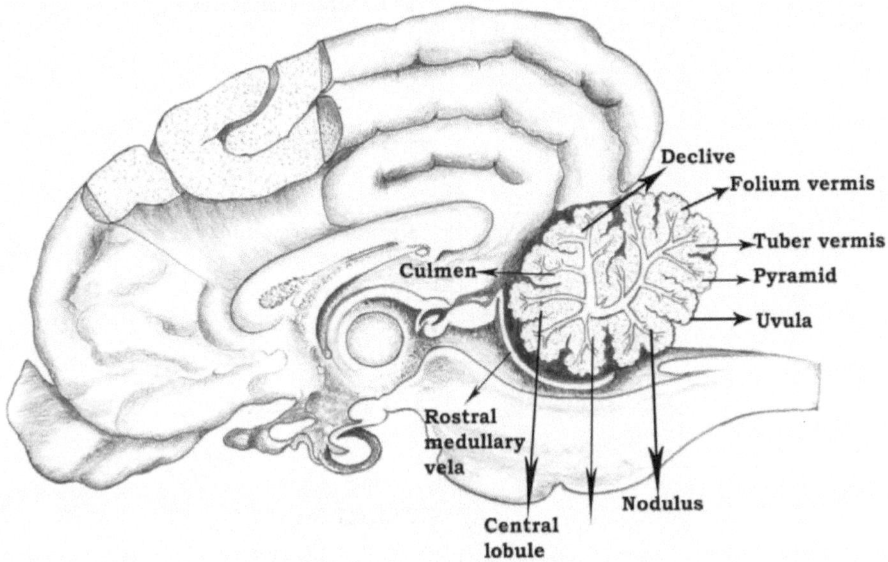

Fig. 3.110: Parts of Cerebellum-sagittal View

The cerebellum is divided into ***lobes***, ***lobules*** and smaller units ***known as folia by fissures*** **(Fig.3.110)**. The **white matter** (medulla) arises from the peduncles and radiates through the various **lobes, lobules and folia** forming a branching structure with resemblance to a **tree**. Because of this appearance and because of an ancient belief that it is the ***seat of the soul***, it is known as the ***arbor vitae*** (***the tree of life***). Gray substance forms a series of nuclei i.e ***fastigial nuclei, lateral cerebellar (dentate) nucleus and nucleus interpositi in the medulla.***

Cerebellar Peduncles: Cerebellum is attached to the brainstem by the **three cerebellar peduncles** on each side and by the caudal and rotral medullary vela. The **caudal cerebellar peduncle** (***restiform body***) connects with the medulla oblongata. The **middle cerebellar peduncle *(brachium pontis)*** extend verolaterally to the pons. The **rostral peduncle *(*brachium conjunctivum*)*** attaches the cerebellum with the mid brain and is largely composed of efferent fibers.

Functions: The cerebellum controls balance and coordination of postural and locomotor activities. The **balance** is located in the **flocculonodular lobe**. The caudal lobe is concerned with the feed back regulation of motor function. The rostral lobe receives an input of proprioceptive information.

Ventricles of Brain: The ventricular system of brain consists of two lateral ventricles, one in each cerebral hemisphere (***in telencephalon***), the unpaired third ventricle ***in diencephalon*** and fourth ventricle in rhombencephalon. Each lateral ventricle communicates with the 3rd ventricle through "***interventricular foramen of Munro".*** The third ventricle is a narrow annular space present around the thalamus. The ***mesencephalic aqueduct*** of the mid brain joins the third and fourth ventricles. The **fourth ventricle** is continuous with the **central canal of the spinal cord (Fig.3.111)**. The fourth ventricle communicates with the cisterna magna (**dilated subarchnoid space**) by a central and two lateral microscopic foraminae, called as ***Megendie and Foramina of Luschka*** respectively.

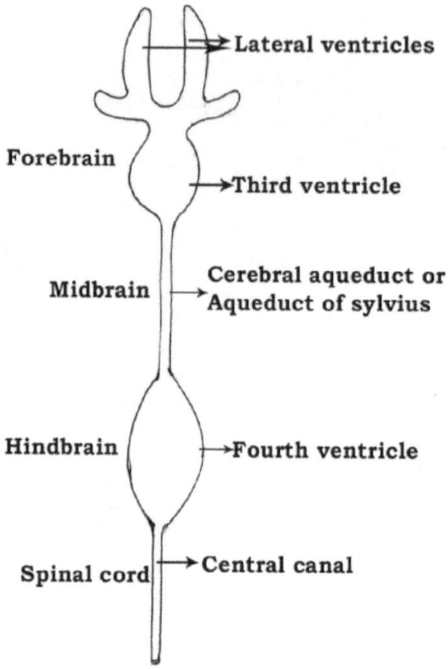

Fig. 3.111: Ventricles of Brain (Schematic)

Boundaries of lateral ventricle: Each lateral ventricle has a **roof, floor and a medial wall. The roof** is formed by the corpus callosum and the medial wall by the ***septum lucidum.*** The **floor is** formed by the two chief nuclei, the **caudate nucleus** in front and the hippocampus behind and the body of the fornix medially and in front.

Boundaries of the third ventricle: The **floor** of the 3rd ventricle is formed by the hypothalamus. The **roof** is formed by the ***tela choriodea*** (*meningeal piamater and underlying ependyma that gives rise to the choroid plexus in each of the ventricle of the brain)* ***and fornix****. The* ***anterior wall*** is formed by ***lamina terminalis***, a thin layer of gray matter stretching from the superior face of the optic chiasma to the rostrum of the corpus callosum.

Boundaries of fourth ventricle: The **floor** is formed by the medulla and the pons. The **lateral wall** is formed by the posterior cerebellar peduncles (***restiform body***) and anterior cerebellar peduncles. The **roof** is formed by the **vermis** of the cerebellum and the **anterior and posterior medullary** *vela*. "***Velum" is a thin layer of white matter prolonged from the vermis of cerebellum***

Cerebrospinal fluid: is normally a clear colourless fluid formed from the blood plasma by the choroid plexus of the brain. The choroid plexus consists of an epithelium and the underlying pia mater. They are adherent to the walls of the ventricles by an attachment of the pia mater. The attachment line is termed the ***tela choroidea*****. One choroid plexus is present in each lateral ventricle and in third and fourth ventricles of brain**. Cerebrospinal fluid flows within the ventricular system and into the central canal. It flows into the subarchnoid space from the fourth ventricle through bilateral recesses and apertures. The major drainage routes for the return of cerebrospinal fluid to the venous blood are arachnoid villi to sinuses of duramater which inturn are drained by ***emissary veins and lymphatics associated with peripheral nerves.***

Functions: The cerebrospinal fluid cushions the CNS and acts as a chemical buffer. It also transports nutrients and waste products, there by taking over the function of the lymphatics lacking in the brain.

Reticular Formation

Diffuse network of white matter (nerve fibers) interspersed with gray matter, located in the brain stem (thalamus, mid brain, pons and medulla oblongata) is called **reticular foramation** due to its **reticulated** (***network***) appearance. It **regulates various autonomic functions, such** as **sleep, waking and sexual arousal.** One of the most important tasks of the reticular formation is regulating the functions of the autonomic nervous system and directly involving with **unconscious functions.** It helps to **regulate the heart beat, breathing and the process of digestion, urination and defecation.**

Pyramidal motor system: The pyramidal tracts are named so because they start from pyramidal neurons of cerebral cortex and pass through the pyramids of medulla oblongata. The pyramidal tract refers to fibers of upper motor neurons that originate in cerebral cortex and terminate in the spinal cord ***(corticospinal tract) or brain stem (cortico bulbar tract).*** The corticospinal fibers descending through the internal capsule to the brain stem, converge to a point from multiple directions giving the impression of ***inverted pyramid.*** Pyramidal system deals with the ***regulation of conscious muscle movements***. The pyramidal tracts include both the **corticospinal and corticobulbar tracts.**

The corticobulbar tract conducts impulses from the **brain to certain cranial nerves**. These nerves control the muscles of the face and neck and are involved in **facial expression, mastication, swallowing and other motor functions.**

The corticospinal tract: conducts impulses from the **brain to spinal cord**. The corticospinal tract is involved in control of **voluntary movements**. The majority of the fibers of the corticospinal tract cross over in medulla, resulting in muscles being controlled by the opposite side of the brain. The cortcospinal tract begins from cells of ***Betz*** (**large pyramidal cells of cerebral cortex**).

The Extrapyramidal Motor System: The *extrapyramidal motor system* is composed of motor fibers which do not pass through the medullary pyramids but which nevertheless exert a measure of control over body movements. The extrapyramidal system **indirectly controls motion.** It is also referred to as the **indirect activation pathway of motor functions**. Primarily, the extrapyramidal system is involved in **maintaining equilibrium, coordination, posture, muscle tone and reflexes**. For example, when a person tries to maintain an erect posture while sitting or standing, many muscles are contracting in a coordinated manner. This coordination is under involuntary control at subconscious level by the extrapyramidal pathways, namely the ***rubrospinal tract, tectospinal tract, reticulospinal tract and vestibulospinal tract.***

Lemniscal System: (***In Greek* "lemniscal" *means -Ribbon or band***) It is an ascending spinal tract, carrying sensory information to the brain. ***The ascending pathways of this group are divided into the Medial lemniscus and Extra lemniscus.*** It carries sensitive impulses relating to **touch, pressure, vibration and joint proprioception.** The leminscal system typically shows a chain of three neurons i.e ***1. First stage neurons, 2. Second stage neurons and 3. Third stage neurons.***

The medial lemniscus: includes the most important ascending tracts. It can be divided into the ***spinal lemniscus*** for the trunk and limbs and the ***trigeminal lemniscus*** for the sensory fibers from the head.The sensory fibers of the **spinal lemniscus** run in the dorsal funiculus of the spinl cord. Those arising from the ***lumbosacral plexus*** and the more caudal part of the trunk occupy the **medial position** (***fasciculus gracilis***). Those from the ***brachial plexus*** and the cranial part of the trunk assume **lateral positions** (***fasciculus cuneatus***). Both the tracts end in the like named nuclei (***nucleus gracilis and nucleus cuneatus***) of the medulla oblongata. After synapsing, the axons of the **second stage** neurons decussate opposite side to reach the nucleus of thalamus where they again synapse. The **tertiary axons** extend to the somesthetic (sensory) area of cortex.

Extra lemniscal system*:* forms a ***second spinothalmic tract***, which convey impulses that are characterised by slower propagation and less precise originating stimuli compared to the medial lemniscus. The primary axons terminate in neurons of the dorsal horn close to their spinal root. After forming synapse, the **second stage neurons** pass into the white matter, where they travel to synapse in the thalamus. The **tertiary neurons** project from the thalamus to the cortical area rostral to that of the medial lemniscal system. ***The spinothalmic tract convey the impulses of pain and temperature.***

CRANIAL NERVES

1. Olfactory Nerve

The olfactory nerve conveys the ***sense of smell.*** It consists of fibres which are the axons of the olfactory cells in the olfactory part of the nasal mucous membrane.The fibres are collected into small bundles, pass through the cirbriform plate of the ethmoid bone to the convex face of the olfactory bulb of the brain.

2. Optic Nerve

Conveys the special sense of vision. This nerve is composed of meduallated fibres which are axons of the ganglion cells of retina. The fibres converge within the eyeball at the optic papilla, where they form the optic nerve.The nerve leaves eye ball at its ***infero-lateral quadrant.*** Then it passes on base of brain and forms ***optic chiasma*** with optic nerve from opposite eye ball **(Fig.3.112).**

3. Oculomotor Nerve

It is a motor nerve controlling eye movements by innervating four extraocular muscles. It arises from the ***ventromedial aspect of the cerebral peduncles*** **(Fig.3.112)**. It leaves the cranium thorugh the ***foramen orbitorotundum*** and divides into **dorsal and ventral branches**. The **dorsal branch** supplies **rectus dorsalis and levator palpebrae superioris muscles**. The **ventral branch** supplies **rectus medialis, rectus ventralis and ventral oblique muscles** and also conveys **parasympathetic efferents** to the ciliary ganglion which after relay in the ganglion are distributed to the ***ciliary muscle and constrictor pupillae of iris***.

4. Trochlear Nerve

It is the **fourth cranial** nerve and is the **motor nerve** to the **superior oblique muscle** of the eyeball. It is the ***finest*** of the cranial nerves. **It is the only cranial nerve arising from the dorsal aspect of the mid brain**, close to and behind the posterior colliculus of corpora quadrigemina. This nerve leaves the cranium thorugh the **foramen orbitorotundum**.

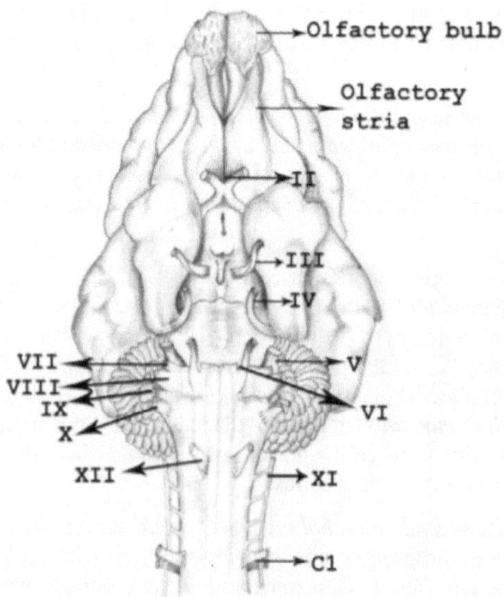

Fig. 3.112: Origin of Cranial Nerves

5. Trigeminal Nerve

It is the fifth cranial nerve and is a **mixed nerve**. It is the ***largest*** of cranial nerves. It is connected to the lateral aspect of the pons by a large sensory root and a small motor root; the **sensory root forms the semilunar ganglion** under which the motor root passes forward. The convex face of the ganglion gives off three branches, the **ophthalmic nerve, the maxillary nerve and sensory part of mandibular nerve.**

The ophthalmic nerve is purely sensory and leaves the cranium through the foramen orbitorotundum and divides into ***frontal, lacrimal and nasociliary branches***. The frontal nerve emerges from the orbit through the supraorbital canal and supplies the upper eyelid and the skin. The ***lacrimal nerve*** supplies the lacrimal gland, skin over the temporal fossa, frontal sinus and gives a long ***cornual branch*** which passes below the lateral border of the frontal bone ***along with the branches of superficial temporal artery and vein to supply the corium of the horn*** **(Fig.3.113)**.

In dehorning operation in cattle, the temporal line is used as palpable landmark to block the cornual nerve which innervates the horn in cattle. The cornual nerve emerges from the orbit and courses towards the base of the horn along the temporal line. The cornual artery which supplies the horn, must also be ligated or its branches cauterized. Additionally, a ring nerve block is sometimes performed by depositing a local anaesthetic around the base of the horn to achieve maximal pain suppression.

The ***nasociliary nerve*** runs between rectus dorsalis, retractor oculi and then between rectus dorsalis and medialis and turns toward the ethmoidal foramen and divides into the **ethmoidal nerve and the infratrochlear nerve. The ethmoidal nerve** pases through the ethmoidal foramen into cranial cavity and leaves it through the cribriform plate of ethmoid and supplies the **nasal mucous membrane.** The **infratrochlear nerve** runs towards the medial canthus and supplies the **conjunctiva, lacrimal ducts, lacrimal sac and the third eyelid.**

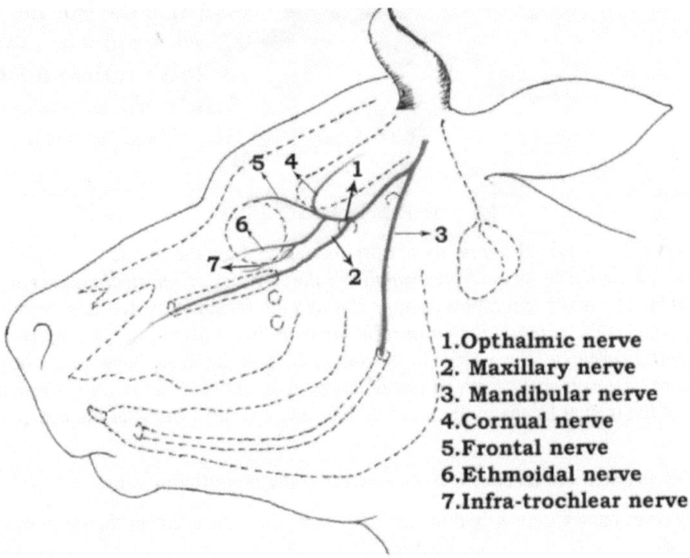

Fig. 3.113: Branches of Opthalmic Nerve

The maxillary nerve is the **largest** of the three branches and is also purely sensory like the opthalmic. It emerges out of the cranium through the foramen orbitorotundum runs forward in the pterygopalatine fossa and gives off the following branches. (a) ***zygomatic or orbital*** **branch** runs to the lateral canthus and supplies **lower eyelid and skin.** (b) ***Sphenopalatine nerve*** is given off in the pterygopalatine fossa and bears the **sphenopalatine ganglion.** It divides into (i) **posterior nasal**, which passes through sphenopalatine foramen to supply nasal mucous membrane;

(ii) **the greater or anterior palatine,** which runs through the palatine canal and groove to supply **hard palate and gums.** (iii) **the lesser or posterior palatine** which passes downward to supply the **soft palate (Fig.3.114).**

The **maxillary nerve continues as the infraorbital nerve** which passes through the infraorbital canal, gives off dental branches to the upper cheek teeth, alveolar periosteum and gums, emerges out of the infraorbital foramen and divides into nasal and labial branches to supply **nostril and upper lip (Fig.3.114).**

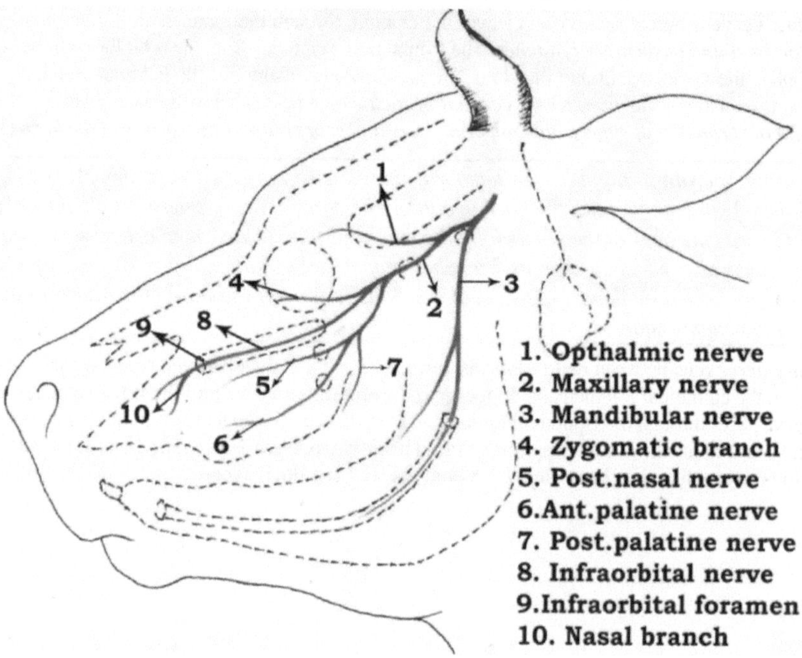

Fig. 3.114: Branches of Maxillary Nerve

The mandibular nerve: It is a **mixed nerve.** Its sensory root arises from the semilunar ganglion soon after which it is joined by the motor root. The motor fibres ***supply all the muscles of mastication except posterior belly of digastricus*** **(Fig.3.115).** The nerve leaves the cranium through the **foramen ovale**, runs downwards between the pterygoideus muscles enters the ***mandibular foramen of the mandible***, runs through the ***inferior dental canal and gains exit at the mental foramen*** **(Fig.3.115).** In its course through the mandibular canal the mandibular nerve supplies dental branches to lower cheek teeth and sends a branch through the incisor canal to supply lower incisors. After emerging out of the mental foramen, the nerve divides into a number of labial filaments to supply the lower lip.

It gives the following branches in its course before entering the mandibular canal.

a. **Masseteric nerve**: passes outwards through the mandibular notch, enters the deep face of masseter and supplies it.

b. **Deep temporal nerve**: passes upward to supply temporalis.

c. **Buccinator nerve**: passes downward and forward on the medial aspect of temperomandibular articulation, runs downwards in the submucous tissue of the cheek and **supplies mucosa of the cheek.**

d. **Pterygoid nerve**: arises in common with the preceding and supplies the **pterygoideus muscles** and gives branches to tensor palate and tensor tympani.

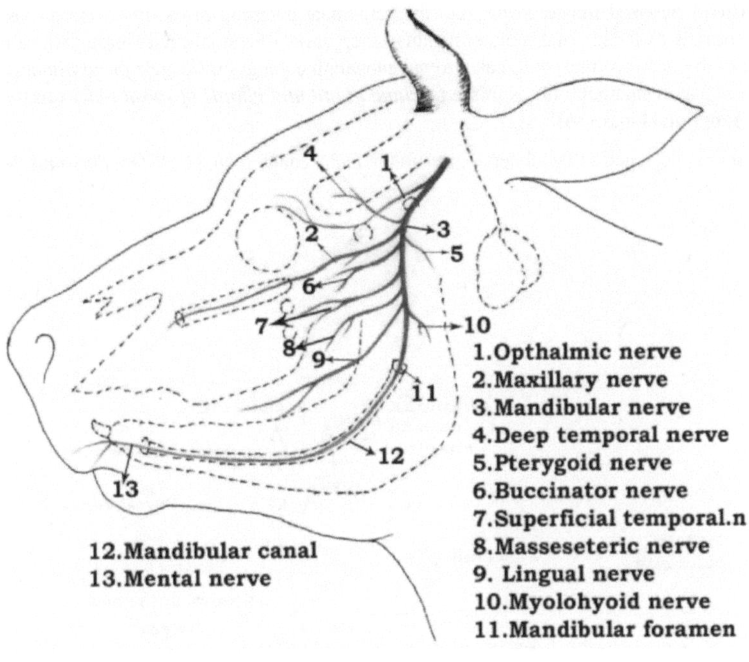

Fig. 3.115: Branches of Mandibular Nerve

e. **Mylohyoid nerve**: passes down to supply the mylohyoideus muscle and also the **anterior belly of digastricus.**

f. **Superficial temporal nerve**: passes backward to the posterior border of the mandible a little below its neck, turns outward and then forward under the parotid lymph gland and divides into **dorsal transverse facial nerve**, supplying **skin of the cheek** and a **ventral branch** which unites with the **dorsal buccal division of the facial nerve**. It also gives a branch to parotid salivary gland which conveys postganglionic secretomotor fibres from otic ganglion

g. **Lingual nerve**: runs downward and forward between the ramus of the mandible and medial pterygoid muscle to the root of the tongue, where it divides into **superficial and deep branches (Fig.3.115). The superficial branch (sublingual nerve)** accompanies the mandibular duct on the deep face of the sublingual gland and supplies the ***mucous membrane of the tongue and floor of the mouth***. The deep branch, runs **between hyoglossus and genioglossus muscles** to the tip of the tongue. **It supplies the mucous membrane of the anterior two third of the tongue.**

6. Abducent Nerve

This is the sixth cranial nerve and is a motor nerve. It arises just behind the pons, lateral to the inferior pyramid of the medulla. It leaves the cranium through the foramen orbitorotundum and supplies the ***lateral rectus and retractor oculi muscles*** of the eye in the orbit.

7. Facial Nerve

This is the seventh cranial nerve and is a **mixed nerve**. It arises from the lateral part of the corpus trapezoideum immediately behind the pons. The bent part of the nerve, genu, bears at its highest point the ***geniculate ganglion*** in facial canal. After its emergence through the stylomastoid foramen, it terminates into ***dorsal and ventral buccal nerves***. The following branches are detached within the facial canal.

The great superficial petrosal nerve arises from the geniculate ganglion in the facial canal, passes backward, reaches the cranial cavity by the internal auditory meatus, emerges out of cranial cavity through the foramen lacerum and is continued as the nerve of pterygoid canal to sphenopalatine ganglion (***largest parasympathetic ganglion***). This nerve conveys parasympathetic fibres to the ***lacrimal gland and glands of nasal mucosa*** **after relay in the sphenopalatine ganglion (Fig.3.116).**

The stapedial nerve is detached as facial nerve turns in the facial canal. It supplies ***stapedius muscle*** of the middle ear.

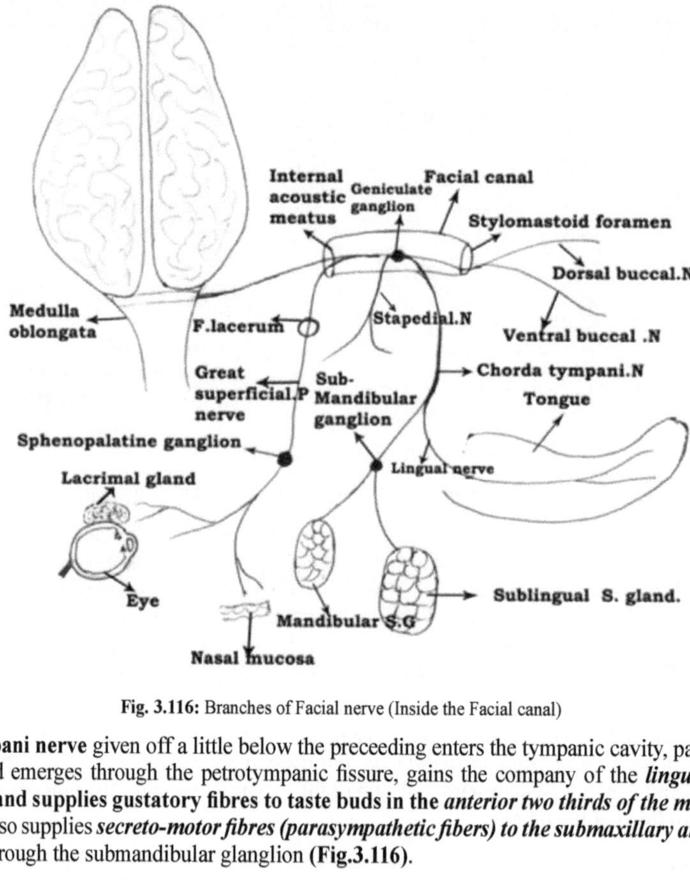

Fig. 3.116: Branches of Facial nerve (Inside the Facial canal)

The chorda tympani nerve given off a little below the preceeding enters the tympanic cavity, passes across it and then descends and emerges through the petrotympanic fissure, gains the company of the ***lingual branch of the trigeminal nerve*** **and supplies gustatory fibres to taste buds in the** ***anterior two thirds of the mucosa membrane of the tongue***. It also supplies ***secreto-motor fibres (parasympathetic fibers) to the submaxillary and the sublingual salivary glands*** through the submandibular glanglion **(Fig.3.116).**

After emerging through the stylomastoid foramen, the facial nerve gives off the following **(Fig.3.117).**

a) **Posterior auricular nerve**: which runs upward and backward under the parotid gland and ***supplies posterior auricular*** muscles.

b) **The internal or deep auricular nerve**: passes through a foramen in the conchal cartilage and supplies ***skin on the internal surface of the external ear.***

c) **Digastric branch**: descends below under the cover of parotid gland and supplies the ***posterior belly of digastricus, occipitohyoideus and stylohyoideus muscles.***

d) **Auriculopalpebral nerve**: passes upward under the parotid gland and divides into anterior auricular branch supplying anterior auricular muscles and palpebral or temporal nerve which runs forward to supply ***orbicularis oculi, corrugator supercili and levator nasolabialis muscles*** **(Fig.3.117).**

> *Auriculopalpebral nerve block can be used for eye examination. The auriculopalpebral nerve block is performed by injection of an anaesthetic agent under the skin midway between the lateral canthus of eye and the base of the ear at the level of zygomatic arch.*

e. **A cervical branch** which passes under parotid gland and parotidoauricularis muscle downward and backward and anastomoses with **cutaneous branches of cervical spinal nerves (Fig.3.117).**

Terminal Branches: After giving the above collateral branches the facial nerve finally divides into ***dorsal and ventral buccal nerves***.

a. **The dorsal buccal** nerve passes forward on the upper part of masseter and is joined by a branch from the superficial temporal division of the trigeminal nerve. It continues forward under **zygomaticus and along the ventral border of dilator naris lateralis** and ramifies on the muscles of the upper lip and nostril. **It also supplies zygomaticus, malaris and buccinator.** It anastomoses with ventral buccal nerve and receives a communicating branch along the anterior border of masseter.

> *The dorsal buccal branch of the facial nerve is vulnerable to damage in lateral recumbency during general anaesthesia when the head is not properly padded.*

b. **The ventral buccal nerve** passes downward obliquely across the lower part of masseter, runs forward along the ventral border of depressor labii inferioris. **It supplies the muscles of the lower lip (Fig.3.117).**

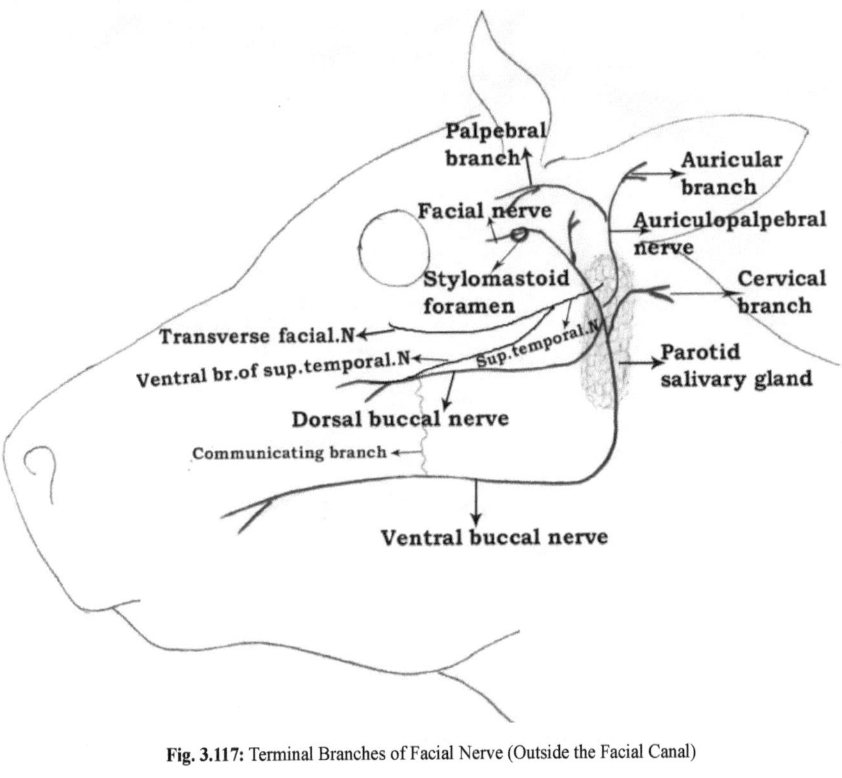

Fig. 3.117: Terminal Branches of Facial Nerve (Outside the Facial Canal)

8. Acoustic Nerve (*Vestibulocochlear Nerve*)

This is the eighth cranial nerve and is the nerve of ***sense of hearing and equilibrium***. This nerve has cochlear and vestibular branches which function as separate nerves. It arises from the **medulla oblongata** at the lateral part of the corpus trapezoideum just behind the preceding (**facial**) nerve. The nerve passes outward along with the facial to **the internal auditory meatus of petrous temporal bone**. Here it divides into two branches an **upper vestibular and the lower cochlear nerves**. In the internal auditory meatus vestibular nerve presents the **vestibular ganglion.** The ***vestibular nerve*** innervates the semicircular canals and its associated structures of internal ear. It transmits the sensation of **position and equilibrium**.

The ***cochlear*** division of the auditory nerve is concerned with ***hearing and it bears a cochlear ganglion in spiral organ of corti.***

9. Glossopharyngeal Nerve

This is the ninth cranial nerve and is a mixed nerve. It is arises from the lateral surface of the medulla oblongata. It leaves the cranium through the ***foramen lacerum (jugular foramen)***. At the level of jugular foramen it bears ***two ganglia i.e proximal (jugular) ganglion and distal (petrosal) ganglion*** **(Fig.3.118).** The ***first branch i.e tympanic nerve arises from petrosal ganglion*** *and* enters the tympanic cavity, where it joins with the branches of facial and internal carotid (sympathetic) nerves in forming plexus from which a nerve ***lesser superficial petrosal nerve*** leads to the otic ganglion to supply the ***parotid salivary gland.*** The glossopharyngeal nerve passes downward, **medial to the great cornu of the hyoid bone (Fig.3.118)** and divides into ***pharyngeal and lingual*** **branches. The former gives branches** to ***stylopharyngeus muscle and pharyngeal mucosa***. The ***lingual branch*** enters the tongue parallel to the **lingual nerve of mandibular nerve and the hypoglossal nerve (Fig.3.118)**. It gives ***sensory branches to taste buds of posterior one third of the tongue*** and motor fibers to the **levator palati muscle and the glands of soft palate.**

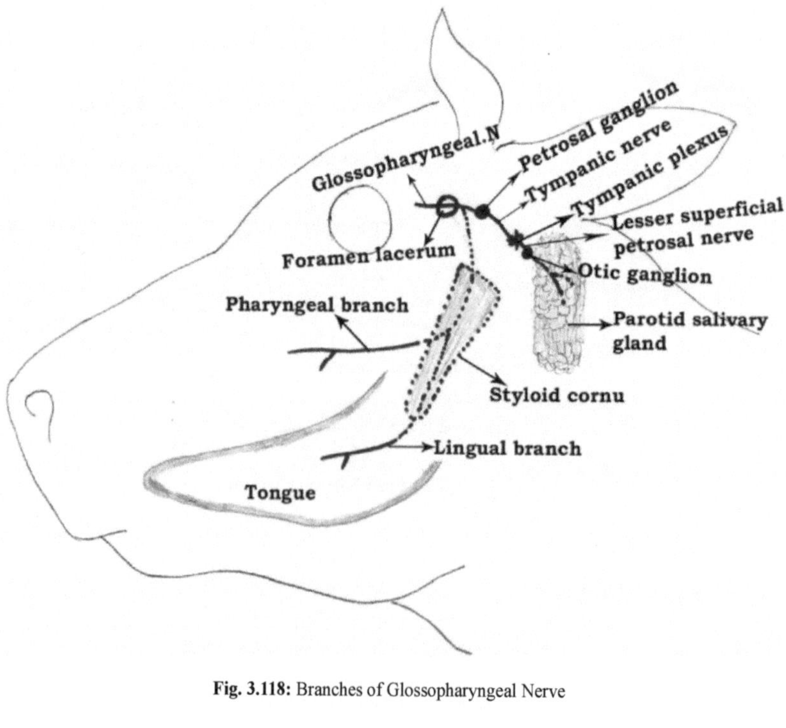

Fig. 3.118: Branches of Glossopharyngeal Nerve

10. Vagus Nerve

This is the tenth cranial nerve and is a mixed nerve. *The vagus nerve is the longest of the cranial nerves and is known as the* ***"wanderer"*** *nerve, because it supplies vast areas of the body from the head to the caudal abdomen.* It arises from lateral aspect of the medulla oblongata by several filaments. It leaves the cranium through the ***foramen lacerum***. In the foramen it bears the ***jugular ganglion***. It descends along with ***cervical sympathetic trunk*** *to form a common cord on the dorsal part of the carotid sheath above common carotid artery and descends on respective surfaces of oesophagus deeply in the jugular furrow and enters the thorax* **(Fig.3.119).** The ***right vagus*** crosses under the ***right brachial artery*** across the trachea, reaches the oesophagus behind the aortic arch and divides into dorsal and ventral branches. The ***left vagus*** enters the thoracic cavity, passes under the arch of left brachial artery and the root of the aorta, reaches the left lung and then across the surface of the oesophagus and divides into ***dorsal and ventral branches***. The two ***dorsal and the two ventral branches*** of the vagi of two sides unite forming two trunks i.e the ***dorsal and the ventral trunks*** **(Fig.3.119).** They pass through the diaphragm into the abdominal cavity to supply the abdominal organs.

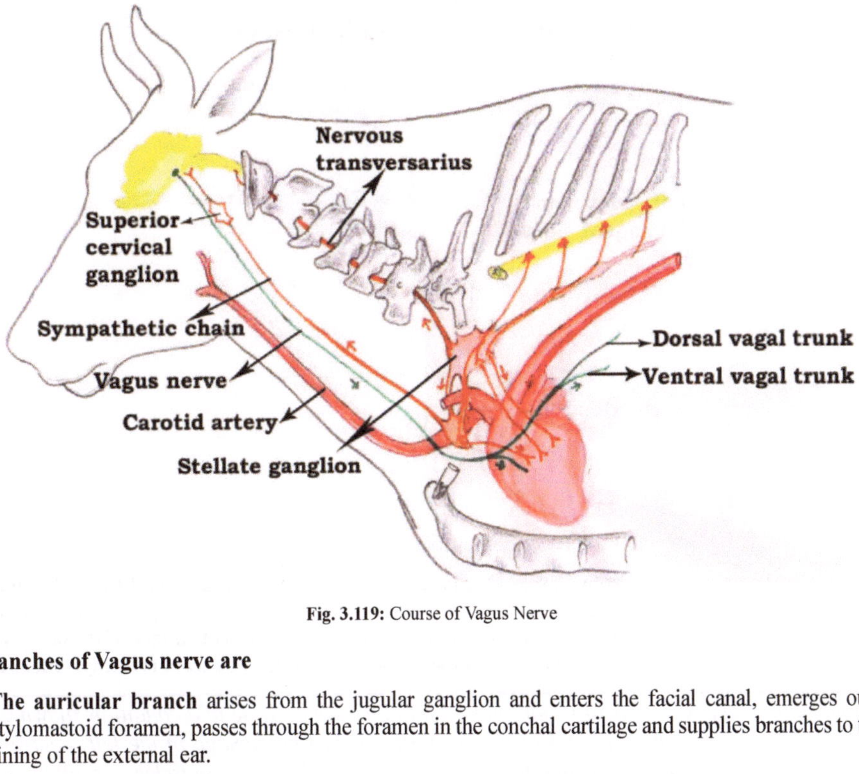

Fig. 3.119: Course of Vagus Nerve

The Branches of Vagus nerve are

(a) **The auricular branch** arises from the jugular ganglion and enters the facial canal, emerges out at the stylomastoid foramen, passes through the foramen in the conchal cartilage and supplies branches to the inner lining of the external ear.

(b) **The pharyngeal branch**: This branch with the pharyngeal branch of glossopharyngeal and the sympathetic fibers form pharyngeal plexus from which motor fibres are supplied to the **pharyngeal constrictors, muscles of soft palate except tensor palati.**

(c) **The anterior laryngeal nerve** arises from the vagus near the tympanic bulla and passes downward across the pharyngeal lymph glands and pharynx to the thyroid foramen of the larynx. It presents ***ganglion nodosum*** at its origin. Here it gives off an external branch to **cricothyroideus muscle. The internal branch enters the larynx through the thyroid foramen and is distributed to the laryngeal mucosa.**

(d) In the neck, the vagus gives off **branches to trachea and oesophagus.**

In the thoracic cavity, the vagus gives off the following branches

(e) **Cardiac branches** to the heart and **Pulmonary branches** to the lungs.

(f) **The posterior laryngeal nerves**: ***These are also called as recurrent laryngeal nerves since they take a backward course after their origin.*** These are right and left recurrent laryngeal nerves. They arise from the vagus at different levels on the two sides.

The **right recurrent laryngeal nerve** arises from vagus ***at the level of posterior border of the first rib.*** It gives sensory branches to the trachea and the oesophagus, leaves the thorax, passes up the neck **in the jugular furrow in the carotid sheath below the common carotid artery (Fig.3.120)** and gives off branches to **all the laryngeal muscles on right side except the cricothyroideus muscle.**

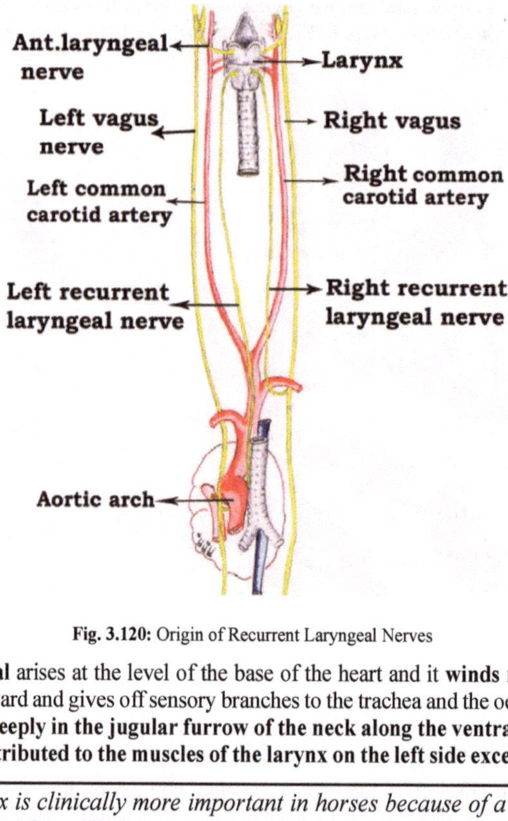

Fig. 3.120: Origin of Recurrent Laryngeal Nerves

The **left recurrent laryngeal** arises at the level of the base of the heart and it **winds round the right face of the aortic arch** then passes forward and gives off sensory branches to the trachea and the oesophagus **(Fig.3.120).** Then it leaves the thorax, passes **deeply in the jugular furrow of the neck along the ventral face of the oesophagus.** It reaches the larynx and is **distributed to the muscles of the larynx on the left side except cricothyroideus muscle.**

Anatomy of the larynx is clinically more important in horses because of a condition known as laryngeal hemiplegia (also called roaring) is mostly caused by damage of the left recurrent laryngeal nerve. This causes partial paralysis of the intrinsic laryngeal muscles, especially the cricoarytenoideus dorsalis muscle.

The dorsal trunk gives off (1) a branch accompanying omaso-abomasal artery and its divisions and **supplies omasum and abomasum** (2) branches which accompany splenic, right and left ruminal arteries supplying corresponding organs (3) branches which accompany the division of anterior mesenteric artery, supplying the **small and large intestines except the terminal colon and rectum and** (4) **branches to kidney. The ventral trunk** passes on the right face of reticulum and terminates on the parietal surface of abomasum. It gives off the ***pyloric branch*** which passes along the lesser omentum to ***supply the liver, first and second parts of duodenum and pyloric part of abomasum.***

When the caudal mediastinal lymph nodes are enlarged by a disease they disturb the functions of oesophagus or vagus nerves causing chronic bloat.

11. The Spinal Accessory Nerve

This is the eleventh cranial nerve and is a motor nerve. It has two roots i.e medullary and spinal roots. ***It is the only cranial nerve having root from spinal cord.*** The ***spinal root*** arises from the ***first five cervical segments*** of the spinal cord between dorsal and ventral roots of spinal nerves and ***enters the cranium thorugh the foramen magnum*** and joins the ***medullary root*** to form spinal accessory nerve. The medullary root arises from the lateral aspect of the medulla oblongata by several rootlets behind and in a series with those of the vagus nerve. The nerve thus formed leaves the cranial cavity along with the glossopharyngeal and vagus nerves through the ***foramen lacerum*** and pass downward and backward and divides into ***dorsal and ventral*** branches. The ***dorsal branch*** passes backward under brachiocephalicus and ramifies on the ***deep face of trapezius***. The ***ventral branch*** passes downward across the oesophagus and trachea and ***supplies strenocephalicus*** **(Fig.3.121).**

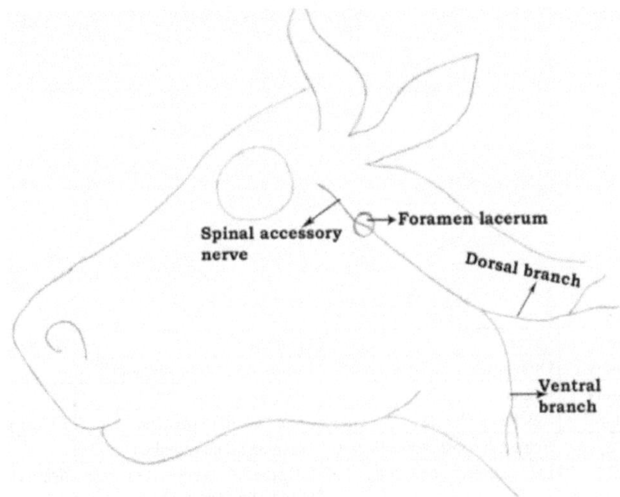

Fig. 3.121: Branches of Spinal Accessory Nerve

12. Hypoglossal Nerve

It is the twelth cranial nerve and is the motor nerve to the muscles of the tongue. Its fibres arise from the ventral face of the medulla in a series lateral to the posterior half of the pyramid. The nerve then emerges through the ***hypoglossal foramen*** runs downwards and backward **parallel to the styloid cornu of hyoid** and related to the atlanto-occipital articulation **(Fig.3.122).** It passes over the glossopharyngeal nerve and common carotid artery. ***It supplies the muscles of the tongue.***

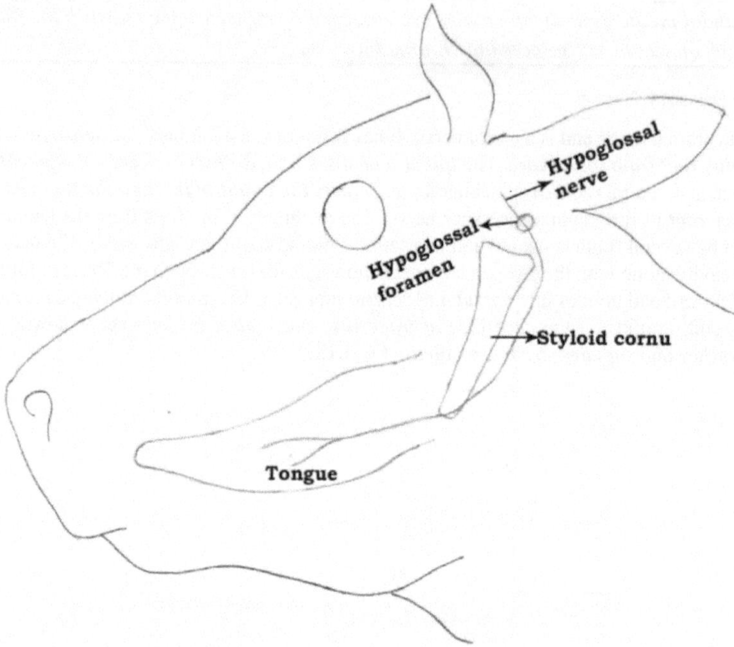

Fig. 3.122: Course of Hypoglossal Nerve

Name	Type	Origin	Foramen	Associated Ganglion
1.Olfactory	Sensory	Olfactory mucous membrane	Cribriform plate of ethmoid	-
2.Optic	Sensory	Retina	Optic formen	-
3.Oculomotor	Motor	Cerebral peduncles	Foramen orbitorotundum	***Ciliary ganglion***
4.Trochlear	Motor	Behind the posterior colliculus	Foramen orbitorotundum	-
5.Trigeminal	Mixed	Lateral aspect of the pons	**a.Opthalmic Nerve**- (Foramen orbitorotundum) **b.Maxillary Nerve**- (Foramen orbitorotundum) **c.Mandibular Nerve** (Foramen ovale)	***Semilunar ganglion***
6.Abducent	Motor	Inferior pryramids of medulla oblonagata	Foramen orbitorotundum	-
7.Facial	Mixed	Corpus trapezoideum	Stylomastoid foramen	***Geniculate ganglion***
8.Auditory	Sensory	Corpus trapezoideum	Interanl acoustic meatus	***Vestibular and Cochlear ganglia***
9.Glosso-pharyngeal	Mixed	Medulla oblongta	Foramen lacerum	***Otic ganglion***
10.Vagus	Mixed	Medulla oblongata	Foramen lacerum	***Jugular ganglion***
11.Spinal accessory	Motor	Medulla oblongata and spinal cord	Foramen lacerum	-
12.Hypoglossal	Motor	Posterior part of pyramids of medulla oblongata	Hypoglossal foramen	-

AUTONOMIC NERVOUS SYSTEM

It controls the activities of **secretory glands**, **smooth muscles** (in the walls of viscera and blood vessels) and **cardiac muscle.**It is nothing but ***visceral efferent (motor) nervous system.***

It consists of fibres emerging from the **midbrain, medulla oblongata** of the brain stem and **thoracic, lumbar and sacral portions of spinal cord.** The efferent part of autonomic system is characterized by interruption in ganglia located outside the central nervous system, so that it consists of **preganglionic and postganglionic parts**. The ***preganglionic fibres are medullated and postganglionic fibres are nonmedullated.***

The **craniosacral** outflow from the brain and sacral segments of spinal cord constitutes the ***parasympathetic system.*** The outflow from the ***thoracic and lumbar parts*** of spinal cord constitutes the ***sympathetic system.***

The parasympathetic system does not pass in any independent pathways, but its fibres are incorporated in the ***III (Oculomotor), VII (Facial), IX (Glossopharyngeal) and X (Vagus)*** cranial nerves and **ventral primary branches of third, fourth and fifth sacral spinal nerves.** The ganglia where the fibres are interrupted are generally located in the walls of the organs supplied (***intramural***) excepting **ciliary, sphenopalatine, submandibular and otic ganglia** in the course of the cranial distribution, which are located outside the organs supplied.

The **sympathetic system** consists of preganglionic fibres emerging from the **thoracic and lumbar parts** of spinal cord and are interrupted in ganglia located close to the vertebral column called as the ***vertebral or lateral ganglia.*** The ganglia situated more peripherally are called the ***collateral ganglia*** (**Coeliac, anterior and posterior mesenteric ganglia**).

The parasympathetic and sympathetic systems are ***mutually antagonistic*** in their actions, physiologically and pharmacologically. The visceral organs are supplied by both the systems, the fibres from each forming networks of plexuses.

Anatomical Differences between parasympathetic and sympathetic nervous systems:

Parasympathetic nervous system	Sympathetic nervous system
Cranio-sacral part	Thoraco-lumbar part
Preganglionic fibers are long and postganglionic fibers are short	Preganglionic fibers are short and postganglionic fibers are long
Increases the secretory activity of glands of digestive and respiratory system	Inhibits the secretory activity of glands of digestive and respiratory system.
Motor to smooth muscles of digestive and respiratory system.	Inhibits the activity of smooth muscles of digestive and respiratory system. But motor to arrectores pilorum muscle of the skin.
Decreases the heart rate	Increases the heart rate.
Inhibits the secretory activity of sweat glands	Increases the secretory activity of sweat glands
Constricts the pupil	Dilates the pupil
Stimulated by Acetylcholine	Stimulated by adrenaline

The Parasymapathetic System

The efferent pathways consists of cranial and sacral parts.

The cranial part: The cranial part consists of efferent fibres present in the ***third, seventh, ninth and tenth cranial nerves*****(Fig.3.123).** The **oculomotor parasympathetic** fibres arise from the ***Edinger Westphal nucleus*** in the mid brain. The preganlionic fibres pass along the nerves in the branches supplying the inferior oblique muscle and enter the **ciliary ganglion**. The postganglionic fibres leave the ganglion by the short ciliary nerves to distribute to the **ciliary muscle and constrictor pupillae of the iris.**

The ***facial nerve*** contains efferent fibres which arise in the **superior salivary nucleus** of the medulla oblongata. These pass along the facial, then in its chorda tympani branch and ultimately reach the lingual nerve and enter the **submandibular ganglion**. The postganglionic fibres from this ganglion supply the **mandibular and sublingual salivary glands**. Some parasympathetic fibers travel in the **great superficial petrosal nerve**, reaching the **sphenopalatine ganglion from which postganglionic fibers** are relayed to the mucous membrane of the nose and palate and to the ***lacrimal gland*** via ***the zygomatic branch of maxillary nerve and the lacrimal nerve*** **(Fig.3.123).**

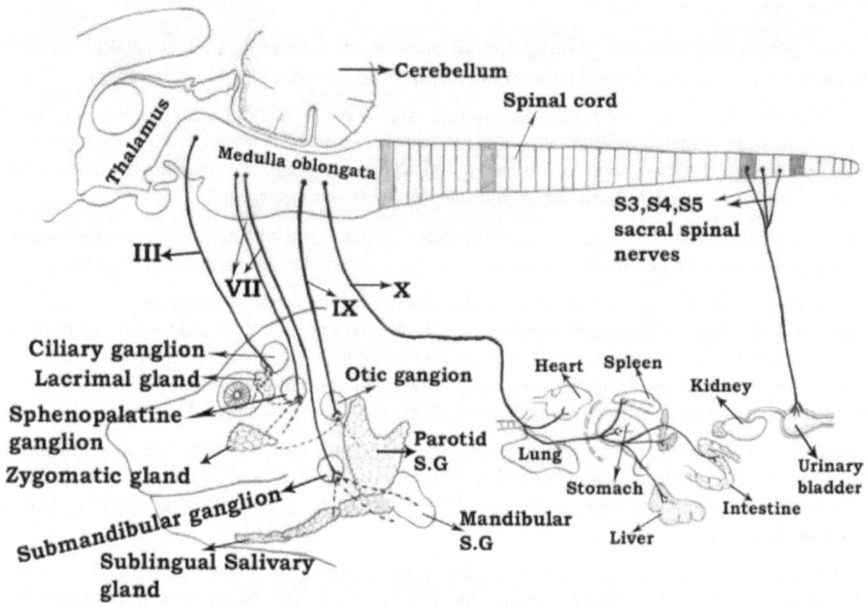

Fig. 3.123: Distribution of Parasympathetic Nerve Fibers

The ***sphenopalatine ganglion*** is the largest of the **cephalic parasympathetic ganglia** and is placed deeply in the pterygopalatine fossa close to the sphenopalatine foramen.

The **glossopharyngea**l nerve contains efferent fibres which arise in the **inferior salivary nucleus** of the medulla oblongata, travel in this nerve and its tympanic branch, traverse the tympanic plexus and enter the lesser superficial petrosal nerve and terminate in the **otic ganglion**. This ganglion is placed immediately below the **foramen ovale** on the internal face of the **mandibular nerve**. From this ganglion the postganglionic fibres are relayed through the superficial temporal nerve and supply secretomotor fibres to the **parotid salivary gland (Fig.3.123).**

The **vagus** contains a very **large proportion of parasympathetic fibres** which arise in the dorsal nucleus of vagus in medulla oblongata, travel in this nerve and in its **oesophageal, pulmonary cardiac, gastric and intestinal branches.** The branches terminate in small ganglia placed in the walls of individual viscera (i.e ***intramural ganglioa eg: Meissner's plexus and Aurebach's plexus***). The **postganglionic fibres are relayed finally in the glands and smooth muscles and cardiac musculature (Fig.3.123).**

Cranial nerve/Spinal nerve	Origin of parasympathetic nerve fibers	Associated ganglion	Structures supplied
Oculomotor nerve	Edinger Westphal nucleus of mid brain	Ciliary ganglion	Constrictor pupillae and ciliary muscle of eye
Facial nerve	Superior salivary nucleus of medulla oblongata	Submandibular ganglion *Sphenopalatine ganglion (Largest parasympathetic ganglion)*	Submandibular and sublingual salivary gland. Lacrimal gland
Glossopharyngeal nerve	Inferior salivary nucleus of medulla oblongata	Otic ganglion	Parotid salivary gland
Vagus nerve	Dorsal vagal nucleus of medulla oblongata	Ganglia present in walls of the viscera *(Myenteric plexus and Aurebach's plexus)*	Heart, Lungs, stomach, Intestine etc.,
S3, S4,S5 sacral spinal nerves	Lateral horn of spinal cord (Sacral part)	Ganglia present in walls of the viscera	Rectum, urinary bladder, uterus and other genital organs

The sacral part: The sacral part of the efferent parasympathetic fibres are contained in the ventral primary divisions of the **third, fourth and fifth sacral spinal** nerves. The visceral branches containing these fibres form a plexus with the sympathetic pelvic plexus. Minute parasympathetic ganglia are located in the walls of the viscera and from here the postganglionic fibres are relayed to **rectum, urinary bladder, uterus, pelvis and external genitalia.**

The Sympathetic System: This is the **larger subdivision** of the autonomic nervous system and includes two ganglionated cords with their branches and plexuses and two collateral ganglia **(coeliaco-mesenteric and posterior mesenteric ganglia)**. It has a much wider distribution, as it **innervates all sweat glands of the skin, arrectores pilorum muscles, muscular walls of blood vessels in addition to viscera.**

The preganglionic fibres of the thirteen thoracic and the first four lumbar segments of spinal cord are interrupted in the ganglia situated on either side of the vertebral column. The ganglia form a ganglionated trunk on either side of the vertebral column extending from the head to the sacrum. The number of ganglia correspond to the number of segments of the **spinal cord in the thoracic, lumbar and sacral regions except in the cervical region** (in the adult). In cervical region generally only two ganglia are present i.e ***superior and inferior cervical ganglia*** and there is only **one (unpaired) ganglion present in coccygeal region (*ganglion impar*)**. In addition to the gangliated sympathetic trunk, the **coeliac, anterior and posterior mesenteric ganglia represent the collateral ganglia** in which sympathetic efferents are relayed **(Fig.3.126).** These *ganglia are present in the abdominal cavity on the walls of the corresponding arteries and the postganglionic fibres supply the viscera of the abdominal and pelvic cavities*

The sympathetic ganglia are connected to the spinal nerve by a ramus communicans. This contains white and gray rami. The **white ramus** contains the **preganglionic** efferents from the spinal cord to the ganglia. The **gray ramus** contains ***post ganglionic fibres*** to ***blood vessels, sweat glands and arrectores pilorum muscles of skin*** **(Fig.3.124).**

The **preganglionic fibres** arising from the lateral horn cells of spinal cord pass via the ventral root of the spinal nerve and enter the ganglion of the sympathetic trunk and from here, **postganglionic fibres** supply the viscera. Some of the post **postganglionic** fibres join back the spinal nerves i.e gray ramus and supply ***blood vessels, sweat glands and arrectores pilorum muscles of the skin*** **(Fig.3.124).**

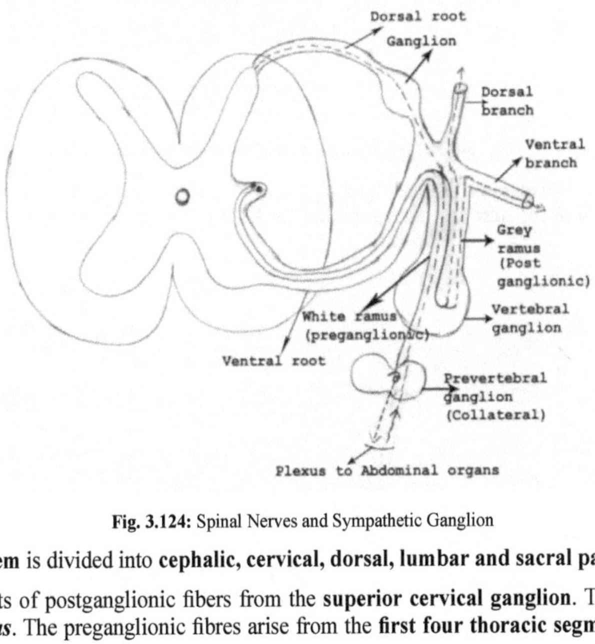

Fig. 3.124: Spinal Nerves and Sympathetic Ganglion

The **sympathetic system** is divided into **cephalic, cervical, dorsal, lumbar and sacral parts.**

Cephalic part: consists of postganglionic fibers from the **superior cervical ganglion**. The ***ganglion is situated below the wing of atlas***. The preganglionic fibres arise from the **first four thoracic segments** of spinal cord and reach the ganglion by the **cervical sympathetic trunk**. The postganglionic fibres from this ganglion supply gray rami to **first cervical spinal and last four cranial nerves** and branches also accompany common carotid artery and its branches to supply the structures of the head.

Cervical part: consists of the **superior and inferior cervical ganglia**, connected by an intervening cord (cervical sympathetic trunk) on either side. The **inferior cervical ganglion** is placed on the internal face of the costal insertion of the scalenus ventralis muscle and against the longus colli. It is usually flattened and ***united with the first thoracic ganglion to form the stellate ganglion.*** This ganglion gives the cervical trunk and detaches anteriorly the ***nervus transversarius*** which **accompanies the vertebral artery in canalis transversarius (Fig.3.125).** This nerve passes through the **canalis transversarius** and supplies smooth muscles of blood vessels. It detaches two or three cardiac branches which with the vagus form a cardiac plexus.

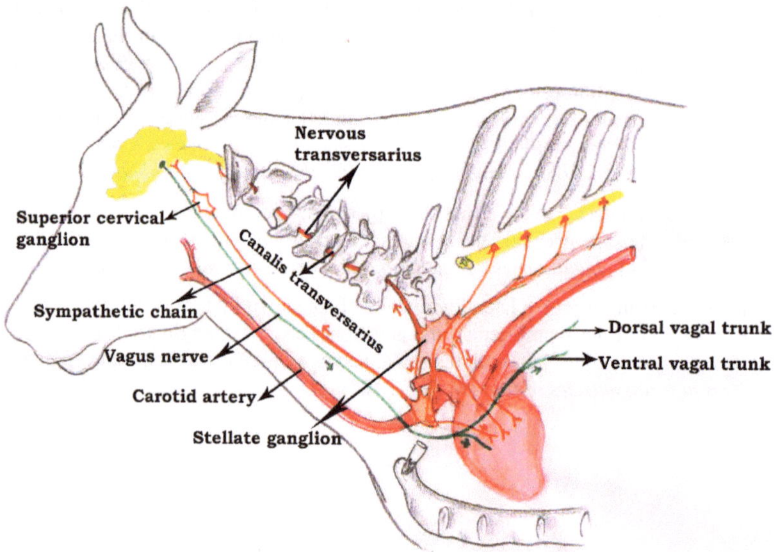

Fig 3.125: Sympathetic Trunk in Neck Region

Thoracic part consists of **thirteen pairs of ganglia** on either side connected by a cord which extends from the **inferior cervical ganglion to the first lumbar ganglion (Fig.3.126).**

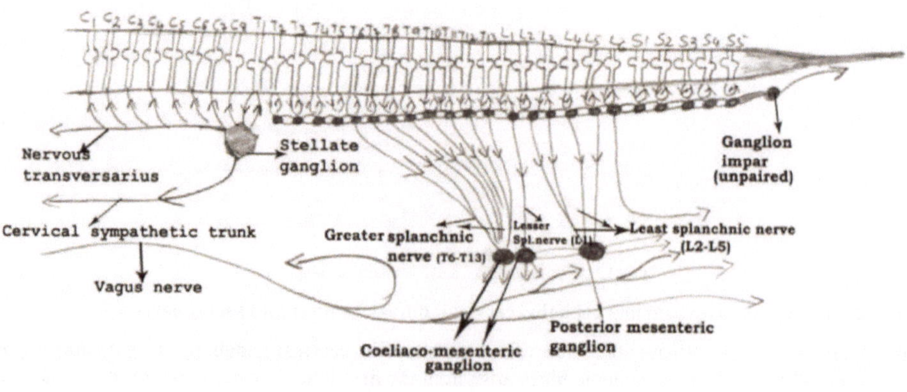

Fig. 3.126: Sympathetic Chain

The first four thoracic ganglia give (a) **aortic branches** (b) **cardiac branches** (c) **pulmonary branches** and (d) **oesophageal branches.** These unite with the respective fibres of the vagus and form plexuses and supply the viscera.

The ***greater splanchnic nerve*** is **formed by preganglionic fibers arising from the fifth thoracic ganglion to the thirteenth thoracic ganglion (T5-T13).** *It passes* backward between the crura of the diaphragm and the psoas minor, enters the abdomen and joins the coeliaco-mesenteric ganglia.

The ***lesser splanchnic nerve*** is formed by fibres from the **first lumbar ganglion (L1)** which joins the coeliac ganglion and adrenal plexus. The ***least splanchnic nerve*** is **formed by preganglionic fibers arising from the 2nd lumbar to 5th lumbar ganglia (L2-L5).**

Abdominal or lumbar part is the continuation of thoracic trunk. It lies along the internal border of the psoas minor muscle above the aorta and posterior venacava and presents ***six pairs* of ganglia** which are connected by rami communicans to spinal nerves. Abdominal part consists of **collateral ganglia. These are *coeliac, anterior mesenteric and posterior mesenteric ganglia* (Fig. 3.126).** They are present along the course of coeliac, anterior mesenteric and posterior mesenteric arteries **and they form coeliac plexus, anterior mesenteric plexus and posterior mesenteric plexus** respectively. The coeliac plexus and its divisions supply the viscera and form **subsidiary plexuses such as gastric plexus, hepatic plexus, splenic plexus and pancreatic plexus** to supply these organs.

The post ganglionic fibres from **anterior mesenteric ganglion** supply subsidiary plexuses to the different parts of **the intestine, except terminal colon and rectum and kidney**. The post ganglionic fibres from **posterior mesenteric ganglion supply rectum, kidney, testis in male and ovary in female.**

Pelvic or sacral part is the continuation of the lumbar trunk. It extends along the inferior face of the sacrum and consists of ***five pairs of ganglia* (Fig.3.126).** The **pelvic plexuses** are formed by branches from the **lumbar and sacral ganglia** and from posterior mesenteric ganglia. From here secondary plexuses supply **rectum, bladder, uterus, vagina, accessory sex glands and cavernous tissue of penis or clitoris.**

The sacral parts of the two sympathetic trunks unite behind, below the last sacral segment to form the ***ganglion impar (unpaired,* Fig.3.126)** which is continued by the coccygeal nerve that accompanies the middle coccygeal artery.

3.7 NERVE BLOCKS AND NEURECTOMIES OF THE HEAD AND NECK

1. Cornual Nerve block: Cornual nerve is a sensory nerve supplying to the horn core and skin around its base. It is a branch of lacrimal nerve which is a division of the opthalmic branch of trigeminal nerve.

The cornual nerve emerges behind the orbit and ascends along frontal crest and placed relatively superficial in the upper third covered by skin and the thin layer of frontalis. The caudal part of the nerve is having close association with the superficial temporal artery.

Indications: for amputation of horn and in certain conditions affecting the horn.Ex: Horn cancer, horn fracture.

Site: *close to frontal crest of the frontal bone about one inch below the base of the horn* midway between eye and horn below the frontal crest **(Fig.3.127).**

> Cornual nerve block in sheep is to be done at caudal border of the root of the zygomatic process and dorsal margin of orbit. In goat both cornual branch of zygomaticotemporal nerve at caudal border of the root of zygomatic process and cornual branch of the infratrochlear nerve at the rostrodorsal margin of the orbit at one third of the distance from medial angle to lateral angle of the eye have to be blocked.

2. Mandibular nerve block: The mandibular nerve is a branch of trigeminal and enters the mandibular foramen on the medical aspect of vertical ramus of the mandible and emerges through mental foramen, on the lateral aspect of the mandible at the junction of body and horizontal ramus. During its course sensory branches are given off to teeth and gums of lower jaw.

Indications: To desensitize the cheek teeth, alveoli and gums of lower jaw.

Site: At the mandibular foramen on the medial aspect of the vertical ramus. The nerve can be blocked by inserting a long needle medial to the mandible to the intersection of the plane of the occlusal surfaces of the cheek teeth and a line from the vascular groove to the temporomandibular articulation **(Fig.3.127).**

3. Mental nerve block: The mandibular nerve gains exit at the mental foramen at the junction of lateral aspect of the body and horizontal ramus of the mandible. The mental foramen and nerve are on the lateral surface of the body of the mandible caudal to the fourth incisor.

Indications: To desensitize the lower lip.

Site: *At the mental foramen of the mandible at the junction of the horizontal ramus and body* **(Fig.3.127).** Mental foramen is palpated caudal to fourth incisor at the level of the rostral end of the mandibular space. This nerve block anaesthetizes incisors, lower lip and chin.

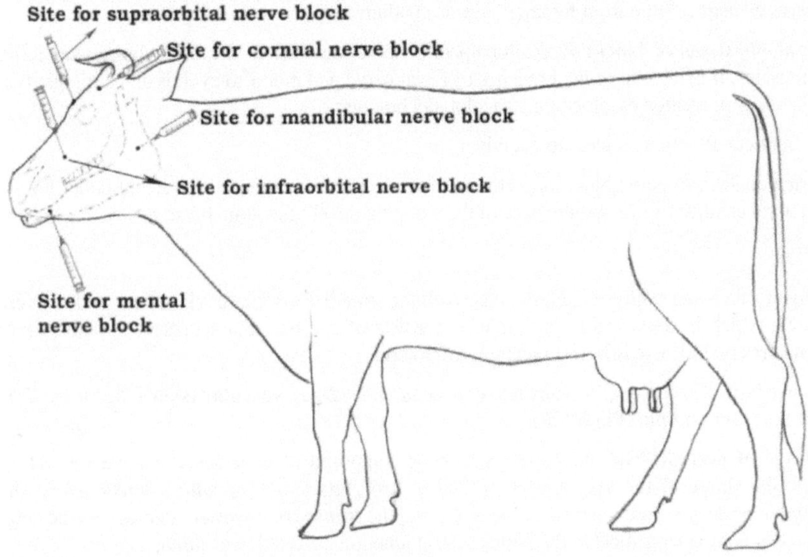

Fig. 3.127: Sites for Nerve Blocks of the Head

4. Maxillary nerve block: The maxillary nerve which is a branch of the trigeminal nerve, is sensory in nature and emerges through the foramen orbitorotundum, passes forwards in the pterygopalatine fossa and enters into infraorbital canal through maxillary foramen. The maxillary nerve gives branches to the teeth of upper jaw.

Indications: To desensitize the teeth, alveoli and gums of upper jaw.

Site: The maxillary foramen to be reached by inoculation needle through the site 2 to 3 cm below the external canthus of the eye and between the posterior border of the malar bone and coronoid process of mandible.

5. Infraorabital nerve block: Infraorbital nerve is the continuation of maxillary nerve and emerges out through infraorbital foramen.

Indications: Surgical interference with the upper lip and nostrils or to place nasal rings in bulls.

Site: *The infraorbital foramen is reached through above the level of the upper 3rd cheek tooth in canines and horses and 1st cheek tooth in ox* **(Fig.3.127).**

6. Supraorbital (frontal) nerve block: Supraorbital (frontal) nerve is one of the terminal branches of the opthalmic division of the fifth cranial nerve. It is accompanied by the supraorbital artery and is sensory to the upper eyelid.

Indications: To desensitize the upper eyelid.

Site: *At the root of the supraorbital process* **(Fig.3.127).**

7. Orbital nerve block (Peterson's block): Opthalmic and maxillary branches of trigeminal nerve are sensory in nature and emerge out from the cranium through foramen orbitorotundum. The opthalmic nerve supplies branches to the eye ball proper, eyelids, conjunctiva, lacrimal sac and third eyelid, while zygomatic branch of maxillary nerve supplies to skin of lower eyelid.

Indications: Evisceration of the eyeball, orbital abscesses, malignant diseases of eye.

Site: Foramen orbitorotundum through behind the middle of the supraorbital process in the temporal fossa. A 12cm curved needle is inserted in the angle between the frontal and temporal processes of the zygomatic bone and is passed across the rostral border of the coronoid process of the mandible to reach III, IV, VI and ophthalmic and maxillary nerves as they emerge from foramen orbitorotundum

8. Auriculopalpebral nerve block: Auriculopalpebral nerve supplies to the orbicularis oculi muscle besides external ear muscles. It is the one of the branches of facial nerve and motor to eyelids and auricular (ear) muscles. Closure of eyelids is prevented by blocking auriculopalpebral nerve.

Indications: Surgical affections related to eyelids.

Site: The auriculopalpebral nerve block is performed by injection of an anaesthetic agent under the skin midway between the lateral canthus of eye and the base of the ear at the level of zygomatic arch.

EYE

Eye is the organ of vision, which is able to receive light stimuli from the environment and convert it into an electrical signal, which is conveyed to the brain. It consists of eye ball and accessory structures (adnexa), The accessory structures include **eye lids and lacrimal apparatus**.

Structure of eye ball: it consists of **fibrous layer** (***cornea and sclera***), **vascular layer** (***choroid, ciilray body and iris***) and **nervous layer** (***retina***, **(Fig.3.128).**

1. Fibrous layer of eyeball: The outer fibrous layer is composed of very dense collagenous tissue, which is responsible for the **shape of the eye**. It is composed of two parts i.e the ***opaque, whitish sclera***, that encloses approximately the posterior three quarters of the globe and the ***transparent cornea***, that covers the anterior part of the globe. The two components meet at the corneoscleral junction, referred to as ***limbus***.

Sclera: The sclera varies in thickness, being thinnest near to the equator (up to 0.5 mm) and gaining in the thickness towards the posterior pole of the eye (up to 2 mm). At the corneoscleral junction, the inner surface of the sclera is marked by a small ridge, where the ciliary muscle attaches. The outer surface is marked by the **scleral groove** (***sulcus sclerae***), which is especially **prominent in carnivores**. The scleral venous plexus, through which the aqueous humor drains, is located between these two structures and is important for the regulation of the ocular pressure.

Cornea: The cornea forms the anterior, transparent segment of the fibrous layer of the eyeball and bulges forward. Its proper substance consists of parallel fibers of collagen, that are arranged in a lamellar form. ***The highest point of the cornea is called the vertex***. The ***cornea of carnivores is rounded, while it is oval in ungulates.***

2. The Vascular Tunic: It lies internal to the fibrous tunic and comprises the ***choroid, ciliary body and iris in caudo cranial sequence.***

The **choroid** is a thin membrane lying between the sclera and retina. It is loosely attached to the sclera by the ***lamina fusca*** except where vessels and nerves pass through. The internal surface is in intimate contact with the pigment layer of the retina. The choroid is generally dark brown in colour but an extensive area above the level of the optic papilla has a **metallic luster**, the colour varying from iridescent blue to green, the tapetum of the chorioid. Posteriorly it is perforated by the optic nerve. It is continuous anteriorly with the ciliary body.

Ciliary body: It is the middle part of the vascular tunic and connects the choriod with the periphery of the iris. The ***body presents on its internal surface the ciliary processes and on its external face the ciliary muscle.*** It consists of 3 parts i.e **(1) ciliary ring (2) ciliary processes and (3) ciliary muscle (Fig.3.128).** The ciliary ring is thicker than the choroid. On its internal face it presents numerous ridges, the union of which form the ciliary processes.There are approximately **70-80 ciliary processes in the dog and more than 100 in the ox and horse.**

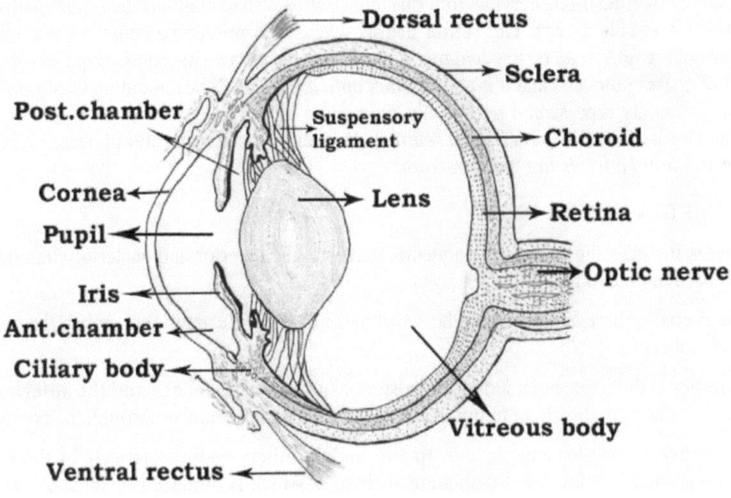

Fig. 3.128: Structure of Eye Ball

The ciliary muscle constitutes the outer part of the ciliary body and lies between the sclera and ciliary processes. It forms a circular band of unstriped muscle and its fibres are directed meridionally. They arise from the inner face of the sclera and ligamentum pectinatum iridis close to the sclero-corneal junction, run backward along the sclera and are inserted to the ciliary processes and ring. When *the muscle contracts, it pulls the ciliary processes forwards, thus slackening the suspensory ligament of the lens and allows the later to become more convex* **(Fig.3.128).** ***This is the mechanism of accommodation of eye for near objects.***

Iris: is the continuation of the ciliary body and constitutes the **most anterior part of the vascular layer**. It is a thin ring of highly vascular tissue that rests against the anterior surface of the lens **(Fig.3.128).** The free margin of the iris borders the pupil through which light enters the posterior part of the eye. ***The pupil is transversely elliptical when constricted and becomes round when dilated. The granula iridis*** *(iridic granules i.e corpora nigra)* ***are more prominent at the upper margin of the pupil.*** *The bovine iris is wide horizontally.* The periphery of the iris is continuous with the ciliary body and irido-corneal angle. ***The iris separates the space between cornea and lens into anterior and posterior chambers of the eye, which communicate through the pupil and contain aqueous humor*** **(Fig.3.128).** The size of the pupil and the amount of light reaching the retina are regulated by smooth ***sphincter (constrictor) and dilator muscles*** in the iris. The ***sphincter lies near the pupillary margin which on contraction narrows the pupil***, while the fibers of the ***dilator are arranged radially and upon contraction enlarge the pupil.***

Iris angle: is occupied by a loose spongy tissue, its outer border forms the inner wall of canal of **schlemm**. The spaces of the meshwork are called ***spaces of Fontana*** and are in communication with the anterior chamber.The ***canal of schlemm*** appears in meridional sections as one or more endothelial lined oval spaces. It communicates with the anterior ciliary veins in the neighbouring scleral tissue. Together with the spaces of the canal forms an exit for the intraocular fluid. The aqueous humor secreted by the epithelium over the ciliary processes, passes from the posterior chamber, through the pupil into the anterior chamber. On reaching the angle of iris, it passes through the spaces of Fontana to the canal of schlemm.

Diseases of the eye in animals include glaucoma (increased intraocular pressure) and cataract (increased opacity of the lens with ageing). Glaucoma can be caused by inadequate drainage of the aqueous humor which is continuously produced by the ciliary body.

3. The Nervous Layer (Retina): The nervous (internl) tunic of the eyeball contains the light sensitive receptor cells and is kown as the ***retina* (Fig.3.128).** The **retina begins** where the optic nerve penetrates the choroid. Only the posterior two thirds of the retina can be reached by light entering the pupil. This part is relatively thick and contains all ten layers including receptor cells and it is called "***pars optica retinae***". The remaining third is ***blind called "pars ceca retinae***" and is mainly represented by the thin pigmented layer that continues on to the ciliary body ***(pars ciliaris retinae)*** and back of the iris ***(pars iridica retinae).*** The edge caused by an abrupt decrease in thickness at the ***junction of optic and blind parts is the "orra serrata".***

REFRACTIVE MEDIA OF THE EYE

The refractive media includes the cornea, the aqueous humor in the anterior and posterior chambers, the lens and the vitreous body between it and the retina.

Chambers of the eyeball: There are three chambers within the eyeball, the anterior chamber, the posterior chamber and the vitreous chamber.

The **anterior chamber** is the space bounded by the posterior surface of the **cornea and the anterior surface of the iris**. The anterior chamber is in direct communication with the posterior chamber through the aperture of the pupil.

The **posterior chamber** is bounded anteriorly by the iris and the ciliary body, posteriorly by the lens capsule. The anterior and posterior chambers are filled with aqueous humor, which is produced by an active secretory process from the epithelium of the ciliary body. **It is a clear and colorless fluid, containing several electrolytes, glucose, amino acids and ascorbic acid**. It is important for the nutrition of the avascular structures of the eye (**cornea and lens**).

In the healthy eye the rate of production balances the rate of drainage, thus keeping intraocular pressure constant. *Impairment of outflow results in an increase in intraocular pressure (**glaucoma**) leading to retinal atrophy and blindness.*

Vitreous body: The vitreous chamber is the **largest of the three chambers** of the eye. It is bounded anteriorly by the lens and ciliary body, the retina encloses the reminder. The vitreous chamber is occupied by the vitreous body, a soft, clear gel, that conforms to the shape of its surroundings. **It is mainly composed of the vitreous humor, a solution of mucopolysaccharides rich in hyaluronic acid (99% water, 1% solids). It is almost acellular, except for a few hyalocytes, that produce protein fibers**. These fibers reinforce the structure of the vitreous body and are essential to its gel characteristics. The **hyaloid canal** traverses the vitreous body from the posterior surface of the lens to the optic disc. It is the remnant of the hyaloid artery, a branch of the retinal arteries, which supply the lens during embryological development. This artery usually degenerates after birth and the lens is then nourished by diffusion. ***The hyaloid canal is present in the ox, pig and carnivores. In the ox, sheep and pig the vitreous body is a relatively dense structure, while in the horse it has a low density*** *and in* ***carnivores*** *it has a dense core, but a low density in the periphery.*

The refractive power of an optical component is determined by its refractive index, thickness and surface curvature. The **cornea is the most powerful refractive** component of the eye, while the **lens has the highest refractive index**, being surrounded by media with similar indices. The lens is the only refractive component, that is capable of changing its refractive index.

Lens: The lens is a transparent, biconvex structure suspended by the ciliary zonule. It has anterior and posterior poles, an equator and a central axis. The posterior surface is usually more convex than the anterior. During accommodation, the convexity of the lens changes. In the adult the lens is avascular and nutrition is provided by diffusion from the aqueous and vitreous humors. Structures of the lens are capsule of the lens, lens epithelium and lens fibers.

The entire lens is covered by the lens capsule, which consists of a semipermeable, basement membrane, secreted by the cells of the lens epithelium. It is highly refractile and elastic. The zonular fibers, suspend the lens, insert into the superficial layers of the lens capsule. The lens rests in a depression in the vitreous humor, which is tightly adherent to the posterior capsule of the lens. The lens substance consists of concentric lamellae or lens fibres which are colourless and transparent. The substance of the lens is enclosed by a ***lens capsule*** and it is highly elastic. The lens substance consists of a softer cortical and a dense central part called the ***nucleus of the lens. The lens is devoid of vessels and nerves.***

Eyelids: are two musculofibrous folds of which the upper one is more extensive and more mobile. The free margins of the eyelids meet at the medial and lateral angles of the eye and bound an opening known as the **palpebral fissure**. The cilia **(eyelashes)** are usually more prominent and numerous on the upper than on the lower lid. ***In lower eyelids of carnivores cilia are absent***. The posterior surface of the lid is lined with conjunctiva, a thin, transparent mucous membrane. The ***palpebral conjunctiva*** is reflected at the base of the lids to continue on the sclera as the ***bulbar conjunctiva***, which ends at the limbus. The potential space between lids and the eyeball is known as the ***conjunctival sac*** and their dorsal and ventral extremities are the ***fornices***. A slight mucosal elevation, the ***lacrimal caruncle***, is present in the medial angle of the eye. Between the lacrimal caruncle and the eyeball is a dorsoventrally oriented ***conjunctival fold present known as the third eyelid.*** The third eyelid is supported by a **T-shaped piece of cartilage**. The stem of the cartilage is surrounded by an additional lacrimal gland, the **gland of the third eyelid**.

THE LACRIMAL APPARATUS: This consists of the **lacrimal gland proper**, the **gland (s) associated with the third eyelid, several small accessory glands** and a **duct system** that conveys the lacrimal fluid (tears), after it has washed over the eye, into the nasal cavity for evaporation.

The lacrimal gland is flat and lies between the eyeball and the **dorsolateral wall of the orbit.** *The broad dorsal end of lacrimal gland lies under the root of the supraorbital process and long thin tail extends around lateral margin of orbit to a point below lateral angle.* Its secretion is drained by many minute ducts into the dorsal fornix of the conjunctival sac, where it mixes with the secretions of the glands and goblet cells of conjunctiva.

The **puncta lacrimalia** are minute slits, one on the edge of each lid next to the caruncle. Each punctum leads to a short, narrow canaliculus through which the fluid flows to the much larger nasolacrimal duct. The beginning of the **nasolacrimal duct is slightly enlarged, forming the lacrimal sac**, which occupies a funnel shaped fossa near the bony margin of the orbit. The nasolacrimal duct runs rostrally, at first within the thickness of the maxilla, then on its internal surface where it is covered by nasal mucosa. In some species it ends at the nostril, in others more deeply in the nasal cavity.

The tear film washing the eye consists of three layers. The **outermost lipid layer** is derived from the secretion of the ***tarsal glands (present in inner surface of the eyelids)***. It helps in spreading the tears evenly and retards the breakup of the film. The **thick middle aqueous layer** is derived **from the *lacrimal glands***. It **moistens and nourishes the cornea**. The **innermost mucinous layer** is produced **by goblet cells in the conjunctiva and holds the tear film intimately to the cornea.**

Fowl: The size of the eye ball in relation to the size of the head is considerably large. The lower eyelid is more movable. The third eyelid is well developed and is moved by two special muscles. The sclera has an inner layer of cartilage and at the anterior margin, shows a ring of small pieces of bone called the ***"scleral ossicle"***.

The ***ciliary muscle is made up of skeletal muscle fibres***. The iris is yellow in colour. The ***sphincter and dilator pupillae muscles are striated. No tapetum lucidum is present in choroid.*** The ***pupil is round***. The retina is devoid of blood vessels. It displays a remarkable outgrowth called ***"pecten"*** over the optic disc. It is a black pleated ridge projecting into the vitreous body. It is rich in blood vessels and is thought to play a role in the nutrition of the retina. The ***retractor oculi muscle is absent*** and the ***superior oblique muscle does not pass through a pulley***. The muscle ***pyramidalis*** *is* **present in nictitating membrane (third eye lid)**. It arises ventrally on the bulbus and its tendon passes through the loop formed by muscle ***Quadratus*** to the anterior surface of the bulbus where it is spread into the nictitating membrane. The *muscule quadratus* of the third eyelid has a broad, flat origin on the dorsotemporal part of the bulbus. Near the optic nerve its tendon makes a loop to allow passage for the tendon of the muscle *pyramidalis.* ***These two muscles move the nictitating membrane.***

The ***tear gland*** lies near the temporal angle of the eye, on the bulbus and is covered by conjunctiva. Its tubular glands are arranged in lobules, each with a collecting duct and numerous lymphocytes surrounding it. Compared with the tear gland, the ***Harderian gland (glandula lacrimalis accessoria)***, is relatively large and is situated dorsally on the posterior surface of the bulbus. Its duct terminates on the inner surface of the nicitating membrane, also in the conjuctival sac.

EAR

The ear consists of external, middle and internal ears. The structure of the **external ear** comprises an **auricle, external acoustic meatus** and framework of cartilages (**which are chiefly elastic i.e *auricular (conchal) cartilage, annular cartilage and scutiform cartilage***), the integument and muscles.

(1) **Auricle**, a funnel-like structure which collects the sound waves together with its muscles. The middle part of the auricle is much wider and less curved than in the horse. The opening is wide and the concave surface presents four ridges; the convex surface presents corresponding depressions.

(2) **External acoustic meatus,** which conveys sound waves to the tympanic membrane, the partition which separates the external ear canal from the cavity of the middle ear. The external acoustic meatus leads from the cavity of the concha to the tympanic membrane. It consists of a **cartilaginous part which is formed by the lower part of the auricular cartilage and the anular cartilage** and an osseous part formed in the temporal bone. These are united by elastic membranes to form a complete tube. Its calibre diminishes medially, so that the lumen of the inner end is about half of that of the outer end.

Cartilages of External Ear

1. **The auricular (conchal) cartilage**: ***determines the shape of the ear***. The basal part is coiled to form a tube, which encloses the cavity of the concha. This part is funnel shaped and curves laterally and a little caudally. Its medial surface is strongly convex, forming a prominence termed the ***conchal eminence***. The lowest part of the medial margin bears a narrow, pointed prolongation, the styloid process. *Caudal to its base there is a foramen through which the auricular branch of vagus nerve passes.*
2. The **anular cartilage** is a **quadrilateral plate**, curved to form about three-fourths of a ring, its ends are about 1 cm apart medially and are united by elastic tissue. It embraces the osseous external acoustic meatus and forms the cartilaginous part of the external acoustic meatus with the lower part of the auricular cartilage
3. **The scutiform cartilage** is an **irregular quadrilateral plate** which lies on the temporalis muscle rostral to the base of the auricular cartilage. Its superficial face is slightly convex from side to side and its deep face is correspondingly concave. The rostral end is thin and rounded, the caudal part or base is wider and thicker and the cartilage moves very freely over the underlying parts.

The middle ear: The middle ear is housed in the **temporal bone** and is essentially the small air-filled space known as the **tympanic cavity**. The lateral wall of the cavity is formed by the **tympanic membrane**. The medial wall is formed by the petrous part of temporal bone, which houses the internal ear and it **contains two windows (fenestrae)**, closed in the natural state, through which the mechanical stimuli produced by the sound waves enter the internal ear for translation into nerve impulses. The **dorsal vestibular window (*Oval window*)** connects the tympanic cavity with the vestibule of the internal ear. The other, the **cochlear window (*Round window*)** leads to the cavity of the cochlea. It is closed by the thin secondary tympanic membrane.

Auditory ossicles: The transmission of sound waves across the tympanic cavity is mediated by the three auditory ossicles known as **malleus, incus and stapes (Latin names for hammer, anvil and stirrup respectively)** in lateromedial sequence **(Fig.129).** They are situated partly in epitympanic recss and partly in the tympanic cavity.

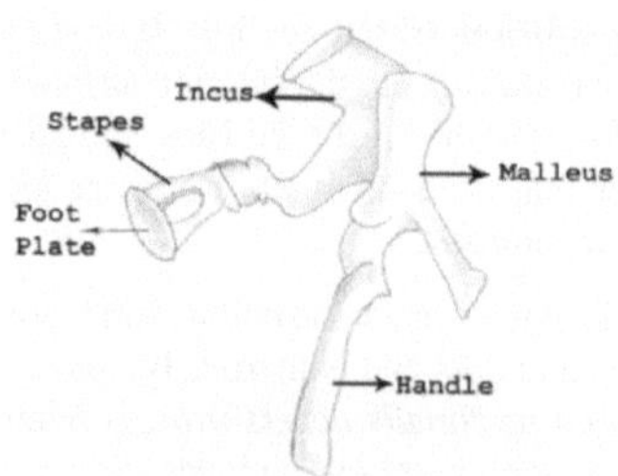

Fig. 3.129: Middle Ear Ossicles

The malleus shows head, neck and manubrium (handle). The head is placed medially and at the junction of neck and manubrium in a muscular process for tensor tympani muscle. The handle (manubrium) of the malleus is embedded in the tympanic membrane so that the head of the malleus protrudes above the membrane by a few millimetres. The medially placed head articulates with the body of the incus. The incus lies caudal to malleus and shows convex body and long and short crura. It articulates with the head of the stapes by means of its long crus. The stapes shows head, neck, 2 crura, a base and small muscular process. The muscular process located at the junction of head and neck is for stepedius muscle. The base (foot plate) of the stapes sits in the vestibular window in the medial wall of the tympanic cavity, thereby ossicles carry vibrations from tympanic membrane to the perilymph of internal ear.

Auditory tube: This structure, often called the **Eustachian tube**, connects the **tympanic cavity with the nasopharynx (Fig.3.130).** It is short with a narrow lumen that is laterally compressed and usually collapsed. The tube is confined by an inverted cartilaginous trough except along its ventral border. The membranous wall of the horse's auditory tube evaginates to form the large, thin walled **guttural pouches** dorsolateral to the nasopharynx.

The **tympanic cavity** is divided into **dorsal, middle and ventral parts. The dorsal part** (tympanic recess) is situated above the level of the tympanic membrane. It contains the **chain of auditory ossicles** and the two associated muscles. The **middle part** includes the tympanic membrane in its lateral wall and opens rostrally into the nasopharynx via the auditory (***Eustachian***) tube**.** The **ventral part** is an enlarged bulbous extension of the temporal bone known as the **tympanic bulla.**

The **tympanic membrane** is a thin partition separating the lumen of the external acoustic meatus from that of the tympanic cavity **(Fig.3.130).** Like the tympanic cavity, it is slanted so that its dorsal part is more lateral than its ventral part and its surface area is thus considerably larger.

The internal ear: The mechanical stimuli produced by sound and by the positional changes of the head are transformed into nerve impulses in the internal ear. It is enclosed in the **very hard petrous temporal bone** for protection and proper functioning.

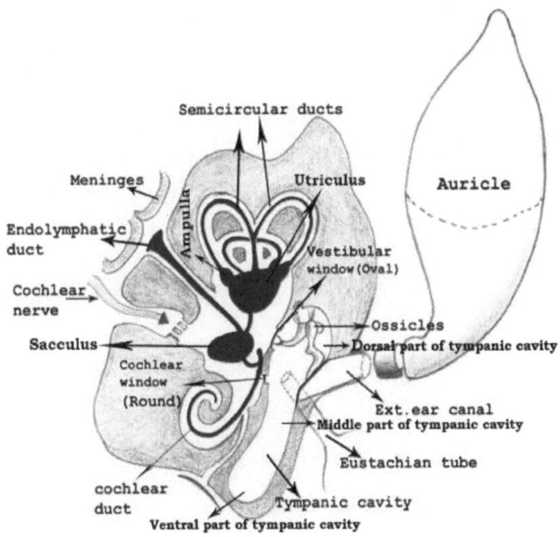

Fig. 3.130: Structure of Ear

The internal ear consists of a closed system of tiny membranous ducts called ***membranous labyrinth***. This ***contains endolymph*** whose movement inside the system stimulates sensory cells in the membranous wall. Two enlargements are present in the center of the membranous labyrinth ***known as the utriculus and sacculus*** **(Fig.3.131).** From the utriculus three semicircular ducts arise and they are concerned with ***balance*** and from the sacculus the ***spiral cochlear duct*** arises which is concerned *with* ***hearing.***

The ***semicircular ducts*** stand roughly at right angles to each other and are designated ***anterior, posterior and lateral*** **(Fig.3.131);** one end of each duct is ampullated close to the utriculus. The endolymph within them is set in motion by movements of the head and this results in pressure on minute barriers present in each ampulla. These pressures deflect the sensory hairs projecting from the receptor cells of the cristae of ampulla, stimulating the individual cells to send impulses to the central nervous system.

Two further receptor areas ***called maculae*** are present in the **walls of the utriculus and sacculus.** They ***monitor the position of the head*** with respect to gravity. The sacculus gives origin to the ***endolymphatic duct*** which ends blindly in the ***epidural space*** **(Fig.3.131).** The membranous labyrinth is housed in a similar but slightly larger osseous labyrinth, a complex excavation in the temporal bone. The center of the cochlea is an osseous pyramid known as the ***modiolus***. Running around the modiolus is the spiral canal, the actual lumen of the cochlea which ends blindly at the apex of the modiolus.

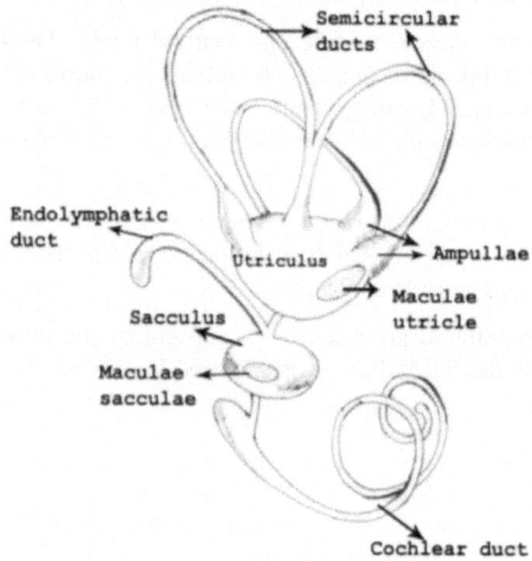

Fig. 3.131: Membranous Labyrinth of Internal Ear

3.8 ORGANS OF THE HEAD AND NECK

MOUTH (*Oral cavity*)

Ox: The oral cavity extends from lips to pharynx and is bounded dorsally by hard palate, ventrally by body of mandible and mylohyoideus muscles, laterally by cheeks, anteriorly by rima oris (anterior opening of mouth bound by lips) and posteriorly it communicates with oropharynx through isthmus faucium.

The ***oral cavity*** is divided into the vestibule and oral cavity proper (***Cavum oris proprium***) by teeth and alveolar processes.

The **vestibule** is the space between teeth and cheeks, while the **oral cavity proper** is the space enclosed by the teeth, gums, hard palate and the floor of the mouth cavity. The two cavities communicate via interdental spaces. Two narrow incisive (nasopalatine) ducts connect the oral cavity with nasal cavity.

Horse : Cavum oris is longer and narrower.

Dog : Rima oris is extensive.

Pig **:** The oral cavity is relatively longer. The rima oris is extensive

Fowl : Cavum oris is triangular and the vestibule is absent.

LIPS

Ox: The upper and lower lips are thick musculomembranous folds surrounding the rima oris and unite on each side at the angle of mouth i.e. commissures, at the level of first cheek tooth. The lips are less mobile and are formed externally by skin and internally by mucosa. The muscle orbicularis oris is placed in between these layers. The area between upper lip and nostrils is bare and without hair, generally black in colour called ***muzzle or nasolabial plate.*** **The muzzle has pebbled surface marked by minute grooves and raised areas.**The philtrum is shallow or absent. The external surface of lower lip has rounded prominence, called ***chin/mentum.***

In **sheep and goat** lips are very mobile and prehensile. The upper lip is divided by a distinct median cleft (philtrum). The skin of upper lip has fine and tactile hairs. The narrow hairless nasal plate between nostrils does not involve upper lip unlike in ox.

Horse: 1. The lips are more mobile and act as ***organ of prehension***. 2. The skin covering both the lips bears fine hairs. Numerous tactile hairs surround the oral cleft. The oral cleft extends to the level of first cheek tooth. 3. The labial glands are numerous and increase in number towards the angle of mouth. 4. The philtrum is shallow or absent. Chin is present.

Pig: 1. The lips are less mobile. 2. There is an area of modified skin (without hair) between nostrils and central portion of upper lip, ***rostral plate***. 3. The philtrum is shallow. 4. The lower lip is noticeably smaller than the upper lip and pointed infront and margin is covered by upper lip. 5. The upper lip presents a transverse notch which accommodates tusk of upper jaw.

Dog: 1. The lips are more mobile. 2. The upper lip is divided by a shallow / distinct median cleft ***viz., philtrum*** depending on breed. 3. The skin covering the lips bears in addition to ordinary hairs many tactile hairs along margins. 4. Lower lip is noticeably smaller than the upper lip. 4. Free edges of both lips are set with rows of short blunt papillae.

Fowl: The lips are absent in fowl.

FLOOR OF THE MOUTH CAVITY

It is free only in the anterior part and rest of the floor is occupied by attached portion of the tongue. Sublingual floor of oral cavity is crescent shaped space that becomes visible when the tongue is raised. It shows prefrenular part lying inside the arch of incisors and supported by incisive part of mandible. The lateral sublingual recesses are bounded laterally by lower cheek teeth and gums and medially by the lateral surface of tongue. ***Caruncula sublingualis / barb*** is a wide, flat and hard/firm papilla with slightly serrated edge **(Fig.3.132).** It lies opposite to or slightly behind the corner incisor tooth, through which the duct of ***mandibular and ventral (monostomatic) part of sublingual salivary gland open into the mouth***. ***Orobasal organ*** is present on a low median ridge just caudal to central incisors and consist of two epithelial grooves ending in a minute depression.They represent remnants of rostral sublingual glands of reptiles.

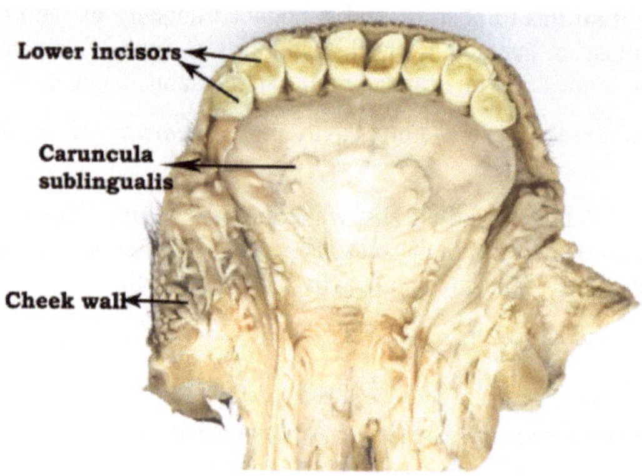

Fig. 3.132: Lower Jaw of Ox

Frenulum linguae is a median fold of mucous membrane of prefrenular part passing to ventral face of the free part of the tongue **(Fig.3.133).** A mucous fold lies on either side of frenulum linguae in the floor of each recess i.e., sublingual fold, under which sublingual salivary gland is placed. It presents series of small papillae along the edge which show the openings of the ducts of dorsal (***polystomatic***) part of sublingual salivary gland. ***Plica pterygomandibularis*** is a vertical fold of mucous membrane connecting the upper and lower jaws behind last cheek tooth.

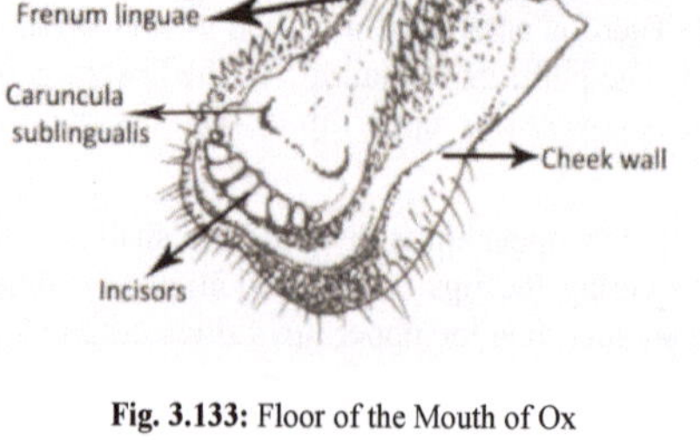

Fig. 3.133: Floor of the Mouth of Ox

Horse: 1. Caruncula sublingualis is opposite to canine tooth and shows opening of mandibular duct only. Small paracaruncular glands are present near caruncla sublingualis. 2. The caruncle is flat and projects laterally from two narrow caruncular folds which are lateral to frenulum. 3. **Orobasal organ** shows two slit like openings leading into minute epithelial canals caudal to central incisors.

Pig: 1. Frenulum linguae is a double fold. 2. ***Orobasal organ*** consists of two solid epithelial sprouts caudal to central incisor. They extend into lamina propria and two minute depressions on the surface of the oral mucosa indicate their position.

Dog: 1. The caruncula sublingualis is a small elevation and located at the base of frenulum linguae and shows openings of Wharton's duct and monostomatic part of sublingual gland. 2. The **orobasal organ** consists of two shallow grooves.

Fowl: The floor of the mouth is a ditch like depression between rami of lower beak.

CHEEKS (Buccae)

Ox: The cheeks form the lateral walls of the mouth cavity and are attached to the alveolar borders of maxilla above and mandible below in the region of cheek teeth.It extends from angle of mouth to the pterygomandibular fold which connects the palate with the mandible behind last cheek tooth. The wall of cheek consists of mucous membrane, intermediate layer of muscles (buccinator muscle and caudally masseter), glands (buccal glands) and skin from within outwards. The mucous membrane presents **large pointed conical caudally directed papillae** and is continuous with the gums of cheek teeth. The size and number of papillae decrease gradually caudally.The ***papilla salivalis*** is at the level of ***upper 5th cheek tooth*** on summit of which ***Stenson's duct opens***. Anterior to masseter it is related to facial artey, vein and ventral buccal nerve.

The buccal glands are arranged in **three rows, dorsal, middle and ventral**. They are located either between mucosa and buccal muscles or between buccal muscles and their ducts open into vestibule. The **dorsal buccal glands** are light yellow lobules opposite the alveolar border of the maxilla and extend from angle of the mouth to the maxillary tuberosity a short distance under the masseter muscle. The **ventral buccal glands** are opposite lower cheek teeth and form a wider and more compact chain of brownish masses from the angle of mouth to rostral border of masseter. The **middle buccal glands** consist of more loosely arranged yellow lobules formed along the dorsal border of the ventral glands and extend from angle of mouth upto first cheek tooth **(Fig.3.134).** ***The lobules lie under and in buccinator muscle.***

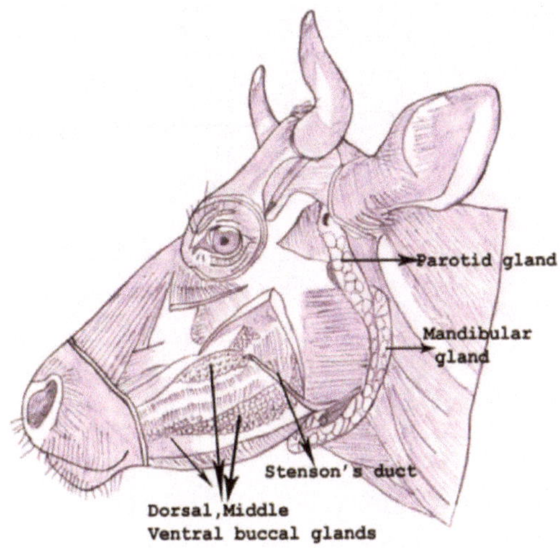

Fig. 3.134: Buccal Glands of Ox

Horse: 1.The buccal glands are arranged in two rows, a dorsal and a ventral row. 2. The mucous membrane is pigmented and papillae are absent on the mucosa, hence it is smooth. 3. The ***papilla salivalis*** is about the level of ***upper 3rd cheek tooth***. 4. The ***dorsal buccal glands*** lie in the submucosa or between bundles of buccinator muscle opposite the upper row of cheek teeth. It consists of rostral part with loose collection of lobules from angle of mouth to rostral border of masseter. The compact caudal part lies on maxilla between masseter and buccinator. 5. The ***ventral buccal glands*** lie along ventral border of buccinator from angle of mouth to rostral border of masseter.

Pig: The buccal glands are in dorsal and ventral rows from angle of mouth to masseter.

Dog: 1. The mucous membrane is pigmented and the papillae are absent on the mucosa. 2. The ***papilla salivalis*** is about the level of ***upper 3rd cheek tooth***. 3. The seromucous globular ***zygomatic (orbital) gland*** located in anterior part of pterygopalatine fossa medial to rostral end of zygomatic arch is homologous to dorsal buccal gland. 4. The ventral buccal glands extend from the level of canine tooth to the level of the third lower cheek tooth. 5. The major and minor (3-4) ducts of zygomatic gland open near the last upper cheek tooth.

Cat: The parotid duct opens opposite to second upper cheek tooth.

Fowl: Cheeks are absent.

Hard Palate

Ox: The mucous membrane of the roof the mouth is termed the hard palate. It is bound infront by dental pad and alveolar arches on the sides. It is continuous behind with soft palate and attached above to the bony palate formed by palatine processes of premaxillae and maxillae and horizontal parts of the palatine bones. The anterior portion forms a prominent ***dental pad*** (thick layer of dense fibrous tissue) covered with horny epithelium.

The oral surface of hard palate is divided by a central median raphe into two symmetrical halves and ***presents 15-18 ridges*** **(Fig.3.135)** ***viz., palatine ridges which are serrated at their free borders.*** The ridges are present only in anterior 2/3rds, while the posterior 1/3rd is smooth. The ***incisive papilla*** lies between the dental pad and first ridge of hard palate **(Fig.3.135)** and bound on either side by fissure which presents the opening of incisive (nasopalatine) duct.

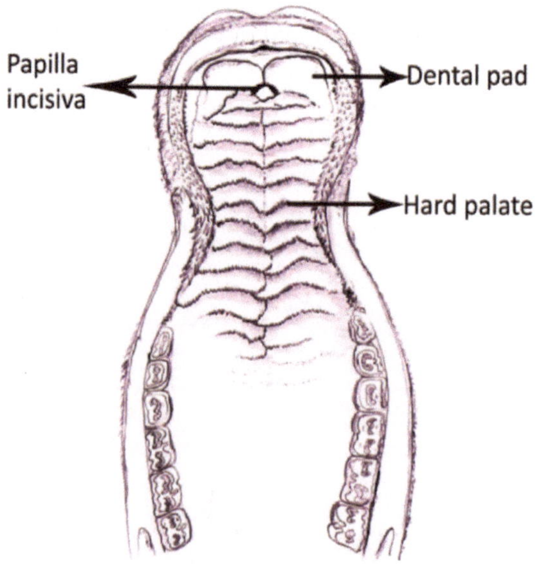

Fig. 3.135: Hard Palate of Ox

Sheep and goat: The sheep shows **14 pairs of ridges,** while in **goat there are 12 pairs.** Glands are present in caudal portion. In sheep it is wide rostrally and caudally with a narrow middle part, while in goat it is of uniform width upto first cheek teeth and then abruptly widens. Palatine raphe is prominent. The ridges end at the level of 3rd and 2nd cheek teeth respectively in sheep and goat

Horse: 1.The total number of ***ridges are 18***, which are curved and nonserrated. 2. They extend the whole length of the hard palate. 3. **Dental pad** is absent, instead ***six alveoli*** for upper incisors are present **(Fig.3.136).** 4. The fissures of incisive papilla *do not show the openings of incisive duct.*

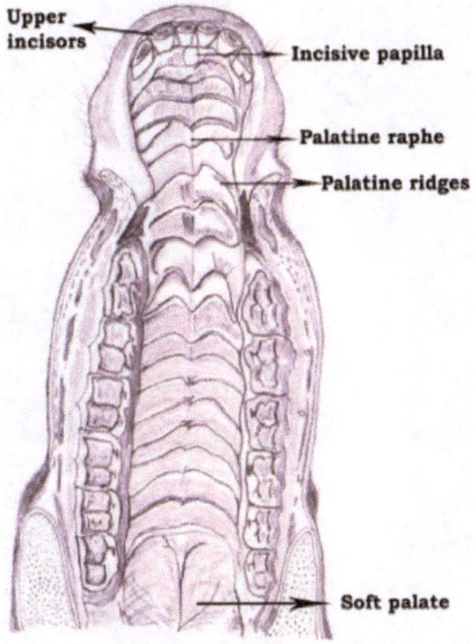

Fig. 3.136: Hard Palate of Horse

Dog: It is widest about the level of 4th cheek tooth. The central raphe is replaced by a median ridge. The number of palatine ridges vary from ***8 to 10*** which are curved and non- serrated. The portion caudal to the level of the last cheek teeth is smooth. The ***incisive papilla*** lies behind the first pair of incisors **(Fig.3.137).** The mucous membrane is pigmented.

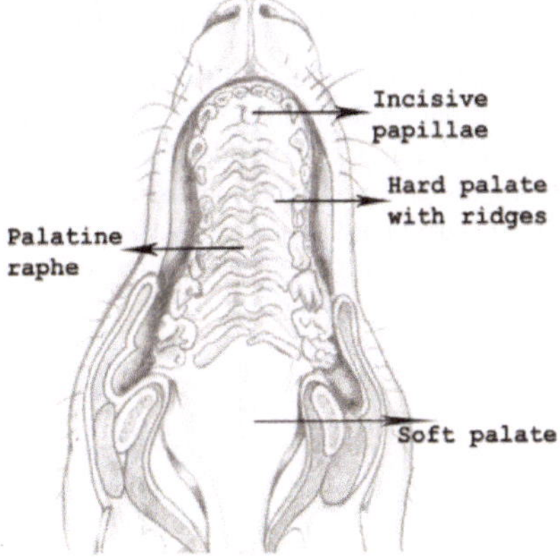

Fig. 3.137: Hard Palate of Dog

Pig: It increases in width upto the level of tusks and then width remains constant. It shows 20-23 pairs of smooth ridges throughout the length. They are high rostrally and gradually lower towards pharynx. Glands are present in rostral portion.Raphe is distinct. Incisive papilla is elongated and nasopalatine ducts open on either side.

Fowl: 1. It is narrow and triangular and presents a median ridge anteriorly and a slit posteriorly which communicates with the nasal cavity. 2. ***Five transverse rows of horny papillae are present behind the median ridge*** **(Fig.3.138).**

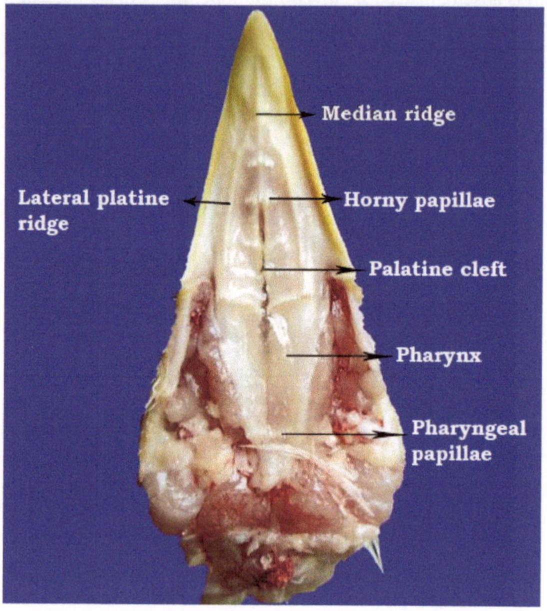

Fig. 3.138: Hard Palate of Fowl

Soft Palate

It is a ***musculomembranous curtain / shelf*** separating the mouth cavity from pharynx except during deglutition. It is caudal continuation of hard palate and extends into pharyngeal cavity from free border of horizontal part of palatine bones. The soft palate subdivides rostral part of pharynx into ***upper nasopharynx and lower oropharynx*** **(Fig.3.139).** The ventral surface forms roof of the oropharynx while the dorsal surface forms floor of nasopharynx.

Ox: It presents oral and pharyngeal surfaces and attached and free borders. The free/caudal border of soft palate lies near the base of the epiglottis except during deglutition so that rostral part of larynx protrude through the intrapharyngeal opening. Two short thick folds run from each side of oral surface to lateral borders of root of tongue, the ***anterior pillars (palatoglossal arches)*** which form lateral boundaries of isthmus faucium. Similarly two folds of mucous membrane extend from the free / caudal border of aboral surface to lateral walls of pharynx, the ***posterior pillars (palatopharyngeal arches).*** Between the diverging anterior and posterior pillars is the ***tonsilar sinus*** housing the bean shaped palatine tonsil.

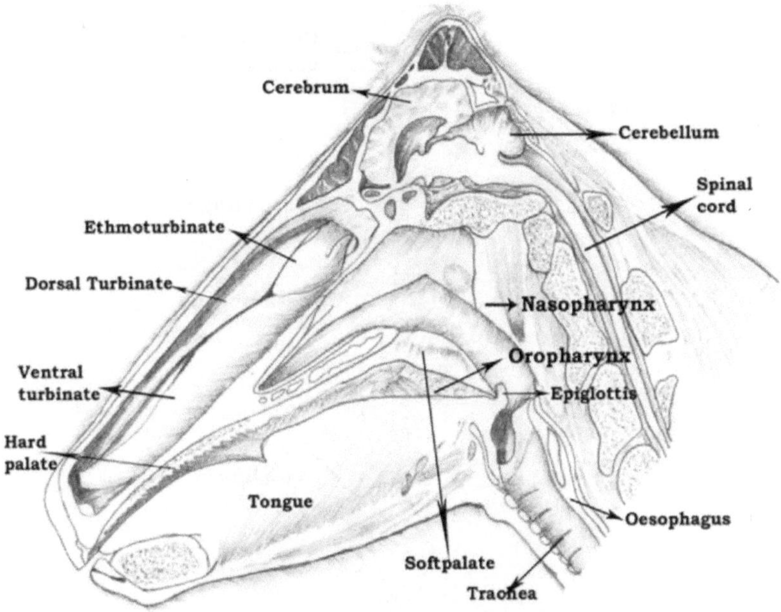

Fig. 3.139: Sagittal Section of Head of ox

Horse: 1. The **soft palate is long precluding oral breathing and vomiting**. 2. The free border is concave and it is in contact with the epiglottis except during deglutition. 3. The posterior pillars unite over the beginning of oesophagus. 3. The tonsil is diffuse.

Pig: The soft palate is short and thick and its caudal border shows a conical projection rudimentary uvula.

Dog: 1. The tonsillar sinus is large. 2. The tonsil is elongated, cylindrical / fusiform and is visible when mouth is opened. 3. The soft palate is long but does not reach base of the epiglottis.

Fowl: The soft palate is absent

Tongue

is situated on the floor of the mouth between the two rami of the mandible. It is supported by a sling formed by the mylohyoideus muscles. ***The tongue consists of root, body and tip.*** The posterior part is the root, attached to hyoid bone, soft palate and pharynx.

The middle part is the body which shows four surfaces. The dorsal (upper) surface or dorsum linguae is free throughout and is in contact with palate except at glossoepiglottic space. An eminence i.e ***torus linguae*** is present on the posterior part of dorsal face of the body and a transverse depression called ***fossa linguae is present infront*** **(Fig.3.140).** The ventral (inferior) surface is related to lingual muscles. The two lateral surfaces are flattened. The free pointed end is the apex or tip of the tongue which is dorsoventrally flattened and shows two (dorsal and ventral) surfaces.

Food tends to collect in the lingual fossa. The fossa is considered a potential site for harboring microbes. It has a delicate mucosa that can easily be pierced by sharp contaminated objects. The torus linguae, the elevation at the root of the tongue, can present an obstacle to passage of a balling gun or cattle mouth speculum

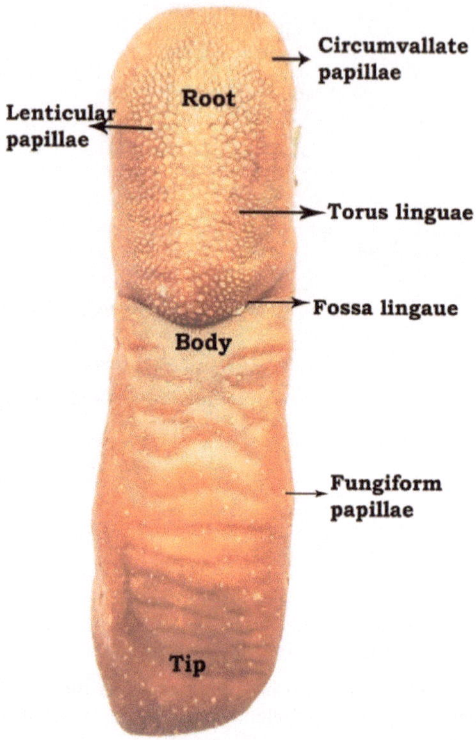

Fig. 3.140: Tongue of Ox

The mucous membrane covering the dorsum of the tongue is variably pigmented. It is thick and dense on the dorsum while on the sides it is thin. The folds of tongue are **1. Frenulum linguae** which passes from lower portion of the free part of the tongue to the floor of the mouth. ***2. Anterior pillars / Palatoglossal arches*** which pass from each side of the edge of the dorsum to the soft palate. ***3. Glossoepiglottic fold*** which passes from the root of the tongue to the base of the epiglottis.

The dorsal surface of the tongue shows five types of papillae i.e **1.** ***Filiform papillae*** are thread like projections located on the dorsum and sides of tip, give rough and rasp like nature to the tongue. **2.** ***Conical papillae*** are large and conical and lie in front of the torus linguae. **3.** ***Lenticular papillae*** are broad horny papillae situated on the torus linguae. Some of these are blunt and conical, while others are round and flattened. **4.** ***Fungiform papillae*** are large and numerous with rounded free ends and a distinct neck. They are scattered on the dorsum and sides of body and tip. **5.** ***Circumvallate papillae are 8 to 17*** in number and arranged in the form of a long narrow group on either side of posterior part of torus linguae **(Fig.3.140).** They are rounded, broader at their exposed surface and sunk in a deep depression bounded by ***annular wall (moat).*** The fungiform and circumvallate papillae are furnished with taste buds.

Horse: 1. The body and root are narrower. 2. Torus linguae is absent. 3.The tip is rounded and spatula like. 4. The mucous membrane is not pigmented. 5. Circumvallate papillae are 2 or 3 in number on posterior part of dorsum.6. Foliate papillae, besides the normal papillae are present **(about 20 mm long**) infront of the anterior pillars of soft palate and contain taste buds.

Dog: 1.The tongue is wide and thin in front and thick posteriorly and more mobile. 2. The mucous membrane is not pigmented and bright red in colour.3. ***The dorsum presents median sulcus linguae*** **(Fig.3.141).** 4. The filiform papillae are found on the entire dorsum and circumvallate papillae are 2 or 3 in number on the posterior part of dorsum. 5. The ***foliate papillae*** are small. 6. The inferior part of the tip of the tongue shows a ***fusiform cord of fibrous tissue, adipose tissue, striated muscle fibres*** and cartilage called, the ***lyssa***.

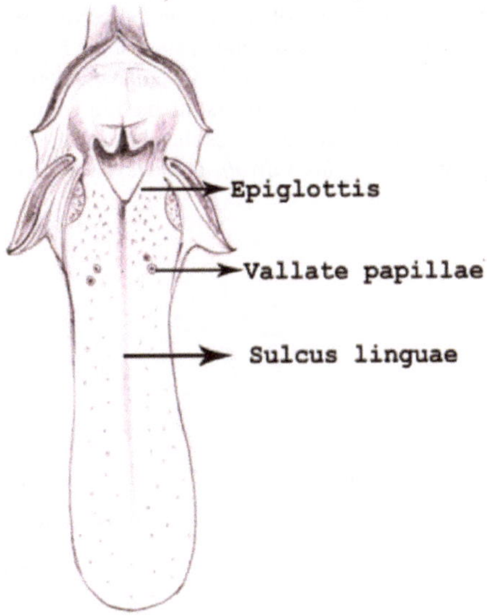

Fig. 3.141: Tongue of Dog

Pig: 1.The tip is long and pointed. 2. The body shows extensive lateral surfaces and an elongated median elevation on dorsum. 3. Circumvallate papillae are two in number. 4. Foliate papillae are present just rostral to palatoglossal arch (7-8mm long), each consists of series of parallel leaves of connective tissue separated fron one another by small furrows.

Fowl: 1.The tongue is narrow and triangular and apex is pointed. The root shows a transverse row of pointed horny papillae **(Fig.3.142).**

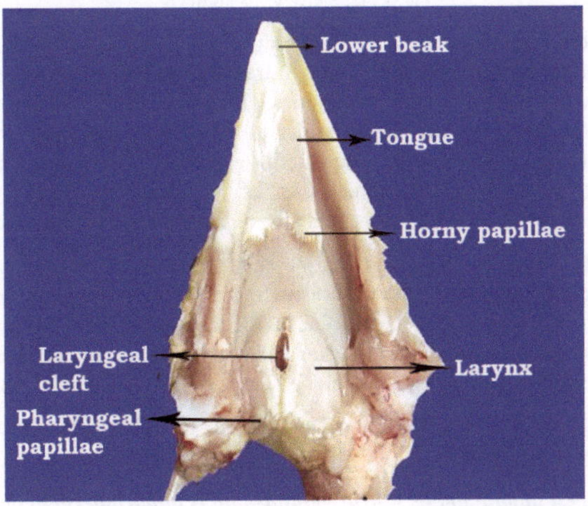

Fig. 3.142: Tongue of Fowl

Salivary Glands

The salivary glands of herbivores are large. The major salivary glands include parotid, mandibular and sublingual glands.

Ox: Parotid salivary gland is **club shaped** and situated between the vertical ramus of mandible and the wing of atlas overlapping posterior part of masseter. Its base is applied against the base of the external ear and the narrow lower part fits into the angle of union of the external maxillary vein and external jugular vein behind the angle of jaw. The anterior border of the gland at its upper part covers the parotid lymph gland **(Fig.3.143).** The ***Stenson's duct*** arising from the lower part of its medial face penetrates the cheek wall opposite the ***upper fifth cheek tooth*** and opens on the summit of large papilla i.e. ***papilla salivalis*** at the level of ***upper 5th cheek tooth into vestibule of mouth cavity*** **(Fig.3.143).**

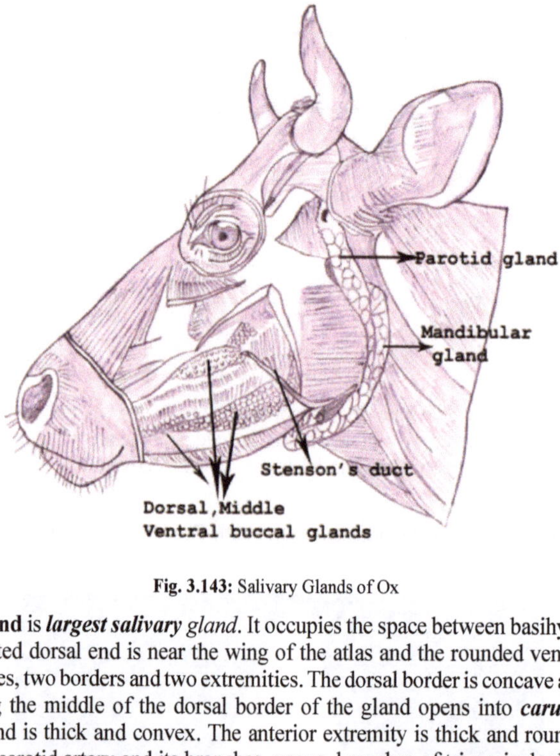

Fig. 3.143: Salivary Glands of Ox

Mandibular salivary gland is ***largest salivary*** *gland.* It occupies the space between basihyoid and the wing of atlas (*fossa atlantis*). The pointed dorsal end is near the wing of the atlas and the rounded ventral end is in mandibular space. It shows two surfaces, two borders and two extremities. The dorsal border is concave and thin. The ***mandibular (Wharton's) duct*** leaving the middle of the dorsal border of the gland opens into ***caruncula sublingualis.*** The inferior border of the gland is thick and convex. The anterior extremity is thick and rounded. The medial surface is related to the common carotid artery and its branches, vagus, branches of trigeminal, pharynx and larynx, while the lateral surface is related to parotid, pterygoideus medialis, digastricus and tendon of sternomandibularis muscle.

Sublingual salivary gland consists of dorsal and ventral parts. The **dorsal part** is long, thin and pale yellow in colour and extends from the anterior pillar (palatoglossal arch) of soft palate to the symphysis of the mandible. It is drained by several ducts which open between the papillae on the floor of the mouth. Hence it is called ***polystomatic part.*** The ***ventral (monostomatic) part*** is shorter, thicker and pink in colour and lies ventral to anterior portion of the dorsal part. It has single duct which opens either along side or joins the Wharton's duct.

Minor salivary glands: include labial, palatine, lingual and buccal glands located in the walls of lips, palate (mostly soft palate), tongue and cheeks respectively.

Horse: 1.The ***parotid is largest among major salivary glands and is quadrilateral*** in outline. 2. It is yellowish red and makes contact with guttural pouch.3. The **Stenson's duct** leaves the gland near anterior border and opens on papilla salivalis about the level **of upper third cheek teeth**. 4. The **mandibular gland is much smaller than the parotid (Fig.3.144).** The Wharton's duct opens alone on caruncula sublingualis.5.Sublingual gland shows ***only polystomatic part,*** which extends from symphysis of mandible to the level of 3rd to fifth lower cheek tooth and the ducts open along the sublingual fold.

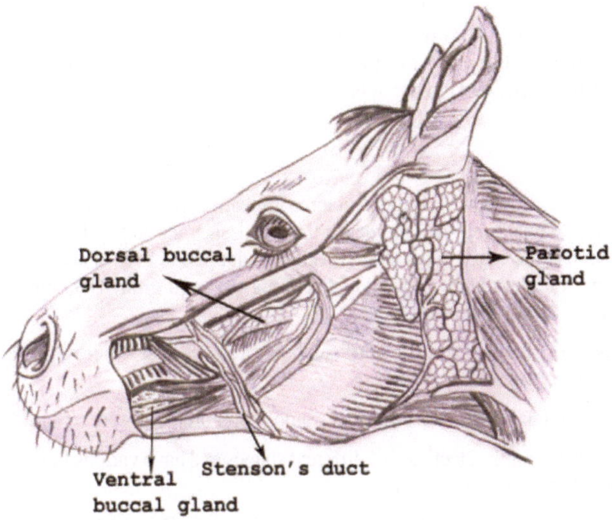

Fig. 3.144: Salivary Glands of Horse

Dog: 1. The ***parotid is irregularly triangular and notched dorsally***. 2. The duct leaves the gland at the lower part of the anterior border of the gland, crosses the lateral surface of the masseter muscle and opens on the ***papilla salivalis opposite upper third or fourths cheek tooth.*** 3. ***Mandibular salivary gland is globular/rounded, larger and lighter in color than parotid*** **(Fig.3.145).** 4. The duct of mandibular salivary gland opens on caruncula sublingualis along with duct of monostomatic part of sublingual gland

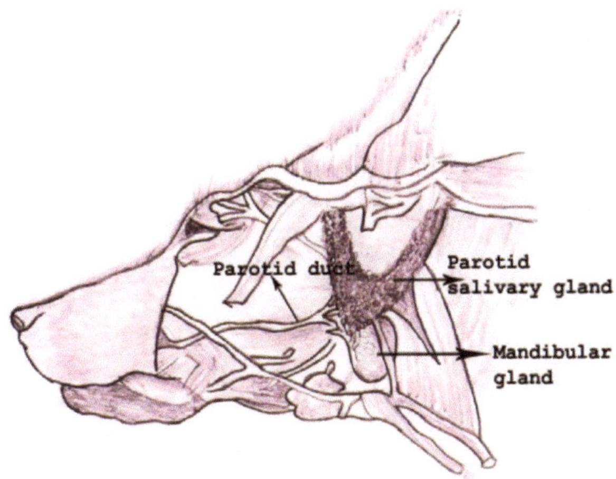

Fig. 3.145: Salivary Glands of Dog

Pig: The parotid gland is triangular and large. **The stenson's duct** opens opposite third or **fourth upper cheek tooth**. The m***andibular salivary gland*** is rounded and smaller than parotid. It is long, narrow and reddish in colour. The duct arises from lateral surface of the gland near rostromedial angle. The ***sublingual salivary gland*** consists of monostomatic (yellowish red) and polystomatic (reddish) sublingual glands. The polystomatic gland is placed rostral to the monostomatic gland.

Fowl: The salivary glands are confined to walls of mouth including palate and pharynx.The submucosa of palate shows **paired maxillary and palatine salivary glands** and at the angle of the mouth in the submucosa **paired triangular salivary glands are present**. In the submucosa of roof of the pharynx also sphenopterygoid salivary glands are present.

Teeth

The teeth are dense, hard white or yellowish white structures implanted in the alveoli of bones of jaws (***Thecodonts***) and project into the mouth. Gums (gingivae) are dense fibrous tissues intimately blended with periosteum of the alveolar processes and blend at the edges of the alveoli with alveolar periosteum of alveoli. The latter fixes the teeth in their cavities. ***Eruption*** of a tooth is the process of **breaking through gum**. The domestic mammals have two sets of teeth (***Diphyodonts***) i.e ***milk and permanent teeth***.

Milk (deciduous / temporary) teeth: The first set of small and few number of teeth, present in early life. Molars are generally absent in deciduous dentition.

Permanent teeth: replace the temporary ones. Incisors, canines and premolars are replaced.

Heterodont teeth: In domestic animlas, teeth are of different shapes and have various functions i.e incisors, canines, premolars and molars in contrast to isodont teeth.

Parts of tooth: The following three parts are present in teeth of animals **(Fig.3.146).**

Crown: Part of tooth seen above the gums.

Root: The portion inside the gums and fixed in the alveolus.

Neck: The line of junction between the crown and the root.

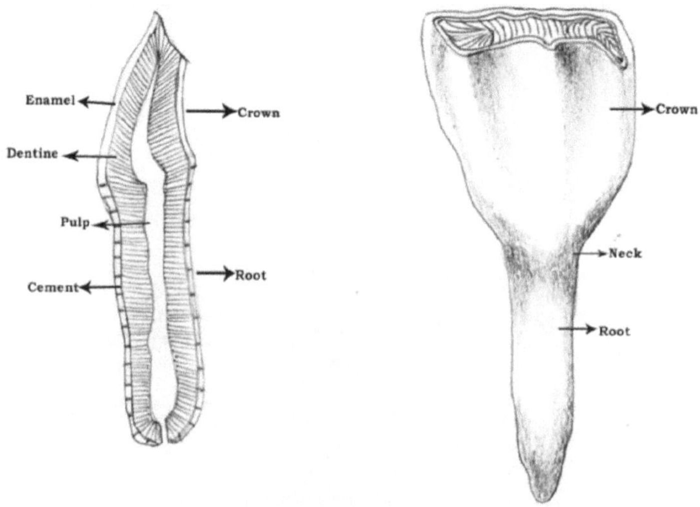

Fig. 3.146: Different Parts of Simple Teeth

According to form and position the teeth are classified as three types in ***heterodonts.***

Incisor (cutting) teeth or nippers: embedded in the alveoli of body of premaxilla and body of mandible.

Canine (shearing) teeth: implanted in the alveoli behind the incisors.

Cheek (grinding) teeth: form the sides of dental arches and implanted in alveoli of maxilla and horizontal ramus of mandible and include **premolars forming rostral group and molars forming caudal group.**

The dentition of domestic animals consists of two dental arches, but the shape, arrangement and number of teeth vary from species to species. The teeth of upper jaw form the upper dental arch and those of lower jaw form lower dental arch. Each dental arch is interrupted between incisors and cheek tooth by a wide interdental space, the ***diastema in ox and horse***. The complete dentition of an animal can be expressed in a condensed form, the **dental formula.**

Dental Formulae of Various Species

	I	C	PM	M	Total
Ox, Sheep and Goat:	0/4	0/0	3/3	3/3	32
Horse:	3/3	1/1	3or4/3	3/3	40 or 42
Dog:	3/3	3/1	4/4	2/3	42
Pig	3/3	3/1	4/4	3/3	44
Cat	3/1	1/1	3/2	1/1	30

In the above formulae the letters indicate the kind of teeth ***i.e I - Incisors, C - Canines, P - Premolars and M - Molars, the number above (numerator) and below (denominator) indicate the number of teeth in the upper and lower jaws respectively on each side.***

Among the domestic mammals the pig has complete dentition.

CLASSIFICATION OF TEETH

1. Basing on structure of tooth:

a) Simple tooth: The cement is confined to root and enamel shows no invagination on crown. The simple teeth are subdivisible into following three types.

Haplodont teeth: which show simple conical crown covered by enamel and simple conical root covered by cement and slightly constricted neck. **eg: Incisors and canines of domestic animals except horse.**

Bunodont teeth: are multituberculate but show flat occlusal surface suitable for crushing the food **eg. cheek teeth of omnivores (Pig).**

Secodont teeth: are multitubercular and capable of shearing or cutting the food **eg: cheek teeth of carnivores (Fig.3.147).**

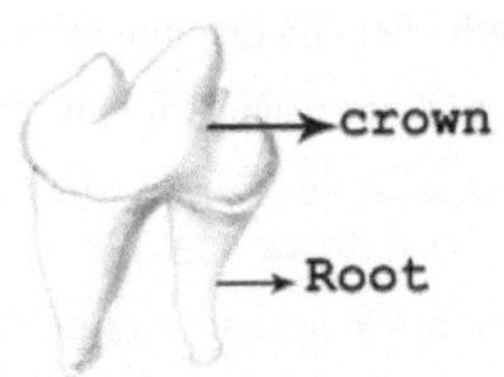

Fig. 3.147: Cheek tooth (Secodont) of Dog

b). Complex tooth: The crown is covered by cement and enamel and invagination of cement and enamel on occlusal surface (infundibulum) into dentine is seen. Hence crown shows central and peripheral enamel and cement. The external enamel forms more or less pronounced folds on the sides of the tooth.

The complex teeth are subdivisible into

Selenodont teeth: Infundibula and dentine surrounding them are semilunar in cross section. **eg: cheek teeth of ox (Fig.3.148).**

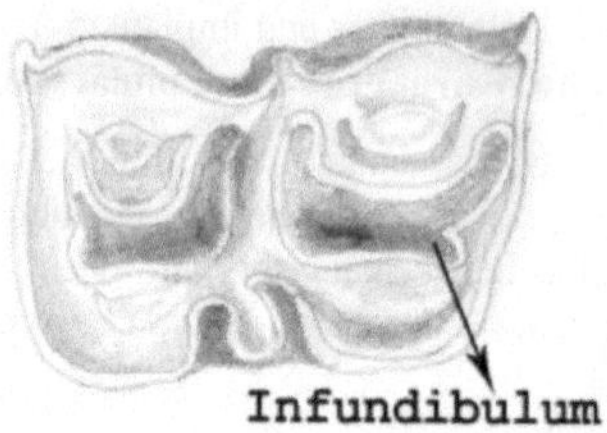

Fig. 3.148: Cheek Tooth (Selenodont)-Ox

Lophodont teeth: The enamel on occlusal surface forms pronounced folds and ridges **eg. cheek teeth of horse (Fig.3.149).**

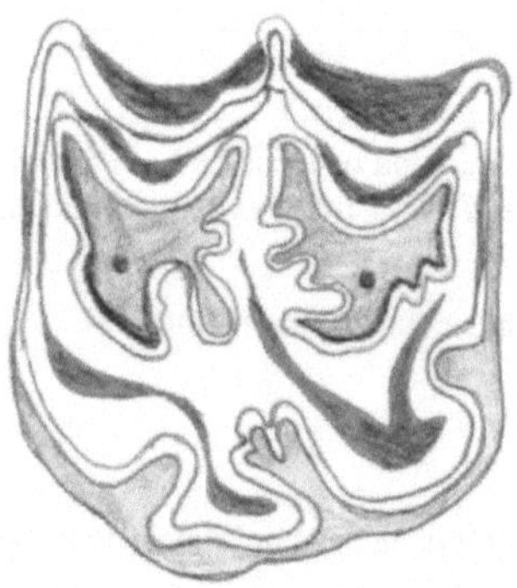

Fig. 3.149: Cheek Tooth (Lophodont)-Horse

2. Basing on growth and length of crown

a) **Brachydont (Short crowned) teeth**: These are simple teeth and show enamel on crown and cement on root. Distinct neck between crown and root is present. **eg: incisors of ruminants, teeth of dog and pig.**

b) **Hypsodont (Long crowned) teeth: These are complex teeth and** the neck is not distinct. The cement surrounds the enamel and teeth continue to grow in height for several years after they erupt resulting in long crown. **eg: canines of pigs, cheek teeth of ruminants and all teeth of horse.**

Basing on alignment of upper and lower jaw teeth the animals are said to be isognathous or anisognathus.

In **Isognathus** condition the upper and lower jaws are of same width and occlusal surface of upper teeth make contact with whole occlusal surface of lower jaw teeth. **eg: Pig.**

In **Anisognathus** condition the lower jaw and dental arch are narrower than the upper eg : **all domestic animals except pig.**

Teeth of Ox: The **incisors** are absent in upper jaw. A thick dental pad replaces the incisors. In lower jaw there are eight incisors which are simple teeth and they are ***termed as central, first intermediate, second intermediate and corner incisors.*** The **crown is sharp, shovel shaped** and shows labial, lingual and masticatory surfaces. The root is single, rounded and permits little /slight movements and neck is very distinct. The **canines are absent.**

The **cheek teeth** are complex (hypsodont) teeth and include premolars and molars. The distance between the right and left lower cheek teeth is less than the distance between the right and left upper cheek teeth (anisognathus). The size gradually increases from first to last cheek tooth. The **crowns are four sided (quadrilateral) except the first which is three sided**. The masticatory surface is not flat and shows prominent enamel folds. The borders are two i.e. lingual and buccal. The lower cheek teeth are slightly rostral to the corresponding teeth in the upper jaw with the result each upper tooth makes contact not only with its corresponding lower tooth but also with latter's caudal neighbour.

The upper premolars show one infundibulum each, while molars show two infundibula per tooth. The infundibula are semilunar in outline with convexity towards the tongue. In lower premolars true infundibula are not formed, while lower molars show two semilunar infundibula each with convexity towards vestibule.

The **buccal borders are lower than the lingual borders** in the upper cheek teeth and reverse is the case in the lower cheek teeth. The wide occlusal surface of the upper cheek teeth slopes toward the hard palate from a high vestibular to a low lingual surface, while occlusal surface of lower cheek teeth is narrow and slopes towards the cheek from a high lingual to a low vestibular surface.

The **upper premolars** are longer laterally than medially, while lower premolars are longer medially than laterally. The cheek teeth have multiple roots. All the upper cheek teeth present three (two vestibular and one lingual) roots while the lower ones show two roots.

Teeth of Horse

Incisors are **six in each jaw**. They are **complex teeth** and show deep invagination, the infundibulum filled with cement. Each tooth is curved, the concavity being towards the tongue. The curvature is well marked in upper incisors than in lower incisors. Each one is three sided in the form of a slender curved pyramid.

Canines are two in each jaw and develop only in male, but vestigeal in the female. They are cone shaped. The upper canines are located at the junction of premaxilla and maxilla, while the lower ones are nearer to the corner incisors.

Cheek teeth are complex (Hypsodont) and there are twelve in each jaw. Like in ox the condition is anisognathus. The ***first rudimentary premolar when present in upper jaw is called wolf tooth.*** The cheek teeth are large, prismatic and quadrilateral in shape except the first and last, which are three sided. The size decreases as it is traced backwards. The **upper cheek teeth are nearly square on cross section**, while those of lower jaw are triangular. The lower teeth are slightly in advance of the upper with the result each one contacts two upper teeth. **The upper teeth are much wider.**

Upper cheek (maxillary) teeth: The buccal surface shows three ridges separated by two longitudinal grooves, while the lingual surface shows a wide rounded ridge separating two shallow longitudinal grooves. The masticatory surface presents two infundibula (anterior and posterior) on each and the surface slopes toward hard palate and the buccal edge is prominent as the vestibular surface is higher than the lingual surface. **They show 3 roots.**

Lower cheek (mandibular) teeth: The buccal surface has a centrally placed distinct longitudinal groove, while lingual face shows one principal distinct groove and several shallow grooves. The masticatory surface slopes towards vestibule and shows a prominent lingual edge as the lingual surface is higher than the vestibular surface. The enamel is arranged in deep longitudinal folds but true infundibula are absent. They show two roots.

Teeth of Dog

Mostly the teeth do not correspond to opposite teeth but to the parts of two teeth of the opposite jaw ***i.e dove tail.*** Incisors are placed vertically and close together. They are six in each jaw.

Canines are two in each jaw. The **upper canine** is separated from the corner incisor by an interval into which the lower canine is received, while the lower canine lies close to the corner incisor.

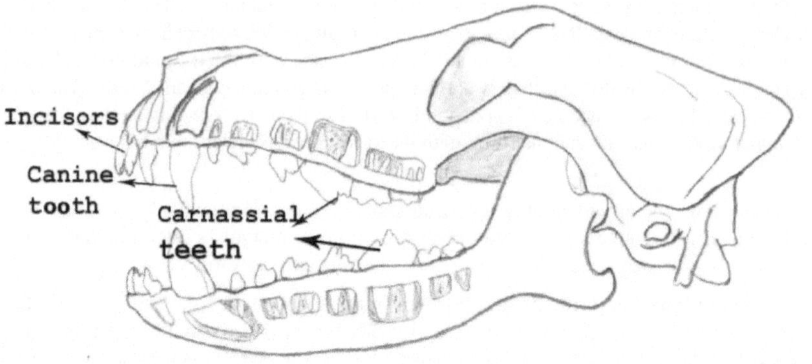

Fig. 3.150: Teeth of Dog

Cheek teeth: are 12 in upper jaw and 14 in lower jaw. The masticatory surface is tuberculate. ***The upper 4th and lower 5th are larger than the rest, termed carnassial or sectorial (Cutting) teeth*** **(Fig.3.150).** Premolars of upper and lower jaws are laterally compressed and show pointed crowns. Both the upper and lower first premolar show single root and short cone shaped crown. Both the upper and lower second and third premolars and also lower fourth premolar show two roots and tricuspid crowns, while upper fourth premolar shows three roots (one lingual and two vestibular) and tricuspid crown. The molars show round cusps. The upper molars show three roots, while first and second lower molars show two roots and lower third molar shows one root and conical crown.

Teeth of Pig: The jaws present isognathous condition. The lower incisors form a shovel like extension of lower jaw for exposing edibles in the ground. The lingual surface of incisors of lower jaw bears longitudinal enamel ridge that is flanked by two grooves. The curved upper incisors show single root. The **canines / tusks** are very large and without roots. The convex surface is covered with enamel the concave with cement. The tusks of sow are much smaller than those of boar and are open at the proximal end for about 2 years after which they develop roots and cease to grow.

The size of premolar and molars increases from rostral to caudal. In the lower jaw P1 and P2 each have two roots P3 has two or three roots and P4 has three roots. P1 has short crown, while remaining each have three cusps. In upper jaw P1 shows two indistinct cusps and P3 and P4 are trituberculate. The P1 has two roots, P2 & P3 each have three roots and P4 has four or five.

The molars are multituberculate and three upper molars show six roots each, while lower M1 and M2 each have four roots and lower M3 has six roots. I_3 appears before other incisors unlike in other animals. Upper teeth erupt about two months later.

Teeth of camel: There are **8 incisors, 6 in lower jaw and two in upper jaw**. The upper incisors are tusk like. The lower incisors show spade shaped crowns. The canines are four in number. **Cheek teeth are 22 in number** 12 in upper jaw and 10 in lower jaw. The **last upper cheek tooth is below the orbit.**

Teeth of elephant: The ***tusks are modified incisors*** and are composed of ivory (dentine).The female Asian elephants are tuskless and even the bulls may or may not have the tusks. Early in development the tusks have enamel cap but this is rapidly worn away leaving only the dentine surrounding the pulp canal. **The cheek teeth are so large that only one is present at a time in each half and six teeth succeed each other instead of occurring simultaneously.**

Fowl: Teeth are absent

PHARYNX

It is a ***funnel shaped*** musculomembranous structure that connects oral cavity with the oesophagus and the nasal cavity with the larynx. It does not extend caudally beyond base of the skull.

The concave **roof** is related to vomer and body of sphenoid (base of cranium) and rectus capitis ventralis and longus capitis muscles. The **lateral walls** are related to stylohyoid and pterygoideus muscles. The floor extends from root of the tongue over and around aditus laryngis to the level of cricoid cartilage of larynx.

The **rostral portion** of pharynx is divided by soft palate into ***upper nasopharynx and lower oropharynx***. The oropharynx extends from the auditus pharyngis to the base of epiglottis. The oropharynx is part of digestive tract. The **roof of oropharynx** is formed by soft palate and floor by root of the tongue. The narrow caudal portion of pharynx is known as laryngopharynx. The laryngopharynx is common to the digestive and respiratory channels and is caudal continuation of oropharynx.

The openings of pharynx: The ***isthmus faucium*** (aditus pharyngis) antero inferiorly between mouth cavity and oropharynx, the ***paired posterior nares*** antero superiorly/rostrodorsally connecting nasal cavity with nasopharynx, ***paired Eustachian openings*** dorsolaterally, ***aditus laryngis*** caudoventrally and ***aditus oesophagi*** at caudal end of pharynx. During swallowing the ***aditus laryngis*** is closed by epiglottis.

Horse: It does not extend beyond base of the skull. It is pushed away from the sphenoid and muscles by guttural pouches hence caudal two thirds of roof of pharynx and latetral walls are related to ***guttural pouches***.

Dog: It is long and extends caudally **to the second cervical vertebra**. The laryngopharynx is long and much of it overlies the larynx.The caudal extent of laryngopharynx is marked internally by an annular fold of mucous membrane. Caudal to pharyngeal opening of auditory tube is a slight mucosal elevation, ***torus tubaricus***.

Pig: The pharynx is long and narrow and extends to the level of axis. The mucous membrane covering the nasal septum is continued into nasopharynx forming pharyngeal septum. Pharyngeal diverticulum is a median blind mucosal pouch in roof of nasopharynx.

Fowl: The pharynx does not show divisions due to the absence of soft palate. The roof shows a longitudinal common opening, the infundibular slit for two **Eustachian tubes**. Infundibular slit is the common opening of the right and left auditory tubes and leads to funnel shaped median infundibular cavity of pharynx. At the junction with the oesophagus on each side of the midline a transverse row of ten large papillae is present.

TONSILS

The lingual, pharyngeal, tubal, palatine tonsils, tonsil of soft palate and paraepiglottic tonsils form a ring of lymphatic tissue around nasopharynx and oropharynx.

Ox: The **lingual tonsil** is present in mucosa of root of tongue. The **spherical palatine tonsil** is 3.5 cm in diameter embedded or concealed in the lateral wall of the oropharynx by connective tissue and musculature of oropharynx. The **tonsil of soft palate** is on ventral surface of soft palate. The **pharyngeal tonsil** is in roof of pharyngeal cavity at the end of septum.The **tubal tonsil** is in lateral wall of the pharyngeal opening of auditory tube **(Fig.3.151).**

Horse: The palatine tonsil lies on the surface of the pharyngeal wall between the base of the epiglottis and the palatoglossal arch **(Fig.3.151).**

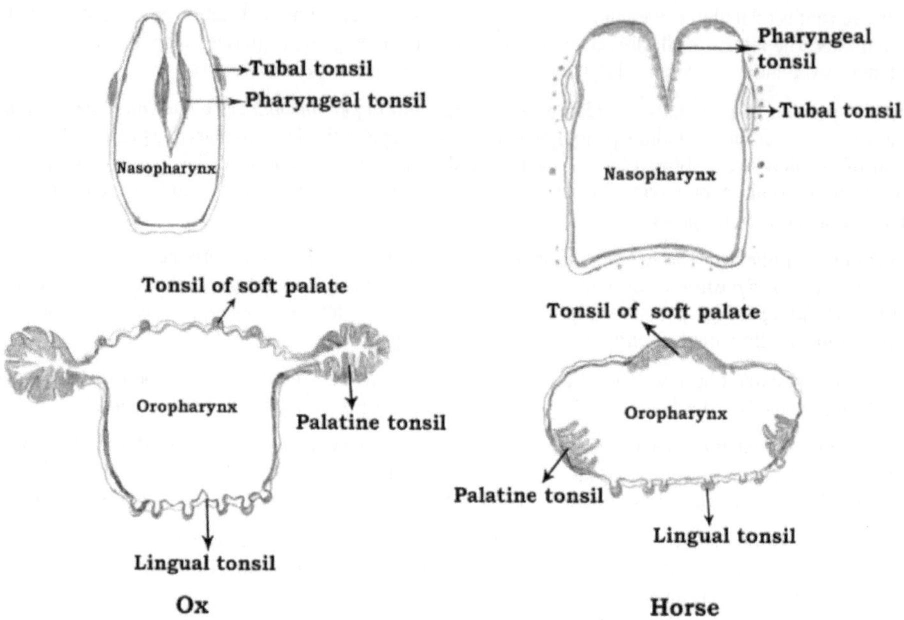

Fig. 3.151: Ring of Lymphatic Tissue in Pharynx of Ox and Horse

Pig: The ***palatine tonsil is absent***.The tonsil of soft palate is large.The paraepiglottic tonsil is present on each side of the base of epiglottis and tubal tonsil is large **(Fig.3.152).**

Dog: The **palatine tonsil** is located on lateral wall of the oropharynx and can be seen when mouth is opened and **tubal tonsil is absent (Fig.3.152).**

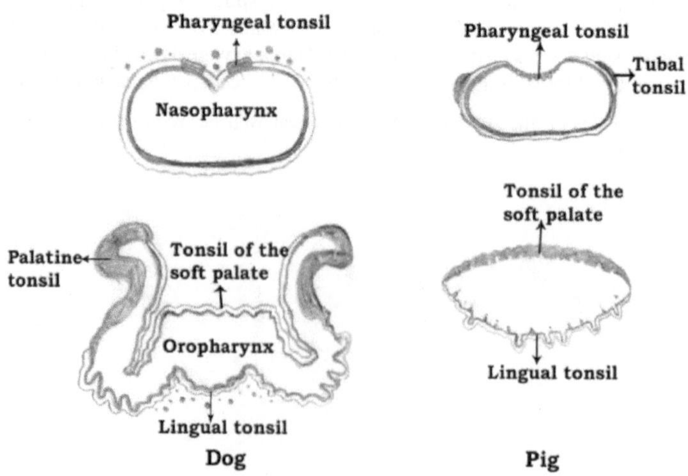

Fig. 3.152: Ring of Lymphatic Tissue in Pharynx of Dog and Pig

Fowl: A well developed lymphoid tissue present in the walls of the infundibular slit of pharynx forms a **pharyngeal tonsil.**

OESOPHAGUS

Ox: It is a long musculomembranous tube extending from pharynx to stomach. It consists of **cervical, thoracic and short abdominal parts**. The cervical part of oesophagus extends from aditus oesophagi of pharynx into thoracic cavity. It is placed on dorsal aspect of trachea upto ***3rd or 4th cervical vertebra***, after which it passes to the left side of trachea and maintains this relation until it reaches to ***6th cervical vertebra*** and then slopes to the dorsolateral surface of trachea at the thoracic inlet **(Fig.3.153).** It is related to left carotid sheath and left recurrent laryngeal nerve, thymus, the tracheal lymphatic trunk and cervical lymph nodes. The **mucosa shows longitudinal folds so lumen presents rosette like appearance in cross section**. The tunica muscularis is striated in throught.

> *On the left side of the neck (at 6th cervical vertebra) in the live cow activity of oesophagus and passage of stomach tube can be seen or palpated here as well as the objects causing the choke.*

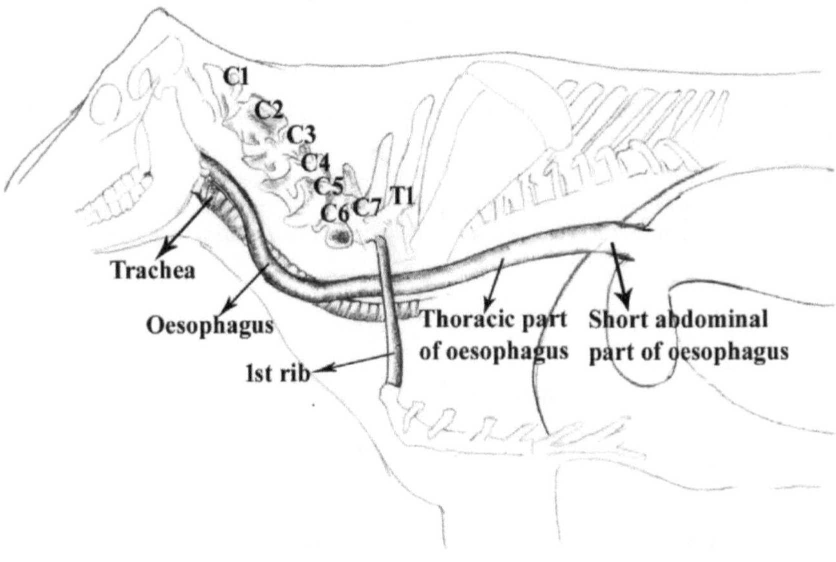

Fig. 3.153: Course of Oesophagus in Ox

Horse: The oesophagus joins the stomach at an acute angle. ***It shows striated muscles upto tracheal bifurcation and caudal third shows smooth muscle fibres.***

Dog: The oesophagus is constricted at the origin as the pharnygoesophageal junction is marked on the inside by an annular fold. The esophagus joins the stomach at the funnel shaped cardia. ***It shows striated muscles.***

Pig: The oesophagus is short and nearly straight. *The mucular coat is striated except at cardia.*

Fowl: It is at first dorsal to trachea and then ***inclines to right and crosses the neck*** without following contour of neck. It presents a diverticulum called "***crop" near thoracic inlet.***

ENDOCRINE GLANDS

The endocrine tissues in the form of separate entities/ distinct organs are described here under. The endocrine glands are devoid of ducts.

THE THYROID GLAND

Ox: It consists of two irregularly triangular lateral lobes and a band like isthmus which connects the posterior ends of the lateral lobes across the ventral surface of the trachea ***at the level of the first or second tracheal ring*** **(Fig.3.154).** Its average weight is 14 to 15 gm.

Horse: The lateral lobes are rounded and located on the most cranial portion of trachea at the junction of the jugular and linguofacial veins.***The isthmus is extremely fine*** **(Fig.3.155).**

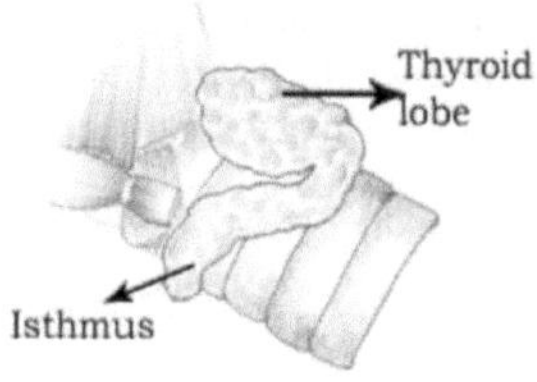

Fig. 3.154: Thyroid Gland of Ox

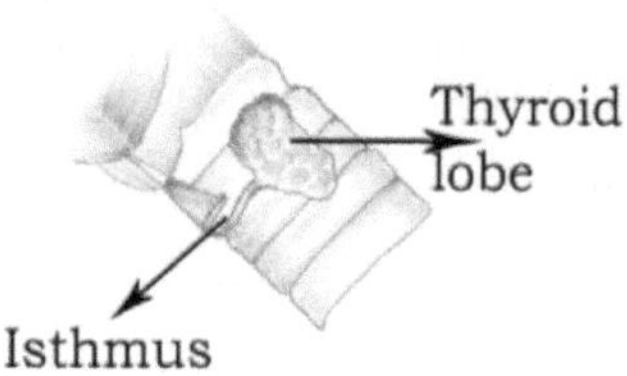

Fig. 3.155: Thyroid Gland of Horse

Dog: The lateral lobes are long, narrow and flattened and situated along the lateral face of trachea from larynx to ***5th or 6th tracheal ring*** **(Fig.3.156).**

Pig: It lies on the midline ventral to the trachea just cranial to the thoracic inlet because of shortness of neck. The lobes are irregularly triangular in outline and measure approximately 5-6 cm in length. The lobes are united for some distance on their ventral surface so that a ***distinct isthmus cannot be identified*** **(Fig.3.156).**

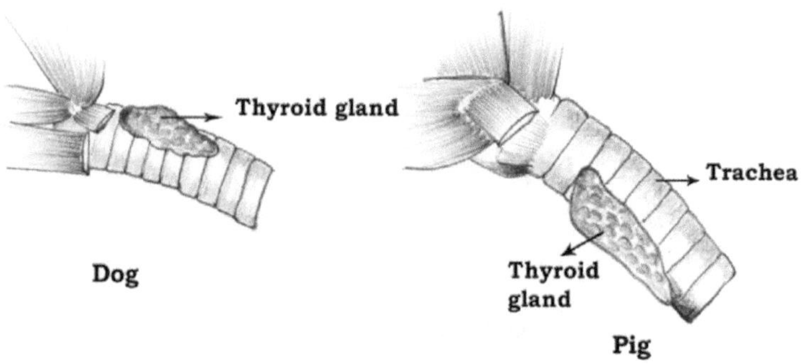

Fig. 3.156: Thyroid glands of Dog and Pig

THE PARATHYROID GLANDS

Ox: are four in number, two on either side i.e., cranial and caudal pairs. The cranial pair occurs near occipital artery, while the caudal pair is in close association with lateral lobes of thyroid gland.

Horse: One parathyroid gland is present on each side in close relation to the dorsal border or anterior extremity of lateral lobe of thyroid gland.

Dog: are four in number. Two are situated on the deep face of thyroid lobes, the others are placed laterally near the anterior extremity of the thyroid lobes.

Pig: Only external or cranial parathyroid glands are present. These glands are located far cranially to the thyroid, embedded in a portion of thymus approximately 3 cm from the paracondylar process near branching of the carotid artery.

THE THYMUS

Thymus is a lymphoid organ believed to secrete hormones. It is well developed in new born and undergoes atrophy or degeneration as age advances.

Ox: is large and lobulated and extends from the larynx to the pericardium in young animals. It shows distinct ***cervical and thoracic parts***. Its cervical part is connected to the thoracic part by a **narrow isthmus** ventral to the trachea. The ***cervical part*** consists of ***right and left lobes*** which extend on the ventrolateral aspects of the trachea from the thoracic inlet to thyroid gland, while the ***single thoracic part*** occupies the anterior mediastinal space **(Fig.3.157)**. The thymus of young animals is *bright pink or red but lightens with age*. ***The thymus grows rapidly during the first six to nine months of postnatal life.*** *Involution begins as early as the eigthth week after birth.*The thoracic part of the thymus is the last part to degenerate and it is quite large in animals for several years old.

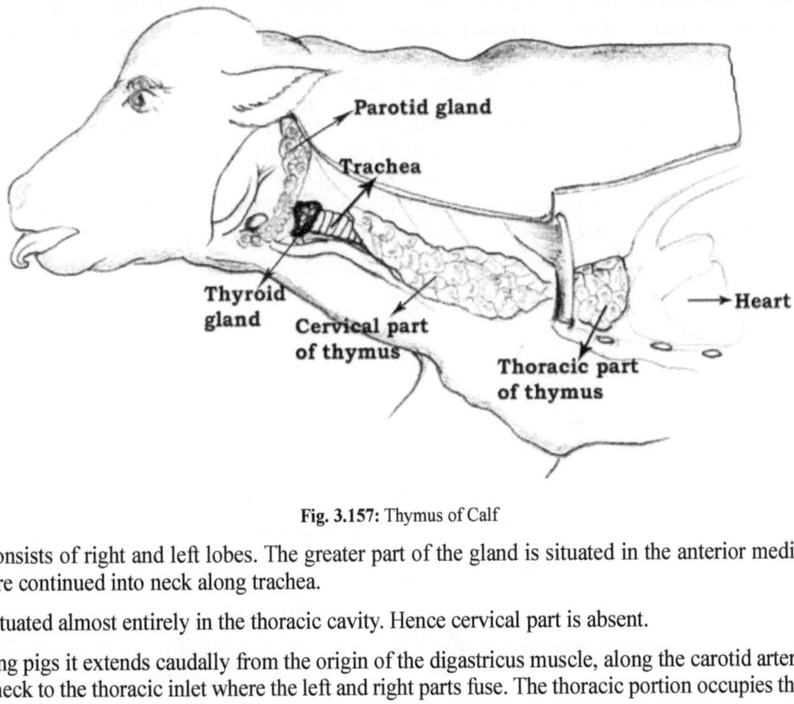

Fig. 3.157: Thymus of Calf

Horse: It consists of right and left lobes. The greater part of the gland is situated in the anterior mediastinum and two lobes are continued into neck along trachea.

Dog: It is situated almost entirely in the thoracic cavity. Hence cervical part is absent.

Pig: In young pigs it extends caudally from the origin of the digastricus muscle, along the carotid arteries on either side of the neck to the thoracic inlet where the left and right parts fuse. The thoracic portion occupies the pericardial mediastinum. It involutes at one year age.

THE PITUITARY GLAND (HYPOPHYSIS CEREBRI)

Ox: It is oval in outline and consists of adenohypophysis and neurohypophysis. It is situated in the hypophyseal fossa on the internal face of the body of postsphenoid and connected by hollow tube of gray matter called infundibulum to the tuber cinereum, a small gray prominence situated between optic chiasm in front and mamillary body behind. A fold of duramater, diaphragma sellae encloses the gland. In cross section the adenohypophysis appears **pink in colour (vascular),** while **neurohypophysis is light gray**. The infundibulum is hollowed by hypophyseal recess.

Horse: It is wider and thinner and infundibulum is shorter.

Dog: It is circular / ellipsoidal and small.

Pig: The pars distalis surrounds the neurohypophysis.

Pineal Gland (Epiphysis cerebri)

Ox: It is a long and fusiform darkly pigmented gland situated dorsally in deep depression **between the thalami and the corpora quadrigemina** of brain. It is attached to posterosuperior quadrant of 3rd ventricle by a short stalk in which a small recess of third ventricle, epiphyseal recess is present.

Horse: It is ovoid or fusiform in shape.

Dog: It is small elongate lancet shaped organ.

Pig: It is elongate cone shaped and greyish white in color

ENDOCRINE GLANDS OF FOWL

Thyroid Gland: The paired thyroid glands are ***deep red*****, oval or elliptical bodies** situated in thoracic inlet in the vascular angle between ***subclavian and common carotid arteries.*** The "***C" or parafollicular cells*** occur in the form of separate glands called ***ultimobranchial glands*** **(Fig.3.158)**. They are ***globular and pink*** in colour and located caudal to thyroid glands in close relation to bifurcation of brachiocephalic artery.

Parathyroid glands: two or three on each side, are minute (1 to 3 mm) irregular spheres and their colour varies from **yellowish brown or brownish-red** structures immediately caudal to the thyroid gland and often one may be attached to that gland. *Because they are small and embedded in connective and adipose tissue, a magnifying glass is useful in identifying them.* The minute **pink ultimobranchial bodies lie next to the parathyroid glands.** ***Topographically the parathyroid and ultimobranchial body form one organ complex*** **(Fig.3.158).**

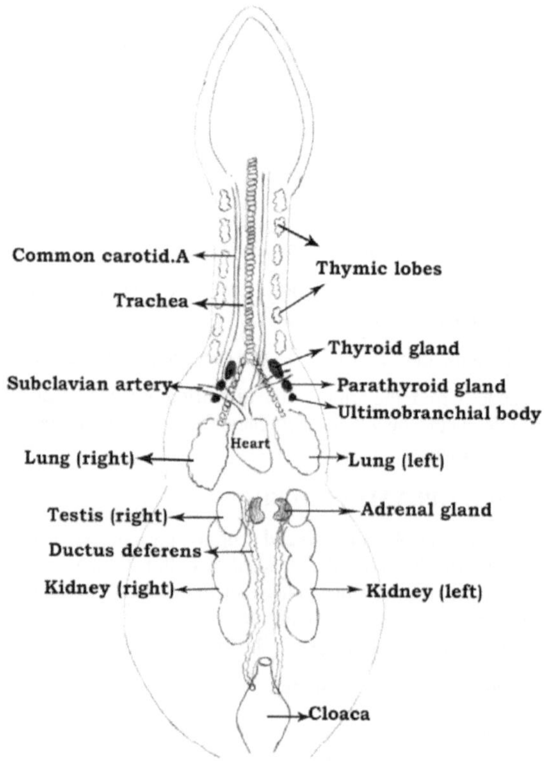

Fig. 3.158: Different Endocrine Glands of Fowl (schematic)

Thymus: The thymus of birds is embedded in the subcutaneous connective tissue of the neck and lies close to the jugular vein. It extends along the neck from the head to the entrance to the thorax. During its development, this organ is divided into completely isolated lobes and ***in the fowl there are 6-8 oval or round, flattened lobes* (Fig.3.158).** In young fowls they measure on the average, 8-15 mm in length, 7-9 mm in breadth and 2-5 mm in depth. The thymus best developed in the young, regresses with the onset of sexual maturity.

Pituitary Gland (Hypophysis cerebri): It was reddish-brown in colour and its weight varies between 10-22 mg in the hen, and 11 -25 mg in the cockerel. The pars distalis of the pituitary has an elongated and flattened appearance and in the fowl, duck and the goose, whereas in the pigeon it is more compressed and rounded. The adenohypophysis extends to the floor of the diencephalon and surrounds the hypophyseal stalk.

Pineal Gland (Epiphysis cerebri): In fowl, it is fusiform shaped reddish brown mass and is measured 2 -2.5 mm in length and 1-1.5 mm in thickness. It lies in the narrow cleft between the cerebral hemispheres and the rostral surface of the cerebellum, attached to the diencephalon by its thin *pineal stalk.*

RESPIRATORY ORGANS OF HEAD AND NECK

The respiratory system comprises of nose including nostrils, nasal cavity, nasopharynx, larynx, trachea, bronchi and lungs of which nose, nasopharynx and greater part of trachea are located in head and neck, while small part of trachea, bronchi and lungs are situated in thoracic cavity.

Nose: The nose in domestic animals is incorporated in the face and forms dorsum nasi rostral to the eyes, while in human it projects distinctly from the face. It is supported by cartilages which are variable in form, size and number.

NASAL CARTILAGES

The free borders of the nasal and incisive bones in mammals provide attachment for the nasal cartilages which support the nostrils.

Ox

Nasal septum: Anteriorly it is cartilaginous, while posteriorly it is formed by perpendicular part of ethmoid. The anterior edge forms medial support of the nostril. Below it is received into groove of vomer bone.

The nasal cartlages are as follows (Fig.3.159)

a) **Dorsal lateral nasal cartilage**: This supports lateral wall of the apex of the nose. Its rostral part extends into the lateral wall of nostril and supports its dorsal part.

b) **Ventral lateral nasal cartilage**: It is *fused with the dorsal lateral nasal cartilage only anteriorly and posteriorly and the gap that remains between the two cartilages in between is bridged by connective tissue* **(Fig.3.159**. This supports lateral wall of the apex and its rostral part extends into lateral wall of nostril and supports it.

c) **Lateral accessory nasal cartilage**: ***It is in the form of an anchor*** **(Fig.3.159)**. It arises from the dorsal lateral nasal cartilage and its branches are directed rostrally and caudally and support the ventral part of the lateral wall of the nostril.

d) **Medial accessory nasal cartilage**: It arises from ventral nasal concha and ventral lateral nasal cartilage and is situated inside the alar fold **(Fig.3.159)**.

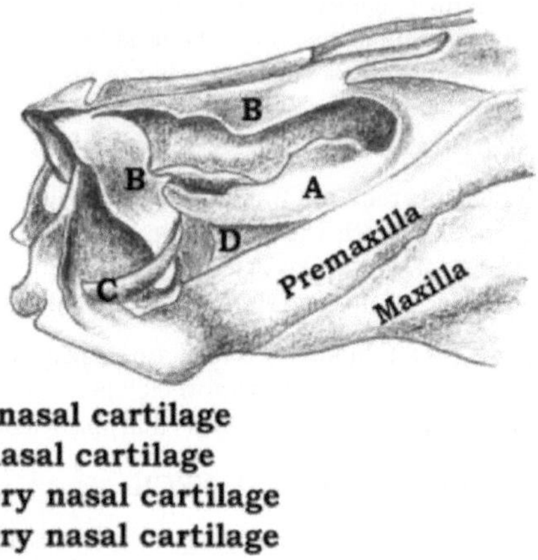

Fig. 3.159: Nasal Cartilages of Ox

Horse: The **lateral accessory nasal cartilage is absent**, while the ventral lateral nasal cartilage is absent or if present it is very narrow. Hence lateral walls of nostrils are without support. The **alar cartilage** is large and attached to anterior border of nasal septum and consists of **lamina dorsally** and a **cornu ventrally**. It supports nostril dorsally, medially and ventrally. The septum nasi does not provide support to medial wall of nostril. The dorsal lateral nasal cartilage is narrow. The medial ***accessory nasal cartilage is 'S' shaped*** **(Fig.3.160)**.

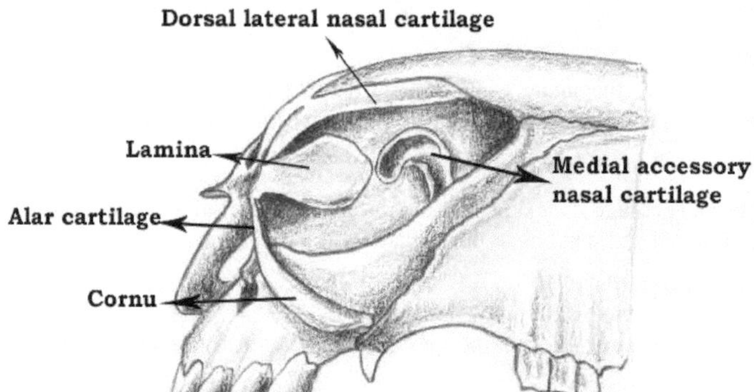

Fig. 3.160: Nasal Cartilages of Horse

Dog: Both dorsal and ventral lateral nasal cartilages are expansive and unite with each other laterally for some distance. The ***lateral accessory nasal cartilage is anchor shaped*** and projects from ventral lateral nasal cartilage and supports the nostril ventrally. The **medial accessory nasal cartilage** arises from the ventral nasal concha and also from ventral lateral nasal cartilage **(Fig.3.161)**.

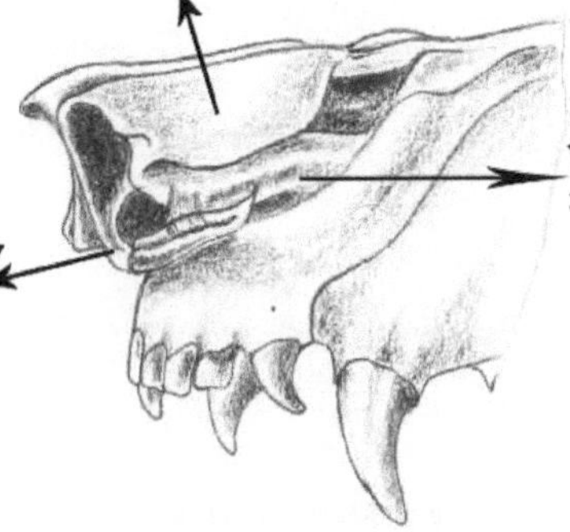

Fig. 3.161: Nasal Cartilages of Dog

Pig: The ***os rostrale*** is a thick transverse plate situated between nostrils and is attached to the rostral border of the nasal septum and incisive bone. It strengthens snout. The dorsal and ventral lateral nasal cartilages extend well into lateral wall of nostrils. The **dorsal lateral nasal cartilage** is divided by a fissure into rostral and caudal parts.The rostral part supports dorsal part of nostril. **Lateral nasal accessory cartilage** is a curved rod arising from the ventral part of os rostrale and extends into lateral wall of nostril. Medial accessory cartilage connects ventral concha with ventral lateral nasal cartilage and supports alar fold. The medial support of nostril is provided by nasal septum and also by os rostrale. The dorsal and ventral lateral nasal cartilages come together lateral to the nostril as in ox and dog and unite along most of their length.

NOSTRILS (NARES)

The nostrils lead into nasal cavity.

Ox: These are ***wider and oval slits*** placed obliquely and bounded by medial and lateral alae or wings, which unite above and below by commissures. The ***lateral one*** is concave, while the ***medial one is convex above and concave below*** **(Fig.3.162)**.

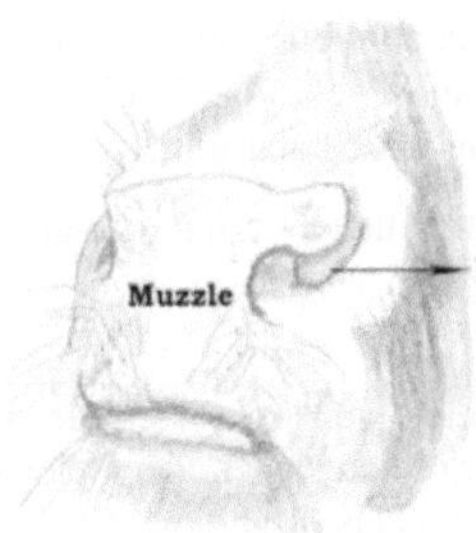

Fig. 3.162: Nostrils of Ox

Horse: The nostrils are ***semilunar in outline*** during normal breathing, highly dilatable and become circular when dilated **(Fig.3.163)**. The nostrils are divided by **alar fold into dorsal and ventral passages.** The ***dorsal passage leads to a blind cutaneous pouch***, the ***nasal diverticulum or false nostril***, while the ***ventral passage (true nostril) leads into nasal cavity.***

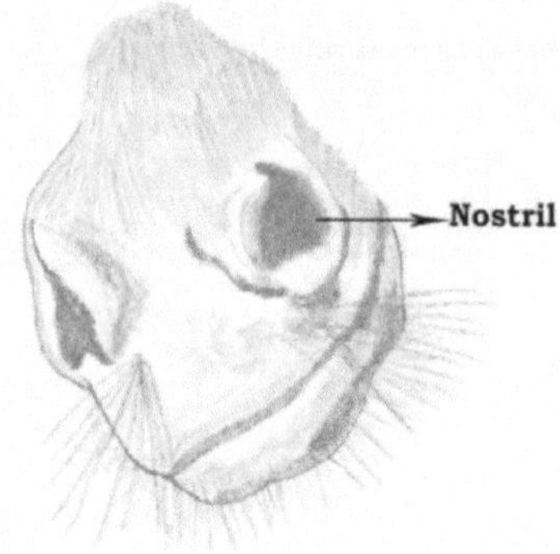

Fig. 3.163: Nostrils of Horse

Dog: The nostrils are ***comma*** shaped.

Pig: Nostrils are oval / circular and supported by Os rostrale and nasal cartilages. The apex of nose is disc shaped fused with upper lip and projects from face as rostrum or snout.

Fowl: The nostrils are narrow, oval and cartilaginous.

NASAL CAVITY

Ox: It is a longitudinal cylindrical passage which extends in front from nostrils to the posterior nares the latter opening into nasopharynx. Nasal septum, an osseo cartilaginous plate divides the nasal cavity into two equal right and left halves. It does not meet the floor throught its length and caudally raises from the floor so the **posterior nares are not completely separated**.

The nasal cavity is bounded dorsally by nasal and frontal bones, ventrally by palatine processes of premaxilla, maxilla and horizontal part of the palatine, laterally by nasal processes of premaxilla, body of maxilla and perpendicular part of palatine bone and turbinate (conchal) bones. The turbinate bones divide each half of nasal cavity into dorsal, middle and ventral meatuses.

Nasal cavity shows **three mucosal folds**. The straight fold is the most dorsal and is continuous with the dorsal concha. Ventral to the straight fold is alar fold which is continuous with ventral nasal concha and contains supporting medial accessory nasal cartilage. The basal fold is the most ventral and unites rostrally with the alar fold. The nasolacrimal duct opens close to the nostril on the medial surface of alar fold.

Horse: The septum nasi meets the whole length of the floor of the nasal cavity so that posterior nares are completely separated. The opening of **nasolacrimal duct** is located on the **floor of nostril** at the junction of skin and mucous membrane and it has several orifices.

Dog: The nasal cavity is almost completely filled with nasal conchae. The caudal part of the septum nasi fails to meet the floor of the nasal cavity so that posterior nares are not completely separated. The nasolacrimal duct opens at the level of canine tooth where the alar fold meets floor of vestibule. The ***lamina transversalis divides caudal part of nasal cavity into upper olfactory and lower respiratory portions.***

Pig: The nasal cavity is long and narrow. Nasolacrimal duct opens on the floor of nostril at the junction of skin and nasal mucosa. This degenerates later and another opening is seen on lateral surface of ventral nasal concha near its caudal end.The septum nasi is present throught the floor of the nasal cavity, **hence the two posterior nares are completely separated**.

Fowl: The nasal cavity opens into the mouth and pharynx by narrow slit like opening. The cavity is cone shaped with apex pointing rostrally.

Posterior Nares (Choanae)

Ox: They are narrow and bounded laterally by pterygoid and perpendicular part of palatine bones and are separated only in upper part by vomer i.e not completely separated.

Horse: The posterior nares are short and divided i.e. **completely separated.**

Dog: They are like in ox i.e not completely separated.

Pig: Completely separated caudally.

THE INCISIVE (NASOPALATINE) DUCT

Ox: It is a paired tube in the floor of nasal cavity directed rostrventrally. It is about 6 cm long and **connects the nasal cavity with oral cavity**. Its nasal opening is hidden in ventral meatus, while the oral opening is in the fissure on either side of incisive papilla caudal to dental pad. The duct of **vomeronasal organ joins incisive duct close to its oral opening.**

Horse: The incisive duct does not open into oral cavity, but **ends blindly under oral mucosa.**

Dog: The **incisive duct receives the duct of vomeronasal organ** and opens into mouth cavity.

Pig: The incisive duct opens into oral cavity.

VOMERONASAL ORGAN (*ORGAN OF JACOBSON*)

Ox: It consists of a pair of ducts about 15-20 cm long, which lie in the floor of nasal cavity on each side of the nasal septum. The **vomeronasal duct joins incisive duct** close to its oral opening and also communicates with ventral meatus of nasal cavity, while the posterior end is blind and lies near **2nd to 4th cheek teeth**.

Horse: The vomeronasal organ does not communicate with mouth though it opens into incisive duct as the latter **ends blindly in mouth cavity**. However it communicates with nasal cavity.

Dog: It joins incisive duct which opens into mouth cavity.

Pig: It is small.

Fowl: Absent.

LATERAL NASAL GLAND

Its duct runs along middle meatus and opens inside the nostril close to straight fold or at the end of it.

Ox: It is absent.

Horse: It lies close to nasomaxillary aperture. The opening is at the level between first and second cheek tooth.

Dog: is located in maxillary recess. Its duct runs along middle nasal meatus and opens near straight fold in nasal vestibule.

Pig: It lies in maxillary sinus

Fowl: The elongated nasal gland (***Salt gland***) extends forward from the dorsal part of orbit in the lateral wall of nasal cavity. Its duct opens into the nasal cavity at the level of the rostral concha.

LARYNX

Ox: It is a short musculo - cartilaginous tube which connects the lower part of the pharynx with the trachea. It consists of cartilages, lined inside with mucous membrane. It is composed of following cartilages.

a) **Epiglottis:** It is an unpaired leaf shaped and most rostral cartilage of larynx situated in front of body of thyroid cartilage and connected to the latter. It shows the base (***posterior part***), apex (***anterior part***) and oral (***anterior***) and pharyngeal (***posterior)*** surfaces. The base shows short process, petiolus which is slightly curved rostrally. The tip (***free rounded part***) curves towards the root of tongue **(Fig.3.164).**

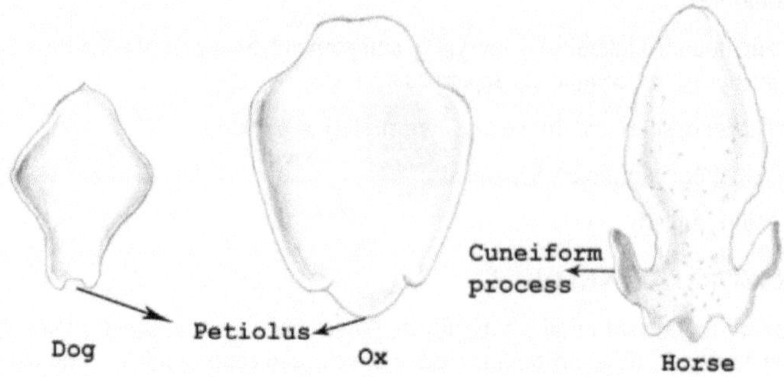

Fig. 3.164: Epiglottis of Different Species

b) **Thyroid cartilage**: It is an unpaired shield shaped cartilage placed ventrally and laterally and consists of two parts, **body and laminae**. The body is the central part attached to base of epiglottis and shows a prominence, the ***laryngeal prominence***. The laminae are the lateral parts which form the sides of larynx and show two cornua on either side, anterior and posterior cornua. The **short anterior cornu** articulates with thyroid cornu of hyoid, while the long posterior cornu curves ventrally and articulates with cricoid cartilage. ***Thyroid fissure*** is present below the anterior cornu bridged by connective tissue to form the ***thyroid foramen***. The rostral and caudal thyroid notches formed at union of two laminae are shallow **(Fig.3.165)**.

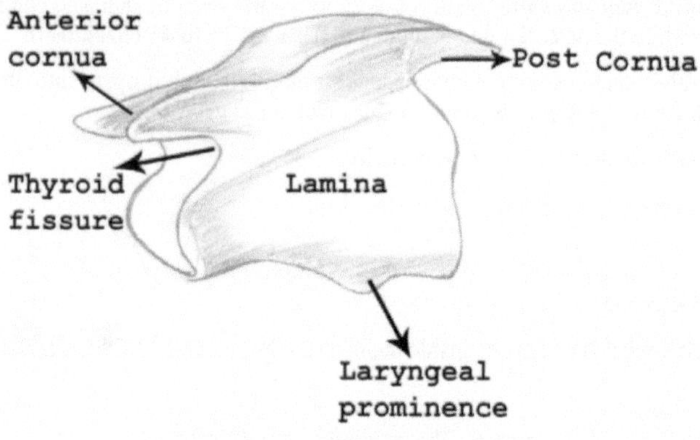

Fig. 3.165: Thyroid Cartilage-Ox

c) **Cricoid cartilage**: It is an unpaired and caudal cartilage. It is joined to the thyroid cartilage and is partly covered by thyroid laminae. **It is signet ring shaped** and consists of a lamina and two arches **(Fig.3.166)**. The dorsal part of lamina is broad and thick and marked by a median crest. On the cranial border of laminae are facets on either side to articulate with arytenoids and at the junction of laminae and arch are articular areas on either side for posterior cornua of thyroid cartilage. The arches form the ventral and lateral parts.

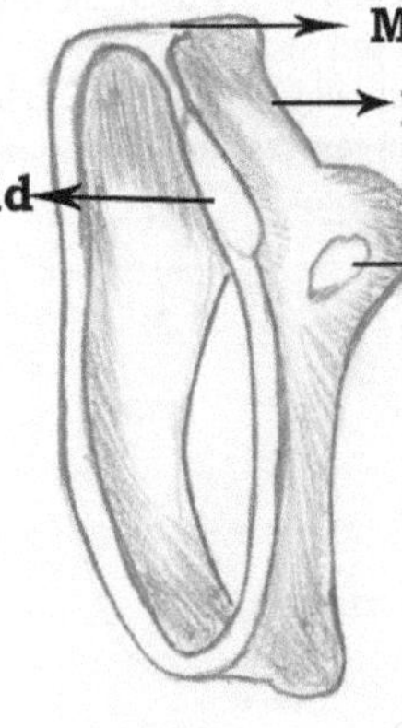

Fig. 3.166: Cricoid Cartilage-Ox

d) Arytenoid cartilages: They are paired and ***pyramidal*** in form. They are situated dorsally in front of cricoid, partly medial and dorsal to lamina of the thyroid cartilage. They show **three surfaces** (medial, dorsal and lateral), **three borders** (anterior, posterior and lateral), a base which faces backwards and an apex which lies in front. The base shows **muscular process** laterally and articular surface for cricoid dorsomedially. The apex consists of horn like **corniculate process** which curves caudally. The anterior and posterior borders form the **vocal process** ventrally **(Fig.3.167)**.

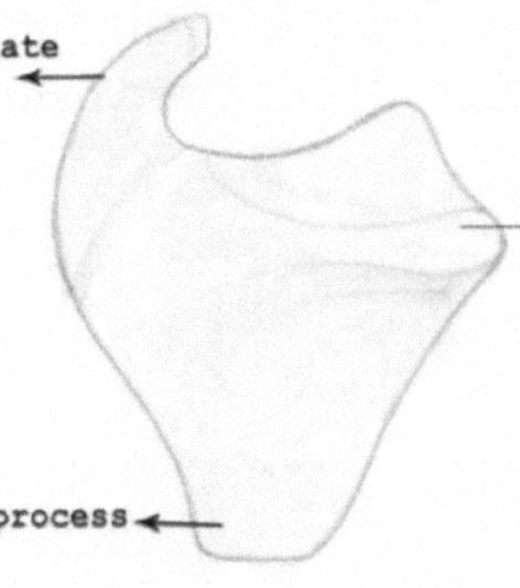

Fig. 3.167: Arytenoid Cartilage-Ox

Aditus laryngis is a large, oval, oblique aperture and is the entrance into the cavity of larynx. **The cavity of the larynx has the following three divisions**:

1. **Vestibule**: It extends between the aditus laryngis and the vocal folds. In front of vocal fold is a depression representing laryngeal ventricle of horse and dog. There is no vestibular fold unlike in horse and dog.
2. **Rima glottidis** (glottic cleft): It is the middle and narrowest part of the cavity, bounded on either side by vocal folds and arytenoid cartilages.
3. **Posterior compartment** (infraglottic cavity): is bounded by cricoid and is continuous with tracheal lumen.

Horse: 1.The **epiglottis is long, pointed and leaf like (Fig.3.164)**. 2. Cuneiform processes extend from the base of the epiglottis upwards and backwards in the vestibular folds. 3. The base of the epiglottis shows a median laryngeal recess in the floor of vestibule. 4. The **thyroid cartilage is incomplete ventrally** as the laminae meet only in the anterior part to form the body. 5. The caudal thyroid notch is very deep and **laryngeal prominence is absent (Figs. 3.168 & 3.169)**. 6. The cricoid cartilage is ring shaped and rostral border of arch is notched ventrally. 7. The laminae are wide **(Fig.3.170)**. 8. The muscular process of arytenoid is prominent. 9. The vocal process is short and rounded. 10. **Laryngeal ventricle (laryngeal saccule) lies between vestibular fold and vocal fold (Fig.3.171).**

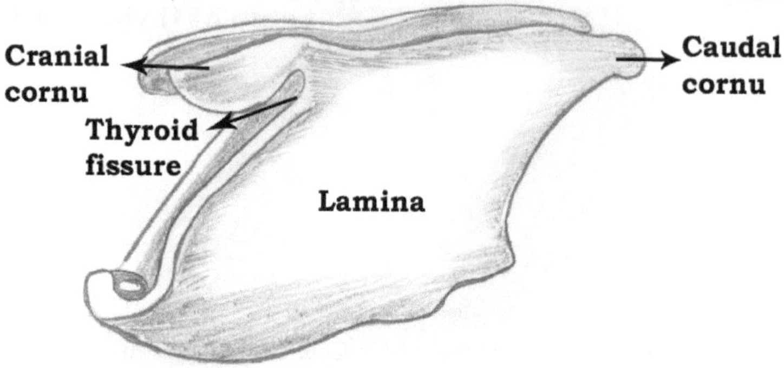

Fig. 3.168: Thyroid Cartilage-Horse (Lateral view)

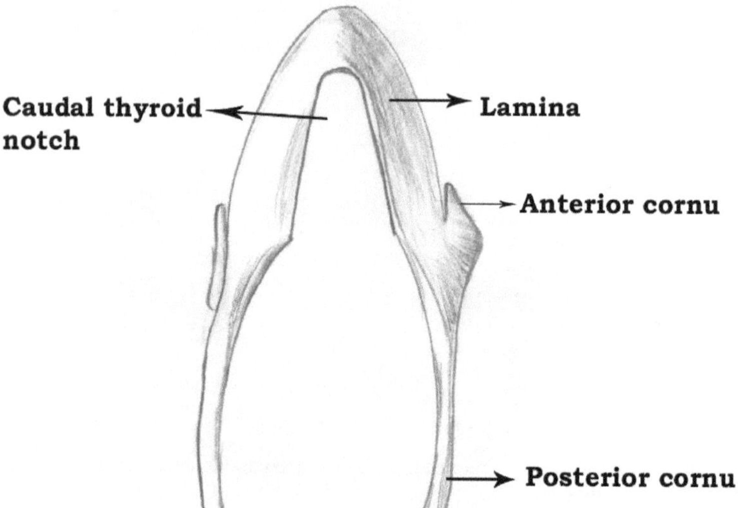

Fig. 3.169: Thyroid Cartilage of Horse (Ventral view)

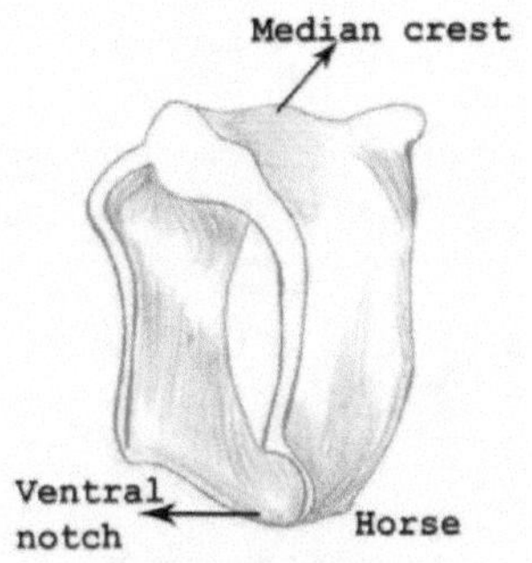

Fig. 3.170: Cricoid Cartilage of Horse

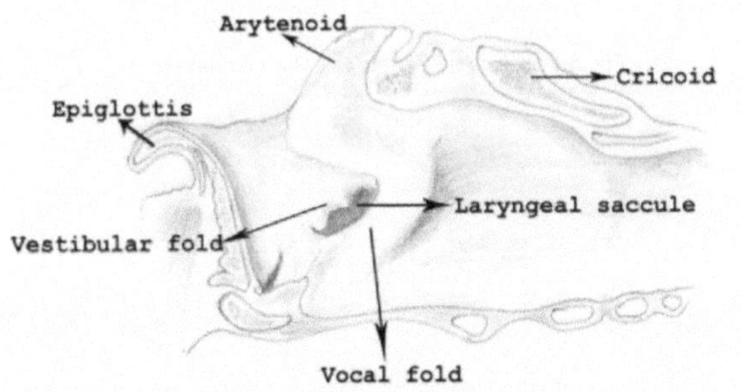

Fig. 3.171: Larynx-Horse (Interior)

Dog: 1.Larynx is very short and epiglottis is quadrilateral. 2. The ***petiolus is slightly forked*** **(Fig.3.164)**. 3. The thyroid cartilage is higher than it is long and laryngeal prominence is present. 4. The thyroid fissure is not converted into thyroid foramen. 5. The caudal thyroid notch is shallow **(Fig.3.172)**. 6. The cricoid is wider dorsally and the cuneiform process is large and arises from the base of the corniculate process and lies in aryepiglottic fold. 7. The ***corniculate process is hook like*** **(Fig.3.173)**.

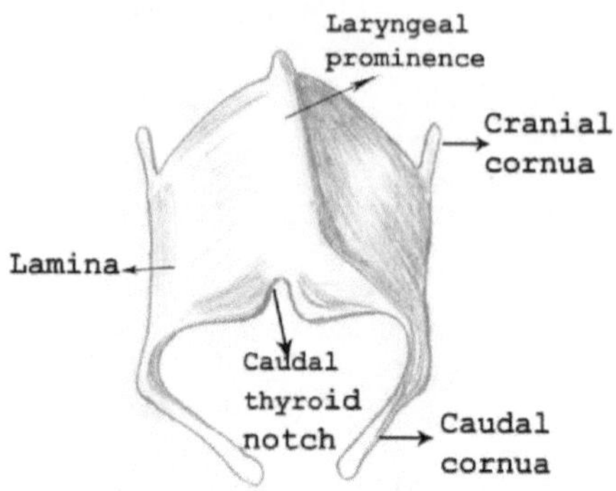

Fig. 3.172: Thyroid Cartilage of Dog (ventral view)

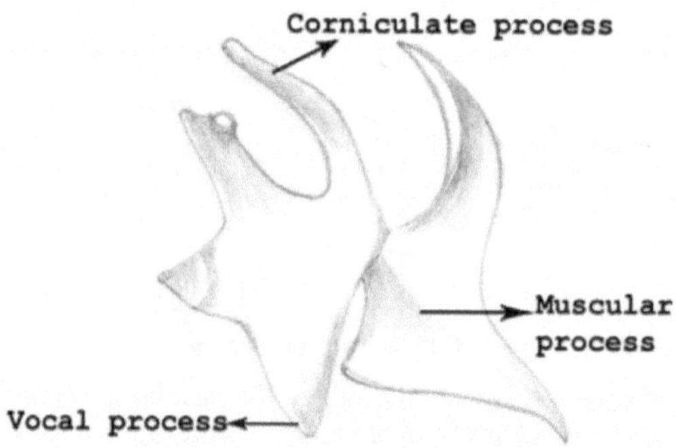

Fig. 3.173: Arytenoid Cartilage of Dog

8. A small **interarytenoid cartilage is present between the arytenoid cartilages**. 9. The vestibular ligament extends from floor of thyroid cartilage to cuneiform process of arytenoid cartilage and contains ventricularis muscle and vestibular ligament. The vocal folds and ligaments are directed cranioventrally. 10. The vocal folds contain vocal ligament and vocalis muscle.

Pig: 1.The larynx is placed more caudally. 2. Thyroid cartilage is very long and shows oblique lines only caudally. 3. Rostral cornu of thyroid cartilage is absent. 4. Ventrally the caudal margin of thyroid cartilage shows a short median projection and the caudal thyroid notch is absent. 5. The lamina of cricoid is long and median crest is prominent. The arches are narrow, directed caudoventrally and drawn out to a point. 6. The corniculate processes are large and show semilunar extension and are fused dorsomedially so as to form an unpaired structure. 7. The muscular process of arytenoid is high. 8. Interarytenoid cartilage is present. 9. The epiglottis forms a deep trough and base is wide and tip is rounded. 10. A median laryngeal recess is present in the floor of the vestibule. 11. The vestibular folds are absent. 12. The laryngeal vestibule is long.

Fowl: The larynx consists of two (cranial and caudal) parts.

Cranial larynx: The anterior part which is made up of **unpaired cricoid and procricoid and paired arytenoid cartilages**.

Caudal larynx or Syrinx (Fig.3.174): is the posterior part and is true organ of voice, situated at the bifurcation of trachea into two bronchi. It involves terminal part of trachea and the first part of two primary bronchi. There are four cartilaginous components.

1. The **cranial cartilages** forming tympanum are comprised of ***four closely apposed cartilaginous rings in male and three in female*** **(Fig.3.174)**. They are slightly greater in diameter than preceeding tracheal rings and their edges blend.
2. The **pessulus** is wedge shaped and lies dorsoventrally. Its sharp cranial edge splits lumen into two primary bronchi **(Fig.3.174)**.
3. The **intermediate** (tracheal syringeal) cartilages are four in number and are 'C shaped .They are attached to pessulus at ventral end and free at dorsal end.
4. **Caudal (bronchial syringeal) cartilages** are 'C' shaped and ***three on each side*** **(Fig.3.174).**

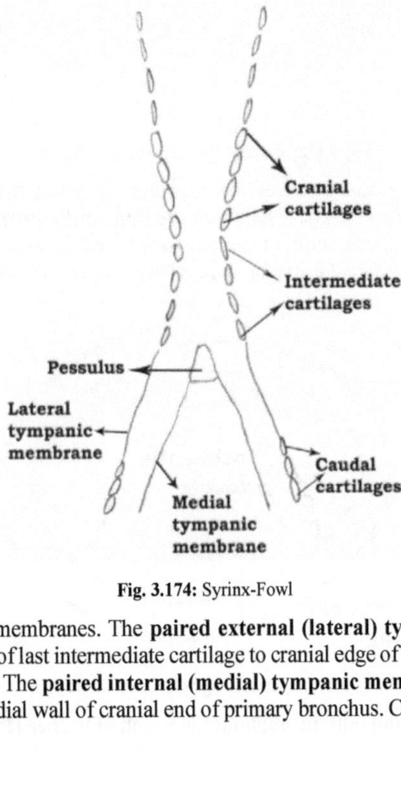

Fig. 3.174: Syrinx-Fowl

There are two pairs of vibrating membranes. The **paired external (lateral) tympanic membrane** lies on lateral aspect of syrinx from caudal edge of last intermediate cartilage to cranial edge of first caudal cartilage being attached dorsally and ventrally to pessulus. The **paired internal (medial) tympanic membrane** stretches between free ends of caudal cartilages and forms medial wall of cranial end of primary bronchus. Cranially it attaches to caudal border of pessulus.

TRACHEA

It is a flexible cartilaginous and membranous air conducting tube extending from the larynx to the hilus of the lungs where it divides into right and left principal bronchi.

Ox: It is made up of about **50-60 'C' shaped cartilaginous rings with open segment of 'C' facing dorsally (Fig.3.175)**. *Tracheal cartilages are not constant in all species and vary even in the animals of the same species. Occasionally, adjacent cartilages are partly or completely fused.* ***It is most often in pig and least often in the ruminants***. The trachealis (smooth) muscle and fibro elastic membrane (membrana transversa) connect the free edges of the tracheal rings. At the beginning of the tube free ends of rings are separated by an interval but further back the ends are in apposition. Caudally the free dorsal ends of the cartilaginous plates form a ***dorsal crest***. The

trachea bifurcates into right and left principal bronchi ***at the level of 5th rib*** and **tracheal (apical) bronchus** is given off from trachea ***at the level of 3rd rib to cranial lobe of right lung.***

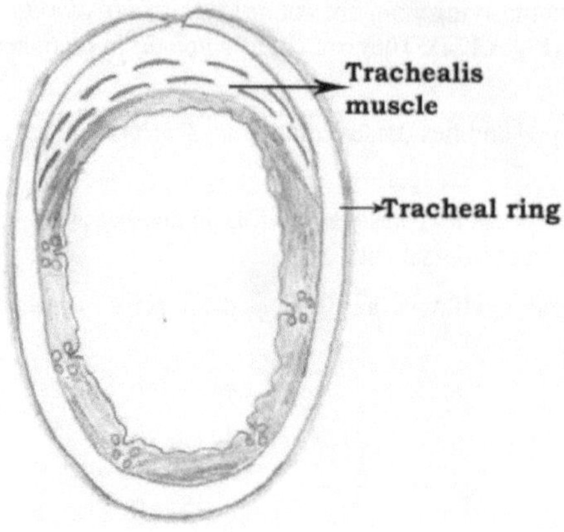

Fig. 3.175: Tracheal Ring of Ox-Cervical Part

Horse: The trachea is longer and flattened dorsoventrally and there are about 48 to 60 tracheal rings. ***The free ends of the tracheal rings overlap slightly in cervical part with the right end overlying the left, while in thoracic part they do not meet*** **(Fig.3.176)**. Several thin **plates of cartilage are found** between the ends of the tracheal cartilages, just cranial to the bifurcation. ***The tracheal bronchus (apical bronchus) is absent.***

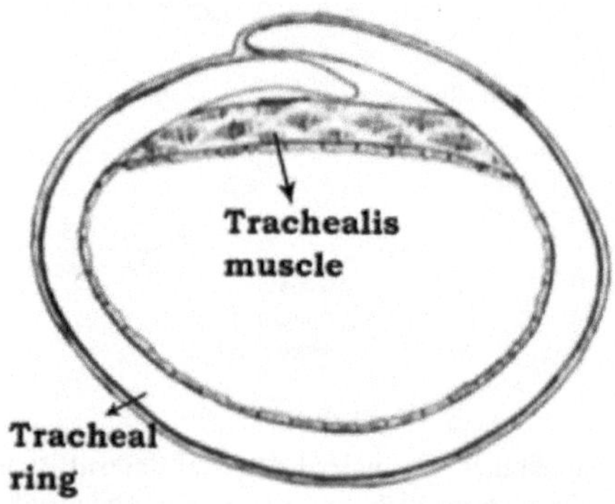

Fig. 3.176: Tracheal ring of Horse-Cervical Part

Dog: The **tracheal rings are open dorsally throughout** the length of trachea **(Fig.3.177)**.

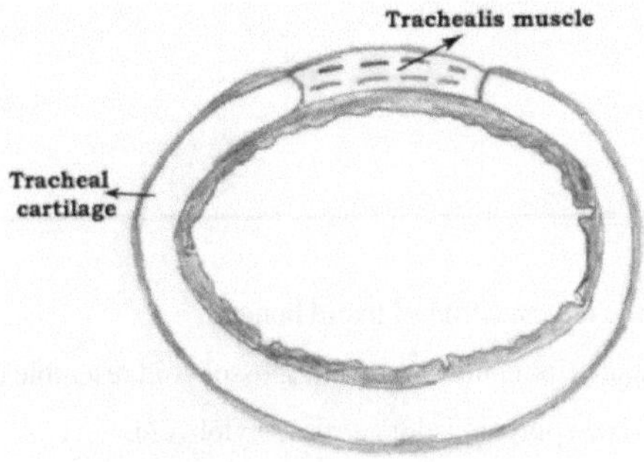

Fig. 3.177: Tracheal Ring of Dog

Pig: Tracheal bronchus to cranial lobe of the right lung is present. The trachea is circular in cross section **(Fig.3.178)**. The ends of cartilages overlap each other and the trachealis is attached to their deep surface.

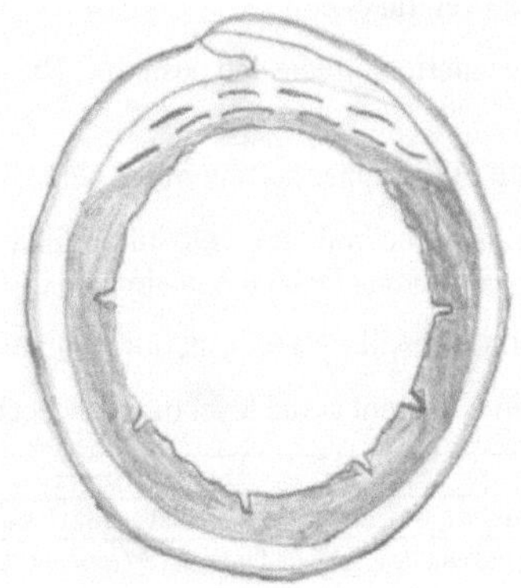

Fig. 3.178: Tracheal Ring of Pig

Fowl: The trachea extends between cranial larynx and caudal larynx and the **tracheal rings are completely closed dorsally**. It does not follow the contour of the neck, instead it crosses neck on right side.

3.9 SUMMARY

In ox and horse the stylohyoid is the largest cornu of hyoid bone.

In horse the body and thyrohyoids are fused and along with glossohyoid resemble a spur or fork.

In dog the glossohyoid is absent. The epihyoid is longer than stylohyoid.

Nasal bone of fowl shows body and frontal, premaxillary and maxillary processes.

In ox the dorsal turbinate is smaller and attached to dorsal turbinate crest of nasal bone. The larger ventral turbinate is attached to ventral turbinate crest of the maxilla.

In horse the dorsal turbinate is larger than ventral one.

In fowl turbinates are three in number i.e anterior, middle and posterior. The posterior is the smallest and the middle one is largest.

In fowl the premaxillae form the skeleton of the upper portion of the beak.

Maxilla is the largest bone of the upper jaw. The body presents infraorbital foramen at the level of the first cheek tooth, while at the level of 3rd or 4th cheek tooth is facial tuberosity in ox.

The maxillary hiatus shows sphenopalatine, maxillary and posterior palatine foramina.

In horse and dog the infraorbital foramen is present at the level of third cheek tooth.

Name of the foramen	Associated bone	Structure passing
Foramen ovale	Temporal wing of post sphenoid	Mandibular division of trigeminal nerve
Foramen orbitorotundum	At the junction of Pre and Post sphenoid i.e. between orbitial wing & temporal wing	*III, IV, VI and maxillary and ophthalmic divisions of trigeminal nerve*
Foramen lacerum	Occipital, Temporal and Post sphenoid	*IX, X, XI cranial nerves.*
Foramen magnum	Occipital	*Spinal cord*
Stylomastoid foramen	Temporal	*Facial nerve*
Ethmoid foramen	Presphenoid and frontal	*Ethmoidal nerve*
Optic foramen	Orbital wing of presphenoid	*Optic nerve*
Maxillary foramen	Maxilla	*Maxillary nerve*
Infraorbital foramen	Maxilla	*Maxillary nerve and Infraorbital artery*
Mandibular foramen	Mandible	*Mandibular nerve, Mandibuloalveolar artery*
Mental foramen	At the junction of body with horizentlal ramus of mandible	*Mental nerve*
Palatine foramen	Horizontal part of palatine	*Greater palatine artery and nerve*

The number of endo and ectoturbinates

ox : 5+18

horse: 6+21

dog : 4+6

pig : 7+13

Lamina transversalis: In dog the lamina lateralis of ethmoid with incurved part of palatine bone and outcurving plate of vomer form a transverse horizontal plate called lamina froms versalio. It divides the nasal cavity into upper olfactory and lower respiratory compartments.

Ox: The frontal sinus is largest and is seen in frontal, parietal, interparietal and supraoccipital bones.

Horse: The maxillary sinus is the largest sinus

Middle Ear: The middle ear is housed in the tympanic cavity. The lateral wall of the cavity is formed by the tympanic membrane. The medial wall contains two windows (fenestrae),

Auditory Ossicles: Tympanic cavity is mediated by the three auditory ossicles known, in lateromedial sequence, as malleus, incus and stapes (Latin name for hammer, anvil and stirrup respectively)

The internal ear enclosed in the very hard petrous temporal bone and shows vestibular and cochlear parts.

Vestibular part: consists of semicircular canals, utricle and saccule and it is concerned with balancing of body.

The semicircular ducts are 3 in number i.e anterior, posterior and lateral.

Cochlear part consists of spiral cochlear duct concerned with hearing.

Endolymphatic duct ends blindly in the epidural space.

Caruncula sublingualis / barb is a wide, flat and hard/firm papilla with slightly serrated edge in which duct of mandibular and ventral (monostomatic) part of sublingual salivary gland open into the mouth.

Orobasal organ is present on a low median ridge just caudal to central incisors. They represent remnants of rostral sublingual gland of reptiles.

Ox: The papilla salivalis is present at the level of upper 5th cheek tooth

Horse: The papilla salivalis is about the level of upper 3rd cheek tooth.

Dog: The papilla salivalis is about the level of upper 3rd cheek tooth.

Zygomatic (orbital) gland: is a seromucous globular gland present in anterior part of pterygopalatine fossa of dog.

The incisive papilla is a diamond shaped papilla which lies between the dental pad and first ridge of hard palate

Torus linguae: is an eminence present on the posterior part of dorsal face of the body of the tongue of ox.

Fossa linguae: is a transverse depression present infront of the torus linguae of tongue of ox.

Circumvallate papillae are 8 to 17 in number on each side in ox.

Horse: Circumvallate papillae are 2 or 3 in number on posterior part of dorsum. Foliate papillae are present infront of the anterior pillars of soft palate .

Dog: Circumvallate papillae are 2 or 3 in number

Lyssa: is a fusiform cord of fibrous tissue, adipose tissue and striated muscle fibres

Pig: Circumvallate papillae are two in number.

In ox mandibular salivary gland is largest salivary gland. The mandibular (Whartons) duct leaving the middle of the dorsal border of the gland opens into caruncula sublingualis.

In horse parotid is largest salivary gland and is quadrilateral in outline. The Stenson's duct opens on papilla salivalis about the level of upper third cheek tooth. Sublingual gland shows only polystomatic part.The momostomatic part is absent.

In dog parotid is irregularly triangular and notched dorsally. Papilla salivalis is opposite to upper third or fourth cheek tooth.

Mandibular salivary gland is globular/rounded, larger and lighter in color than parotid.

In pig parotid gland is triangular and large. The stenson's duct opens opposite third or fourth upper cheek tooth.

Carnassial or sectorial (Cutting) teeth: In dog the upper 4th and lower 5th are larger than the rest, termed carnassial or sectorial (Cutting) teeth.

Pharynx: Pharynx contains 7 openings. They are isthmus faucium (aditus pharyngis), paired posterior nares, paired Eustachian openings, auditus laryngis and aditus oesophagi

Oesophagus: is placed on dorsal aspect of trachea upto 3rd or 4th cervical vertebra in ox.

UNIT 4
THORAX

4.1 BONES OF THE THORAX

Thoracic Vertebrae

Ox: Thoracic vertebrae characterized by **well developed neural spines, short bodies with capitular facets** and transverse processes with tubercular facets for articulation with the ribs (**Fig.4.1).**

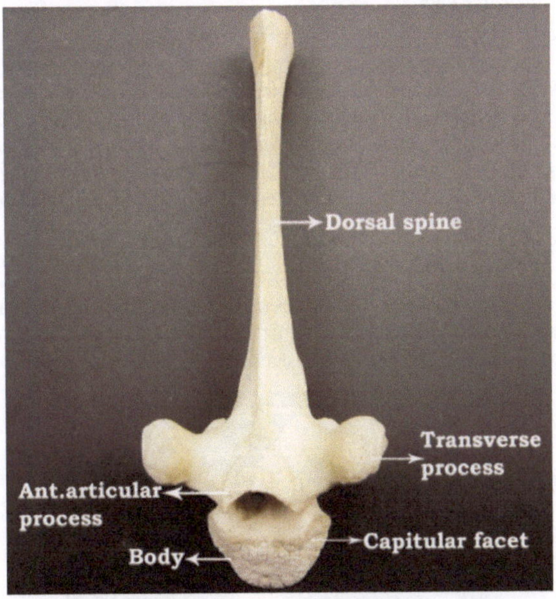

Fig. 4.1: Thoracic Vertebra of Ox

The anterior notches of the pedicles are shallower. The posterior ones are converted into foramina in the posterior series. The articular processes are small, oval and present on the anterior part of the neural arch. The posterior ones spring from the base of the spinous process.

Special features: The spine of the first thoracic vertebra is very long and pointed. The spines of the next two are the longest and behind these gradually diminish in height. The backward slope of first is slight but increases to 10th. ***The last dorsal (13th) has a vertical spine hence it is called*** as ***anticlinal vertebra.*** The tubercular facets articulating with the tubercle of the rib of same number gradually decrease in size from before backwards. The capitualar facets of adjacent vertebrae form complete cavity for articulating with heads of ribs. The last dorsal has no posterior capitular facets.

Horse: The spine of the 1st is shorter and curved backward. The bodies are shorter. The length of the spinous process increases to the 3rd and 4th then gradually diminishes to the 15th beyond which they are about the same height. The backward inclination of the dorsal spine is most pronounced in the second. ***The spine of 16th is vertical (anticlinal)*** and those of the last two are directed slightly backward. The last four or five show distinct mammillary processes.

Dog: The bodies are wider and compressed dorsoventrally. The transverse processes in the posterior of the series bear mammillary processes and in the last three accessory processes also. The posterior facets for the heads of the ribs are absent on the last two or three. The ***11th is the anticlinal vertebra.***

Pig: The thoracic vertebrae are commonly **14 or 15 in number**. Their bodies are relatively long, constricted in the middle and are without ventral crests. There are mamillary processes except on the first two. Small accessory processes occur in the caudal part of the region. The first spinous process is broad, very high and inclined a little cranially. The others diminish gradually in length to the tenth, beyond which they are about equal. The second to the ninth are inclined caudally, the tenth is the "diaphragmatic" and the ***eleventh is vertical (anticlinal)***. The width decreases from the fourth to the tenth, beyond which there is a gradual increase.

Fowl: The **first and 6th vertebrae are free** while **second to the 5th are fused** into one piece. The **seventh is fused to the lumbosacral mass.** Each vertebra presents a complete capitular cavity for the corresponding rib. The superior and inferior spines are well developed and are fused from 2nd to the 5th. The transverse processes are plate like and present tubercular facets at their free ends.

RIBS

Ox: There are **13 pairs of ribs** and these are elongated curved bones. Each rib articulates dorsally with the bodies of the two adjacent thoracic vertebrae and is continued ventrally by a costal cartilage. Those that articulate with the sternum individually by means of costal cartilage are termed **sternal (true) ribs (8 pairs**). The **remainder are asternal (false) ribs** whose long and slender costal cartilages are attached to each other by elastic tissue to form costal arch and have common attachment to sternum. Except in the case of the first the cartilage does not continue direction of ribs but forms with the latter an angle which is open in front.

Note: Number of sternal ribs = No. of sternebrae + 1

Each rib presents a **shaft and two extremities.** The shaft is most curved at its upper part called **angle** while its lower part is twisted and incline inwards. The lateral face is marked by a **wide groove** in its anterior part. The medial surface shows a distinct groove (***costal groove***) at its posterior part (**Fig.4.2).**

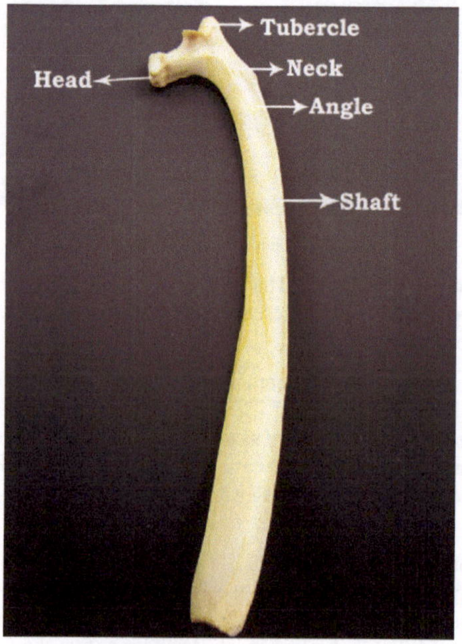

Fig. 4.2: Rib of Ox

The **upper (vertebral) extremity** is made up of a head, neck and a tubercle. The **head** consists of anterior and posterior facets separated by a non-articular groove. The facets articulate with capitular facets of preceeding vertebrae and vertebrae of same number. The neck joins the head to the shaft. The **tubercle** is situated above and behind the head at the junction of the head and neck. Dorsally it presents a transversely placed concave facet for articulation with **tubercular facet** of the transverse process of thoracic vertebra of the same number. The **tubercular facets are absent** in the last two or three ribs. The **lower (sternal) extremity** is smooth and articulates with costal cartilage.

Special Features of 1st Rib:

1. It is the **shortest and least curved** and its sternal end widens very greatly. 2. The lateral surface and the **anterior border present a rough area** about its middle for the **scalenus ventralis muscle**. 3. At the lower part of anterior border is a vascular impression for brachial vessels. 4. The groove on the lateral surface and the costal groove are absent. 5. The tubercle is **larger than that of any other rib (Fig.4.3).**

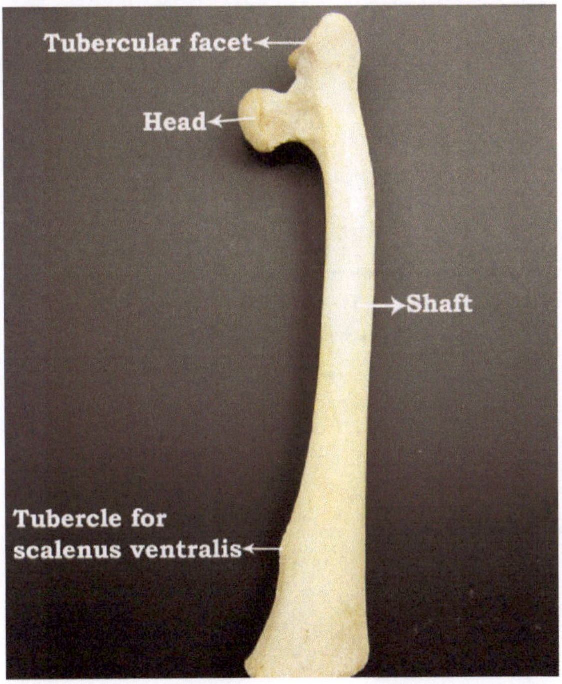

Fig. 4.3: 1st Rib of Ox

The **8th, 9th and 10th ribs are the longest and widest**. The costal cartilages are rods of hyaline cartilage. The first costal cartilage is the shortest.

Horse: There are **18 pairs of ribs, 8 sternal and 10 asternal**. They are shorter, narrower, thicker and more curved. The length increases upto the 10th and then diminishes. The anterior borders of the ribs from 2nd to 8th are sharp and rounded and thick from 9th to 18th. The lower ends of ribs are slightly enlarged and roughened at the junction with the costal cartilages. The first pair of costal cartilages articulate with each other and with sternum.

Dog: There are **13 pairs of ribs. 9 sternal and 4 asternal**. They are **strongly curved, narrow and thick**. The **last rib** is usually **floating** i.e. it does not reach sternum at all. The costal cartilages are long and curve ventrally and forward.

Pig: There are ***14 or 15 pairs***, of which **seven are usually true or sternal** and **seven or eight are false or asternal**. The first rib is prismatic and has a large ventral end and a very short cartilage. The **width is greatest in the third to the sixth and the length is highest usually in the sixth and seventh.**

Fowl: There are **7 pairs of ribs** and are totally bony unlike mammals (i.e no costal cartilage.). Each rib is made up of an **upper vertebral rib** and a **lower sternal rib**. The **1st, 2nd and sometimes 7th do not have sternal ribs (these are floating)**. The head of a rib articulates with the capitular cavity of a single dorsal vertebra of same number. Except the first and the seventh the posterior border of each vertebral rib presents an ***uncinate process*** directed backward to overlap the succeeding rib (**Fig.4.4).**

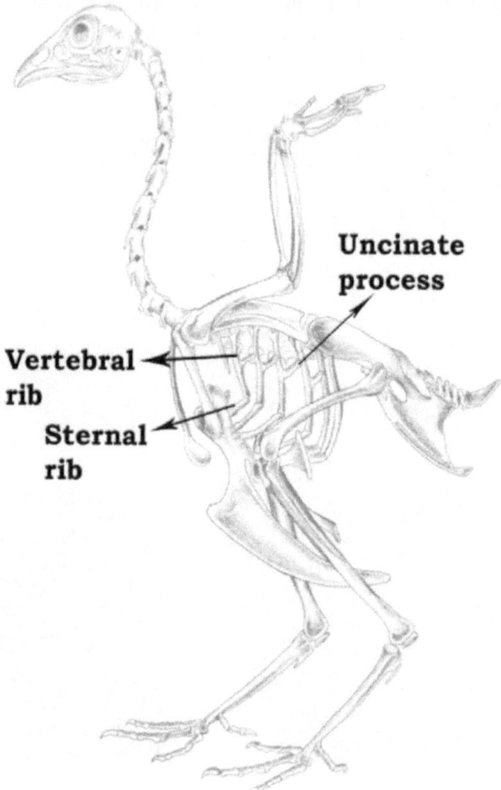

Fig. 4.4: Skeleton of Fowl

STERNUM

Ox: It is made up of **seven bony segments** (sternebrae). It **presents two surfaces, two borders and two extremities.** The **dorsal face** is narrow in front but becomes gradually wider behind. The **ventral face** is strongly convex in front but more or less concave behind the second sternebra. **The lateral borders** are thick in front but become thinner gradually behind. Each border presents eight articular cavities for articulation with the ventral extremities of the costal cartilages.

The **anterior extremity** is the anterior end of the first sternebra which forms the **manubrium sterni or presternum.** The **posterior extremity or metasternum** is formed by the **xiphoid cartilage** which is thin, flexible and nearly circular. Between the pre and metasternum is the **body or mesosternum (Fig.4.5).**

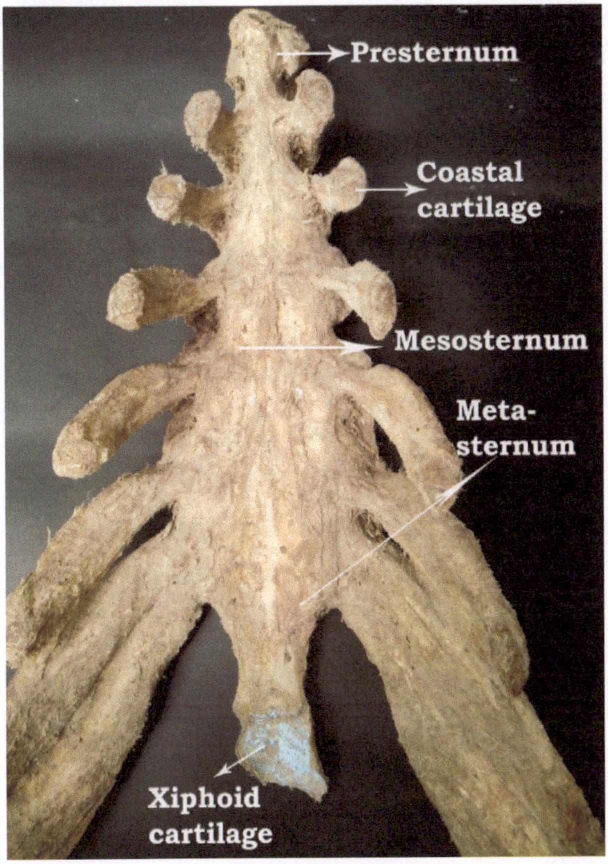

Fig. 4.5: Sternum of Ox-Dorsal View

Horse: 1. Is composed of **7 sternebrae**. 2. It is ***canoe or boat shaped*** and presents **three surfaces, three borders and two extremities**. 3. The superior face is triangular and narrow. 4. The two lateral surfaces are convex above, slightly concave below and present costal cavities on their upper parts. 5. The **two dorso lateral borders** separate the dorsal and lateral surfaces. The inferior border is the keel. 6. The anterior extremity presents a ***laterally compressed cariniform*** cartilage which presents a deep notch superiorly for articulation with the first ribs **(Fig.4.6).**

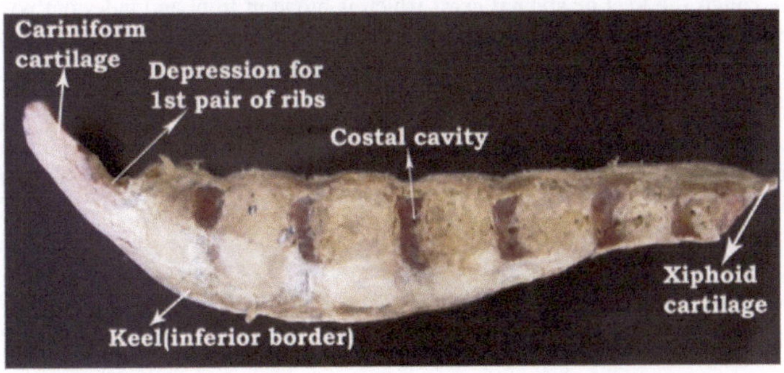

Fig. 4.6: Sternum of Horse-Lateral View

Dog: It is composed of **8 sternebrae**. Each sternebra is slightly compressed from side and constricted in its middle. The **anterior end presents a small presternal cartilage. The xiphoid cartilage is narrow (Fig.4.7).**

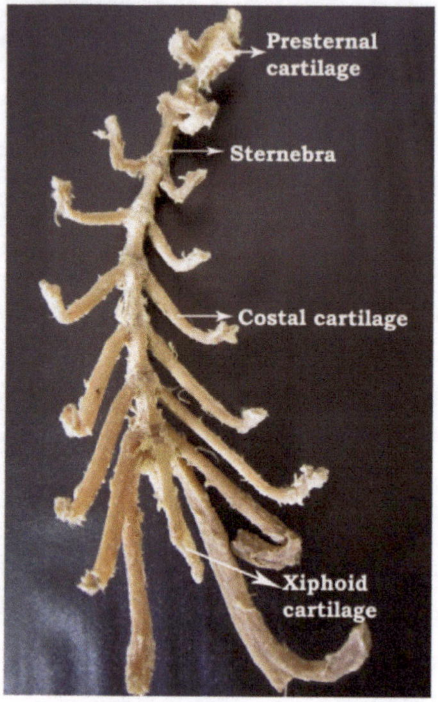

Fig. 4.7: Sternum of Dog

Pig: The sternum consists of **six segments** and resembles that of ox in general form. The first segment (manubrium) is long, flattened laterally and bears a blunt-pointed cartilage on its cranial end; its caudal end forms a synovial joint with the body. The last segment has a long, narrow xiphoid process which bears the xiphoid cartilage.

Fowl: It results from the **fusion of five pieces**. The central wide part forms the body of the bone. Infront of this is the short anterior process, the **rostrum or manubrium** and behind is the **posterior process or metasternum**.

The dorsal surface of the body is pierced by a foramen. The **rostrum** shows on either side of its root an elongated facet for articulation with the coracoid bone. The **metasternum** is very long and extensive and carries ventrally a **thin plate of bone called the keel or sternal crest** which is broad in front and fades out posteriorly **(Fig.4.9).** United to each lateral border of body are the **anterolateral or costal process** in front and the **postero-lateral process** behind, the latter is divided into medial and **lateral xiphoid processes (Fig.4.8).**

The lateral xiphoid process is broad plate like and covers the last two or three ribs. The medial xiphoid process is longer and projects backwards parallel to the lateral border of the metasternum. Between the **anterolateral and posterolateral processes** the lateral border of the body shows four depressions on either side for articulating with the **3rd to 6th ribs (Fig.4.8).**

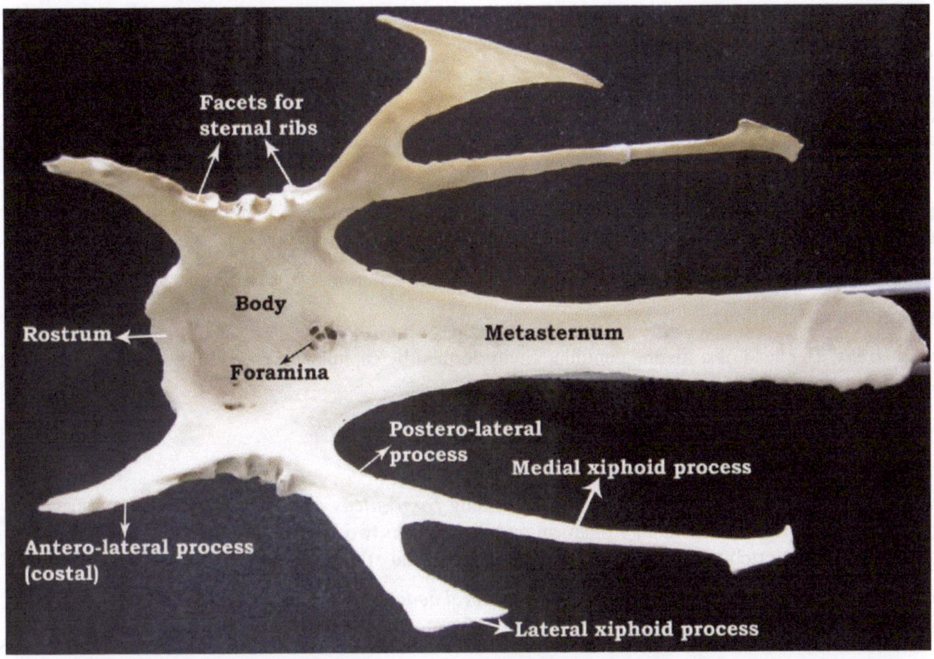

Fig. 4.8: Sternum of Fowl-Dorsal view

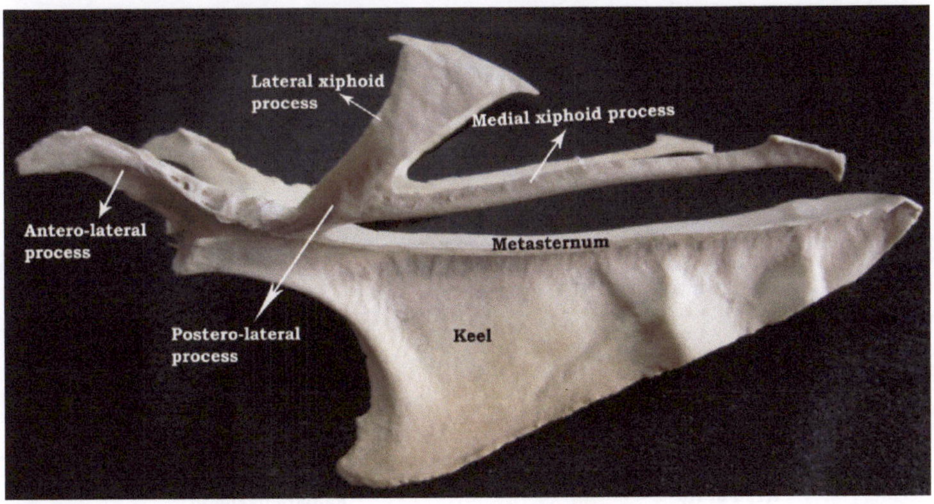

Fig. 4.9: Sternum of Fowl- Lateral View

4.2 JOINTS OF THE THORAX

The joints of the thorax consist of 1) Costovertebral 2) Costochondral 3) Chondrosternal and 4) Intersternal articulations

1.Costovertebral articulation: They are composed of **costo-central and costo-transverse articulations.**

i. Costo-central articulation:

Articular areas: The head of a rib and capitular cavity formed by capitular facets of bodies of adjacent thoracic vertebrae.

Type: Composite, diarthrodial (Trochoid).

Ligaments: a).Capsular ligament,

b) **Conjugal ligament (*Intraarticular ligament*)** extending ***from sulcus of head of a rib*** passes transversely in vertebral canal under dorsal longitudinal ligament and divides into two branches. One of these is attached to the body of the preceding vertebra and the other is attached to the head of the opposite rib **(Fig.4.10).**

c) **Radiate ligament** extending ***from neck of rib to vertebral bodies and the intervertebral disc*** **(Fig.4.10).**

Movements: Rotation, during inspiration and expiration increasing and decreasing size of chest cavity respectively.

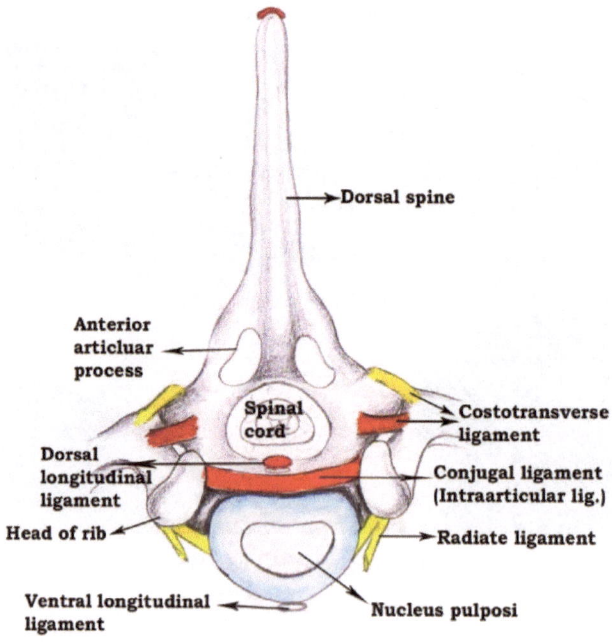

Fig. 4.10: Costovertebral Articulation (Anterior aspect)

b. Costo-transverse articulation

Articular areas: facets of transverse processes of thoracic vertebrae and tubercular facet of ribs of same number.

Type: Simple, diarthrodial (Arthrodia).

Ligaments: a) Capsular ligament. b) **Costo-transverse ligament** is a distinct strong band which arises from the transverse process and ends on the non articular part of the tubercle. It is covered by levator costae muscle.
Movements: Gliding

2. Costochondral articulation: are diarthrodial (arthrodia) type formed between ribs and the costal cartilages

Articular areas: ventral ends of sternal ribs and costal cartilages

Type: Simple, diarthrodial (arthrodia).

Ligaments: Capsular ligament.

Movements: Gliding.

3. Chondrosternal articulation: are diarthrodial (trochoid) type formed between the cartilages of sternal ribs and the sternum.

Articular areas: Costal cartilages of sternal ribs and articular cavities between adjacent sternebrae.

Type: Simple, diarthrodial (trochoid).

Movements: Rotation

Ligaments: 1.**Capsular ligament** (2) and (3) **Superior and inferior chondrosternal ligaments** extending from the cartilage to the sternum on the superior and inferior aspect of the joint. 4. **Cruciate ligament unites the ventral ends of** the first pair of ribs.

Interchondral ligaments: The asternal cartilages are united by their free ends to those in front by elastic fibers. The ninth costal cartilage besides being attached to the eight costal cartilage is also attached to inferior face of the xiphoid cartilage by **chondroxiphoid ligament**.

4. Intersternal articulation: The intersternal articulations except the first are synchondroses, the adjacent strernal segments are connected to one another by discs of cartilages. The first sternebra is articulated to the second by diarthosis which permits limited movements. The different sternal segments are connected on their dorsal aspect by a common internal sternal ligament which is narrow infront and becomes wider posteriorly and ends on the last segment.

Articular areas: adjacent sternebrae

Type: Simple, amphiarthroses while between first and second it is **diarthrodial.**

Ligaments: Dorsal sternal ligament connecting different segments (sternebrae) which becomes wider behind.
Movements: Not appreciable

4.3 MUSCLES OF THE THORAX

1. **Levatores costarum:** These are 10 or 11 pairs, located at the upper part of the intercostal spaces.
2. **External intercostals: These muscles are located in the intercostal spaces, but** donot extend into interchondral spaces.
3. **Internal intercostals:** These muscles are situated internal to the external intercostal muscles and also **extend into the interchondral spaces.**
4. **Retractor costae:** It is a **small triangular muscle** situated behind the last rib under the cover of last digitation of serratus dorsalis posterior.
5. **Rectus thoracis:** This is a thin **quadrilateral muscle** lying on the lateral face of first few ribs and their cartilages under cover of deep pectoral.
6. **Transversus thoracis:** It is a **small triangular muscle** situated on the **dorsal face of the sternum inside the thorax.**
7. **Diaphragm:** It is a ***chief inspiratory*** muscle. It is a large dome shaped, unpaired muscle which forms partition between the thoracic and abdominal cavities. Its **thoracic surface is convex** and is covered by **pleura** and the **abdominal surface** is **concave and is covered by peritoneum.** It consists of **a. *Muscular*** **b. *Lumbar*** ***and c. Tendinous parts*** **(Fig.4.11).**

    a. ***Muscular part:*** consists of **costal and sternal** parts. **Costal part** is attached from the **last rib** to the **junction of the eighth rib** and its cartilage. **Sternal part** is attached along the cartilage of the eighth rib and across the abdominal surface of the xiphoid cartilage.

    b. ***Lumbar part:*** consists of the right and left crura. The **right and left crura are** attached to the body of the first lumbar vertebra by **ventral longitudinal ligament.** The ***right crurs*** is the larger of the two which divides into two divisions circumscribing the ***hiatus oesophagi*** for the passage of the **oesophagus and the vagus nerves.** Between the right and left crura ventral to the last thoracic vertebra is the ***hiatus aorticus*** for the aorta, the **vena hemiazygos and the cistern chyli.** Thoracic duct doesn't pass through hiatus aorticus but through the right crus of the diaphragm.

    c. ***Tendinous part:*** The tendinous centre is pierced on the right by ***foramen venacavae*** for the passage of posterior venacava.

Openings of the Diaphragm: The following **three openings** are present in the diaphragm **(Fig.4.11).**

a. ***Hiatus oesophagi*** **-for passage of oesophagus and vagus nerves.**

b. ***Hiatus aorticus*****- for passage of aorta.**

c. ***Foramen venacavae for passage of posterior venacava.***

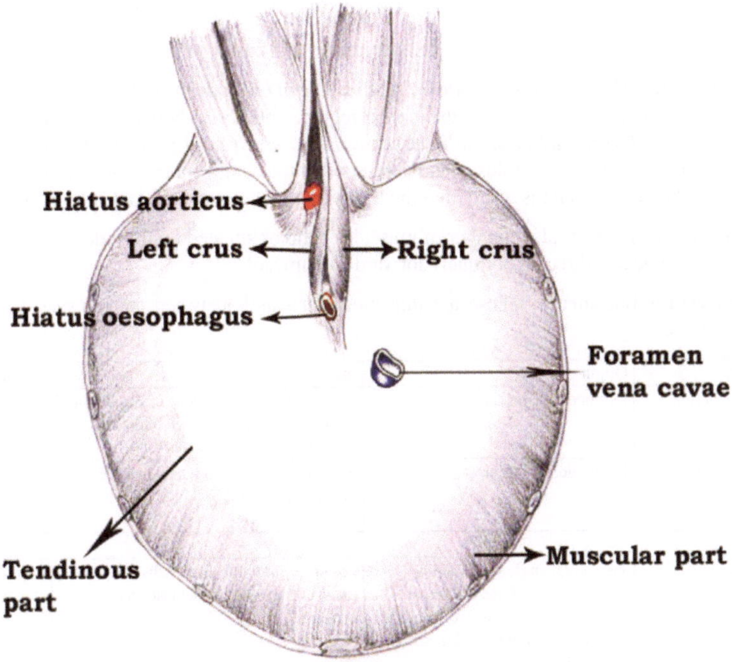

Fig. 4.11: Different Openings in Diaphragm

Name of the muscle	Origin	Insertion	Action
1.Levatores costarum	Transverse process of thoracic vertebrae	Anterior border of the ribs of same number	To aid in inspiration
2.External intercostals	Posterior border of ribs except last rib	Anterior border and external surface of the ribs behind.	To aid in inspiration
3.Internal intercostals	Anterior border of ribs and its cartilage except first.	Posterior border of preceeding rib and its cartilage.	Assist in forced expiration
4.Retractor costae	Transverse process of first 2 or 3 lumbar vertebrae	Caudal border of last rib	To aid in forced expiration
5.Rectus thoracis	Lateral surface of the 1st rib.	Costal cartilages	To aid in inspiration
6.Transversus thoracis	Sternal ligament	Cartilages of the ribs from the 2nd to 8th and adjacent parts of the ribs.	To aid in expiration
7. Diaphragm	As described above		Chief inspiratory muscle

MUSCLE OF THE BACK AND LOIN:

First layer: 1. Trapezius thoracalis 2. Latissimus dorsi

Second layer

1. Rhomboideus
2. Serratus dorsalis anterior**:** This muscle is situated under the serratus thoracis.
3. Serratus dorsalis posterior: Inserts on posterior borders and lateral surfaces of the ***last three ribs***

Third layer

1. **Longissimus costarum:** This muscle has distinct lumbar and costal parts.
2. **Longissimus dorsi:** This is the ***largest and longest muscle in the body***. It is situated medial to the preceeding and is not distinctly separable from it in the lumbar region. Anteriorly about the level of the 7th **rib** it divides into two parts the ***dorsal part or spinalis et semispinalis and vental part or Longissimus cervicis***; The **dorsal part** passes under the complexus and is inserted to the neural spines of the last three or four cervical vertebrae and the **ventral part** is inserted to the transverse processes of the **last four cervical vertebrae.**
3. **Multifidus dorsi:** These are also number of muscular bundles situated on the sides of the spines of lumbar and dorsal vertebrae and directed obliquely forward and upward.
4. **Intertransversalis lumborum:** These are thin muscular stands between the transverse processes of the lumbar vertebrae.

Name of the muscle	Origin	Insertion	Action
1.Serratus dorsalis anterior	Lumbodorsal fascia	By three fleshy digitations to the anterior borders and lateral surface of the ribs from the ***fifth to the seventh***	Inspiratory muscle
2. Serratus dorsalis posterior	Lumbodorsal fascia	Posterior borders and lateral surfaces of the ***last three ribs.***	Expiratory muscle
Third layer:			
1.Longissimus costarum	The lateral angle of the ilium, transverse processes of lumbar vertebrae and the anterior broders and *lateral surfaces of last six or seven ribs*	Posterior border of all the ribs and the transverse process of the last cervical vertebra.	Expiratory muscle
2. Longissimus dorsi	Crest and the lateral angle of the ilium, summits of sacral spines, lumbodorsal spines and supraspinous ligament.	The **dorsal part** is inserted to the neural spines of the last three or four cervical vertebrae and the **ventral part** is inserted to the transverse processes of the **last four cervical vertebrae.**	To extend the back and loin and to flex it laterally.
3. Multifidus dorsi	Lateral part of sacrum, oblique processes of lumbar vertebrae and transverse processes of dorsal vertebrae	Posterior border of neural spines of lumbar and thoracic vertebrae in front.	To extend the back and loin and flex it to a side
4.Intertranversalis lumborum	Present between the transverse processes of the lumbar vertebrae.		To aid in lateral flexion of loin region.

4.4 BLOOD SUPPLY TO THE THORAX

THE HEART OF OX: The heart of the adult ox has an average weight of about 2.5 kg or about 0.4 to 0.5 percent of the body weight.

The Right Atrium

The right atrium forms the right anterior part of the base of the heart and is above the right ventricle. It consists of a posterior ***sinus venarum*** **in to which the veins open** and a **blind diverticulum, the auricle or the auricular appendix**. The latter is a muscular appendage extending forward across the right surface of the aorta and is curving to the left with its apex adjacent to the the origin of the pulmonary artery.

There are **four chief openings** in the right atrium. The opening of the ***posterior vena cava*** returning blood from the posterior parts of the body ***is in the posterior part and just above the coronary groove.*** The opening of ***anterior vena cava*** bringing blood from the anterior parts of the body ***is on the dorsal side just anterior to that of the posterior vena cava.*** The ***coronary sinus*** is the opening of the **great cardiac vein and vena hemiazygos** into the sinus venarum present below the opening of the posterior vena cava. The ***right atrioventricular orifice*** is in the ventral part and leads into the right ventricle (**Fig.4.12).**

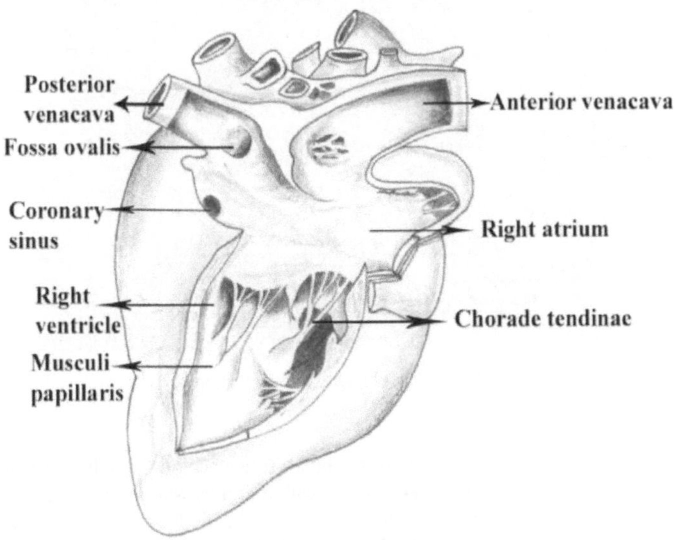

Fig. 4.12: Interior of Heart-Right side

The ***intervenous crest*** is a transverse muscular ridge present in front of the opening of the posterior vena cava. This tends to direct flow of blood from the anterior vena cava towards the atrio-ventricular opening. The ***fosa ovalis*** a remnant of the **fetal foramen ovale,** is an oval depression present in the interatrial septum just behind the ***intervenous crest***. The interior of the auricle is not smooth but crossed in various directions by muscular ridges called ***musculi pectinati***. The ***musculi pectinati terminate*** above on a curved crest, called as "***crista terminalis***".

The Right Ventricle

The right ventricle forms the **anterior part of the ventricular mass** and forms the **anterior border of the heart.** It **does not reach the apex** of the heart. Its cavity is triangular in outline and **crescentic** on cross section. The ***conus arteriosus*** is the cone shaped part of the ventricular cavity leading to the origin of pulmonary artery. The ***crista supraventricularis*** is a thick ridge separating the *atrioventricular orifice from the conus arteriosus*

The **right atrioventricular orifice** is oval, guarded by the tricuspid valve made up of three cusps of ***which two are on the interventricular septum and one on the anterior wall of the right ventricle.*** The ***large moderator band (septomarginal trabecula)*** extends from the base of the great papillary muscle to the ventral part of the anterior wall of right ventricle (**Fig.4.13**). It prevents over distension of the right ventricle. ***Trabeculae carneae*** are muscular ridges present in ventricle except at conus arteriosus. A variety of these in the form of somewhat conical flattened projections are called ***musculi papillaris (papillay muscles)*** and these are **three** in number. ***Two of these are on the interventricular septum and third one is on lateral wall of right ventricle*** (**Fig.4.13**). The ***chordae tendineae*** are fibrous cords attaching at their ends to the cusps of the atrio ventricular valve and to the papillary muscles. Each cusp receives chordae from the musculi papillaris (**Fig.4.13**). The ***pulmonary orifice*** is circular and present at the summit of the conus arteriosus. It is guarded by the pulmonary valve, composed of three semilunar cusps ***i.e medial (anterior), lateral (anterior) and posterior.***

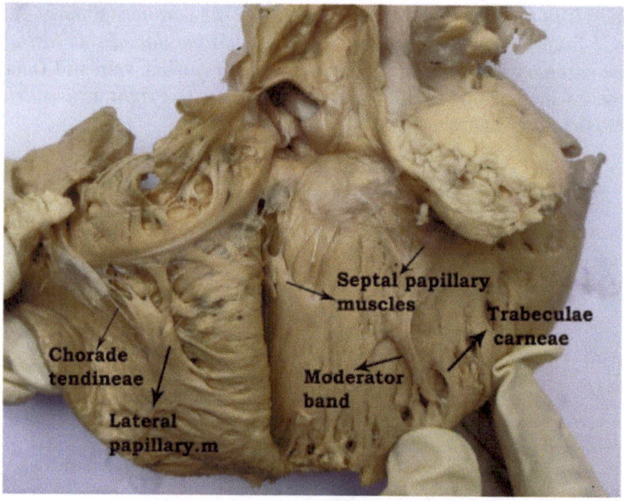

Fig. 4.13: Structures of Right Ventricle of Heart of Ox

The Left Atrium

The left atrium forms the posterior part of the base of the heart. It lies behind the pulmonary artery and aorta and above the left ventricle. It presents a **posterior venous** part with a fibrous wall **in to which 6-7 pulmonary veins open**. The **larger of the pulmonary veins,** from the caudal lobes of the lung, open on the **posterodorsal part of the atrium**. The veins from the **right cranial lobes and middle lobes** cross the posterior vena cava to open into the **dorsal surface** and those from the lobes of the **left lung open into the dorsolateral surface**. A strong, muscular band is present at the entrance of the auricle and form ***musculi pectinati*** as in the right auricle. The left atrioventricular orifice is almost **circular** and is below the posterior half of the atrium.

The Left Ventricle

The left ventricle forms the left posterior part of the ventricular mass. It is thicker than the right ventricle. It forms apex of the heart. The base is continuous with the left atrium and the aorta. **It is circular on cross section.** The cavity is smaller than that of the right ventricle (**Fig.4.14**).

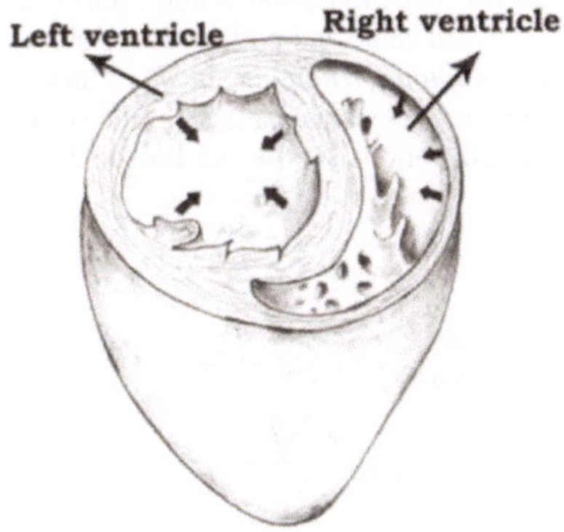

Fig. 4.14: Cross Section of Heart (Ventricles)

The left atrioventricular orifice is oval and smaller than that of right side. It carries the ***bicuspid or mitral valve***. One of the two main cusps is on the lateral margin of the orifice and the other is medial and adjacent to the aortic orifice. The **small accessory cusps** are present between the main cusps. The **aortic opening** is guarded by the **aortic valve, composed of three semilunar cusps**. One cusp is anterior and the others right and left posterior in position. ***Two papillary muscles (musculi papillaris***) are present on ***anterior and posterior walls of the left ventricle*** and these are larger than those of the right ventricle. The ***chordae tendinae*** from each muscle passes to both cusps of the atrioventricular valve. Each chord divides into a number of bands, the majority of which attach to the margin of the cusps but a few attach to the ventricular surface. The **moderator bands (*septomarginal trabeculae*)** are commonly **two large ones** which are more tendinous and **branched**. The **trabeculae carneae** are fewer in left ventrcicle (**Fig.4.15**).

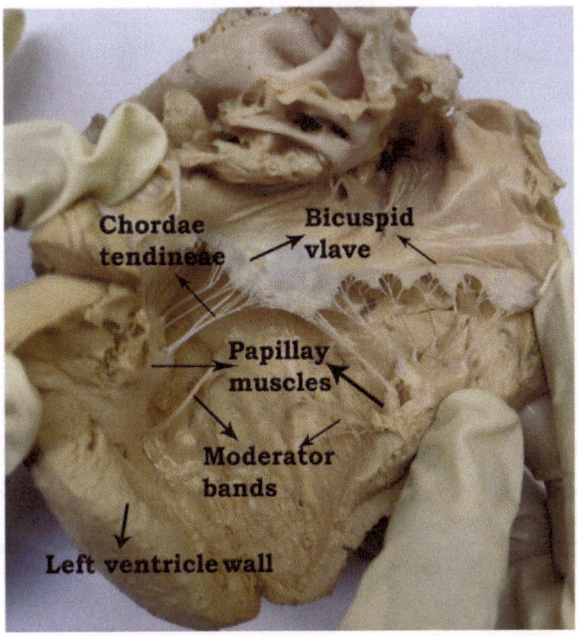

Fig. 4.15: Structures of Left Ventricle of Heart of Ox

Ossa cordis (***ossa-pleural of os***) are two irregulary triangular, semiosseous structures in the aortic ring and adjacent part of the ventricular wall of the heart in old cattle and buffalo. It appears to be entirely cartilaginous in young animals. The **right bone** is larger and is ***irregulary triangular in shape*** and it is about **4 cm in length (Fig.4.16)**. The **left face is concave** and attached to the right semilunar cusp of the aortic valve.The **right surface is convex** craniocaudally. The base is dorsal. The **left bone is smaller and inconstant.** It is present at the junction of the anterior and left posterior cusps.

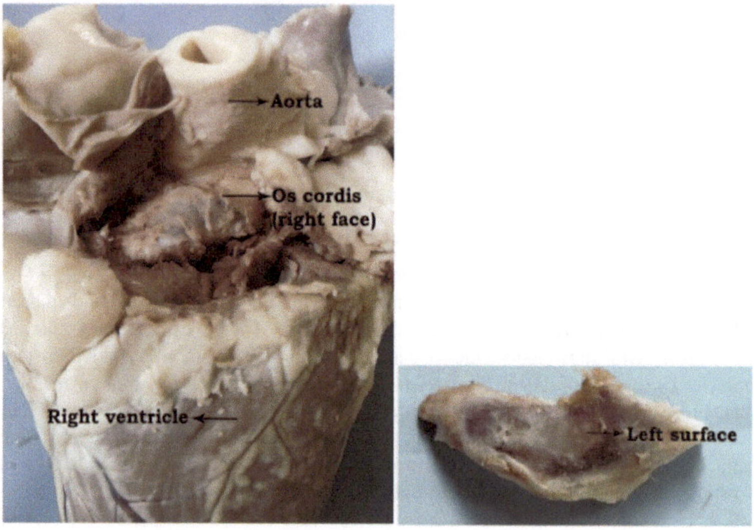

Fig. 4.16: Os cordis of Buffalo

Differences between Right and Left ventricles of Heart

Structure	Right Ventricle	Left Ventricle
Border	Forms the anterior part of the ventricular mass and forms the anterior border of the heart.	Forms the left posterior part of the ventricular mass.
Shape	It is triangular in outline and **crescentic** on cross section.	It is **circular** on cross section.
Thickness	Thin	Thick
Lumen	Large	Small
Apex	It dooes not reach apex of the heart.	It forms apex
Moderator bands	Single and unbranched	2 or 3, branched
Valve	Tricuspid valve	Bicuspid or Mitral valve
Musculi papillares	Three in number	Two in number
Trabeculae carneae	More in number	Few in number
Major vessel	Pulmonary artery arises	Aorta arises
Type of blood	Deoxygenated blood is present	Oxygenated blood is present

CONDUCTING SYSTEM OF THE HEART

The conducting system of the heart mainly consists of ***sino-atrial node, atrio ventricular node and the atrio-ventricular bundle.*** The S.A node initiates the rhythmic contractions in the heart and is named as ***pace maker of the heart***. The **sino-atrial node** is a small collection of vascular neuro-myocardium situated in the wall of the right atrium at the upper end of ***crista terminalis*** (**Fig.4.17**).

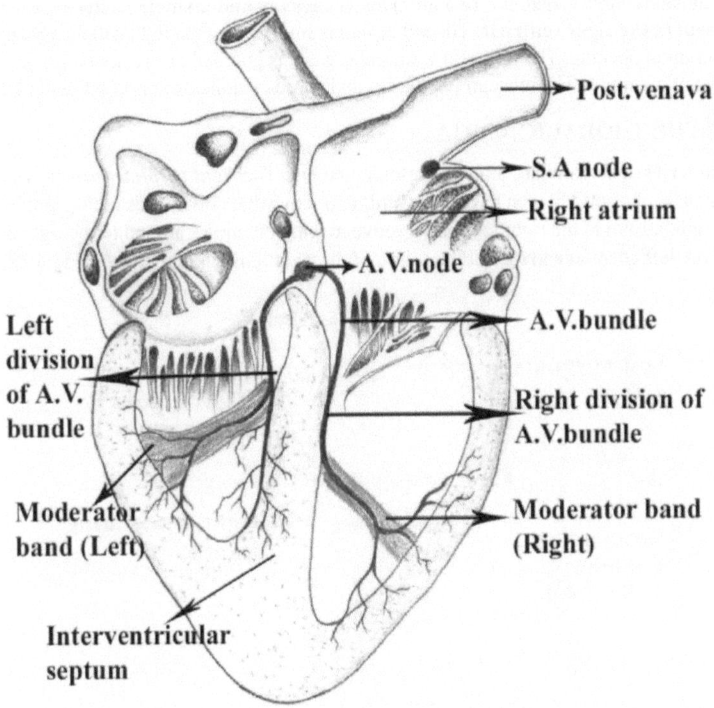

Fig.4.17: Conduction System of Heart

The **atrio ventricular node** is a nodule of the same kind of vascular tissue, situated in the septal wall of the atrium immediately above the opening of the coronary sinus.

The **atrio ventricular bundle** is a pale bundle of the special muscle fibres with which the nerve fibres are associated. It springs from the AV node, runs forward on the septum and reaches the upper border of the ventricular septum. From here it continues as two chief divisions. One of these descends on the right side of the ventricular septum and passes by the moderator band to the lateral papillary muscle. The other branch descends on the left side of the septum passes by moderator band and ramifies on the wall of the ventricle through the bases of the papillary muscles. The bundle and its branches are surrounded by a fibrous sheet and are subendocardial.

Horse: ***The average weight is about 4.0 kg, about 0.7 per cent of the total body weight of the animal.*** The **intermediate groove** is absent. Instead of os cordis, the aortic ring contains on the right side a plate of cartilage. Some times smaller plate is present on the left side.

Dogs: It is ovoid in shape. The apex is blunt and rounded. The long axis is very oblique. The base faces the thoracic inlet. The apex is in close relation to the diaphragm at its sternal part. The left (ventral) and the right (dorsal) longitudinal grooves meet. An intermediate groove is present. The weight of the heart of a dog of medium size is 150 to 180 gms. The tricuspid valve has two chief cusps and three or four small ones. There are four musculi papillares in the right ventricle, all springing from the septal wall. The bicuspid valve consists of two large cusps and four or five small ones. There are two musculi papillares in the left ventricle, both arise from the lateral wall. The pericardium is attached to the sternal part of the diaphragm by fibrous band the ***pericardiophrenic ligament***.

Pig: The heart is broad, short and blunt. The weight of the heart is 0.23 to 0.28 per cent of total body weight (240-500gm).The ventral border of the left auricle is marked by several notches. The intermediate groove is present on left ventricular border. The fossa ovalis is large. The aortic arch is strongly curved. The left subclavian artery and the brachiocepahlic trunk arise separately from the aortic arch.

Fowl: It is proportionately large. There are **two anterior venacavae and a single posterior vena cava. Musculi papillares are absent in the right ventricle**. The left atrium is smaller than the right and the **two pulmonary veins** open into it by a common opening. The left atrio ventricular valve is guarded by membranous cusps corresponding to the bicupid valve of mammals.The musculi papillaries and chorda tendinae are present in the left ventricle.

BRANCHES OF THE THORACIC AORTA

1. The coronary arteries: The coronary arteries are right and left. The ***right coronary artery*** is small and it arises from the anterior sinus of the aorta. It then passes forwards and somewhat downwards to the right between the conus arteriosus and the right atrium to the right coronary groove in which it curves around to the right and backwards to **anastomose with the left coronary artery** at the origin of the right longitudinal groove (**Fig.4.18**).

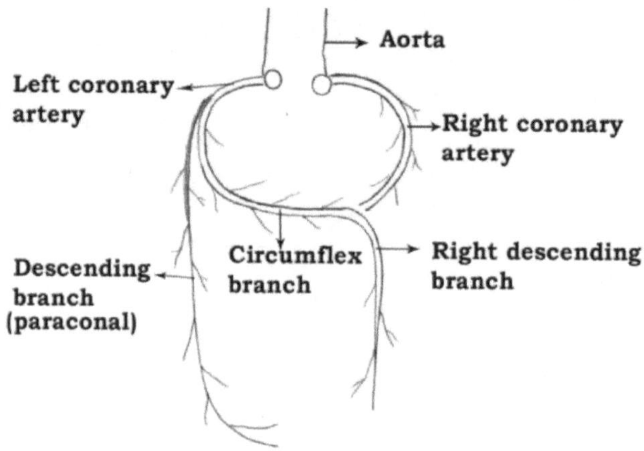

Fig. 4.18: Branches of Coronary Arteries

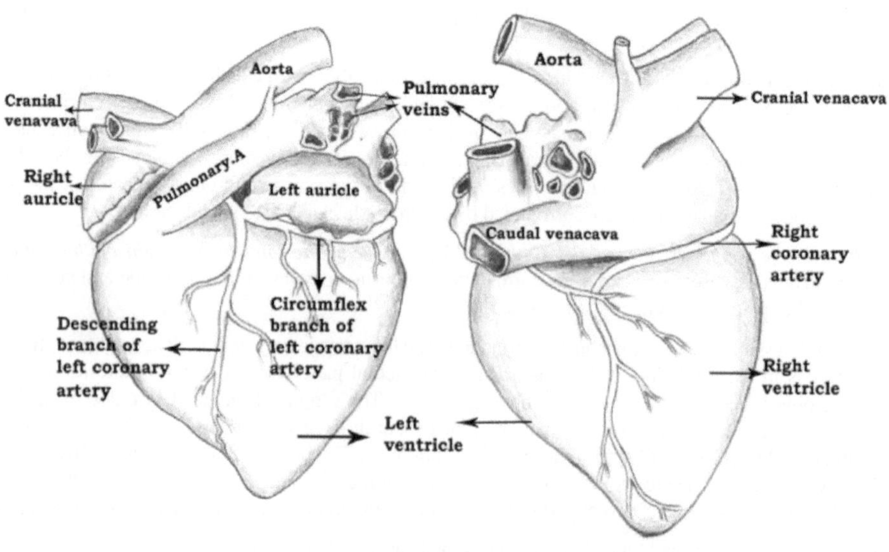

Fig. 4.19: Coronary Arteries of the Heart

The ***left coronary artery*** is larger and it arises from the left posterior sinus of the aorta, emerges behind the origin of the pulmonary artery and divides into two branches. It gives off in its course dorsal and ventral branches to the wall of the heart, emerges behind the origin of the pulmonary artery and divides into two branches i.e ***descending and circumflex branches***. The ***descending branch*** passes down the left longitudinal groove towards the apex supplying branches to both the ventricular walls. The ***circumflex branch*** runs backwards in the coronary groove, gives off a branch which descends in the intermediate groove, curves to right and descends into the right longitudinal groove, after anastomosing with the branches of the right coronary artery, it supplies branches to the artria, ventricles and the origin of the great blood vessels (**Fig.4.19**).

The cardiac veins: The venous blood from the myocardium is returned through two large veins i.e **right and left ascending coronary veins**. These accompany the descending branches of the left coronary artery and join to form the **great cardiac vein,** which joins the vena ***hemiazygos*** and opens into the **coronary sinus** of the right atrium. The ***right coronary artery has no satellite vein***. Several ***vena cordis parvi*** (**small veins**) receive blood from the area supplied by the right coronary artery. They are mostly vertical in direction and cross the right coronary artery to open in the ***recess between the musculi pectinati***.

2. Common brachiocephalic trunk: This is a large vessel which arises within the pericardium from the **convexity of the aortic arch.** It measures about 10 to 13 cm. It divides opposite the **second intercostal space** into ***brachiocephalic and left brachial arteries.*** The **brachiocephalic artery** is directed forwards and upwards beneath the trachea. Opposite to the ***first rib*** it gives off the ***right brachial artery*** and is continued as the ***bicarotid trunk***. The bicarotid trunk divides into ***two common carotid arteries i.e right and left*** (**Fig.4.20**) at thoracic inlet.

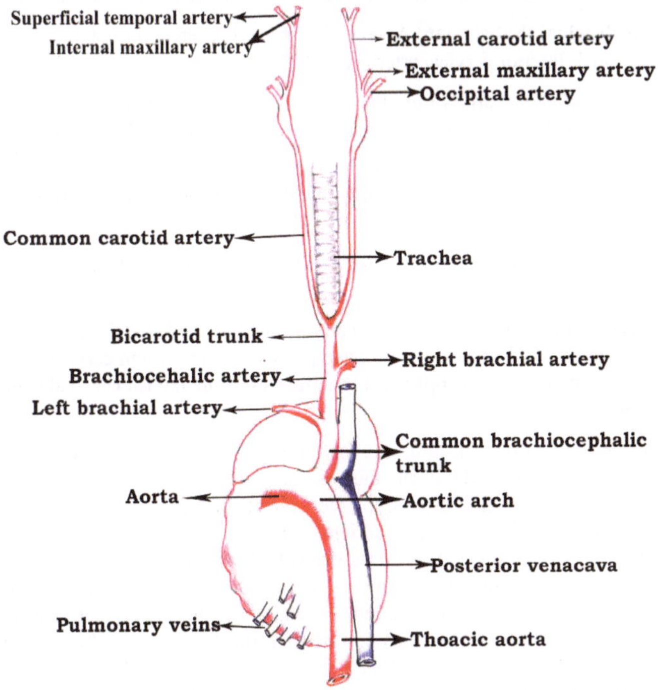

Fig. 4.20: Branches of Common Brachiocephalic Trunk

3. Bronchial artery: It is visceral unpaired. It is the ***nutrient artery of the lungs***. It arises from the posterior face of the aorta. It divides into **right and left bronchial arteries** of which the **right is larger**. Each artery reaches the root of the corresponding lung and detaches small branches to the bronchial lymph glands.

4. Oesophageal artery: It is **visceral unpaired.** It arises from the posterior face of the thoracic aorta and passes downwards and divides into branches to supply the **thoracic part of the oesophagus and posterior mediastinal lymph gland.**

5. Intercostal arteries: These are **parietal paired.** Of the 13 pairs of intercostal arteries the **first pair of intercostal arteries arises from dorsal artery,** the **next four or five from the subcostal artery** and the **rest from the thoracic aorta.** Each intercostal artery gives off branches to the pleura and vertebra and divides into a **dorsal spinal and ventral intercostal branch.** The **dorsal spinal branch** divides into **spinal and muscular branches** the former reinforce the inferior spinal artery by entering into vertebral canal and the latter supply the spinal **muscles. The intercostal branch runs between the external and internal intercostal muscles and supplies these muscles.**

6. Phrenic artery: It is parietal unpaired. Besides there are two or three branches which arise from the thoracic aorta, a little in front of the hiatus aorticus and these supply the crura of the diaphragm.

Brachial (Subclavian) Arteries: The left brachial artery is a branch of the **common brachiocephalic trunk** while **the right is a branch of the brachiocephalic artery.**

Each brachial artery after its origin is directed forwards between the two layers of the anterior mediastinum and the trachea towards the thoracic inlet. The **left artery** is related medially to the **oesophagus, trachea and thoracic duct.** Both the arteries are related below to the **vagus, cardiac and recurrent laryngeal nerves.** Each brachial artery leaves the thoracic cavity by winding round the anterior border of the first rib below the insertion of **scalenus ventralis** and above the brachial vein to reach the axilla, thus leaving an impression on the first rib. The brachial artery gives rise **intrathoracic branches within the thorax** and **extrathoracic branches** outside the thorax.

Intrathoracic Branches of Brachial (Subclavian) Artery: These are 1. Common trunk (*Costocervical trunk*), 2. The internal thoracic artery and 3. Inferior cervical artery (**Fig.4.21**).

1. Common trunk (***Costocervical trunk***) arises from the dorsal face of the brachial artery close to its origin and soon divides into subcostal, dorsal, deep or superior cervical and vertebral arteries (**Fig.4.21**).

(a) **The subcostal artery** passes upwards and backwards along the ventral aspect of the bodies of the thoracic vertebrae and gives off the ***second to the fifth intercostal arteries*****, occasionally first intercostal artery (Fig.4.21).**

(b) The **dorsal artery gives off first intercostal artery.** It then passés deeply into the serratus cervicis and trapezius.

(c) The ***deep cervical artery*** (**superior cervical artery)** arises usually outside the thorax from the superior face of the vertebral artery about the level of the transverse process of the seventh cervical vertebra and passes on the deep face of the complexus and **supplies all the muscles of the lateral cervical group, ligamentum nuchae and skin** (**Fig.4.21**).

(d) **The vertebral artery** is large. It runs upwards and forwards, the left crossing the oesophagus and the right, the trachea, within the thorax (**Fig.4.21**). Each emerges out of the thorax between the scalenus and longus colli muscles, passes under transverse process of the seventh cervical vertebra, detaches the **superior cervical artery,** then enters the foramen transversarium of the sixth cervical vertebra and passes through the series of foramina transversaria of the cervical vertebrae with the satellite vein and ***nervous transversarius of sympathetic trunk***, covered by the intertransversales colli muscles, reaches the intervertebral foramen between the second and the third cervical vertebrae detaches a thick muscular branch and enters the spinal canal and divides in the ring of the atlas into **medial and lateral branches. The medial branch,** the cerebrospinal artery passes on the cranial floor and joins the ***rete mirabile cerbri*** (***a vascular network around the pituitary gland***). **The *lateral branch*** contributes a branch to to retemirabile cerebri and emerges out through the intervertebral foramina of atlas and supplies muscles in this region.

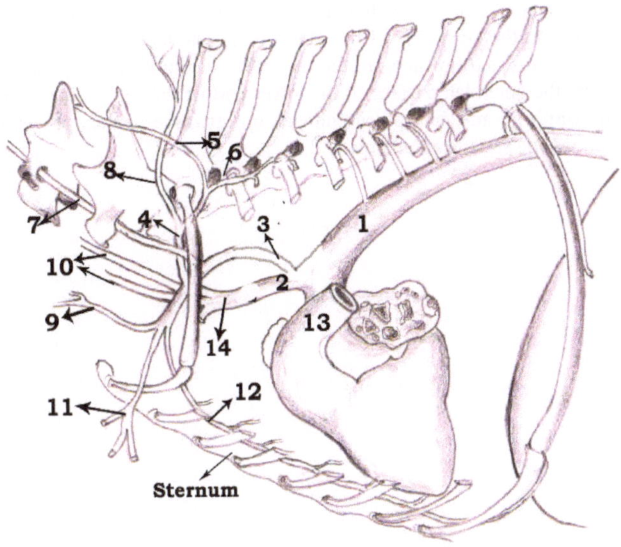

1.Aorta	**7.Vertebral artery**
2.Brachiocephalic trunk	**8.Superior cervical artery**
3.Left brachial artery	**9.Inferior cervical artery**
4.Common trunk	**10.Commmon carotid arteries**
5.Dorsal artery	**11. Brachial artery**
6.Subcostal artery	**12.Internal thoracic artery**
14. Brachiocephalic artery	**13.Pulmonary trunk**

Fig. 4.21: Intrathoracic Branches of Brachial Artery

The **vertebral artery** in its course gives branches to **the intertransversales colli** and opposite to each intervertebral foramen givs off spinal branch to the spinal cord and its meninges. The **spinal branches** enter the spinal canal and reinforce the ventral spinal artery on the ventral face of the spinal cord.

2. The Internal Thoracic Artery: This is a large vessel which arises from the ventral face of the brachial artery **opposite the first rib**. It curves downwards and backwards passes under the transversus thoracics muscle to the eighth costal cartilage and **terminates in to *musculo-phrenic and anterior abdominal arteries* (Fig.4.21)**.

a. The ***musculophrenic or asternal artery*** passes along the groove between the **8th and 9th costal cartilages** and then continues along the costal attachment of the diaphragm and transversus abdominis and gives off muscular branches to the **intercostal muscles, transversus abdominis and diaphragm** and anastomoses with the intercostal branches of aorta.

b. ***The anterior abdominal artery*** passes between the ninth costal cartilage and xiphoid cartilage, passes backwards on the deep face of the **rectus abdominis, supplies this muscle** and the ventral wall of the abdomen and anastomoses with the branches of the **posterior abdominal artery**.

Collateral Branches: At each intercostal space it gives off **dorsal and ventral branches**. The former ascend the intercostal spaces and anastomose with the intercostal arteries of the aorta and supply the intercostal muscles. The **ventral branches** give off small branches to the **transversus thoracics, pleura, pericardium** and pass out between the coastal cartilages as perforating intercostal arteries.

3. Inferior cervical artery: It arises from the brachial artery. It is directed downwards and forward on the lateral face of the jugular confluence on the deep face of the scalenus muscle among posterior cervical lymph glands (**Fig.4.21**). It runs further forwards and upwards on the deep face of the brachiocephalicus between it and the omotransversarius and enters the anterolateral face of the lower part of the supraspinatus. **It supplies branches to the posterior cervical lymph glands, brachiocephalicus, omotransversarius, prescapular lymph glands, supraspinatus and sometimes the sternocephalicus.**

4.5 NERVE SUPPLY TO THE THORAX

Dorsal spinal nerves: There are **thirteen pairs of dorsal (thoracic) spinal nerves** and their arrangements are almost similar. Each nerve is divided into ***dorsal and ventral branches***. The ***dorsal branch*** is further divided into **medial and lateral branches** of which the former supply the spinal muscles and skin of that region. The **lateral branches** are directed upward pass through the longissimus dorsi and appear between it and the intertransversales costarum. They break off into filaments to supply to the skin. The ***ventral branches*** (***intercostal nerves***) are much larger than the dorsal branch and descend to the intercostal spaces in company with the vessels. They ***supply intercostal muscles*** and give off branches which perforate the muscles and supply the cutaneous muscle and skin of the thorax and abdomen. The ventral branches of first and second dorsal spinal nerves enter into the formation of ***brachial plexus***.

Phrenic nerves: The phrenic nerve is the ***motor nerve*** to the diaphragm. It is formed by the union of ventral primary branches of the ***fifth, sixth and seventh cervical spinal nerves***, The root from the **fifth is the largest and the longest** and is on the deep face of the scalenus ventralis muscle and crosses its face obliquely to the thoracic inlet and enters the thoracic cavity below the insertion of the scalenus ventralis. The **root from the seventh is the shortest and the finest**. The common cord of the sixth and seventh unites with the fifth inside the thoracic cavity at the first intercostal space and forms the phrenic nerve.

The ***right phrenic nerve*** continues backward on the right face of anterior vena cava, gains the company of the posterior vena cava runs on its ventral face in venacaval fold and reaches the right half of the tendinous centre of the diaphragm and is distributed to it.

The ***left phrenic nerve*** runs backward with left vagus in the anterior mediastinum. It then diverges from it, runs over the pericardium on the base of the heart in the middle mediastinum, then passes backward, enters the left half of the tendinous centre of the diaphragm and is distributed to it.

4.6 VISCERAL ORGANS OF THE THORACIC CAVITY

Thoracic part of Oesophagus

Ox: At the junction of neck and thorax the oesophagus undergoes a slight curvature, **convex ventrally**. At the first rib the oesophagus is in contact with the cervicothoracic ganglion, the costocervical trunk and the thoracic duct. In the mediastinum, the oesophagus passes dorsally over the base of the heart and the trachea forming **second curvature** which is **convex dorsally**. It crosses the right face of the aortic arch, then passes straight back in the caudal mediastinum, ventral to the aorta, through the **oesophageal hiatus of diaphragm at 8 or 9th intercostal space**. In caudal mediastinum the oesophagus is accompanied by the dorsal and ventral trunk of the vagus on dorsal and ventral aspects respectively and is related dorsally to the large caudal mediastinal lymph node.

Horse: The thoracic part of oesophagus passes dorsally and caudally through the thoracic inlet between the left face of the trachea and 1st rib and **reaching the dorsal surface of the trachea at the level of 3rd thoracic vertebra**. Here it continues in the mediastinum between the lungs, caudally and little dorsally, inclining gradually to the left and reaches the oesophageal hiatus of the diaphragm and terminates at the cardiac orifice of the stomach in the abdomen.

Dog: The thoracic part continues **dorsal to the trachea and ventral to the left longus colli** to the base of the heart. Here it inclines medially, on the aortic arch and passes back over the bifurcation of the trachea and continues caudally between the lungs and passes through the oesophageal hiatus and joins the stomach **at the cardia at the level of 11th or 12th thoracic vertebra**.

Pig: is **short and nearly straight**. It has a calibre in the adult nearly **7.0 cm at either end and about 4.2 cm in its middle part**. The oesophageal hiatus is a long slit.

Fowl: Thoracic part of oesophagus is shorter than the cervical part. It extends caudally dorsal to the trachea and the base of the heart. Dorsally and ventrally it is covered by the cervical and clavicular air sacs respectively. Caudal to the 5th rib it passes between the cranial thoracic air sacs to the medial surface of the left lobe of the liver and joins proventriculus.

TRACHEA

It is a flexible cartilaginous and membranous air conducting tube extending from the larynx to the hilus of the lungs where it divides into right and left principal bronchi.

Ox: The trachea bifurcates into right and left principal bronchi at the level ***of 5th rib** and **tracheal (apical) bronchus*** is given off from trachea at the level of **3rd rib to** cranial lobe of right lung.

Horse: The free ends of the tracheal rings **overlap slightly in cervical part,** while in **thoracic part they do not meet**.

Dog: The tracheal rings are **open dorsally** throughout the length of trachea.

Pig: The trachea is circular in cross section. The ends of cartilages overlap each other and the trachealis is attached to their deep surface.

Fowl: Tracheal rings are completely closed dorsally.

BRONCHI

Ox: Trachea bifurcates into the **left and right principal bronchi** which enter the hilus of corresponding lung. The **left principal bronchus** gives off two branches, the left cranial bronchus to the two divisions of cranial lobe and left caudal bronchus to caudal lobe. The ***tracheal (apical) bronchus*** is given off from trachea at the level of **3rd rib to** cranial lobe of right lung. The **right principal bronchus** gives off two branches i.e **middle bronchus to middle lobe and right caudal bronchus to caudal lobe.** The **accessory bronchus** originates from **right principal bronchus** ventromedial to middle bronchus and enters accessory lobe **(Fig.4.22).**

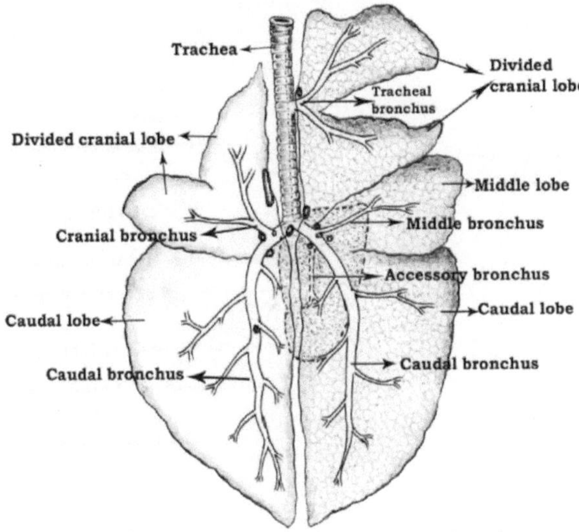

Fig. 4.22: Lobation and Bronchial Tree of Lungs of Ox

Horse: The two primary bronchi divide into cranial and caudal bronchi. The **accessory bronchus** arises a short distance caudal to tracheal bifurcation from right primary bronchus **(Fig.4.23).**

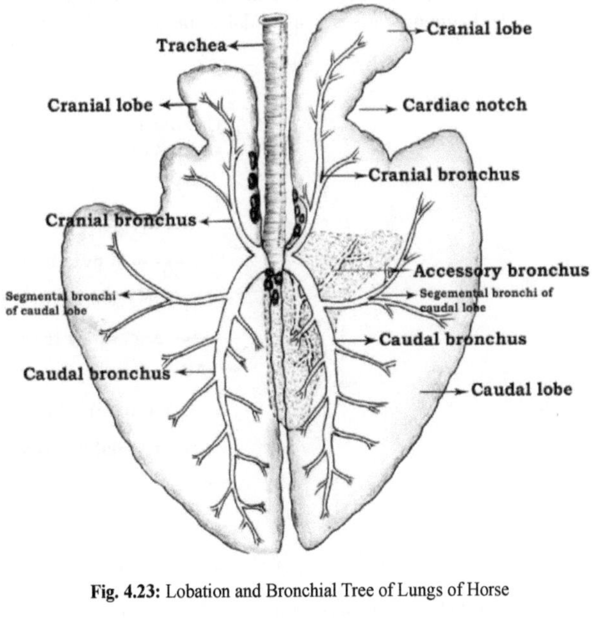

Fig. 4.23: Lobation and Bronchial Tree of Lungs of Horse

Dog: Each bronchus divides into two branches, **cranial and caudal bronchi**. The **cranial bronchus** serves two parts of cranial lobe of left lung and undivided cranial lobe of right lung. The middle bronchus arises a short distance caudal to origin of right cranial bronchus and passes to middle lobe. The **accessory bronchus** arises from right caudal bronchus (**Fig.4.24**).

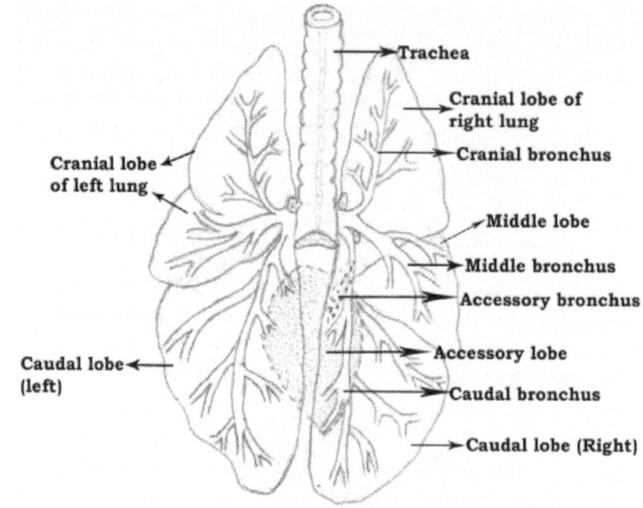

Fig. 4.24: Lobation and Bronchial tree of Lungs of Dog

Pig: The ***tracheal bronchus*** (*right cranial bronchus*) is present for right cranil lobe **as in ox**. The left cranial bronchus divides into cranial and caudal segmental bronchi each serving one of the parts of the cranial lobe. The left and right caudal bronchi give off four dorsal and four ventral segmental bronchi which ventilate caudal lobe. The ***tracheal bronchus serves undivided right cranial lobe***. The **middle bronchus** arises close to tracheal bifurcation and serves middle lobe. **Accessory bronchus** arises just caudal to the middle bronchus and passes ventrally to accessory lobe (**Fig.4.25**).

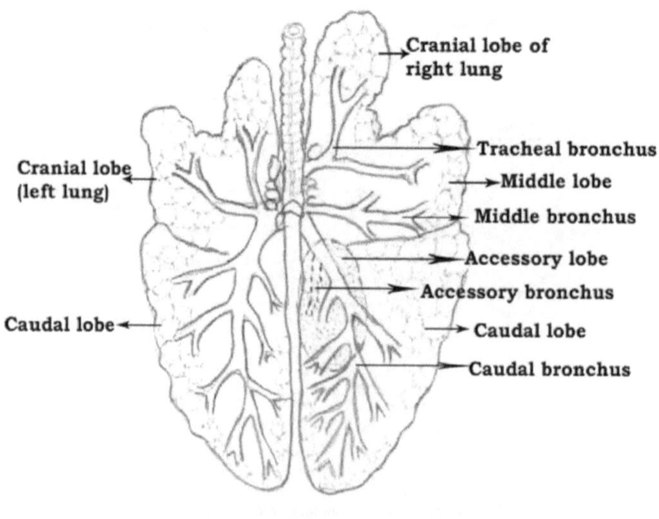

Fig. 4.25: Lobation and Bronchial Tree of Lungs of Pig

Fowl: The stem bronchus opens into the abdominal air sac and while passing through the lung it gives off secondary bronchi which enter the cervical, clavicular and thoracic air sacs.

LUNGS

Ox: Each lung is soft and spongy to touch and crepitates when pressed. Its colour is bright pink in life and it floats in water, while foetal lung is smaller, pale gray in colour, firm to touch, does not crepitate and does not float in water.

Each lung presents three surfaces (**medial, costal and diaphragmatic surfaces**), three borders (**dorsal, ventral and basal borders**) a base and an apex. The ***costal surface*** is convex and lies against the lateral wall of thorax and presents the impressions of ribs. **The *medial (mediastinal) surface*** is less extensive and moulded on to the mediastinum and its contents. It presents hilus, where **bronchus, pulmonary and bronchial vessels and nerves pass from mediastinum to the organ (Fig.4.26)**.

Two impressions are present behind the hilus, the **dorsal one is aortic impression for aorta** and the **ventral one is oesophageal impression for oesophagus (Fig.4.26)**. The **cardiac impression** adapted to heart and pericardium is located in front of the root of lung.

The right lung shows groove for caudal vena cava. A special fold of **mediastinal pleura called pulmonary ligament** caudal to root of each lung connects mediastinal surface of lung with mediastinum and diaphragm. The **diaphragmatic surface** which is at the base of the lung is concave and lies on the diaphragm.

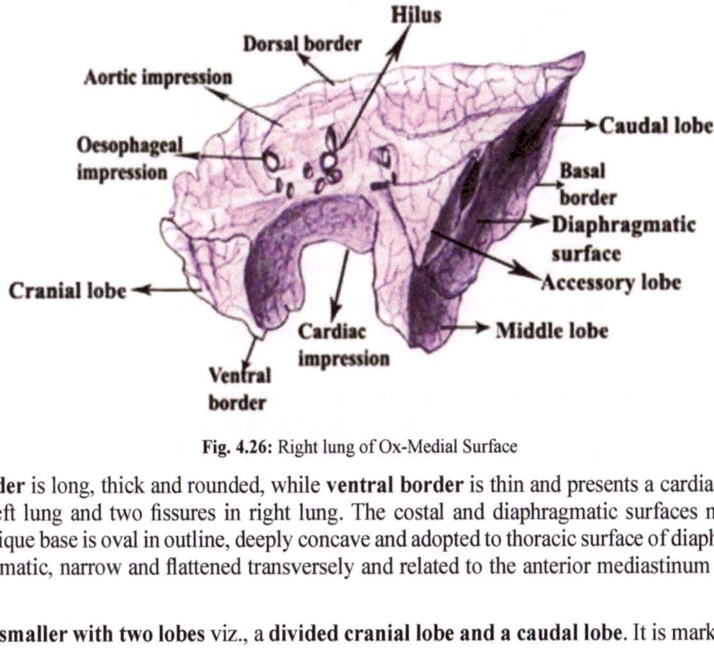

Fig. 4.26: Right lung of Ox-Medial Surface

The **dorsal border** is long, thick and rounded, while **ventral border** is thin and presents a cardiac notch. It shows one fissure in left lung and two fissures in right lung. The costal and diaphragmatic surfaces meet at the **basal border**. The oblique base is oval in outline, deeply concave and adopted to thoracic surface of diaphragm (**Fig.4.26)**. The apex is prismatic, narrow and flattened transversely and related to the anterior mediastinum and anterior part of pericardium.

The **left lung is smaller with two lobes** viz., a **divided cranial lobe and a caudal lobe**. It is marked by one fissure (**Fig.4.27**). The **right lung** is larger and shows four lobes divided by two fissures i.e. the divided cranial lobe (supplied by tracheal bronchus), a middle lobe, a caudal lobe and an accessory lobe (**Fig.4.27)**. The accessory lobe is mainly attached to middle lobe. The lobulation of the lungs is conspicuous. The cardiac impression is more deeper on the left lung than on the right.

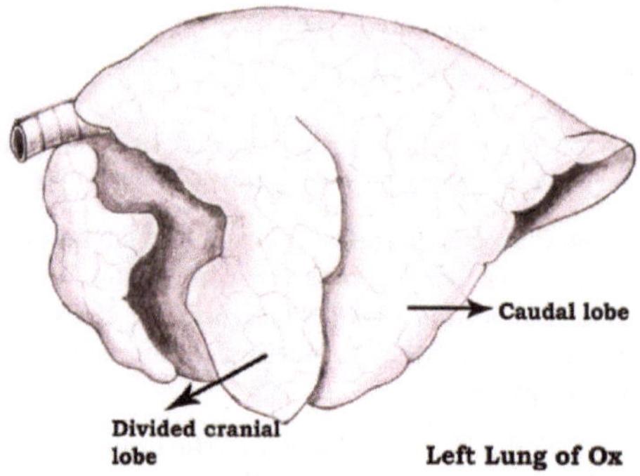

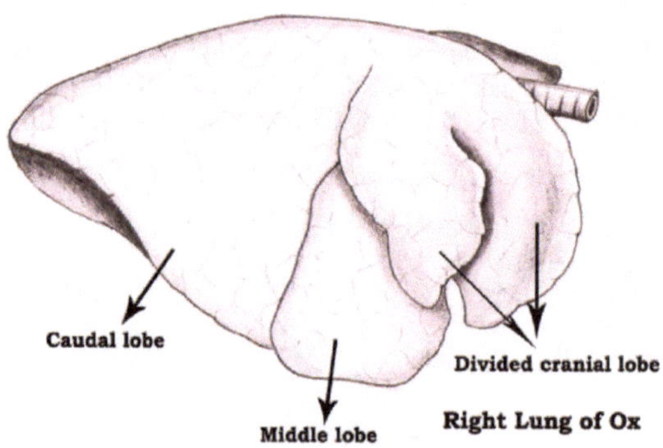

Fig. 4.27: Different Lobes in Right and Left Lungs of Ox

The well marked cardiac notch of the left lung extends from **3rd intercostal space to 5th rib or intercostal space.** The **right cardiac notch is smaller** than that of the left and is restricted to lower parts of 3rd and 4th intercostal spaces.

Horse: There is **no external evidence of lobation** as fissures are absent. Each lung shows a cranial and a caudal lobe while the right lung in addition has an accessory lobe which is attached to medial surface of caudal lobe. ***The lobulation is not distinct due to small amount of interlobular tissue*** (**Fig.4.28**).

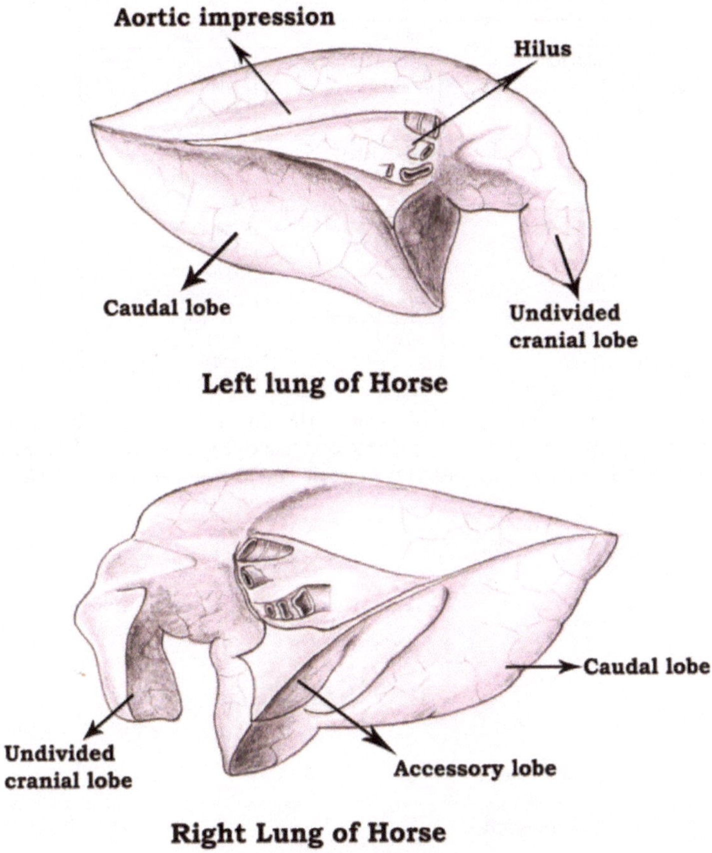

Fig. 4.28: Lungs of Horse

Dog: The inter lobar fissures are deep and extend to the root. The left lung consists of a divided cranial lobe and a caudal lobe. The right lung consists of the undivided **cranial lobe, the middle lobe, the caudal lobe and an accessory lobe**. The **accessory lobe is attached to caudal lobe. Cardiac notch is more extensive on the right side**. The lobulation is not distinct.

Pig: The fresh lungs are bluish pink. The left lung shows divided **cranial lobe and caudal lobe, while the right lung shows undivided cranial lobe, middle lobe, caudal lobe and an accessory lobe**. Lobulation is evident but not quite distinct as in ox.

Different Lobes of Lungs in Domestic Animals

Species	Left Lung	Right Lung
Ox, Sheep and Goat	Divided cranial lobe Caudal lobe	Divided Cranial lobe Middle lobe Caudal lobe Accessory lobe
Horse	Cranial lobe Caudal lobe	Cranial lobe Caudal lobe Accessory lobe
Dog and Cat	Divided cranial lobe Caudal lobe	Cranial lobe Middle lobe Caudal lobe Accessory lobe
Pig	Divided cranial lobe Caudal lobe	Cranial lobe Middle lobe Caudal lobe Accessory lobe

Fowl: The lungs are located in the dorsal part of the thorax. The lobes are absent and the costal impressions are deeper. The stem bronchus passes through the entire lung to communicate with a system of air sacs. **There are 9 air sacs** i.e. **clavicular, cervical, anterior and posterior thoracic and abdominal**. The **clavicular being unpaired (Fig.4.29).**

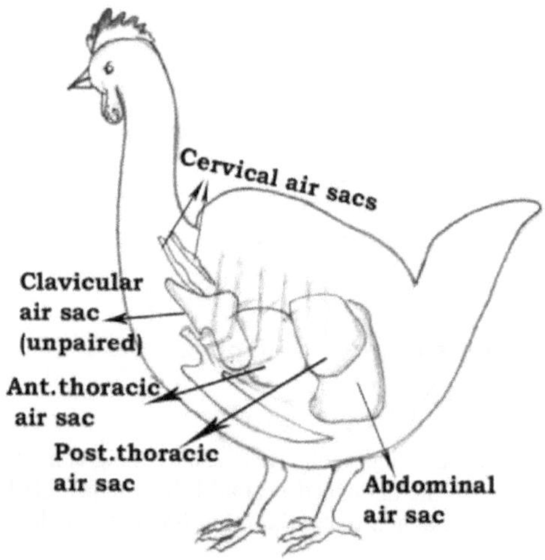

Fig. 4.29: Air Sacs of Fowl

The air sacs permit an unidirectional flow of air through the lungs. The air moving through bird lungs is largely "**fresh air'** and has a higher oxygen content. In contrast, air flow is bidirectional in mammals, moving back and forth into and out of the lungs. As a result, air coming into a mammal's lungs is mixed with old air and this mixed air has less oxygen. **So in lungs of birds more oxygen is available to diffuse in to blood.**

4.7: SURGICAL OPERATIONS OF THE THORAX

The ausculataion and percussion are usually done in the thoracic region clinically to determine the functional state of the heart, lungs and other organs.

Auscultation: The sounds produced by the functional motility of organs of thoracic cavity and intra abdominal portion of the digestive tract are detected by using instruments like stethoscope.

Percussion: Hearing of sounds, produced artificially by using fingers or instruments over the area of observation.

Area of auscultation and percussion for ***heart is 4th and 5th inter costal space on left side***, since heart is asymmetrical in position and in contact with left chest wall here.

Auscultation and Percussion of lungs: A triangular area is marked for this purpose. The boundaries of the triangle are

a. Posterior angle of scapula anteriorly

b. Olecranon process of ulna below

c. 11th intercostal space behind.

Note: Thick layer of subcutaneous fat is a formidable barrier to palpation and auscultation in pigs.

4.8 SUMMARY

Ox: Thoracic vertebrae are characterized by **well developed neural spines, short bodies with capitular facets. The last dorsal (13th) has a vertical spine hence it is called as *anticlinal vertebra.***

Horse: The spine of *16th is vertical (anticlinal)*

Dog: The ***11th is the anticlinal vertebra.***

Fowl: The **1st and 6th are free** while **2nd to the 5th are fused** into one piece. The **7th is fused to the lumbosacral mass.**

Ox: There are **13 pairs of ribs.**

Those that articulate with the sternum by means of costal cartilage are termed **sternal (true) ribs (8 pairs**). The **remainder are asternal (false) ribs (5 pairs)**

Note: Number of sternal ribs = No. of sternebrae + 1

Special features of 1st Rib:

1. It is the **shortest and least curved**
2. The lateral surface and the **anterior border present a rough area** about its middle for the **scalenus ventralis.**

Horse: There are **18 pairs of ribs, 8 sternal and 10 asternal.**

Dog: There are **13 pairs of ribs. 9 sternal and 4 asternal.**

Fowl: There are **7 pairs of ribs**

The **1st, 2nd and sometimes 7th do not have sternal ribs** (**floating**).

Except the first and the seventh the posterior border of each vertebral rib presents an ***uncinate process*** directed backward to overlap the succeeding rib.

Ox: Sterinum is made up of **7 bony segments** (sternebrae). The **anterior extremity** is the anterior end of the first sternebra which forms the **manubrium sterni or presternum.**

The **posterior extremity or metasternum** is formed by the **xiphoid cartilage.** Between the pre and metasternum is the body or **mesosternum**.

Horse: It is composed of **7 sternebrae**. It is **canoe or boat shaped**. The anterior extremity presents a **laterally compressed *cariniform*** cartilage

Dog: It is composed of **8 sternebrae**.

Fowl: The **metasternum** is very long and extensive and carries ventrally a **thin plate of bone called the keel or sternal crest**

Longissimus dorsi: This is the ***largest and longest muscle in the body.***

Anteriorly about the level of the 7th **rib** it divides into two parts i.e ***dorsal part (spinalis et semispinalis) and vental part (longissimus cervicis).*.**

In ox, the tracheal (apical) bronchus is given off from trachea at the level of **3rd rib to** cranial lobe of right lung.

In **ox** the tracheal rings in **cervical part** are ***open***, but in **thoracic part rings** are in **apposition**.

Horse: The free ends of the tracheal rings **overlap slightly in cervical part** while in **thoracic part they do not meet. The tracheal bronchus is absent.**

Dog: The tracheal rings are **open dorsally** throughout the length of trachea.

Pig: Tracheal bronchus to cranial lobe of the right lung is present. The trachea is circular in cross section.

Fowl: All tracheal rings are completely closed dorsally.

Lungs:

Ox: The **left lung is smaller with two lobes** viz., a **divided cranial lobe and a caudal lobe**. The ***right lung is larger*** and shows four lobes.

Horse: There is **no external evidence of lobation** as fissures are absent. ***The lobulation is not distinct due to small amount of interlobular tissue.***

The ***middle lobe is absent in right lung of horse.***

Dog: The interlobar fissures are deep and extend to the root.

Fowl: The lungs are located in the dorsal part of the thorax. There **are no lobes** and the costal impressions are deeper. There are **9 air sacs** i.e. clavicular, cervical, anterior and posterior thoracic and abdominal, the ***clavicular being unpaired.***

The area of auscultation and percussion for ***heart is 4th and 5th inter costal space on left side in ox.***

UNIT 5
ABDOMEN

5.1 BONES OF THE ABDOMEN

LUMBAR VERTEBRAE

Ox: The lumbar vertebrae are **characterized by elongated flattened transverse processes** (projecting outwards) and large, strongly curved articular processes **(Fig.5.1a).** The body is constricted in the middle and expanded at the extremities. The anterior extermity is less convex and posterior is less concave. The posterior vertebral notches are much deeper. The **intervertebral foramina are often double** in the anterior part of the series and are very large further back.

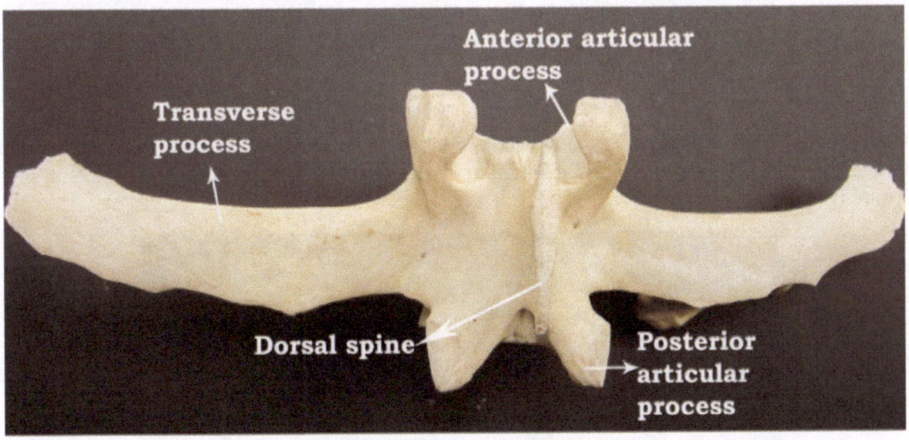

Fig. 5.1a: Lumbar Vertebra of Ox- Dorsal View

The articular processes are placed further apart. The transverse processes are shortest in the first and the length gradually increases to the 5th and in the 6th they are shorter than those of the 5th. The spines are broad flattened plates, resemble that of last thoracic vertebra and are of the same height as the last thoracic vertebra. That of the last is the narrowest of all.

Horse: The transverse process of the 5th lumbar vertebra at its medial part has an **oval facet posteriorly** which articulates with corresponding facet on anterior border of the transverse process of 6th lumbar vertebra. Sometimes the 5th has small facet anteriorly for the fourth also. The transverse process of 6th is thick at the base and thin and narrow elsewhere and curves forward. **It articulates by a large concave facet with the corresponding facet on the wing of the sacrum (Fig.5.1b).**

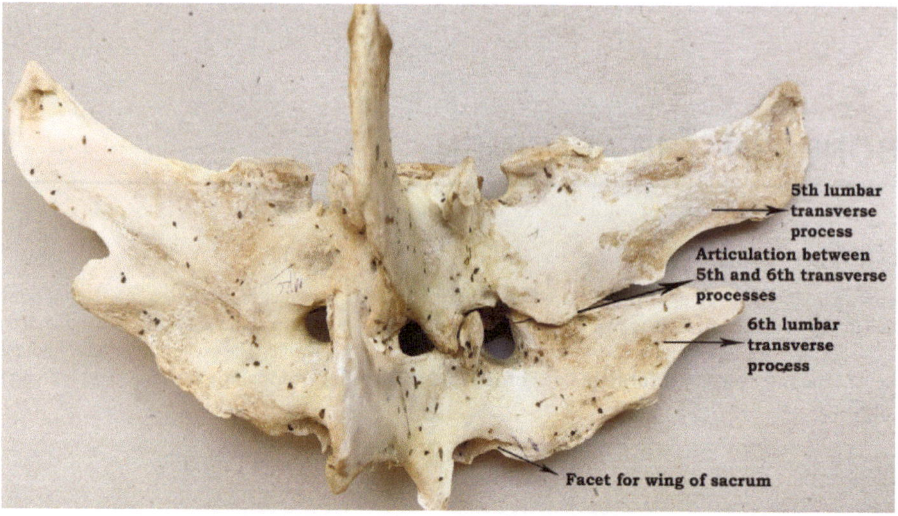

Fig. 5.1b: Fifth and Sixth Lumbar Vertebrae of Horse

Dog: The bodies increase in width from first to last. The transverse processes are plate like and are directed downward and forward. The **accessory and mammillary processes are present** and spinous processes incline a little forward **(Fig.5.2).**

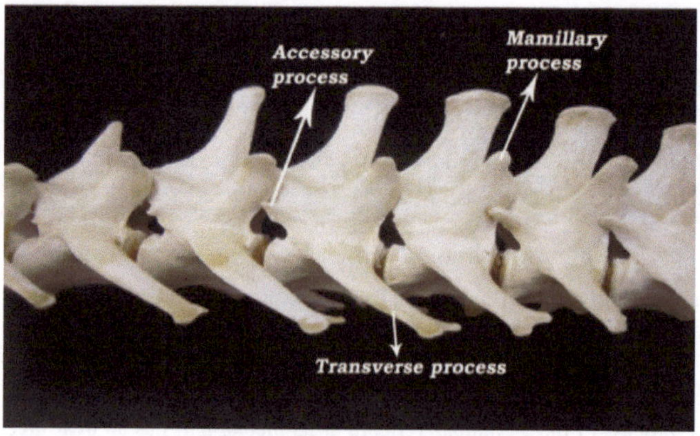

Fig. 5.2: Lumbar Vertebrae of Dog

Pig: The lumbar vertebrae are ***six or seven in number***. The bodies are longer than in the thoracic region and bear a ventral crest.

Fowl: The ***fourteen lumbar and sacral vertebrae are fused together and form lumbosacral mass.*** This with the ***7th dorsal and 1st coccygeal, altogether 16, are fused into one mass called synsacrum***. The spines form a crest in the anterior third but absent posteriorly. The transverse ridges on the ventral face indicate the position of the transverse processes.

5.2 MUSCLES OF THE ABDOMEN

There are four abdominal muscles viz., 1.Obliquus abdominis externus; 2. obliquus abdominis internus; 3. Rectus abdominis and 4. Transversus abdominis. The rectus abdominis muscle is entirely fleshy and is situated along the floor of the abdomen. The other muscles have each a muscular part laterally and an aponeurotic part ventrally. The aponeurotic part of the two side muscles meet in the median line and form a median fibrous raphe-the **linea alba which presents little behind its middle the umbilicus.**

1. Obliquus abdominis externus: It is the **largest and the most superficial** and extensive of all the abdominal muscles. The fibres of this muscle are **directed downwards and backwards (Fig.5.3).**

The aponeurosis of this muscle at its insertion to the prepubic tendon detaches a fibrous expansion the ***poupart's or inguinal ligament*** which extends upwards and forwards on the medial face of the thigh and is inserted to the lateral angle of the ilium. It forms the **posterior wall of the linguinal canal.** In front of the pubis and about 5 cm from the median line its aponeurosis is perforated by the subcutaneous or external inguinal ring for the exit of the spermatic cord.

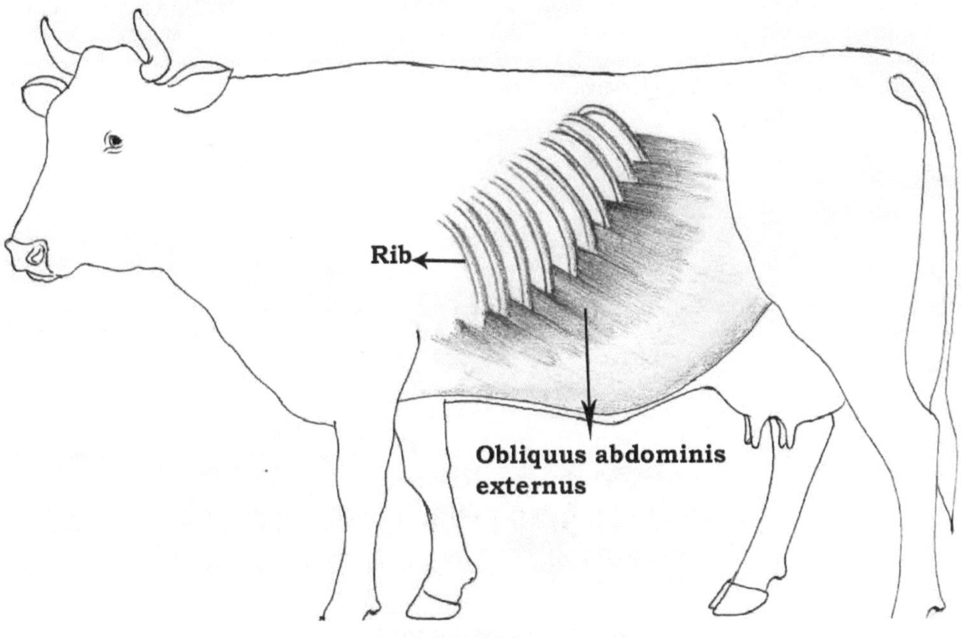

Fig. 5.3: Obliquus Abdominis Externus Muscle

2. Obliquus abdominis internus: It is situated under the preceeding and it extends from the **lateral angle of the ilium to the last rib**; its fibres pass **downwards and forwards (Fig.5.4).** The medial part of the muscle forms the anterior wall of inguinal canal. The slit like upper opening of the canal, the abdominal or internal inguinal ring is present here.

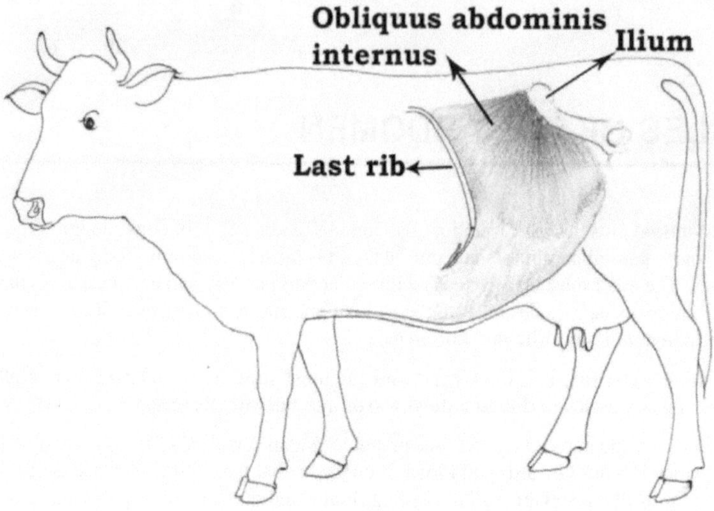

Fig. 5.4: Obliquus Abdominis Internus Muscle

3. Rectus abdominis: This muscle is confined to the **floor of the abdomen and extends from the sternum to the pubis (Fig.5.5).** The two muscles are separated except at the pelvis by an interval of about 2 to 4 inches, so that the abdominal wall here is entirely fibrous, consisting of the aponeuroses of the oblique and transverse muscles and abdominal tunic. *It shows on its superficial face five tendinous inscriptions (linea transversae) near the second of which is a foramen* ***for the passage of subcutaneous abdominal vein.***

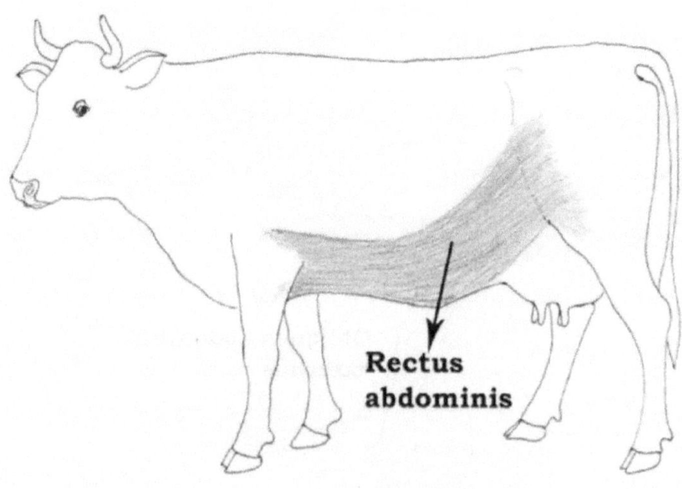

Fig. 5.5: Rectus Abdominis Muscle

4. Transversus abdominis: arises from the transverse process of last four lumbar vertebrae and inserts on linea alba on ventral aspect of the abdomen **(Fig.5.6).**

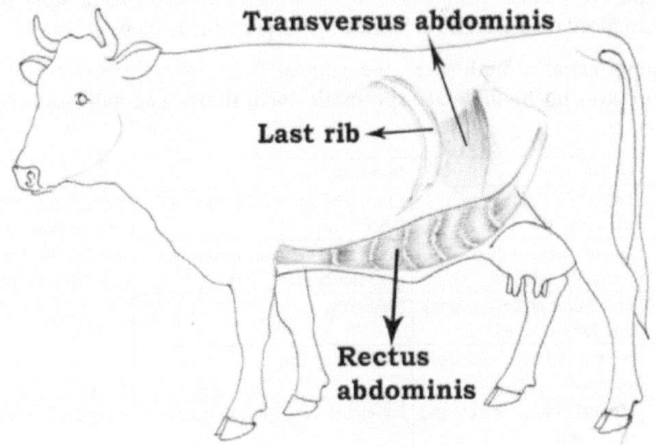

Fig. 5.6: Transversus abdominis Muscle

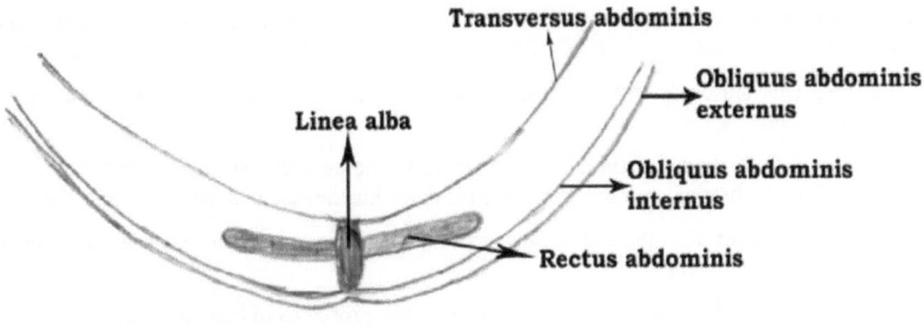

Fig. 5.6a: Schematic Representation of all Abdominal Muscles

Prepubic tendon: This is the tendon of ***insertion of the two recti abdominis muscles*** which are inserted to the anterior borders of the two pubic bones between the iliopectineal eminences. It is directed downwards and forwards and receives on its lateral borders the insertion of the two oblique abdominal muscles.

Cremaster externus: This is a narrow flat band of muscle detached from the internal oblique muscle of the abdomen. It passes into the inguinal canal along with the spermatic cord. It is covered externally by the cremasteric fascia and is attached to the lateral or dorsal surface of the finger like process formed by the tunica vaginalis. Under certain stimuli, it ***raises the tunica vaginalis and thus brings testes and epididymis closer to the external inginal ring.***

Inguinal canals: The inguinals canals are paired, slit like passages through the posterior part of the abdominal floor on either side of the prepublic tendon.They are equally well developed in both sexes and extend from the deep inguinal ring to the superficial inguinal ring.

The **anteromedial wall** of the inguinal canal is formed by the posterior part of the **internal oblique muscle of the abdomen.** The **posterolateral wall** is formed by a portion of the **aponeurosis of the external oblique muscle** ***and it is called as inguinal or poupart's ligament.***

The **abdominal or internal inguinal ring** is formed by the free borders of the **internal oblique muscle** anteriorly and the upper border of the inguinal ligament posteriorly. Its **medial angle** is formed by the **lateral margin of the prepubic tendon**. The **lateral angle** is formed by the attachment of the internal oblique to the inguinal ligament.

The external inguinal ring is a slit like opening in the aponeurosis of the **external oblique muscle of the abdomen and it is 15cm long.** Its rounded medial angle is formed by the prepubic tendon.

The structures of inguinal canal in both sexes: the external pudic artery, vein, the inguinal nerves and lymph vessels. **Additional structures in the male are spermatic cord, tunica vaginalis and the cremaster externus muscle.**

Name	Origin	Insertion	Action
Obliquus abdominis externus	Lateral face of the ribs from 5th-13th	Linea alba, prepubic tendon and tuber coxae	Reduce the size of the abdominal cavity and put pressure on the abdominal viscera and help in "***micturition, defecation, forced expiration and parturition***".
Obliquus abdominis internus	Lateral angle of ilium and poupart's ligament	Linea alba, prepubic tendon and posterior border of last rib.	
Transversus abdominis	Transverse processes of last four lumbar vertebrae.	Linea alba	
Rectus abdominis	Ventral and lateral parts of sternum.	Prepubic tendon	
Cremaster externus	Internal oblique muscle and iliac fascia.	Parietal layer of tunica vaginalis	To raise the tunica vaginalis

SUBLUMBAR MUSCLES

These are situated below the bodies and the transverse processes of the lumbar vertebrae

1. **Psoas minor:** This muscle lies along the ventrolateral aspect of the bodies of the last dorsal and all the lumbar vertebrae.
2. **Psoas major:** This muscle is larger than the preceding and is situated ventral to the lumbar transverse processes and ilium.
3. **Iliacus:** This muscle is situated on the anterior part of the pelvic surface of the ilium lateral to the ilio-pectineal line. It has two parts forming a groove to receive the preceding muscle with which it forms iliopsoas.
4. **Quadratus lumborum:** This muscle is partly covered by the psoas major and placed under transverse processes of lumbar vertebrae.
5. **Intertransversales lumborum:** present between transverse processes of lumbar vertebrae.

Name	Origin	Insertion	Action
1.Psoas minor	The intervertebral disc between the 12th and 13th thoracic vertebrae and all lumbar vertebrae.	Psoas tubercle of the ilium	To flex the pelvis on the loin and incline it laterally
2. Psoas major	Upper posterior borders of the last two ribs and the transverse processes of the lumbar vertebrae.	In common with the iliacus to the trochanter minor of the femur.	To flex the hip and rotate the thigh outwards
3.Iliacus	Iliac surface and shaft of ilium	Trochanter minor of the femur	To flex the hip and rotate the thigh outwards
4.Quadratus lumborum	Ventral surface of the upper part of the last two or three ribs and transverse processes of lumbar vertebrae.	The anterior border of the first five lumbar transverse processes and wing of sacrum.	To flex the loin laterally.
5.Intertransversales lumborum	Present between the transverse processes of the lumbar vertebrae.		To aid in lateral flexion of loin region.

5.3 BLOOD SUPPLY TO THE ABDOMEN

Branches of the abdominal aorta: Some are paired and some are unpaired. ***All branches are visceral except lumbar arteries and external iliac arteries which are parietal.***

I. Coeliac Artery: It is visceral unpaired. This artery arises from the ventral face of the abdominal aorta as it enters the abdominal cavity. The coeliac ganglia are on the lateral face of the artery and the coeliac plexus encloses the artery along its course. It is about 7 to 9 cm long, runs downwards on the left face of the rumen, turns forward to the right, related to the rumen, pancreas on the left and the right crus of the diaphragm and posterior vena cava on the right and is ***continued as omaso-abomasal artery***.

Collateral branches

(1) The **hepatic artery** arises from the **coeliac artery** as it crosses the posterior vena cava. It passes to the right and somewhat downwards and forwards above the portal vein to the portal fissure and gives off the following branches: (a) **Pancreatic branches** to the pancreas. (b) **Dorsal and ventral hepatic branches** to the corresponding lobes of the liver, of which latter is large and gives off ***the right gastric artery*** which runs in the lesser omentum and supplies initial part of duodenum, pylorus and anastomoses with the branches of the dorsal branch of the **omaso-abomasal artery (left gastric artery)**. (c) **Cystic branch to gall bladder.**

(2) **The gastroduodenal artery** divides into **pancreatico-duodenal and right gastro-epiploic arteries.** The former supplies **the pancreas and second part of duodenum** and anastomoses with the first intestinal branch of the anterior mesenteric artery. The **right gastro-epiploic artery supplies the pylorous and anastomoses** with the **left gastroepiploic artery** (**continuation of ventral branch of omasoabomasal artery**).

(3) **The right ruminal artery** arises usually by a common trunk with the **splenic artery**. It forms a sharp curve and runs downward and backwards in the right longitudinal groove of rumen, giving off numerous branches to it, reaches the posterior transverse groove, passes in it, reaches the left face of the rumen and anastomoses with the left ruminal artery. **It supplies the right face and the posterior one-third of the left face of the rumen (Fig.5.8).**

(4) **The left ruminal artery** descends at first on the anterior part of the right face of the rumen, enters the anterior transverse groove, passes to the left face of the rumen, runs backward in the left longitudinal groove and anastomoses with the branches of the right ruminal artery. **It supplies the anterior two thirds of the left face of the rumen (Fig.5.7).** After its origin it gives off a ***reticular artery*** which passes along the dorsal curvature of rumen, turns downward in rumino-reticular groove and passes to the right and **supplies the reticulum (Fig.5.7).**

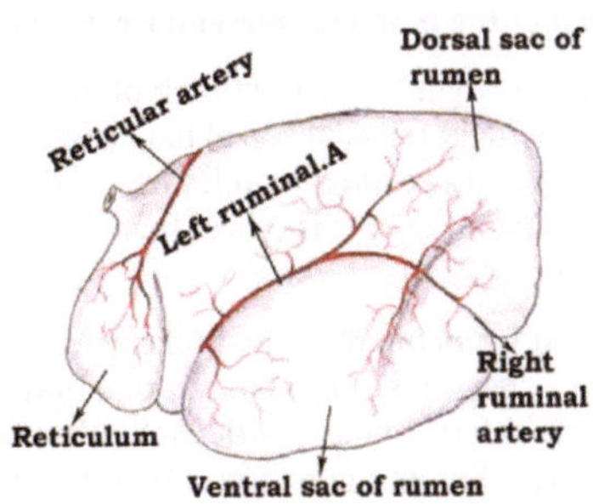

Fig. 5.7: Branches of Coeliac artery-Left View

(5) **The splenic artery** arising in common with the ***right ruminal artery*** passes forwards, crosses the dorsal curvature of the rumen, reaches the hilus of the spleen and is distributed in it.

(6) **The omaso-abomasal artery** is the continuation of the coeliac artery. It is 10 to 13 cm long, passes downwards and forwards to the greater curvature of the omasum and divides into **dorsal and ventral branches. The dorsal branch** (*left gastric artery*) passes backwards over the greater curvature of the omasum then along the lesser curvature of the abomasum, supplying branches to these compartments and beyond the pylorus it anastomoses with the right gastric artery. **The ventral branch** (***left gastro epiploic aretery***) passes downwards and forwards over the greater curvature of the abomasum giving branches to this compartment and **anastomoses with the right gastro-epiploic artery (Fig.5.8).**

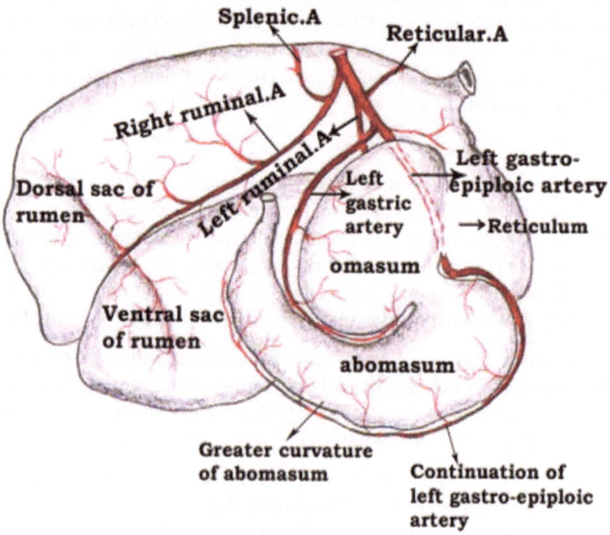

Fig. 5.8: Branches of Coeliac Artery

II. Anterior Mesenteric Artery: It is visceral unpaired and arises from the ventral face of the abdominal aorta ***at the level of 2nd lumbar vertebra*** immediately behind the origin of coeliac artery. The lateral face of the artery is enclosed by the anterior mesenteric ganglia and the mesenteric plexus. It gives off the following branches:

1. **Pancreatic branches** to the pancreas.
2. The **middle colic artery** is short and arises from the cranial surface of the anterior mesenteric artery and supplies **transverse and descending colon.** It runs backward on the dorsal face of descending colon to **anastomose with the short colic branch of the posterior mesenteric artery (Fig.5.9).**
3. The **Ileocaeco-colic artery** is covered on the right by the right limb of the distal loop of the colon. It gives branches to **distal loop of colon and centrifugal turns of spiral loop (Fig.5.9).** The **distal part gives** colic branch to **centripetal turns of spiral loop and proximal loop.**It then continues to ileocaecal fold gives off ileal branch and continued on caecum as caecal artery. The Ileal branch anastomoses with ileal branch of terminal part of anterior mesenteric artery.
4. **The Jejunal branches:** About **15 jejunal branches** arise at regular intervals from the convex surface of whole length of anterior mesenteric artery**, beginning proximal to the middle colic artery. The adjacent jejunal branches of anterior mesenteric artery connect with each other by anastomoses forming two series of superposed arches to supply jejunum and mesenteric lymphnodes (Fig.5.9).** The first and last jejunal arteries anastomose with duodenal branch of pancreatoduodenal branch of gastroduodenal artery of hepatic artery and ileal branch of ileocaeco-colic artery respectively.

5. **The collateral branch** is given off from the inside of the curve of the anterior mesenteric artery distal to ileocaecocolic artery and passes obliquely across the mesentery to join anterior mesenteric artery.

6. **Ileal artery** arises from concave surface of terminal branch of anterior mesenteric artery and anastomoses with ileal branch of ileocaeco-colic artery **(Fig.5.9).**

Anastomoses between various branches of anterior mesenteric artery ensure continuous blood supply in the event of blockade in any part of the artery.

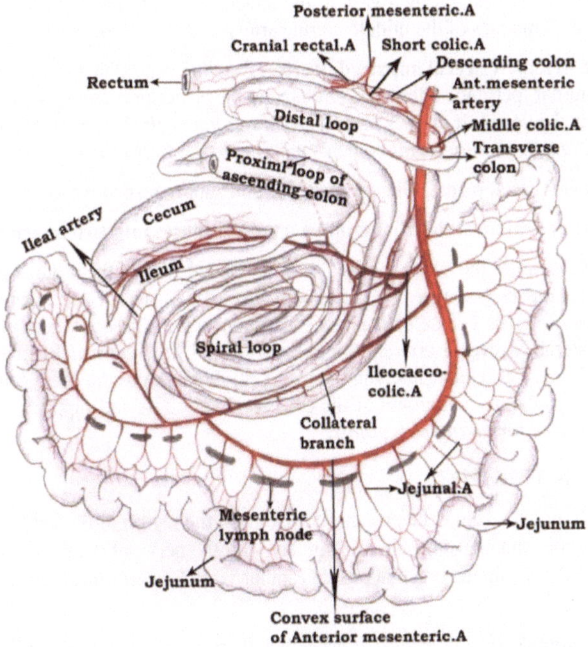

Fig. 5.9: Branches of Anterior Mesenteric Artery of Ox

III. Renal Arteries: Visceral paired: These are right and left and arise close together from the inferior face of the abdominal aorta about 8 cm behind the origin of the preceding branch. The **right renal artery is shorter but large,** while the **left renal artery is longer but narrow**. The right artery pushes forward, outward and downward over the posterior vena cava and enters the hilus of the right kidney. The left artery usually passes forward and downward to the hilus of the left kidney. In addition **each renal artery gives off small branches to the ureter, renal lymph gland and adrenal.**

IV. Lumbar Arteries: Parietal paired: There are **6 pairs of lumbar arteries** of which the first five arise from the aorta and sixth arises from the internal iliac artery. They arise from the dorsal face of the aorta pass across the bodies of lumbar vertebrae, gain the inter- transverse spaces and divide into dorsal and ventral branches. The **dorsal or lumbar spinal branches are larger**. They supply spinal branches to reinforce the ventral spinal artery and muscular branches to supply the muscles of the loin region. The **ventral branches supply the abdominal muscles and skin.**

V. Internal Spermatic/Ovarian Arteries: Visceral paired: arise at the level of the fifth lumbar vertebra from the ventral face of the aorta close together near the posterior mesenteric artery.

In males each is very long slender branch. It is at first directed backward in the sublumbar region and then downward a little lateral to the pelvic inlet and reaches the internal inguinal canal as one of the constituent structures of the spermatic cord. In anterior border of spermatic card it exhibits a remarkable tortuous disposition. It forms numerous coils **surrounded by the *pampiniform plexus of veins*** and closely associated with the spermatic nerves and lymphatics and unstriped muscle fibres. The artery reaches the upper extremity of the testis and gives epidydimal branch and first branch of ductus deferens and penetrates the tunica albuginea to supply the parenchyma.

In the female, this ***vessel is the ovarian artery***. It is a slender flexuous vessel which passes backwards and outwards in the sublumbar region and then turns downward on the posterior part of the abdominal wall to the anterior part of the broad ligament of the uterus. ***It* gives branches to uterine tube *and anterior uterine branches*** to the part of the **the horn of the uterus.** After giving anterior uterine branch it enters the ovary by dividing into several tightly coiled branches forming a cone with its base on the ovary at the attachment of the mesoovarium. The anterior uterine branch anastomoses with the branches of the middle uterine artery in the mesometrium.

VI. Posterior Mesenteric Artery: Visceral unpaired: It arises from the ventral face of the aorta near its termination behind the origin of the internal spermatic arteries. It is related to the posterior mesenteric ganglion and the posterior mesenteric plexus encloses the vessel. It divides into an ***anterior, short colic*** branch to supply the ***terminal part of the colon*** and a ***posterior, longer cranial rectal*** branch supplying to the **first part of rectum**.

VII. External Iliac Artery: Parietal paired. One on each side and supply respective hind limbs.

At the level of the **5th lumbar vertebra, the abdominal aorta terminates into two internal iliac arteries.**

Middle Sacral Artery: It continues the aorta. It arises from the dorsal face of the aorta at the angle of divergence of the internal iliac arteries, passes backward on the ventral face of the sacrum and is **continued as the middle coccygeal artery**. It gives off in its course spinal branches, branches to the coccygeal muscles and two lateral coccygeal arteries. The lateral coccygeal arteries **divide into dorsal and ventral branches** and are connected with the middle coccygeal artery at regular intervals. They supply branches to the coccygeal muscles. The ***middle coccygeal artery*** runs through the haemal arches of the coccygeal vertebrae and supplies coccygeal muscles. ***The middle coccygeal artery is used for taking pulse in ox.***

VENOUS DRAINAGE IN ABDOMEN

The External Thoracic Vein: This vein is inconstant. It arise from the region of the flank and the abdominal wall and passes forwards under the cutaneous muscle in company with the nerve of the same name and joins the deep brachial vein in the axilla. It may join the brachial or subscapular vein. ***It is very large and is always present in the horse as the spur vein.***

The Subcutaneous Abdominal Vein: In the male, it is small and drains the venous blood from the inguinal region. It passes forwards under the cutaneous muscle, passes through a foramen in the rectus abdominis and joins internal thoracic vein.

The Azygos vein: is **unpaired vein** in the upper part of the thorax posterior to the heart. In the **horse and dog** the right vein, the ***vena azygos*, is present**. In the **ox, sheep and pig** the **left vein is present** and is called ***vena hemiazygos***, whichever vein is present has its ***tributaries, the intercostal veins from the the fourth to the last.***

The Vena Hemiazygos: This is a ***large unpaired vein*** situated on the ***left side of the roof of thoracic cavity***. This begins in the region of the last thoracic vertebra and passes forward, along the bodies of the vertebrae and close to the aorta, to the fifth vertebra. Here it turns downward across the aorta and pulmonary artery. On reaching the left atrium it turns backward and to the right and joins the great coronary vein on the posterior surface of the heart. It receives, the intercostal veins *except first three on the left and the first six on the right*, blood from the dorsal spinal muscles and diaphragm.

The Posterior Vena Cava: is ***largest vein and unpaired vein,*** receiving blood from the pelvis, hind limbs, mammry gland (in part), the abdominal wall (except anterior wall), urogenital system, the digestive system and spleen. It is slightly to the right of the median plane in the abdomen and further to the right in the thorax. It is formed under the body of the **fifth lumbar vertebra** by the union of the **two common illiac veins** (each common illiac vein is formed by the union of the external and internal illiac veins). It passes forwards below the bodies of the lumbar vertebrae slightly to the right of the median plane and the abdominal aorta. It leaves the company of the aorta about the level of hiatus aorticus, runs downwards and forwards, reaches the upper part of the dorsal border of the liver, runs forwards partly embedded along the dorsal border of the gland receiving hepatic veins, then passes through the **foramen vena cavae (*foramen dextrum*)** of the diaphragm, enters the thoracic cavity passes in the groove between the mediastinal and diaphragmatic lobes of the right lung in company with the right phrenic nerve enclosed in a special fold of the pleura and opens into the posterior part of the sinus venosus of the right atrium. Its tributaries are ***middle sacral vein, internal spermatic veins (in male), uteroovarian vein (in female), renal veins, lumbar veins, hepatic and phrenic veins.***

THE PORTAL VEIN

It is a large venous trunk ***returning the blood from the splanchnic area*** and contains the digested nutrients which are absorbed from the small intestine and destined to reach the liver. After detoxification in liver this blood reaches the posterior vena cava through hepatic veins.

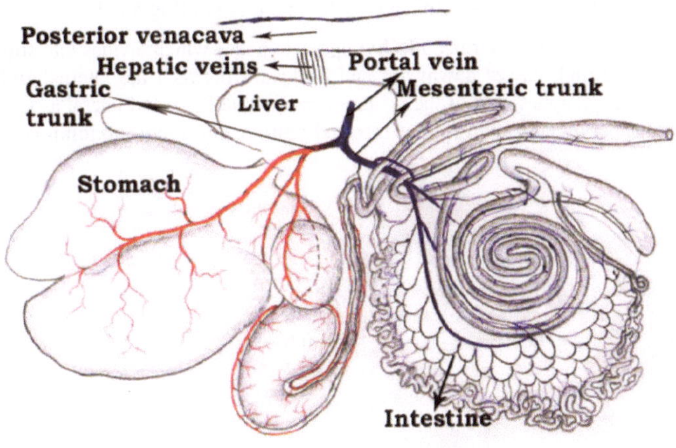

Fig. 5.10: Portal Vein

The portal vein it is ***formed by the union of two trunks i.e gastric and mesenteric* (Fig.5.10).** The ***portal vein is characterised by two sets of capillaries unlike other veins, one set (1st set) at beginning i.e in wall of alimentary canal and another set in the liver (2nd set,* Fig.5.11*)*** The ***gastric trunk*** is formed by the union of the right ruminal, splenic, left ruminanl, reticular and omasoabomasal veins. It also receives the gastro-duodenal and pancreatic veins. The ***mesenteric trunk*** is formed by the union of ***anterior and posterior mesenteric veins.***

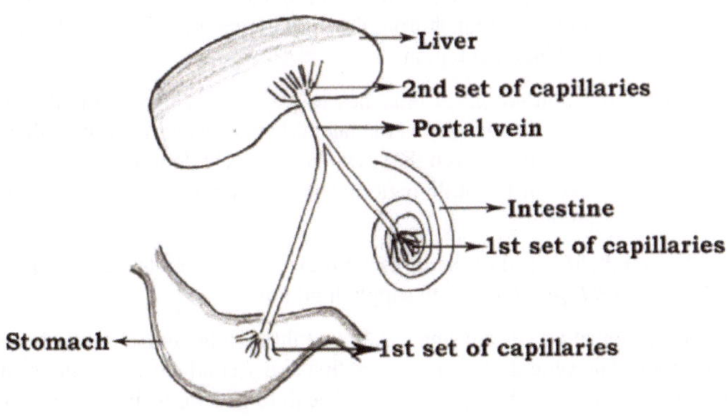

Fig. 5.11: Two sets of Capillaries of Portal View

5.4 NERVE SUPPLY TO THE ABDOMEN

The Lumbar Spinal Nerves

There are six pairs of nerves. Each lumbar spinal nerve divides into **dorsal and ventral branches**. The **dorsal branches** are distributed to the muscles and the skin of the loin. The **ventral branches** slightly differ in their distribution. They pass under the psoas minor and psoas major and emerge at the lateral border of the latter. They supply branches to the sublumbar muscles, abdominal muscles and the skin **(Fig.5.12).**

The **ventral branch** of the first lumbar is termed **ilio-hypogastric nerve** which divides into **superficial and deep branches**. The **superficial branch** passes downward and backward between the internal and external oblique muscles, perforating the latter, supplies skin of the posterior part of the flank and lateral aspect of the thigh. The **deep branch** runs under the peritoneum and **supplies internal oblique and rectus abdominis muscles (Fig.5.12).**

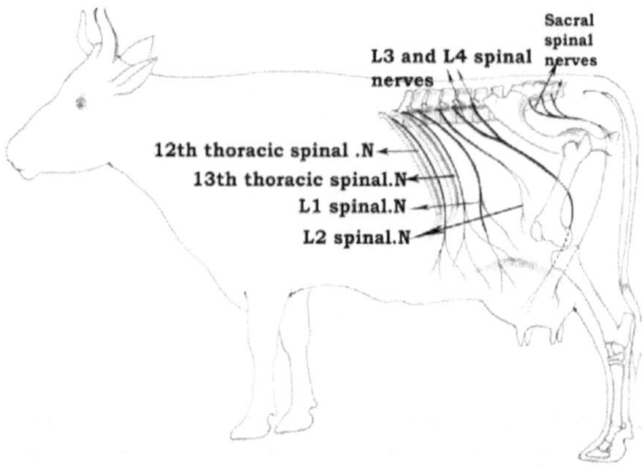

Fig. 5.12: Thoracic and Lumbar Spinal Nerves

The **ventral branch of the second lumbar** supplies psoas major and continues ***as the ilio-inguinal nerve***. This also divides into a superficial branch supplying skin infront of thigh and lateral face of the stifle. The **deep branch supplies abdominal muscles**, unites with a branch from the third lumbar nerve, passes through the inguinal canal, supplies external genitalia and skin of inguinal region.

The **ventral branch of the third lumbar** gives branches to psoas muscles and **divides into superficial and deep branches**. The **superficial branch** continues as the lateral cutaneous nerve of the thigh passes outward and backward emerges below the point of hip, between iliacus and obliquus abdominis externus, under cover of tensor fasciae latae and ramiflies on the skin of the stifle region. The **deep branch** forms the external spermatic nerve which descends into the inguinal region.

The ventral branches of the **fourth, fifth and sixth lumbar spinal** nerves enter into the ***formation of the lumbosacral plexus*** along with ***1st and 2nd sacral spinal*** *nerves* to supply hind limb.

The dorsal branches of sacral spinal nerves are small, gain exit through the dorsal sacral foramina and supply the muscles and skin of the croup. The ventral branches of the first and second enter into the formation of the lumbo-sacral plexus along with 4th, 5th and 6th lumbar spinal nerves.The third generally gives off a branch to the plexus and the rest unites with the fourth and divides into pudic and posterior haemorrhoidal nerves.

5.5 VISCERAL ORGANS OF THE ABDOMINAL CAVITY

Abdominal Part of Oesophagus

Ox: The abdominal part of oesophagus is very short and opens into the stomach on a sort of dome, the ***atrium ventriculi***. The mucosa shows longitudinal folds so lumen presents rosette like appearance in cross section. The tunica muscularis is striated.

Horse: The oesophagus joins the stomach at an acute angle. The wall shows striated muscles upto tracheal bifurcation only and caudal third shows smooth muscle fibres.

Dog: The esophagus joins the stomach at the funnel shaped cardia. The wall shows striated muscles.

Pig: The oesophagus is short and nearly straight. The mucular coat is striated except at cardia.

Fowl: The wall of the oesophagus increases in thickness caudally. An **oesophageal tonsil** is present at the junction with the provenriculus.

STOMACH (ventriculus)

The stomach is a sac like enlargement of the alimentary canal between the oesophagus and duodenum.

The stomach of ruminants (ox, sheep and goat) is much larger, more complex and has four compartments viz., rumen, reticulum, omasum and abomasum.

RUMEN

Ox: It occupies nearly 3/4th of the abdominal cavity particularly the left half of abdominal cavity from cardia at the 8th rib to caudal blind sac at the pelvic inlet. It is a huge, laterally compressed sac. It presents two surfaces, two borders and two extremities. The **parietal (left) surface** is convex, faces to left and related to diaphragm, left abdominal wall and spleen. ***Atrium ventriculi*** is a dome like area situated at the vertebral extremity of **8th and 9th ribs** slightly to the left of the midline where the oesophagus enters the stomach.

The **visceral (right) surface** is irregular, faces to right and related chiefly to the intestines, liver, omasum, abomasum, pancreas, left kidney, left adrenal, aorta and posterior venacava. The dorsal curvature (border) is convex and lies against the diaphragm and roof of abdominal cavity. The ventral curvature (border) is also convex and related to abdominal floor.

The left and right longitudinal grooves are shallow. The left longitudinal groove extends on the left face of the rumen from anterior transverse or cranial groove to the posterior transverse or caudal groove. It gives an accessory groove extending for a short distance along the left surface of dorsal sac **(Fig.5.13).**

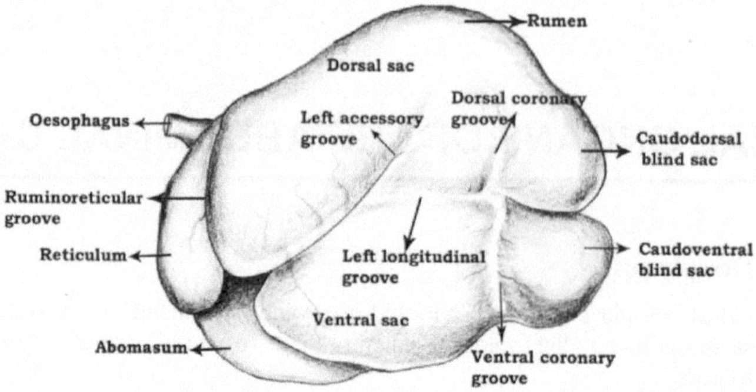

Fig. 5.13: Rumen of Ox (Exterior- Left view)

The ***right longitudinal groove*** which lies on the right face of the rumen gives off dorsally a right accessory groove that rejoins the main groove and with it surrounds an elongated bulge, the ***insula ruminis***. It divides into dorsal prominent dorsal limb and ventral limb and the greater omentum attaching to the latter. The ***cranial and caudal transverse grooves*** are two deep transverse grooves connecting the right and left longitudinal grooves cranially and caudally and these four grooves divide the rumen into dorsal and ventral sacs **(Fig.5.14).**

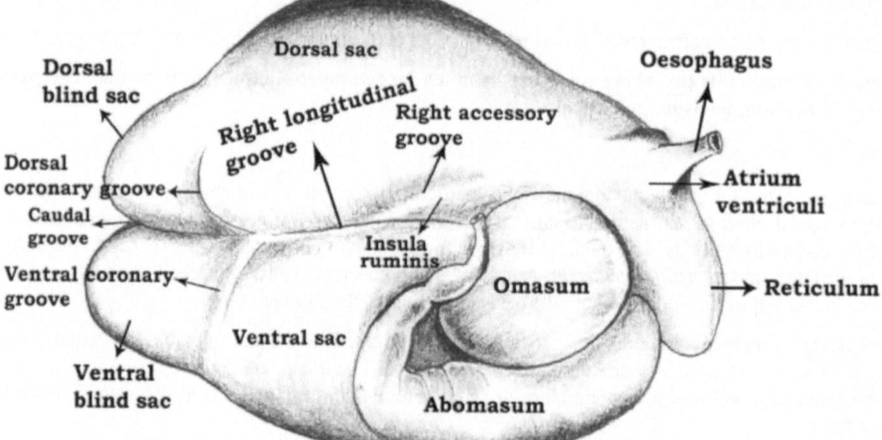

Fig. 5.14: Rumen of Ox (Exterior-Right view)

The **dorsal and ventral coronary grooves** extend in opposite directions from the caudal end of the right and left longitudinal grooves and along with posterior transverse groove mark off the caudodorsal and caudoventral blind sacs in posterior extremity.

The anterior extremity is divided ventrally by a transverse groove into two sacs i.e ***dorsal and ventral***, of which dorsal sac is continuous with the reticulum while the ventral one is blind. The ruminal grooves contain fat, blood vessels, lymph nodes and nerves.

The cranial sac of rumen communicates in front with the reticulum by a wide ***ruminoreticular*** opening marked externally by a ***ruminoreticular groove*** which lies opposite to cardia and represented by ruminoreticular fold inside. This groove separates rumen from reticulum.

The oesophagus enters the stomach at the junction of rumen and reticulum and the opening of oesophagus is the cardia which is located on a dome like projection of rumen ***viz., atrium ventriculi.***

Interior appearance: The grooves dividing the rumen externally are represented on the inside by ***pillars (muscular folds)*** of corresponding names, which project like shelves to varying degree into the interior of the rumen as cranial and caudal pillars, right and left longitudinal pillars surrounding the intraruminal opening through which the dorsal sac communicates with the ventral sac. The ***mucosa is studded with number of papillae which are absent on pillars. The papillae are foliate, filiform or club shaped*** **(Fig.5.15).**

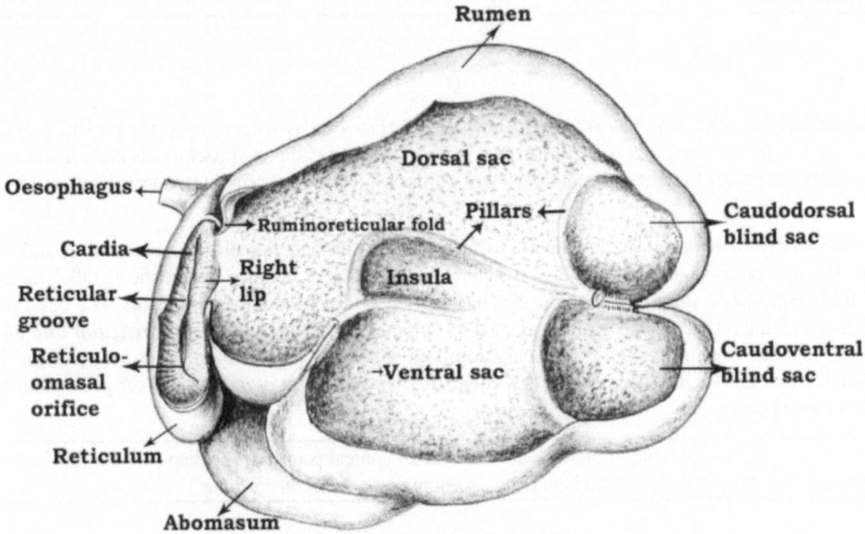

Fig. 5.15: Rumen of Ox Interior (Left view)

The **ruminal pillars** along with rest of musculature act to mix the contents. The coarse forage on the surface of rumen contents at the level of cardia stimulates receptors near the cardia that reflexely increase motility of stomach through vagus nerves and coarse material is regurgitated in **rumination, a process which includes a) regurgitation b) remastication c) reinsalivation and d) reswallowing**. The reswallowed cud is finely saturated with saliva.

Rumen acidosis results in lowered pH and lead to ruminal parakeratosis, a condition characterized by hardening and enlargement of the papillae of the rumen. Bloat is another condition that could result from excessive gas accumulation in the rumen resulting from fermentation. Temporary relief can be achieved by trocarization of the rumen on the left paralumbar fossa.

RETICULUM

Reticulum is most **cranial and smallest of the four compartments**. The **greater part of reticulum is on left side (Fig.5.13).** It extends from the level of **6th rib to 8th rib**. It is spherical but slightly flattened cranio-caudally. It shows two surfaces, two curvatures and two extremities. The **parietal surface** faces forwards and is convex, while the **visceral surface** is flattened, faces backwards and joins the rumen dorsally. The lesser curvature faces to right and is connected with omasum, while the greater curvature faces to left and is ventral. The right extremity forms the blind sac (fundus reticuli). ***Reticulum can be auscultated at the ventral ends of left 6th and 7th intercostal spaces.***

Elevation of dorsal part of left flank indicates **acute bloat with free gas in rumen**. Distension of entire left contour and ventral part of right abdominal wall is caused by rumen overloaded with ingesta.

Interior appearance: The mucous membrane lining the reticulum is studded with horny papillae and raised into folds which enclose 4-6 sided spaces or cells giving the **honeycomb appearance (Fig.5.20).** These cells are subdivided by smaller folds. The reticulo-omasal orifice is situated at the lesser curvature of the reticulum.

> Cattle may ingest sharp objects such as nails and wires. Metal objects could drop to the bottom of the reticular floor and become lodged within the reticulum. The contractions of the stomach could cause sharp objects to penetrate the wall of the reticulum and diaphragm and reach the heart. This can lead to a condition known as traumatic reticulopericarditis or traumatic reticuloperitonitis commonly known as ***hardware disease.***

OMASUM

It is ellipsoidal and extends from ***7th to 11th rib***. It shows two surfaces and two curvatures. The parietal surface faces to right and is directed forward. The visceral surface faces to left and is directed backwards and related to rumen. The greater curvature faces to right and is directed backwards, while the lesser curvature faces to left and is directed forwards.

Interior: The cavity of omasum communicates with reticulum through reticulo-omasal opening and with the abomasum through omasoabomasal opening. It is filled with about a hundred crescentic parallel longitudinal muscular folds **(*omasal laminae*)** of varying sizes and are studded with papillae **(Fig.5.16)**. The omasal groove is less distinct than the reticular groove and ***is devoid of laminae and is continuous with reticular and abomasal grooves.*** The laminae arise from the greater curvature and sides and their free edges project into the interior. Between the laminae are the interlaminar recesses **(Fig.5.17)**. ***The function of a omasum is to press food between the laminae and absorb water.***

> The interior of the omasum has laminae dotted with small conical papillae. The disposition of the laminae is similar to the pages of a book and hence the common name ***" butcher's bible"***

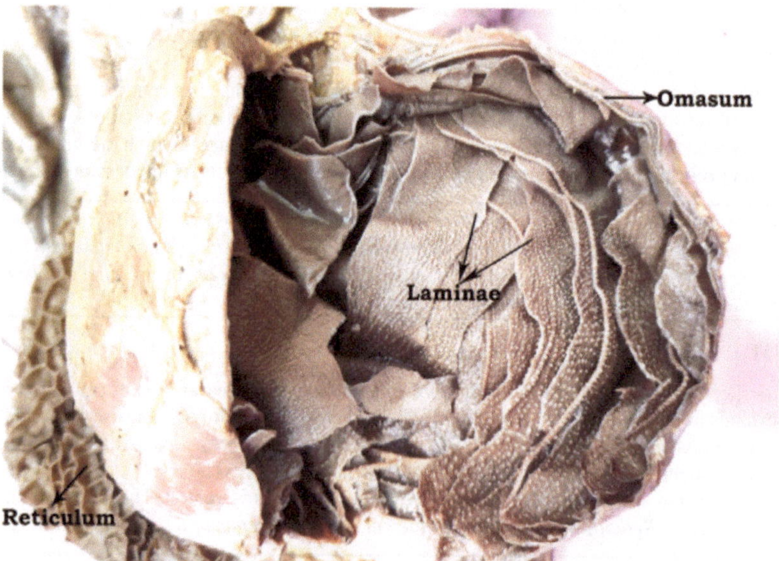

Fig.5.16: Omasum of Ox (Interior)

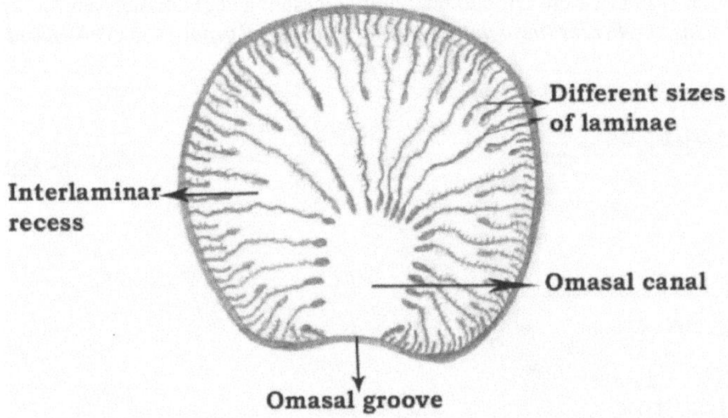

Fig. 5.17: Omasum of Ox-Interior (Schematic)

ABOMASUM

It is most distal and true **glandular compartment** of ruminant stomach. It is in the form of an **elongated or pear shaped** thin walled sac ***(often"J" shaped in appearance)***. It lies on the floor of the abdomen mostly to the right of the median plane. It lies chiefly on abdominal floor from the xiphoid cartilage backwards. It is divided into three parts, a ***fundus*** (anterior blind end), ***a body and a pyloric*** part. The body is constricted in the middle and shows a larger (anterior) part and a smaller pear shaped (posterior) part. The pyloric part of abomasum joins the duodenum. The abomasum presents two (greater and lesser) curvatures and two (parietal and visceral) surfaces. The **smaller pyloric part of abomasum** lies at the ventral part of ***9th or 10th rib*** and joins the duodenum.

Interior Appearance: The cavity of abomasum is divided into two parts by a constriction corresponding to regions of proper gastric glands and pyloric glands. The first part (including fundus and body) presents a dozen or more permanent spiral folds and mucosa is greyish red, while in second part the mucosa is lighter and in the vicinity of pylorus forms irregular transient folds. ***Torus pyloricus*** is a round protuberance on the inside of lesser curvature near pylorus **(Fig.5.18).**

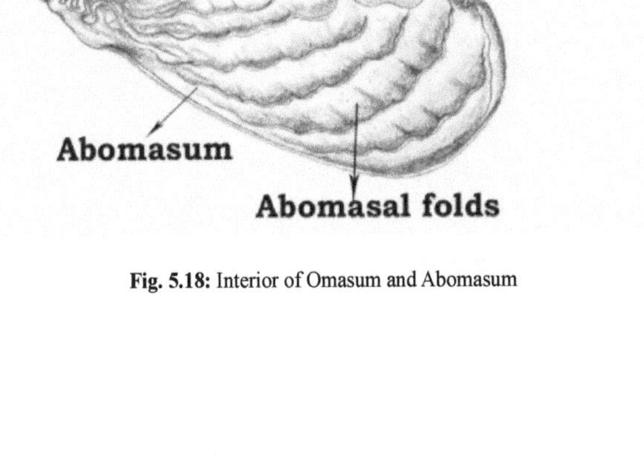

Fig. 5.18: Interior of Omasum and Abomasum

Gastric Groove: It extends from cardia through reticulum, omasum and abomasum almost to the pylorus and is divided into three segments a) ***reticular (oesophageal) groove b***) ***omasal groove*** and **c)** ***abomasal groove*** **(Fig.5.19).**

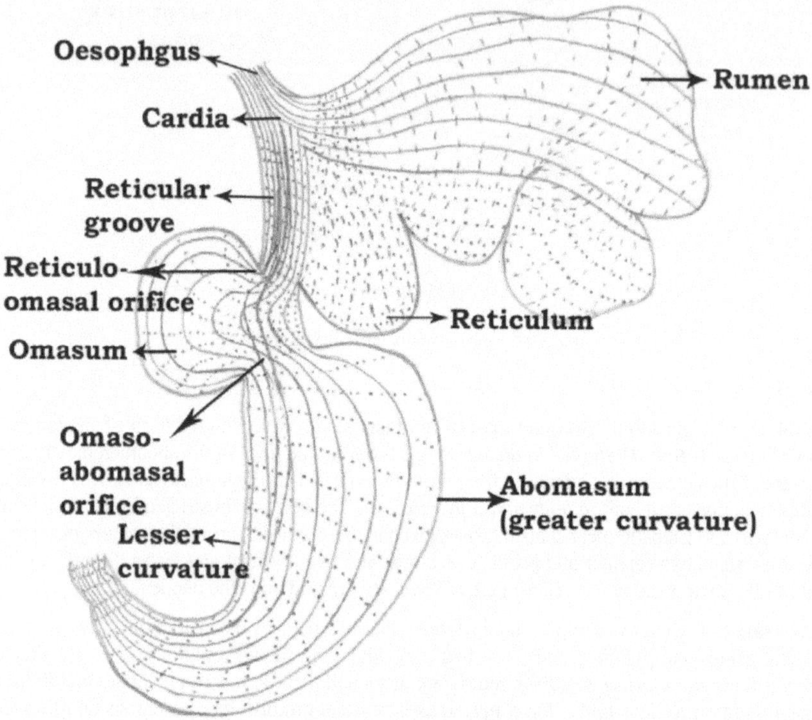

Fig. 5.19: Gastric Groove of Ox

The ***reticular groove*** is formed by two right and left muscular ridges or lips twisted in a clock wise direction in dorsal view. It extends from cardia to the reticulo-omasal opening from left to right. It is 15-20 cm long in ox and 7-10 cm in sheep and goat. The muscular layer of the stomach wall takes part in the formation of the lips and floor of the groove **(Fig.5.20).**The floor of the reticular groove presents longitudinal folds and is marked by horny papillae at the reticulo-omasal opening which are thin and curved. ***A reflex triggered by the presence of salts in liquids passing through pharynx and proximal portion of oesophagus brings the lips of the reticular groove together to form a tube. In suckling calves closure of reticular groove conducts milk directly to abomasum bye passing rumen and reticulum.***

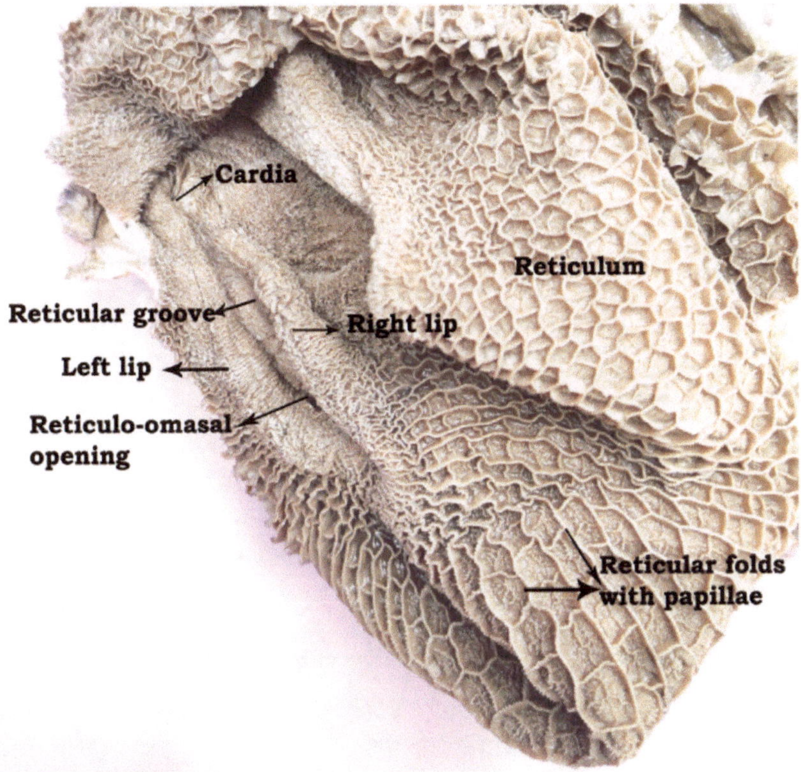

Fig. 5.20: Reticular (Oesophageal) Groove of Calf

The ***omasal groove*** at the base of omasum is free from laminae and connects the reticulo-omasal opening with omaso-abomasal opening. It is flanked by two mucosal ridges covered with papillae. The muscular omasal pillar crosses the omasal groove near the omasoabomasal opening, which is flanked by two mucosal folds, ***vela abomasa***.

The ***abomasal groove,*** the third segment of gastric groove, is a band like area located along the lesser curvature and is free of folds.

Horse: The stomach is simple and bent sharply to form a **'U' shaped sac**, so that cardia and pylorus lie close to each other. It is **located in left dorsal part of abdominal cavity**. The parietal surface faces craniodorsally and to the left applied against the diaphragm, liver and spleen. The visceral surface faces caudoventrally and to the right related to jejunum, descending colon, the diaphragmatic flexure and right dorsal segment of ascending colon and the left lobe of pancreas.

The greater curvature is extensive and is related to spleen and great colon. The lesser curvature is short and faces dorsally to the right. The ***left dorsal extremity is the blind sac, saccus cecus*** which is the most dorsal and caudal part of the stomach, while the right extremity is continued by duodenum **(Fig.5.21).**

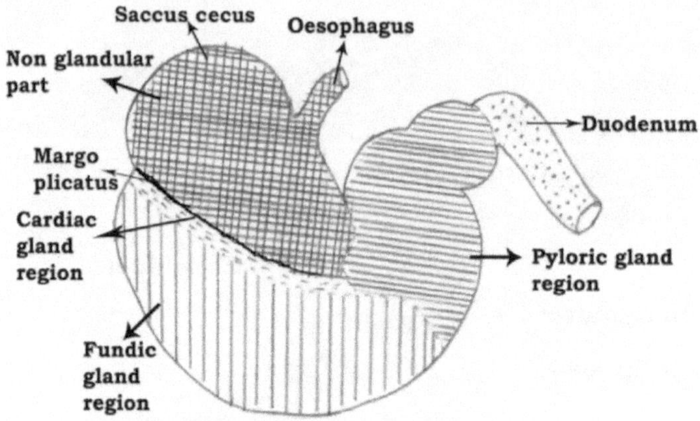

Fig. 5.21: Stomach of Horse (Schematic)

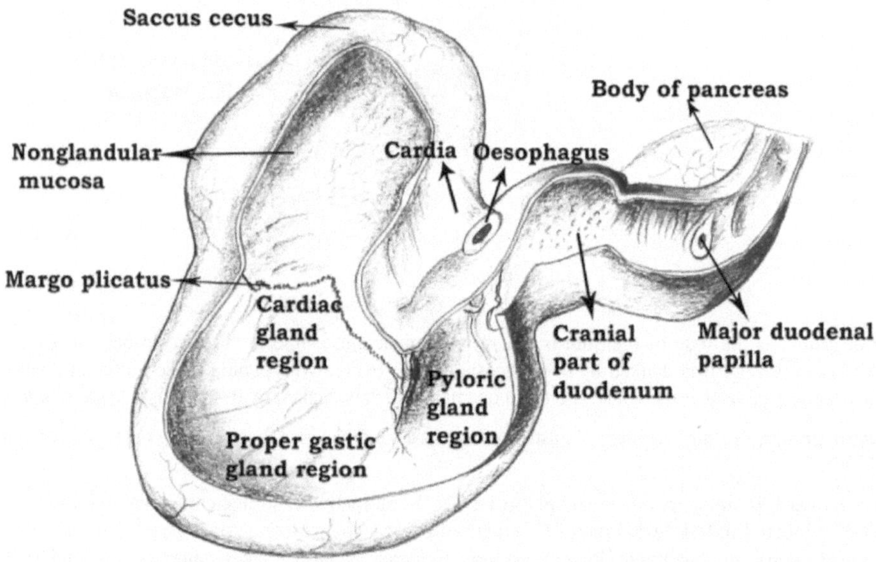

Fig. 5.22: Stomach of Horse (Interior)

In the interior ***margo plicatus*****, a sinuous ridge** divides the mucous membrane into two parts, non-glandular and glandular. The latter is **softer and velvety to touch** and is below and to the right of ridge, while the **former is whitish** and lines greater part of left sac **(Fig.5.22).**

Dog: The stomach is "***pyriform***" shaped and flattened craniocaudally. **The mucosa is folded and totally glandular.** The **parietal surface** is extensive faces forwards, downwards and to the left and is related to liver, diaphragm, left lateral and ventral abdominal walls. The **visceral surface** is less extensive and related to intestine and pancreas. The fundus and body are on the left side of the abdomen and pyloric part is ventral and to the right turning dorsally and slightly cranially. The extensive **greater curvature** is related to spleen, while the **lesser curvature** is less extensive and nearly straight. *The empty stomach cannot be palpated because it lies entirely in the intrathoracic part of* *abdominal cavity and fails to make contact with abdominal wall.* The greater omentum covers ventral and lateral aspects of abdominal organs except spleen and descending colon on left and duodenum on right, liver cranially and urinary bladder caudally. It shows superficial and deep walls.

The **cardiac gland region** is a narrow annular zone at the cardia. The **proper gastric gland region** lines about two-thirds of stomach i.e fundus and almost entire body. The **pyloric gland region** takes up about one third of stomach and is mainly found in pyloric part but extends also into body reaching cardia in the vicinity of lesser curvature.

Pig: It has **both glandular and non-glandular** parts. The latter is small. The fundus shows a small flattened conical diverticulum pointing to right caudally distinguishing it from other species. It is set off from the fundus by an annular groove. The **cardiac gland** region is extensive and occupies fundus including diverticulum and most of the body. The **proper gastric gland** region lines distal portion of body near greater curvature. The **pyloric gland** region lines most of pyloric part except for a small area near greater curvature. The cardiac gland region is soft, smooth and light red or grey, the proper gastric glands region is brownish red and shows folds and the pyloric region is devoid of folds and is pale pink to yellowish, while **nonglandular mucosa** is white. The muscular coat is like in horse. The ***cardia is at the level of 12th thoracic vertebra.*** The **greater curvature** is directed towards the left and ventrally, the **lesser curvature** is directed towards the right and dorsally. The empty and moderately full stomach lies within intrathoracic part of abdominal cavity mainly to left of median plane and pyloric part is on the right. The lesser curvature is related to pancreas and visceral surface is in contact on left with spleen and coiled ascending colon and on right with jejunum.

Fowl: The stomach consists of two parts ***i.e cranial glandular compartment or proventriculus and a caudal muscular compartment or gizzard.*** Between the two compartments is the intermediate zone which is marked by a constriction called ***isthmus*** **(Fig.5.23).** The ***proventriculus*** *(**glandular stomach**)* is an elongated fusiform thin walled tubular organ ***related to liver on the lateral*** *and* ***ventral aspects and spleen on its superoposterior aspect.*** It is ***connected infront with oesophagus and behind with gizzard*** **(Fig.5.23).**

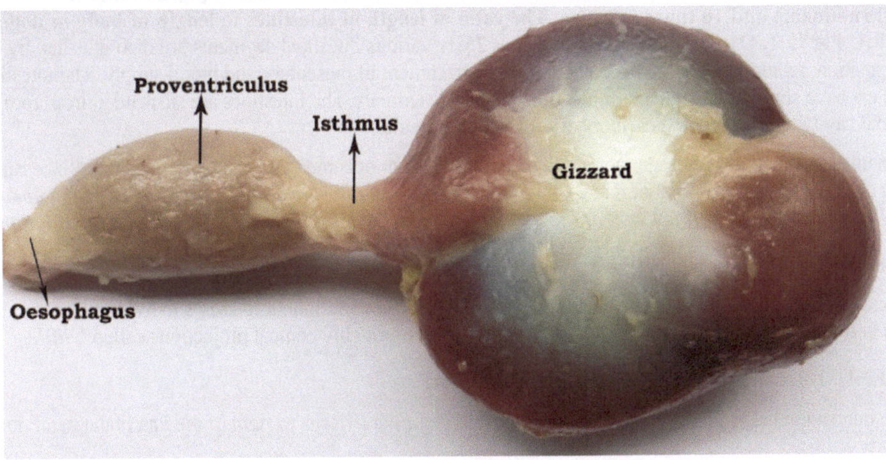

Fig. 5.23: Stomach of Fowl

The ***gizzard (muscular stomach)***: is a thick walled ***muscular disc*** like organ situated behind and partly *between the two lobes of the liver*. It is made up of ***smooth muscles rich in myoglobin.*** These are dark coloured ***caudodorsal and cranioventral thick muscles*** and the ***light coloured craniodorsal and caudoventral thin muscles***. The muscles attach to the ***right and left tendinous centers in the lateral wall of the gizzard*** **(Fig.5.24).** Because the muscles are asymmetrically arranged, rotator as well as crushing movements are set up when the gizzard contracts. The inner surface of the ***gizzard is lined by a hardened membrane, the cuticle called the "Koilin" layer***, which is carbohydrate-protien complex secreted by the gizzard. It shows two orifices on its **antero-dorsal aspect one each for proventriculus and duodenum.**

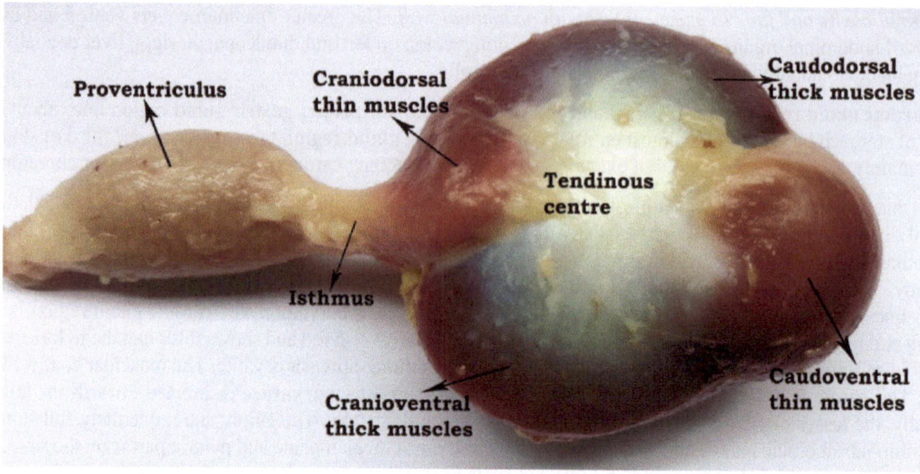

Fig. 5.24: Muscles of Gizard of Fowl

INTESTINE

It extends from pylorus to anus. It is divided into two parts i.e. small intestine and large intestine. ***The proximal part because of its relatively small lumen is called small intestine and because of wider lumen distal part is called as the large intestine.*** The total length of intestine and its segments differ with species, breed and animal to animal. **The length is generally 5 times to the body length in dog, 15 times in pig, 20 times in ox, 25 times in small ruminants and 10 times in horse. The ratio of length of intestines to length of body in dog is 5:1, horse 10:1, Pig 15:1, Ox 20:1 and sheep and goat 25:1.** Various intestinal segments are distinguished by shape, length, position, relations with other organs, mode of attachment of mesentery and blood supply. The intestines of dog and cat have simple arrangement unlike other domestic animals. The intestines are suspended from roof of the abdominal cavity by a common mesentery, **a fold of peritoneum**.

In ruminants intestinal mass fills supraomental recess to the right of rumen and caudal to omasum. Since ruminant stomach occupies greater part of abdominal cavity ***intestines are confined to a small part of right half of abdominal cavity. The large stomach fills left half of the abdominal cavity and displaces intestines entirely to the right.***

SMALL INTESTINE

Small intestine begins at the pylorus and terminates at the caecocolic junction. It is subdivided into duodenum, jejunum and ileum. The mucosa is velvety in appearance due to roughly conical projections called ***'villi'.***

DUODENUM

Ox: The duodenum is the first part of small intestine and begins at pylorus to right of median plane in all domestic animals.

The duodenum begins at the pylorus close to the ends of the ninth to eleventh ribs and two flexures divide the duodenum into three parts. The ***first (cranial) part*** extends to right cranially from pylorus along visceral surface of liver near portal fissure and forms the **"S" shaped curve, sigmoid loop** (***ansa sigmoidea / cranial flexure***). The **bile duct opens into second bend of "S" shaped curve, while the pancreatic duct opens into the duodenum about 30 cm further back (Fig.5.25).**

The first part is attached to liver by means of hepatoduodenal ligament. The ***second (descending) part*** passes caudally from cranial flexure towards right kidney on the right face of root of mesentery and forms the iliac (caudal) flexure near tuber coxae. Caudal to right kidney it turns to left and cranially and is attached medially to coils of colon. The ***third (ascending) part*** passes cranially high in common mesentery ventral to pancreas on the left face of root of mesentery in the vicinity of left kidney and continues as the jejunum by turning ventrally at duodenojejunal flexure. At the duodenojejunal flexure the duodenum is attached to the descending colon by duodenocolic fold. The mesoduodenum is short.

b) JEJUNUM: is the longest part of the small intestine.It begins at the duodenojejunal flexure at the cranial end of the duodenocolic fold. The mesentery is long and allows great range of movement of jejunum. The disc shaped ascending colon is sagittally placed and surrounded on the ventral, cranial and caudal aspects by tightly coiled jejunum.The coils of jejunum are arranged very closely ***forming a festoon (garland like)*** at the free edge of mesentery surrounding spiral loop of ascending colon **(Fig.5.25).** The cranial loops lie deep within supraomental recess and are related to liver, pancreas, omasum, abomasum and rumen through the deep wall of greater omentum. Ventrally the coils are related through greater omentum to abdominal floor. The caudal coils usually project from the supraomental recess.The ***mesenteric lymph glands*** are located along the visceral border of mesentery.

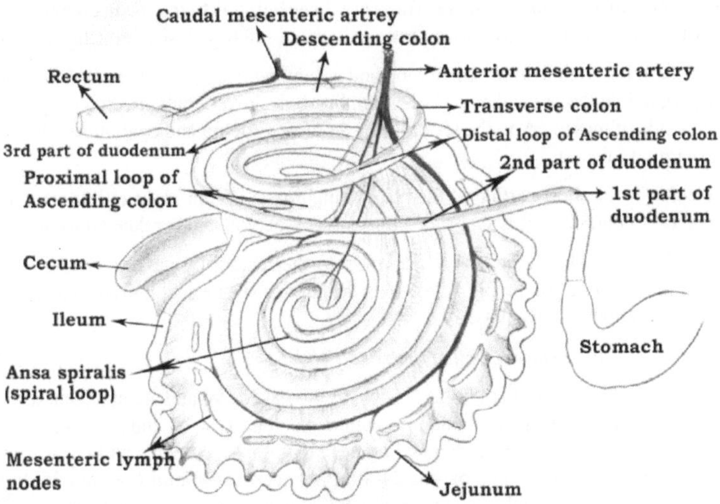

Fig. 5.25: Intestine of Ox

c) ILEUM: is the shortest straight and terminal segment of the small intestine and connects it to large intestine passing cranially ventral to caecum.It enters large intestine on ventromedial surface of caecocolic junction forming ileal orifice **(Fig.5.25).** It is *suspended by mesoileum.* The ileocaecal fold is present between antimesenteric border of ileum and caecum. The ileal orifice is at the level of fourth lumbar vertebra. ***Peyer's patches occur on antimesenteric wall*** and are visible on mucosal surface as irregularly raised plaques or bands.

LARGE INTESTINE

The large intestine extends from the termination of ileum to the anus and consists of caecum, colon and rectum. It is only slightly wider than small intestine with the exception of caecum and proximal part of colon.

CECUM: It is the initial blind part or great cul-de-sac of large intestine and joined to colon at ileal orifice. It is slightly **S-shaped and lies on right side of abdominal cavity (Fig.5.25).** The base lies high in right flank. It has greatest diameter among different parts of intestine. It extends caudally from ileocolic junction. **It consists of base, body and an apex.** The initial portion which joins the colon is the base, while the apex is the free blind end protruding from supraomental recess and **lies at the pelvic inlet.**

COLON: The colon shows three parts ***i.e ascending, transverse and descending parts*** and continues cranially from caecum. Its diameter is at first the same as that of caecum but soon diminishes.

a. **Ascending colon** is the **longest of the colic segments** and is divided into i) **proximal, ii) spiral and iii) distal loops.**

i) **The proximal loop** (**s-shaped curve**) consists of three parts. The **first part** of proximal loop runs cranially from caecocolic junction and doubles back on itself dorsolaterally ventral to right kidney at about the level of 12th rib as **second part** which passes caudally along the right abdominal wall separated from it by greater omentum, parallel and ventral to descending duodenum and doubles on itself once more but mediodorsally and continues as third part. The **third part** of proximal loop lies on left face of mesentery and related to ascending duodenum and descending colon and left kidney.

ii) **The spiral loop** is arranged in the form of an elliptical flat disc shaped loop and consists of **1.5-2.0 centripetal turns** towards centre of coil, central flexure where it reverses direction and **1.5-2.0 centrifugal turns** towards the periphery of the coil. Centripetal turns equal the number of centrifugal turns **(Fig.5.25).** The coils are best appreciated from left side of mesentery. The last centrifugal turn is followed by distal loop at the level of 1st lumbar vertebra. There are **3 centrifugal turns in sheep and 4 in goat** and distal half of last centrifugal turn spirals away from coil and continues close to attachment of jejunal coil.

iii) **The distal loop** lies medial to proximal loop and ascending duodenum and consists of an upper caudally directed part, a tight flexure at the level of 5th lumbar and a lower cranially directed part. The latter passes along right side of mesentery to the level of 13th thoracic vertebra and continues as transverse colon after turning sharply to the left.

b. **Transverse colon** is the short portion of the colon which passes **from right to left cranial to the anterior mesenteric artery (Fig.5.25).** It is suspended by short mesocolon and is related dorsally to pancreas.

c. **Descending colon**: It connects the transverse colon to the rectum by passing caudally on left and shows sigmoid curve near pelvic inlet. **(Fig.5.25).** It is suspended by mesocolon and passes caudally in close proximity to roof of abdominal cavity.

Rectum and Anus: *Described in Unit -6 i.e Hind limb and Pelvis.*

Lymphoid Tissue of Gut: The solitary nodules are visible to the naked eye and are abundant throughout the small intestine **(Figs.5.26, 5.27)**, but occasionally found in cecum and colon of the ox and are absent in cecum and colon of small ruminants. The patches of aggregate lymph nodules are upto 2.0 cm wide and reach a length of 25 cm in ox and of 15 cm in the sheep and goat. **The ox has 24-40, the sheep 18-40 and the goat 25-30 lymph nodules.** The most distal patch of aggregate nodules extends through the ileal opening a short distance into the cecum. It is composed of large follicles, many with very distinct fossulae, which render the surface of the patch uneven and pitted. A similar patch is regularly observed at the distal end of the proximal loop of the ascending colon. It is 7-20 cm long in ox and 4-20 cm long in the small ruminants. No other patches of aggregate nodules are present in the colon of ruminants.

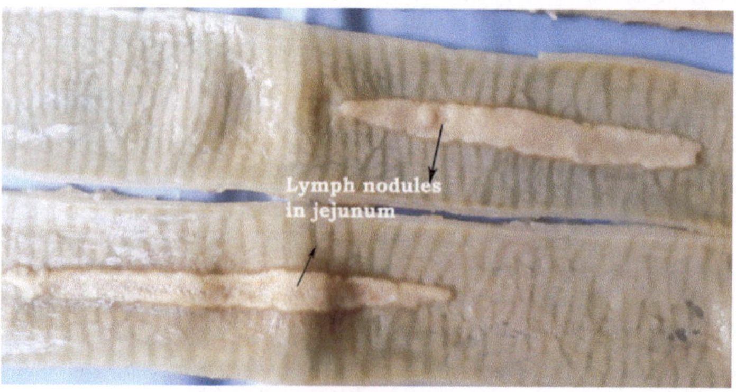

Fig. 5.26: Lymph Nodules in Jejunum of Ox

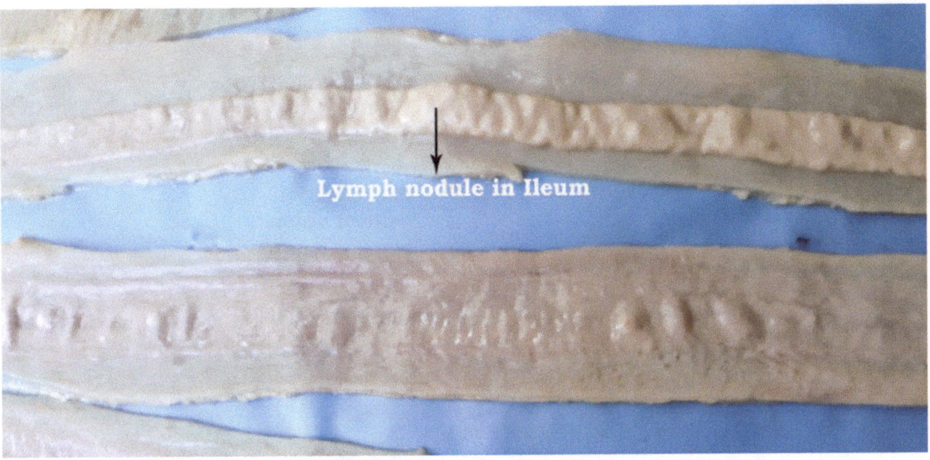

Fig. 5.27: Lymph Nodules in Ileum of Ox

HORSE

Duodenum: The duodenum gives **horse shoe like** appearance. The cranial part of the duodenum presents sigmoid loop and shows a dilatation called ***duodenal ampulla or diverticulum duodeni.*** It is located 12 to 15 cms from the pylorus in which there is **major duodenal papilla on which bile duct and major pancreatic duct open**. The **minor duodenal papilla located opposite to diverticulum duodeni** is a projection on which minor pancreatic duct opens.

Jejunum: The jejunum mingles with large coils of descending colon. The mesojejunum is extensive allowing more mobility of coils. The mesenteric lymph glands are located at the root of mesentery. Due to great length of mesentery loops of jejunum are not confined to particular area of abdominal cavity though they are **found mostly in left dorsal quadrant**.

Ileum: The ileum joins the caecum of large intestine. The ileal orifice is in the center of the papilla ilealis. The ileocaecal fold attaches dorsal band of caecum with antimesenteric border of ileum.

Large intestine: The large intestine of horse is characterized by the **longitudinal muscular bands** (*Taeniae*) and **sacculations** (***Haustra***). The former is due to thickening of outer longitudinal muscle layer of tunica muscularis, while the latter is due to thickening or constriction of the inner circular muscle layer of tunica muscularis.

Cecum: The large caecum and ascending colon are chambers for bacterial fermentation of cellulose. The caecum is very large, comma shaped and lies on right side of abdominal cavity and is **sacculated (4 rows of sacculations) by four *longitudinal bands of smooth muscles* (*ventral, dorsal, medial and lateral*) *viz., taenia* (Fig.5.28).** It occupies large part of **right half of abdominal cavity.** It presents a base, body and an apex. The **base is bulbous**, most dorsal part, strongly curved and shows greater curvature dorsally and lesser curvature ventrally and lies in the right paralumbar fossa. **The base extends from pelvic inlet lying against paralumbar fossa to fifteenth rib.**

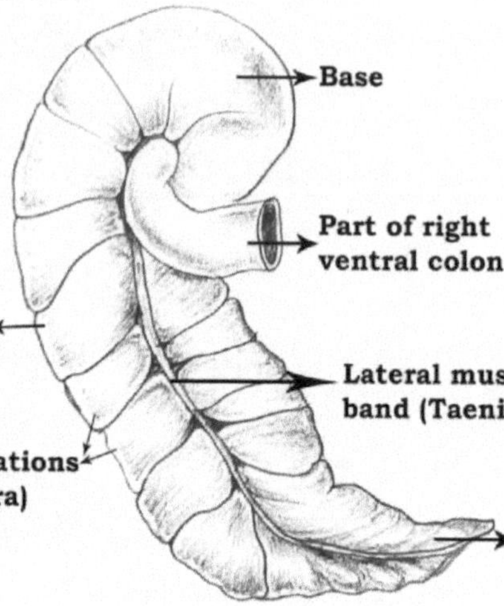

Fig. 5.28: Cecum of Horse

The **body** which tapers to apex lies against abdominal floor and has 4 longitudinal muscular bands one each on dorsal, ventral, lateral and medial surfaces. Between adjacent saccules of caecum and colon semilunar folds project into the interior of gut and increase internal surface area. The **apex** lies 20 cm caudal to xiphoid cartilage. The caecocolic fold attaches lateral band of caecum with right ventral colon. The lesser curvature of base of caecum shows ileal opening and distal and caudolateral to it is caecocolic opening near center of circle described by greater curvature of base of caecum.

Colon: Like caecum the colon is also sacculated and shows longitudinal muscular bands (***taenia***). The ***ascending colon is also called great colon*** **because of its large size** It extends from caeco-colic orifice to transverse colon **(Fig.5.29).** The beginning and the end of the ascending colon are to the right of the root of the mesentery. It is doubled on itself twice and hence consists of two parallel parts arranged in large **horse shoe shaped loop** occupying ventral half of abdominal cavity. These loops are open caudally and lie in dorsal planes one on top of the other and consist of the following parts.

Part	**Number of Taenia (Muscular bands)**
Right ventral colon	4 (2 dorsal 2 ventral)
Sternal flexure (lies in xiphoid region)	4
Left ventral colon	4 (2 dorsal and 2 ventral)
Pelvic flexure (lies near pelvic inlet)	1
Left dorsal colon	1 at the beginning, latter 3
Diaphragmatic flexure (lies near diaphragm)	3
Right dorsal colon	3 (2 dorsal and 1 ventral)

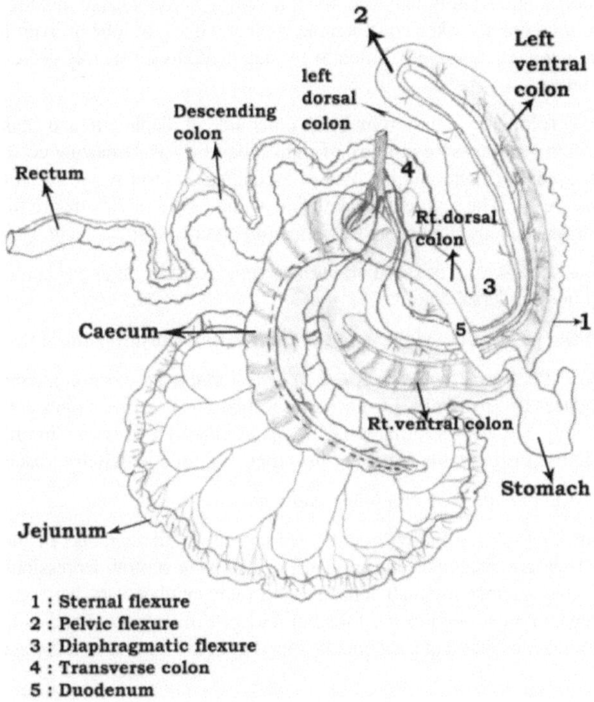

Fig. 5.29: Intestine of Horse

The **first part, right ventral colon** runs cranially from cecum and ends at sternal flexure. The **second part, the left ventral colon** passes caudally from sternal flexure on the left side of abdomen and doubles back on itself in front of the pelvic inlet forming pelvic flexure. The **third part, the left dorsal colon** passes cranially dorsal to the left ventral colon to the diaphragmatic flexure continuing on right as the short but very wide **fourth part, the right dorsal colon (Fig.5.30).**

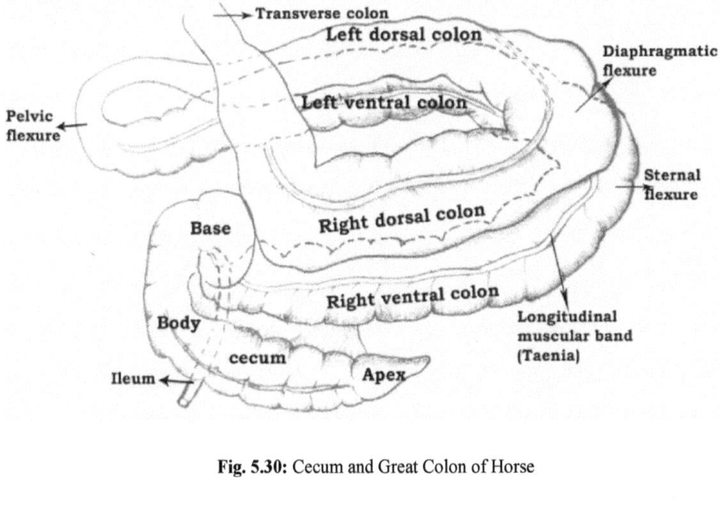

Fig. 5.30: Cecum and Great Colon of Horse

The **left dorsal colon** is dorsal and slightly lateral to the left ventral colon. Diaphragmatic flexure is craniodorsal to sternal flexure. **Right dorsal colon** makes considerable contact with right lobe of liver. It has greatest diameter among four parts. It is continuous as transeverse colon by turning medially by sharply decreasing in diameter **at the level of 18th thoracic vertebra.**

When distended right dorsal colon may press on lungs on other side of diaphragm and cause respiratory difficulty and chronic distension resulting in pressure atrophy of right lobe of liver. At narrow cecocolic orifice and initial portion of ascending colon, pelvic flexure and junction of ascending and transverse colon flow of ingesta may be impeded and impaction may result. The segments on left side including pelvic flexure are free and are supported by ventral abdominal wall only. Hence these parts are subjected to volvulus /displacement.

Right and left ventral colons show 4 rows of sacculations between 4 bands. Left dorsal colon shows no sacculations while they are not distinct in right dorsal colon.

Transverse colon is short and passes from **right to left cranial to anterior mesenteric artery.**

Descending colon is also called ***small colon because of small diameter*** when compared to great colon. It is deeply sacculated and produces two rows of semispherical sacculations in which faeces are divided into balls. The descending mesocolon is long and allows formation of loops of small colon with wide range of movement **like jejunum but should be distinguished from latter by presence of taenia which are absent in jejunum.**

Rectum and Anus: *Described in Unit -6 i.e Hind limb and Pelvis.*

Lymphoid Tissue of Gut: The solitary lymph nodules are present in all segments of the intestines, varying in number and distribution. They are about 1-2 mm in diameter and have central depressions. Patches of aggregate lymph nodules occur in large number in small intestine and their number vary between 100-200. In the large intestine, patches of aggregate lymph nodules are found at the apex of the cecum and in the pelvic flexure of the great colon. The prominent patches found at the ileocolic junction in the ruminants and pig are absent in the horse.

DOG

Duodenum: The **major duodenal papilla lies about 5 to 8 cm** from the pylorus on which bile duct and minor pancreatic duct open. The major pancreatic duct opens 2.5 cm further back. The descending deodenum is not covered by greater omentum and lies directly against the right dorsolateral abdominal wall. Mesoduodenum of descending duodenum encloses right lobe of pancreas.

Jejunum: The mesentery is long. The jejunum consists of about **six to eight large loops (Fig.5.31).** The mass of jejunal loops occupies the ventral part of abdominal cavity covered by greater omentum and lies against lateral and ventral abdominal walls. The rest of the intestine is crowded against roof of abdominal cavity.

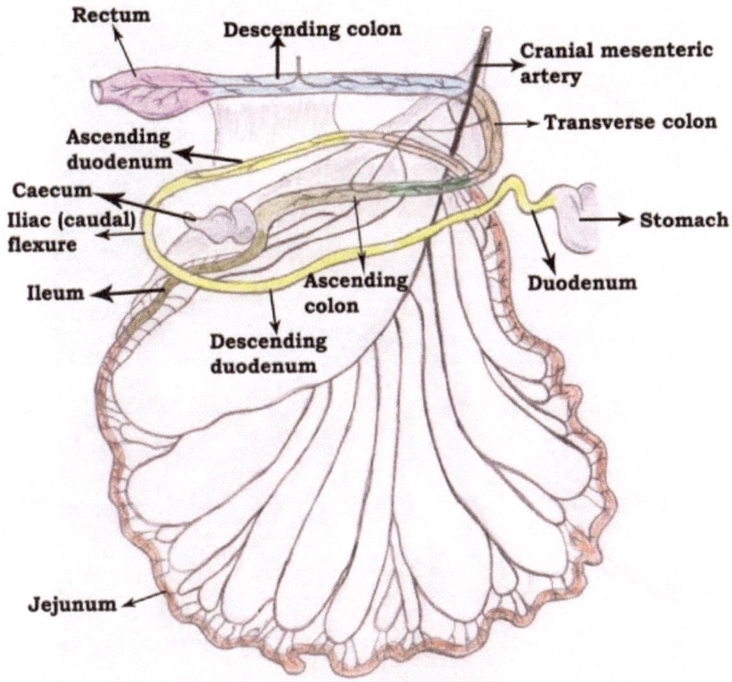

Fig. 5.31: Intestine of Dog

Ileum: opens into proximal end of ascending colon, the orifice being surrounded by a ring like mucosal fold.

Cecum: It is irregularly twisted and its blind end is bent and often pointed cranially. It opens into colon by caecocolic orifice **(Fig.5.31).**

Colon: The colon is short and consists of three clear parts ascending, transverse and descending colon. The colon first passes cranially on the right side of abdominal cavity as ascending colon turns to left from right and crosses medial plane cranial to anterior mesenteric artery as transverse colon and then posterior-caudally on the left side as the descending colon. The **descending colon**, the **longest part of three** follows a straight course before it joins rectum **(Fig.5.31).** The colon shows a loop open caudally, while in case of duodenum the loop is open cranially.

Rectum and Anus: *Described in Unit -6 i.e Hind limb and Pelvis.*

Lymphoid Tissue of Gut: The solitary nodules are present throughout the small intestine, but they are rarely noticed with naked eye because mostly they are submucosal. In the colon they are visible as small whitish gray nodules. Patches of aggregate lymph nodules about 20-25 are present in dog throughout the small intestine in the wall opposite mesenteric attachment. They are round, oval or elongated with a pitted or nodular surface and are raised above the mucosa **(Fig.5.32).**

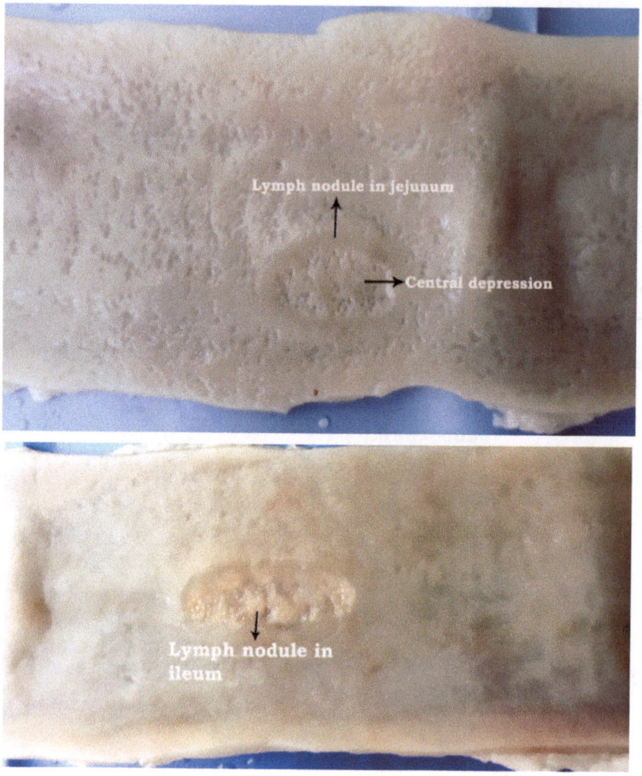

Fig. 5.32: Lymph Nodules in Jejunum and Ileum of Dog

PIG

Duodenum: The cranial part of duodenum presents sigmoid loop. The pancreatic duct opens into duodenum 12-20 cm distal to that of bile duct.

Jejunum: The jejunum is found mainly in ventral part of right half of abdominal cavity but may extend along floor into left half and lies ventral to coiled ascending colon and caecum.

Ileum: The **Peyer's patches measure upto 3.5 m long.** Numerous deep irregular depressions give the mucosal surface an unevenly pitted appearance.

Cecum: It lies on the left side of abdominal cavity and shows ***sacculated*** appearance (**three rows of sacculatations**) and **shows 3 bands** (***lateral, medial and ventral)***. It is cylindrical and is along left abdominal wall with apex in inguinal region.

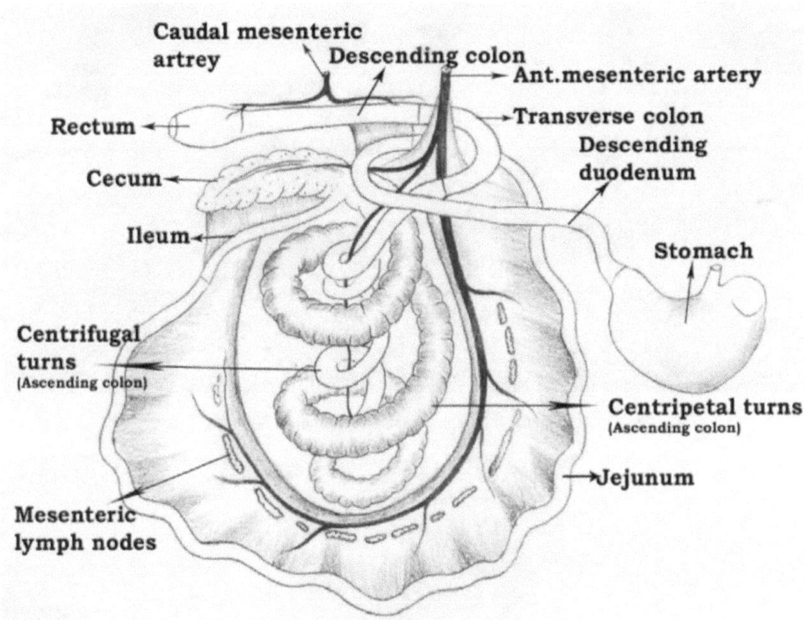

Fig. 5.33: Intestine of Pig

Colon: The ascending colon forms a cone shaped coil. The ascending colon shows centripetal turns, central flexure and centrifugal turns. The **ansa spiralis** is between caecum and transverse colon and its turns are piled up to form a thick cone. There are no proximal and distal loops. The ascending colon shows sacculated appearance and shows bands, while **there are no bands in descending colon (Fig. 5.33).**

The ileal orifice is at the summit of papilla ilealis which is bent slightly toward the caecum.The papilla is connected to wall of colon by mucosal folds. Ascending colon is greatly enlarged and forms conical mass of **spiral coils forming apex, centripetal turns (*spiralling towards the centre of coil i.e clockwise*), central flexure and centrifugal turns** (*towards the periphery of the coil i.e counter clockwise*). At central flexure colon reverses direction from centripetal to centrifugal course (**Fig. 5.33).**

Rectum and Anus: *Described in Unit -6 i.e Hind limb and Pelvis.*

Lymphoid Tissue of Gut: Both solitary and aggregate nodules are present in large number in small intestine. The solitary nodules are whitish and have a diameter of 1-2 mm. The patches of aggregate lymph nodules are found mostly in the small intestine, which are 20-30 averaging about 10 cm in length (**Fig.5.34**). Numerous deep irregular depressions give their surface an unevenly pitted appearance.The most distal patch has the extraordinary length of 1.5 to 3.2 m (**Fig.5.35**). It extends along the entire ileum including papilla ilealis. No patches are present in cecum and colon, but occasionally small patches are found in ascending colon.

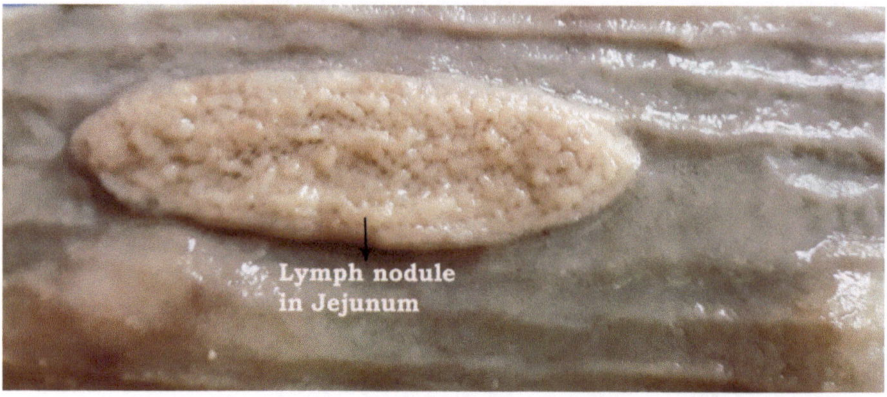

Fig. 5.34: Lymph Nodule in Jejunum of Pig

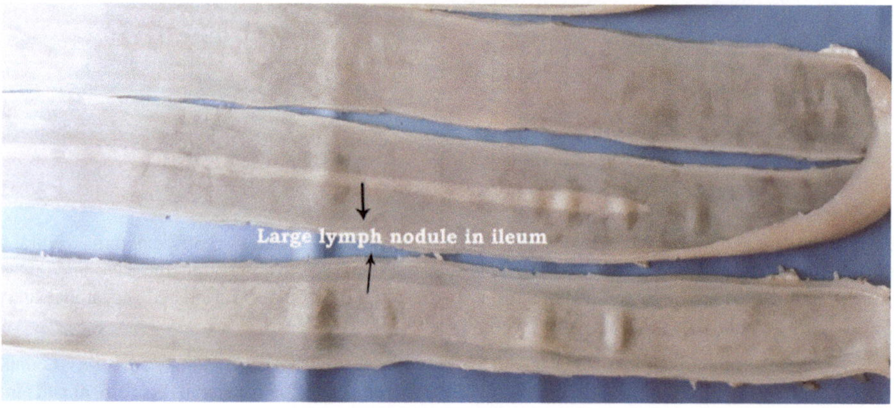

Fig. 5.35: Lymph Nodules in Ileum of Pig

FOWL

Duodenum: The duodenum is in the form of a loop with closely related descending (proximal) and ascending (distal) parts with the pancreas wedged between them. The **two bile ducts and two or three pancreatic ducts** empty near each other at the termination of duodenum.

Jejunum and ileum: The duodenum is continued as jejunoileum coiled between abdominal air sacs. ***Meckel's diverticulum*** is a rudimentary structure a **remnant of yolk stalk** and sac is found on the convexity of the jejunum usually at the beginning of distal half of the jejunum. It is about **12.5 cm long and 0.5 cm in diameter**.

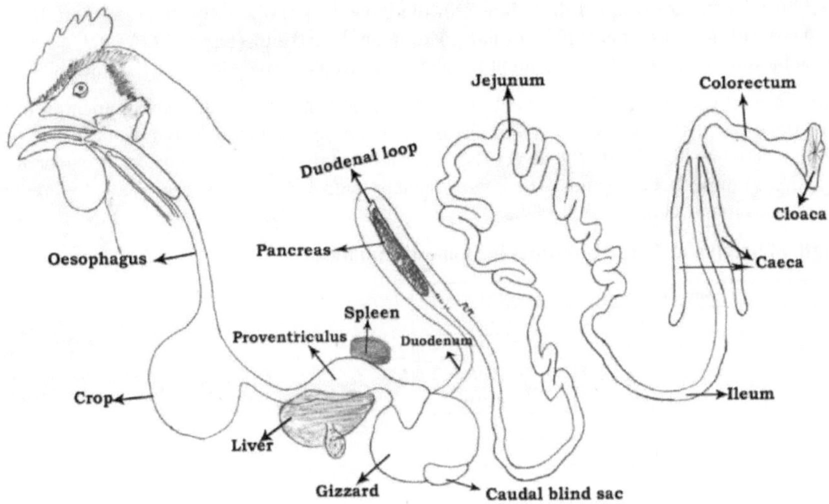

Fig. 5.36: Digestive System of Fowl

Cecum and colon: A pair of blind ended caeca about 7 inches long run cranially parallel to ileum. They open into the intestines at the junction of the ileum and colorectum. The **colon / colorectum** extend from ileum and opens into coprodeum of cloaca (**Fig.5.36**).

Cloaca: is a common passage to the digestive and urogenital systems and opens to the exterior at the vent. Colon, ureters and deferent ducts in male and left oviduct in female enter into it at various levels. The **cloaca is divided sequentially in to coprodeum, urodeum and proctodeum** by two or more or less complete annular folds (**Fig.5.37**).

Coprodeum: is the ***continuation of the colon in which feces are stored***. It is bounded caudally by the coprourodeal fold which may be stretched by the pressure of the feces so that its central opening is everted through the vent (**Fig.5.37**).

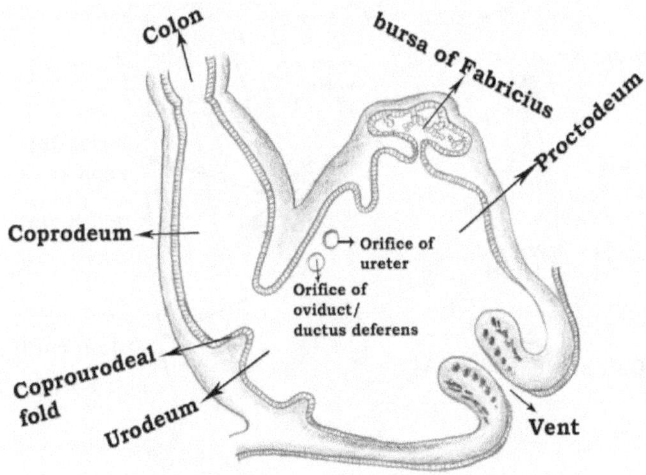

Fig. 5.37: Different Parts of Cloaca of Fowl

Urodeum: The **ureteric orifice is in the dorsolateral wall above the papilla of the deferent duct**. In the **female, the slit like opening of the oviduct occupies similar position on the left side (Fig. 5.37).** A small patch of vascular tissue in the lateral wall of the urodeum is thought to supply the lymph for the tumescence of the phallus.

Proctodeum: is a short and most caudal segment of the cloaca, ending at the vent. **A small opening in its dorsal wall leads to the cloacal bursa (Bursa of Fabricius).** It is an accumulation of lymphatic tissue performing immunological functions **(Fig. 5.37)**. ***Bursa*** consists of a lobulated wall surrounding an irregular lumen. The lobules are similar to those of the thymus. The bursa gradually regresses from the age of two to three months. A small nodule remains in the adult.

Average length of Small and Large Intestines in Domestic animals

Species	Small intestine	Large intestine
Ox	25.0-40.0 m	11.0 -11.5 m
Sheep and goat.	20.0-25.0 m	4.0-6.5 m
Horse	19.0-22.0 m	7.5 - 8.0 m
Dog	2.0-4.0 m	0.3-0.9 m
Pig	15.0-20.0 m	4.0-4.5 m
Fowl	22.0-35.0 cm	85.0-120.0cm

LIVER

Ox: Liver is the largest gland in the body. It is situated entirely in the **right half of abdominal cavity** (except for a small portion) from lumbocostal angle to ventral end of 7th or 8th rib obliquely downwards and forwards (**Fig.5.38**). **Percussion of liver in ox** is limited to **last four intercostal spaces caudoventral to lung**. In well nourished & young animals, it is light brown and dark reddish brown in emaciated and older animals. Its average weight is 4.5 -5.5 kg.

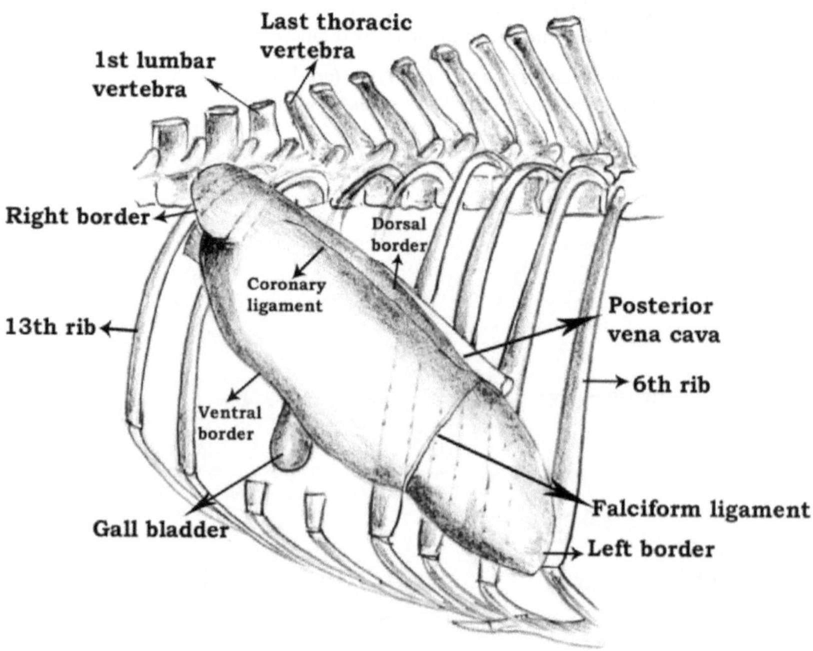

Fig. 5.38: Orientation of Liver in Ox

It presents two surfaces and four borders. The **diaphragmatic (parietal) surface** is convex and applied against the diaphragm, last two ribs and lumbo costal angle. The **visceral surface** is concave and very irregular. It is **related to the reticulum, omasum, abomasum duodenum, pancreas and gall bladder**. Among these reticulum, omasum, abomasums and gall bladder leave distinct impressions *i.e. reticular, omasal, abomasal and cystic impressions* respectively. The ***portal fissure*** is the area where the portal vein and hepatic artery enter the liver and bile duct leaves the liver (**Fig. 5.39**).

The **right border** presents renal impression formed by caudate process and right lobe for right kidney and right adrenal. The **dorsal border** lodges posterior vena cava and presents oesophageal notch below its middle. The **ventral border** is thin and presents gall bladder and the **umbilical notch for round ligament** (**Fig.5.39**). The left border is thin and convex.

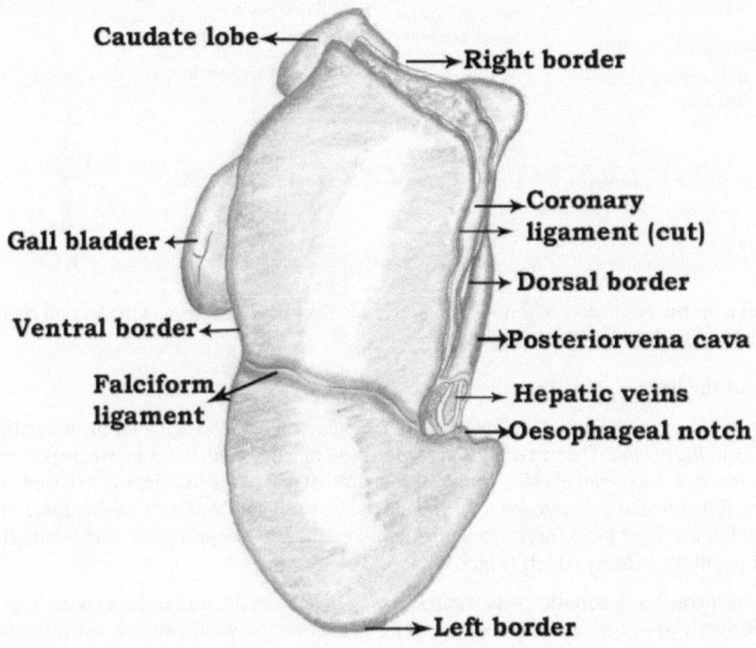

Fig. 5.39: Liver of Ox (Parietal Surface)

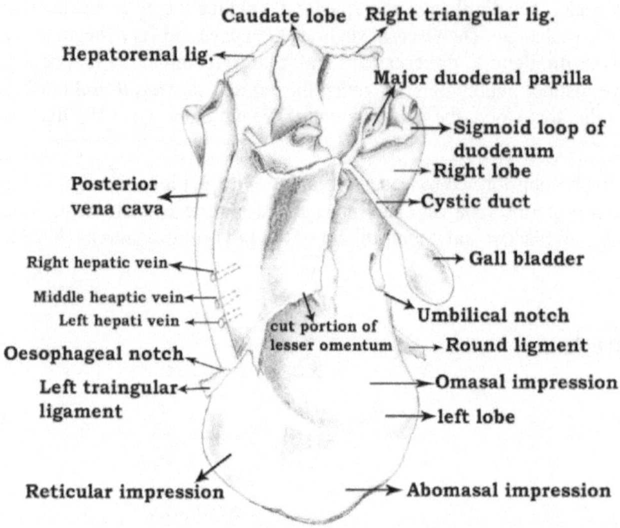

Fig. 5.40: Liver of Ox (Visceral surface)

The **hepatic duct** joins the cystic duct to form the common bile duct which opens into the second bend of S-shaped loop of duodenum about 50-70 cm distal to pylorus.

Different lobes of the liver

Left lobe: The part of liver to the left of the line from the oesophageal notch to notch for the round ligament and it is ventral in position. ***Right lobe***: The part of the liver to the right of a line from the point where posterior vena cava crosses dorsal border to fossa of gall bladder. ***Quadrate lobe***: is that part of the liver between the left and right lobes ventral to the portal fissure and between notch for round ligament and gall bladder. ***Caudate lobe*:** The part of the liver between the left and right lobes, dorsal to the portal fissure. It ***has two processes***, **large caudate process on right and small papillary process on left (Fig.5.40).**

Hepatic veins: The **three large hepatic veins** (***vena hepatica dextra, media and sinistra***) open in to the posterior vena cava just before it passes through the foramen vena cava. They lie within the parenchyma of the liver and their openings into the vena cava are best seen from the lumen of posterior vena cava. They receive blood after detoxification from the liver carried to it by the portal vein and hepatic artery. The ***right hepatic vein*** draining right lobe and caudate lobes joins the vena cava between the right and caudate lobes. The ***middle hepatic vein*** joins the vena cava close to the left hepatic vein. The ***left hepatic vein draining*** left lobe joins the vena cava near the oesophageal notch (**Fig.5.40**).

Ligaments of liver: ***Right triangular (lateral) ligament***: attaches the right border of liver to the dorsolateral abdominal wall. ***Left triangular (lateral) ligament***: attaches the liver to the diaphragm in the region of oesophageal hiatus. ***Caudate ligament (Hepatorenal ligment)*:** attaches the caudate lobe to the right kidney. ***Falciform ligament***: attaches the parietal surface of liver to the sternal part of diaphragm. ***Round ligament***: extends from umbilical notch to the umbilicus (**Fig.5.40**). ***Coronary Ligament***: extends from the right triangular ligament along the diaphragmatic surface of the liver to the right of the caudal vena cava and passes ventral to the vein before reaching the left triangular ligament at the oesophageal notch.

Lesser omentum is a peritoneal fold extending from the oesophageal notch to the portal fissure of liver and it passes over the parietal face of omasum to lesser curvature of abomasum.

Horse: Its average weight is **5.0 kg and in large breeds it weighs upto 10.0 kg.** The liver of horse extends from right parachondriac to the left parachondriac region in a sloping direction from right to left. It consists of **left, right, quadrate and caudate lobes.** The **left lobe** is subdivided into **left lateral and left medial lobes,** while the right lobe is undivided **(Fig.5.41).**

The quadrate lobe presents several notches on its border and is separated from right lobe by a deep notch. The **caudate lobe has only caudate process but no papillary process.** The **renal impression** is formed **by right lobe and caudate process.** The ***visceral surface shows gastric impression in front and duodenal and colic impressions behind the portal fissure*** (**Fig.5.41).** The **ventral border** presents two large notches and many small notches. The **gall bladder is absent.** The bile duct opens into the diverticulum duodeni 12-15 cm distal to the pylorus.

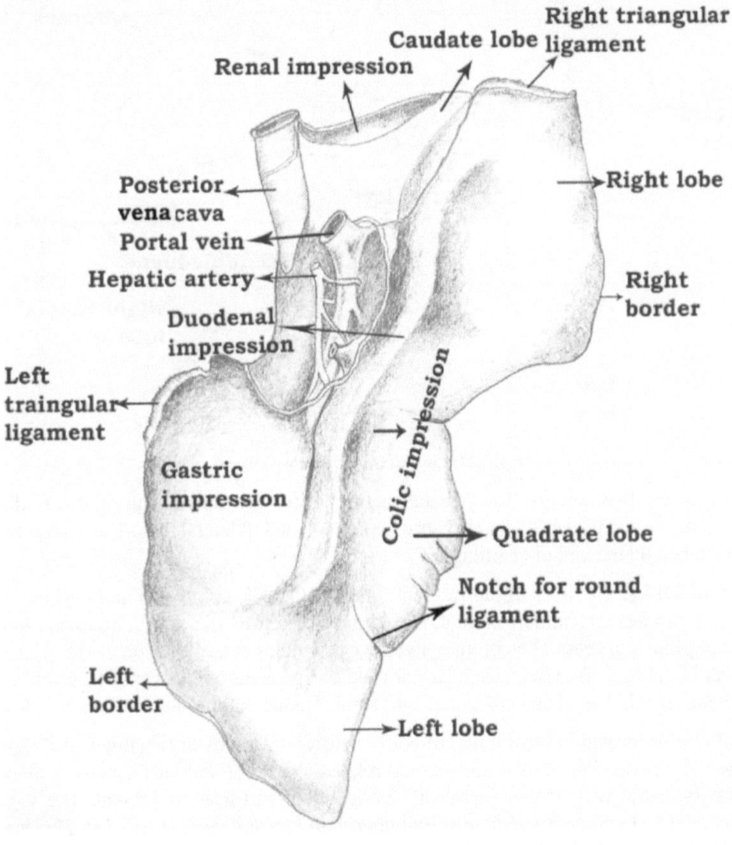

Fig. 5.41: Liver of Horse (Visceral surface)

The ***right triangular ligament*** attaches the right lobe to the dorsal abdominal wall and the ***left triangular ligament*** attaches the left lobe to the tendinous center of the diaphragm **(Fig.5.41)**, while two laminae of ***coronary ligament*** pass on either side of posterior venacava from right and left triangular ligaments to diaphragm. The laminae unite ventral to posterior venacava where falciform ligament begins.

Dog: It **weighs 3% of total body weight.** The liver of dog is divided into ***right lateral, right medial, left medial, left lateral, quadrate and caudate lobes*** (**Fig.5.42**) by deep notches which converge towards the root of liver. Between the two medial lobes and ventral to porta is quadrate lobe. **The deep renal impression for right kidney is formed by caudate process and right lateral lobe.** The caudate lobe is dorsal to porta and has caudate process on right and papillary process on left. The ***left medial lobe*** is prismatic, while the ***left lateral lobe is the largest lobe*** of liver and is oval in shape. The ***gall bladder lies in fossa between quadrate and right medial lobe*** (**Fig.5.42**).

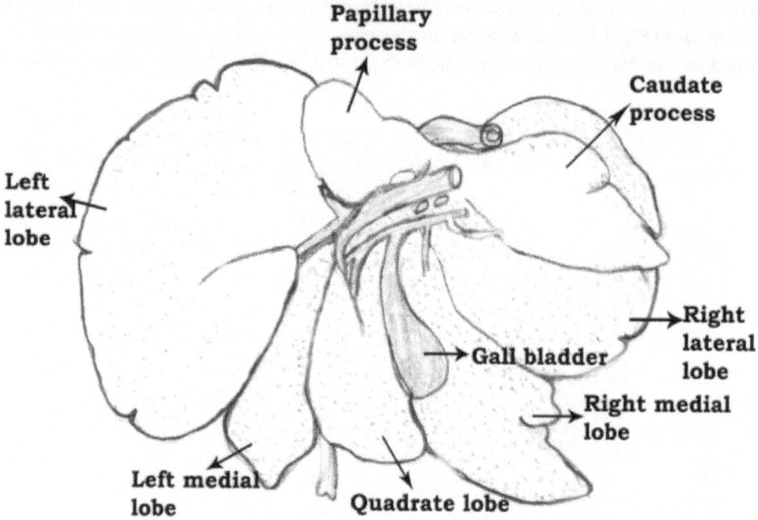

Fig. 5.42: Liver of Dog (Visceral surface)

It shows two surfaces and two borders. The parietal surface is strongly convex and related to diaphragm, while visceral surface is concave and presents a large gastric impression on left lateral lobe. The ventral border lies on the floor of the abdomen behind the xiphoid cartilage.

Pig: It **weighs 1.5 to 2.0 kg**. The liver of pig resembles that of the dog in lobation and position. It exhibits deep fissures that divide it into **left lateral, left medial, right lateral, right medial lobes, quadrate lobe and caudate lobe. There is no papillary process.**The coronary ligament resembles that of the horse. The falciform ligament is very short or absent in the adult. Neither triangular nor caudate ligaments are present. The caudate process fails to make contact with the right kidney. High content of interlobular tissue outlines minute liver lobules on the surface.

Fowl: The liver of fowl is located in ventral part of body cavity and consists of **two lobes, the right and left**. The ***right lobe is large***. The parietal surface is convex and related to ventral and lateral body walls. A deep cardiac impression on cranio-ventral part of this surface for pericardium and heart is present. The visceral surface is irregular and concave. ***The left lobe is subdivided into lateral and medial parts*** (**Fig.5.43**). *The impressions left by proventriculus and gizzard on the left lobe and spleen and small intestine on right lobe are present.*

The **bile ducts are two in number**. The hepatoenteric duct from left lobe of liver and cysticoenteric duct from gall bladder enter the intestine near the distal part of the ascending duodenum.

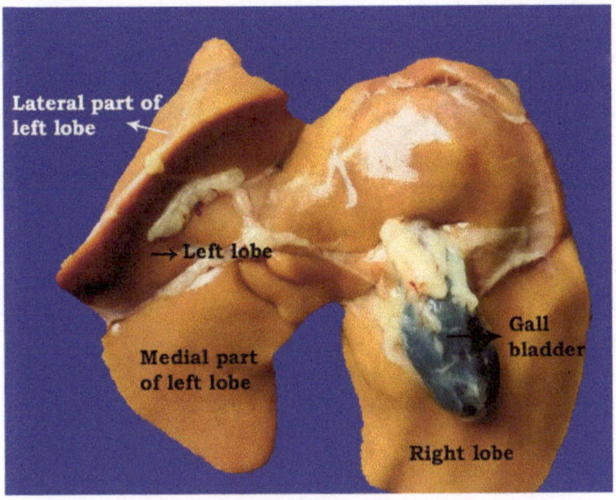

Fig. 5.43: Liver of Fowl

Average weight of Liver in various Domestic animals

Species	Average Weight
Ox	3.0-5.5 kg
Sheep and goat.	0.35 kg
Horse	2.5-5.5 kg
Dog	127gm-1.35 kg
Pig	1.5 to 2.0 kg
Fowl	50.0 -80.0 gm

GALL BLADDER

Ox: It is pear shaped and has **fundus, body and neck**. It lies on the visceral surface of liver and projects beyond ventral border of liver and contacts the abdominal wall at the ventral part of ***10th or 11th*** intercostal space. The cystic duct is continuation of the neck of the gall bladder.

Horse: The gall bladder is absent.

Dog: It lies in fossa between the **quadrate and right medial lobe**. It is visible on visceral as well as diaphragmatic surface of liver and is in contact with diaphragm.

Pig: It is in fossa between the quadrate and right medial lobes. Its fundus does not reach the ventral border of the liver. The **common bile duct opens on papilla duodeni about 2.5 to 5.0 cm from the pylorus.**

Fowl: It lies on the visceral surface of the right lobe of liver and is elongated.

PANCREAS

It is a lobulated gland resembling salivary glands in gross appearance.

Ox: It is a reddish cream and **irregularly quadrilateral** gland. It weighs about 350 gms. It consists of body and right and left lobes. The **body** is relatively small and lies against the cranial part of duodenum. The **right lobe** is long and extends from the body to the right along the descending duodenum, while the **left lobe** is wide and extends from the body to the left **(Figs. 5.44 & 5.45).**

It shows two (dorsal and ventral) surfaces, four borders and four angles. The **borders are right, left, posterior and anterior**. The **posterior border is irregular and presents a deep notch** (***insisura pancreaticus***) on body for portal vein. The angles are **anteromedial, antero-lateral** (***duodenal***), **posteromedial** and **posterolateral**. The **pancreatic duct is single** and leaves the gland at its posterolateral angle and **opens into duodenum about 30.0 cm distal to the opening of bile duct.**

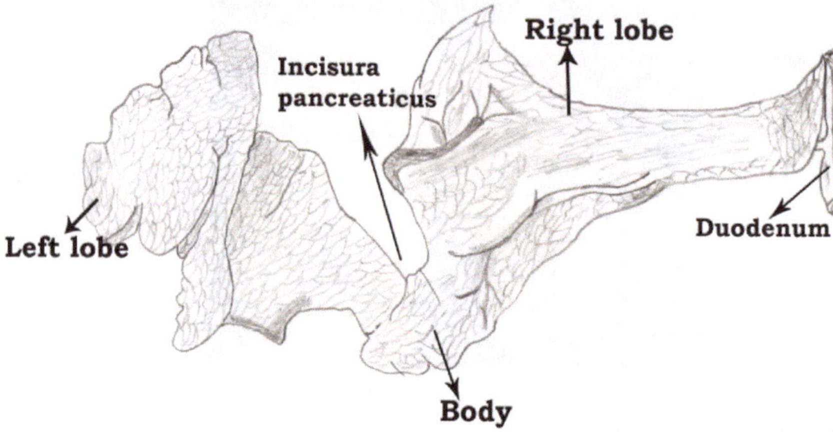

Fig. 5.44: Pancreas of Ox (Schematic)

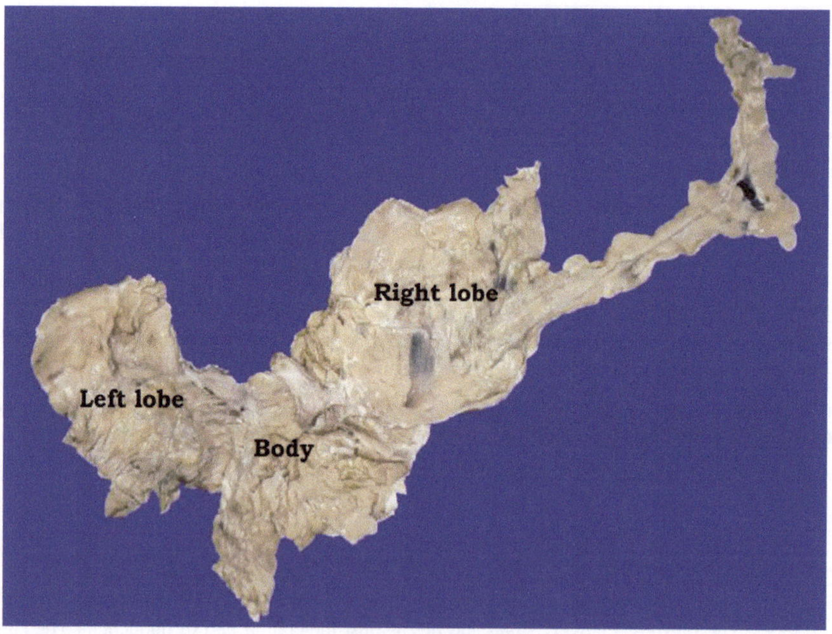

Fig. 5.45: Pancreas of Ox

Horse: It is ***triangular in outline***. It has a large body with perforation (***annulus pancreaticus***) a small right lobe and a long left lobe **(Fig. 5.46).** The ventral surface is related to the caecum, great colon and small colon. The angles are anterior (duodenal), left (splenic) and right. There are two pancreatic ducts. i.e. **major pancreatic duct and minor (*accessory*) pancreatic duct**. The **major pancreatic duct** opens along with the bile duct **into diverticulum duodeni** about 15 cm distal to the pylorus, while the **minor pancreatic duct opens into the duodenum on minor duodenal papilla opposite to the diverticulum duodeni.**

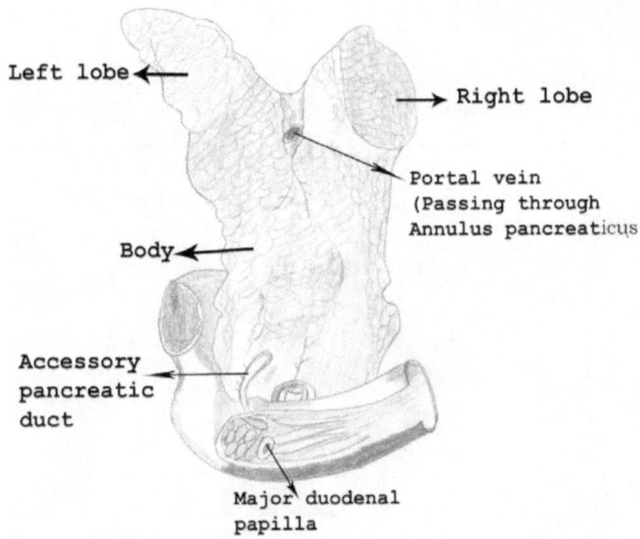

Fig. 5.46: Pancreas-Horse

Dog: It is ***'U' or 'V' shaped*** with a centrally placed body with pancreatic notch, right and left branches **(Figs. 5.47 and 5.48).** The pancreatic ducts are two, the minor duct unites with bile duct and opens into duodenum about 5 to 8 cm distal to the pylorus, while the major duct opens into duodenum a few centimetres distal to the opening of minor duct.

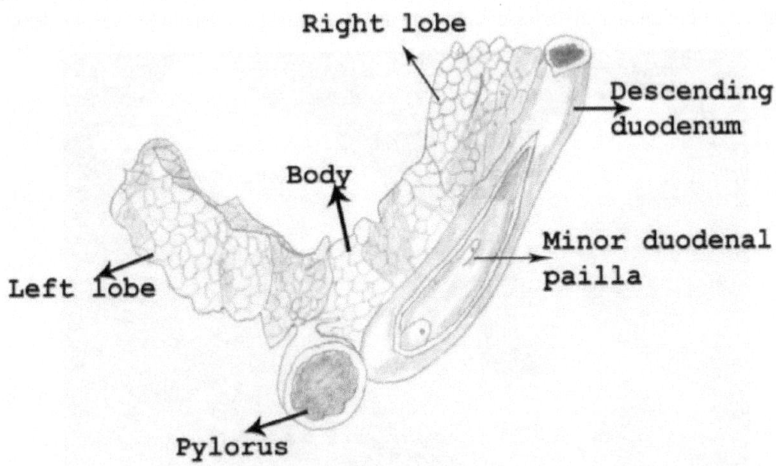

Fig. 5.47: Pancreas of Dog (Schematic)

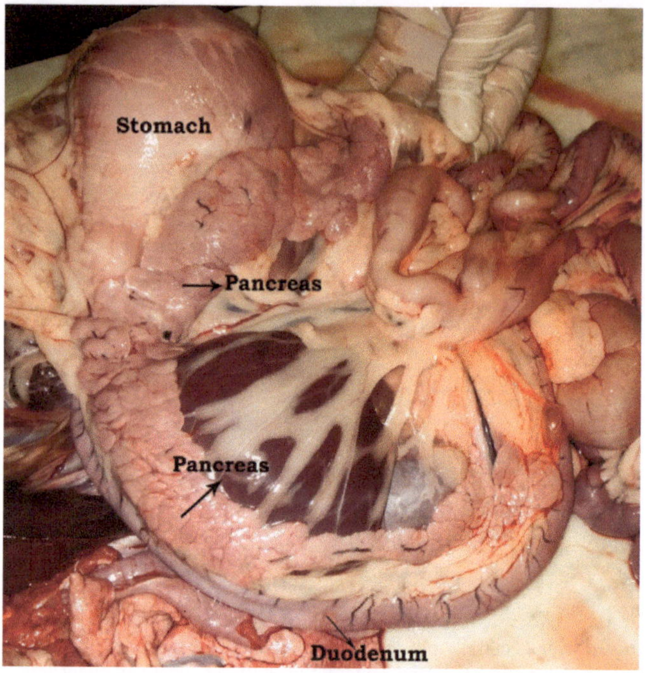

Fig. 5.48: Pancreas of Dog

Pig: It consists of a small right and large left lobes connected by centrally placed extensive body which forms a ring of tissue (**annulus pancreaticus**) for passage of portal vein **(Fig. 5.49).** Only accessory pancreatic duct is present which leaves right lobe of the gland. The body lies against lesser curvature of stomach and cranial part of duodenum. The ***left lobe*** is related to transverse colon and base of cone shaped ascending colon. The ***right lobe*** accompanies cranial part of duodenum in lesser omentum and descending duodenum in mesoduodenum.

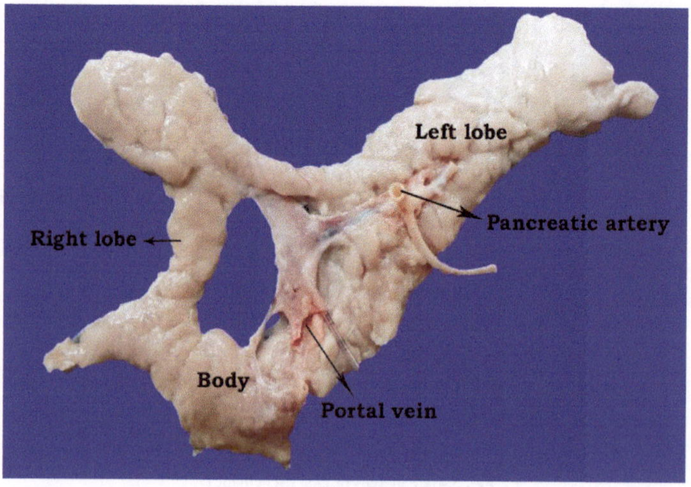

Fig. 5.49: Pancreas of Pig

Fowl: The pinkish, ribbon like **pancreas** of birds is situated between the two limbs of the duodenum and enclosed within the ***lig. pancreatico-duodenale***, a double serous lamella which connects the two intestinal segments. It shows dorsal, ventral and splenic lobes. The **splenic lobe** is very narrow strip running towards the spleen, which is particularly rich in islets of Langerhans. The dorsal and ventral lobes are connected by a parenchymal bridge of varying width. There are three efferent pancreatic ducts two of which arise from the ventral and one from dorsal lobe. All these ducts empty into the ascending limb of the duodenum.

SPLEEN

Ox: It is an elongated flat lymphoid organ related to dorsal sac of rumen. Its long axis is oblique extending from dorsal ends of last two ribs to the ventral end of **8th or 9th rib** about hands breadth above its sternal end. It is bluish red and purple and weighs approximately 900g. It is **elliptical and flattened.** It has two surfaces, two borders (anterior and posterior) and two rounded extremities i.e dorsal and ventral. The **ventral extremity** of spleen varies with state of contraction.The surface is marbled by prominent splenic corpuscles. **The hilus lies on the dorsal third of the visceral surface nearer to anterior border (Fig. 5.50).**

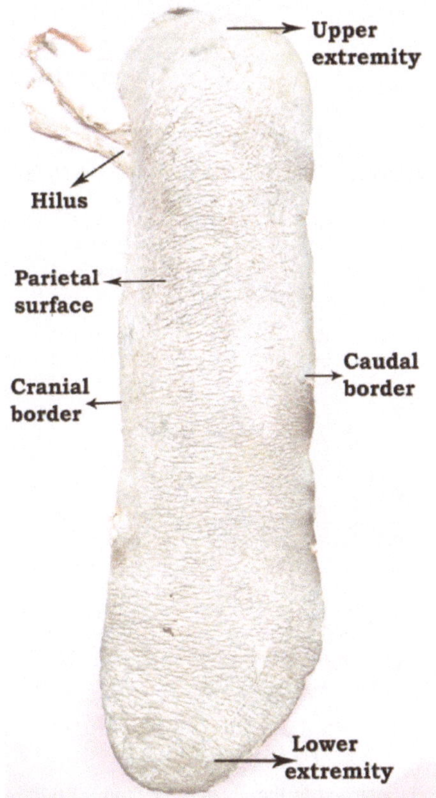

Fig. 5.50: Spleen of Ox

Horse: It is **scythe or triangular shaped** and weighs about 1 kg. A ridge divides the visceral surface into two unequal areas i.e. **gastric impression and colic impression** which are present in front and behind the ridge respectively. The **base presents a renal impression** for left kidney. The **hilus is an elongated groove**. The gastrosplenic omentum extends between visceral surface of spleen and greater curvature of stomach **(Fig. 5.51).**

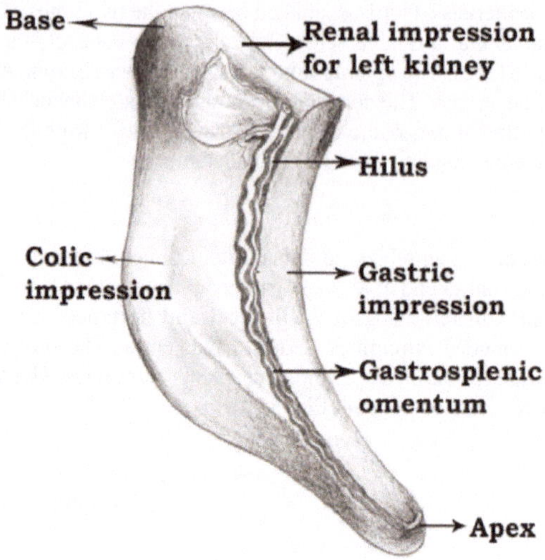

Fig. 5.51: Spleen of Horse

Dog: It is **falciform shaped**, long and narrow. The ventral end is wider. The hilus is like a **longitudinal ridge (Fig. 5.52).**

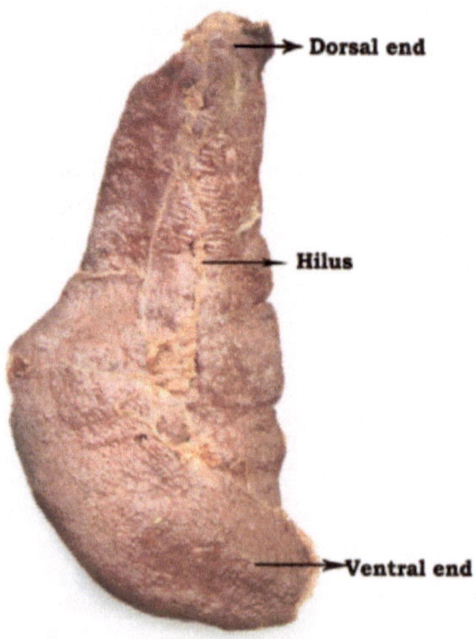

Fig. 5.52: Spleen of Dog

Pig: It is **elongated** and it is loosely attached to the greater curvature of the stomach by a wider gastrosplenic ligament. It has dorsoventral orientation.

Fowl: is a small organ of **brownish-red colour**. It is ***round or egg-shaped***, in the aquatic birds more triangular with a flattened dorsal and a convex ventral surface and in the pigeon it is oval. The spleen of the fowl and duck weighs 1.5-4.5 g. It lies against the dorsal surface of the right lobe of the liver in a space formed dorsally by the gonad, ventrally by the liver and laterally by the gizzard.

PERITONEUM

Peritoneum: is a thin serous membrane which lines the abdominal cavity and pelvic cavity (in part) and viscera contained therein. The peritoneal cavity, the potential space between parietal peritoneum and visceral peritoneum contains a thin film of serous fluid. In front of pelvic inlet the parietal peritoneum dips into inguinal canal to form tunica vaginalis to cover the spermatic cord and the testicles.

Pelvic peritoneum: is continous cranillay with abdominal part. It lines the pelvic cavity for variable distance caudally and is then reflected onto the viscera and from one organ to another **(Fig. 5.53).** Since part of the pelvic cavity caudally is not lined by peritoneum that part of the pelvic cavity is ***retroperitoneal***.

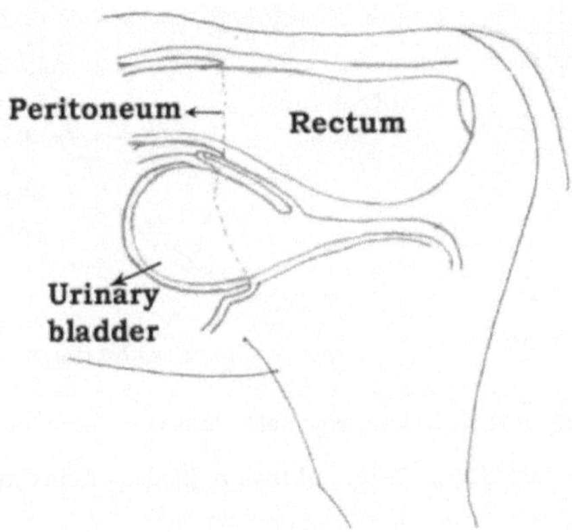

Fig. 5.53: Pelvic Peritoneum

Greater omentum is a double fold of peritoneum passing from stomach to other viscera which is a pathway for the vessels and nerves. It conceals ventral sac of rumen, most of the intestine and pregnant uterus. It consists of ***superficial and deep parts***.The **superficial part** of greater omentum extends from left longitudinal groove of rumen to right side by passing below the ventral sac of rumen to greater curvature of abomasum, caudal border of first part of duodenum and ventral border of second part of duodenum **(Fig. 5.54).**

The **deep part** extends from right longitudinal groove of rumen to visceral surface of liver, ventral surface of descending duodenum and first bend of proximal loop of ascending colon by passing around ventral aspect of intestines and turns dorsally. The two walls are continuous along the posterior transverse groove of rumen. The superficial and deep layers of greater omentum form a sac to contain intestinal mass. The two layers of greater omentum enclose a space, the ***omental bursa*** (***lesser peritoneal sac***) which is completely separated from the greater peritoneal cavity except at the ***epiploic*** **(*Omental / Winslow*)** ***foramen. Epiloic (omental) foramen a sagittal slit present between the caudate process of liver and pancreas is the opening to omental bursa.***

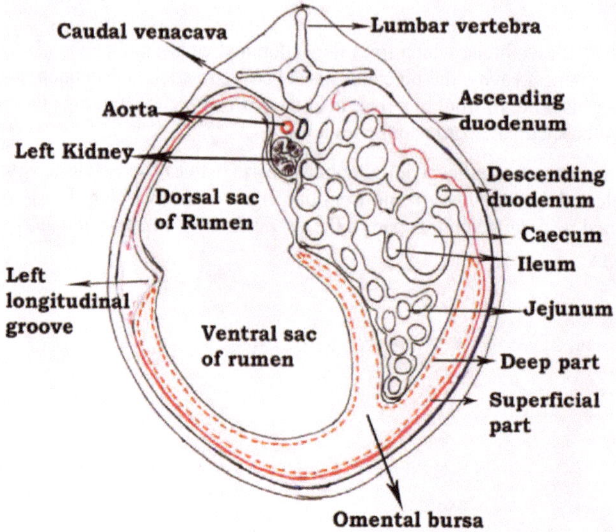

Fig. 5.54: Abdominal Peritoneal Reflections in Ruminants

The ***lesser omentum*** extends from the visceral surface of liver to the lesser curvature of abomasum and first part of duodenum. **(Fig. 5.55).**

A free slip of the lesser omentum has the appearance of an ear of pig and is known as the ***"pig's ear"***. This can be used in omentoplexy and in identifying the abomasum in cases of left abomasal displacement.

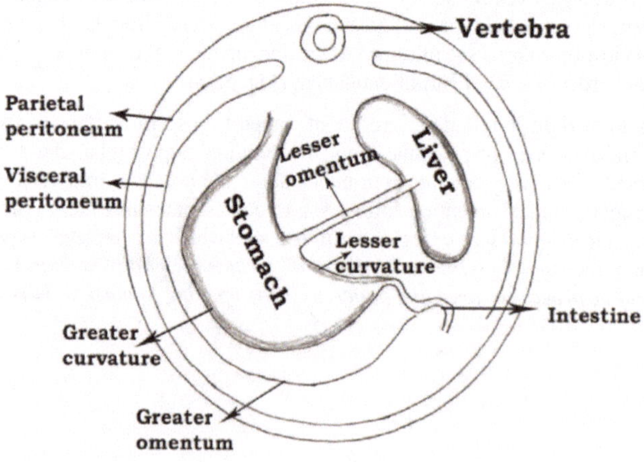

Fig. 5.55: Abdominal Peritoneal Reflections in Monogastric Animals

Parietal peritoneum is reflected from the sacrum onto the rectum forming visceral peritoneum. A transverse fold of peritoneum extending from the lateral pelvic wall lies between rectum and urinary bladder and is ***termed genital fold***. The ventral layer of this fold is reflected onto the dorsal surface of the bladder. Thus there is a pouch between the rectum and genital fold called ***rectogenital pouch*** and another between the genital fold and the bladder called ***vesicogenital pouch*** **(Figs. 5.56, 5.57).**

The ***genital fold*** **inmale contains ductus deferens**, part of the **vesicular glands and the uterus masculinus** (***fetal remnant***). The peritoneum from ventral surface of the bladder forms pubovesical pouch. While passing from bladder to pelvic floor the peritoneum forms middle ligament of bladder. It also passes from each side of the bladder to the lateral pelvic wall forming lateral ligament of bladder **(Fig. 5.56).** This contains in its edge the round ligament of bladder.

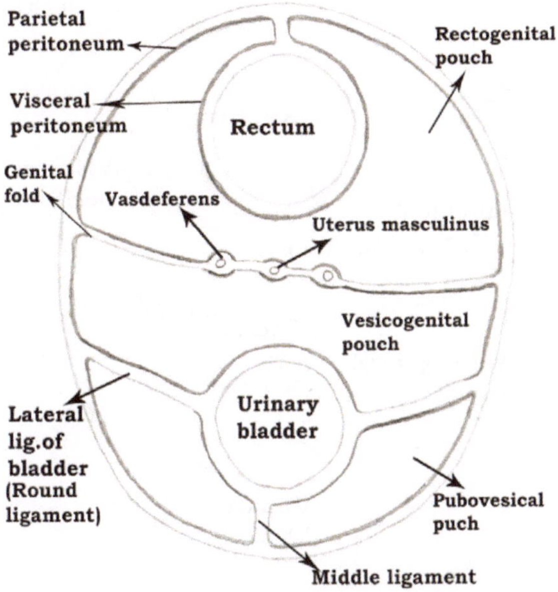

Fig. 5.56: Pelvic Peritoneal Reflections of Male

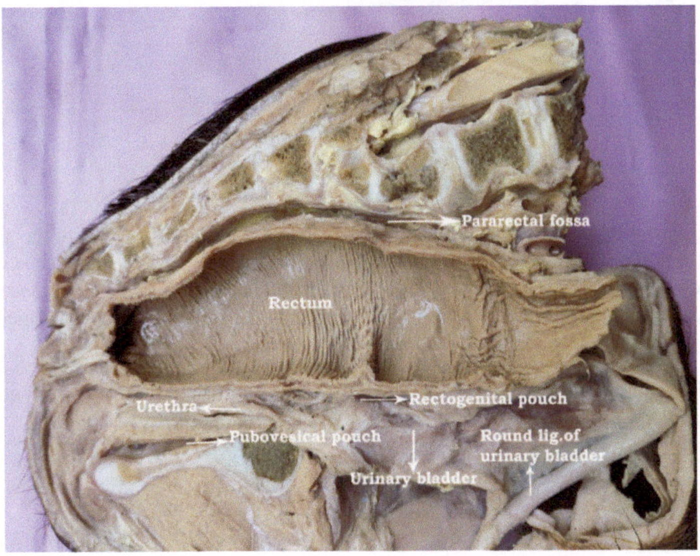

Fig. 5.57: Peritoneal Cavities in Male

In female the arrangement is modified by the presence of uterus. The **genital fold is enlarged to enclose the uterus and a small part of vagina.** It forms two extensive folds, the broad ligaments of the uterus, which attach the uterus to the sides of pelvic cavity and lumbar part of abdominal wall **(Fig. 5.58).** It divides the pelvic peritoneal cavity completely into dorsal rectogenital pouch and the vesicogenital pouch. The peritoneum is reflected from the floor of the pelvis onto neck of the bladder forming a shallow pubovesical pouch.

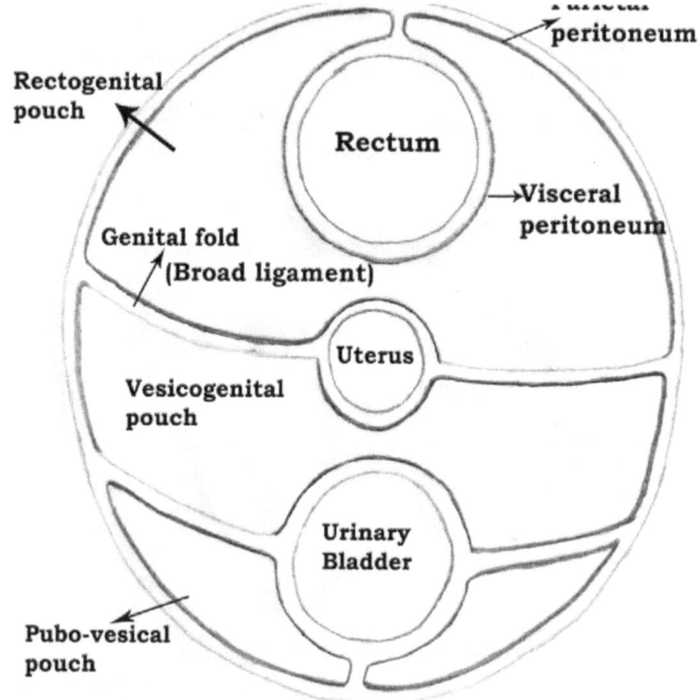

Fig. 5.58: Pelvic Peritoneal Reflections of Female

Mesentery is a peritoneal fold which attaches the jejunum and ileum to the dorsal wall of the abdomen. Specific names are applied to the peritoneal folds attached to various portions of the digestive tube such as mesoduodenum, mesocolon and mesorectum etc. The mesoduodenum suspends the duodenum, while the mesocolon suspends the descending colon from sublumbar region. The coils of the jejunum are suspended by the mesojejunum around the root of the mesentry. The mesojejunum is also called the ***great mesentery***.

Ligaments are folds which pass between viscera other than parts of the digestive tube or connect them with the abdominal wall, but donot contain blood vessels and nerves **eg:** ***lateral ligaments of bladder.***

URINARY ORGANS

The urinary system consists of paired kidneys and ureters and unpaired urinary bladder and urethra.

KIDNEYS

Ox: The kidneys are **lobated (18-20 lobes)** glands located in sublumbar region. If distended with pyelonephritis lobation of kidneys is obliterated. The **right kidney is retroperitoneal, while the left kidney is surrounded by peritoneum.** There is much perirenal fat in cattle and it is ***known as "suet" in meat trade****, is of hard consistency.* The **kidneys are multipyramidal type (Fig. 5.59).**The frontal section of the kidney reveals cortex and medulla. **The *cortex* (outer part)** is rich in *renal or Malphigian corpuscles* which give granular appearance to cortex. **The *medulla*** is the inner part made up of only tubules and is in the form of renal pyramids.

The bovine kidney on longitudinal section shows 20 medullary pyramids one for each lobe. ***The apex of each papilla projects into a calyx minor*** **(Fig. 5.59).** The ***calyces minors form two calyces major,*** *one from cranial half and another from caudal half which meet at hilus to form ureter.*

The complete fusion of the cortical tissue of neighbouring lobes result in a kidney with a smooth surface like in pig, horse, carnivores and small ruminants, while incomplete fusion results in a kidney that is superficially divided by fissures as in ox. In unipyramidal kidney renal papillae also fuse forming a ridge like common papilla, renal crest and calices are not formed as in horse, dog, cat and small ruminants. In multipyramidal kidney there are cup shaped calices one for each papilla as papillae are not fused which are located at the end of a branch of ureter and renal pelvis is absent (ox) or present (pig).

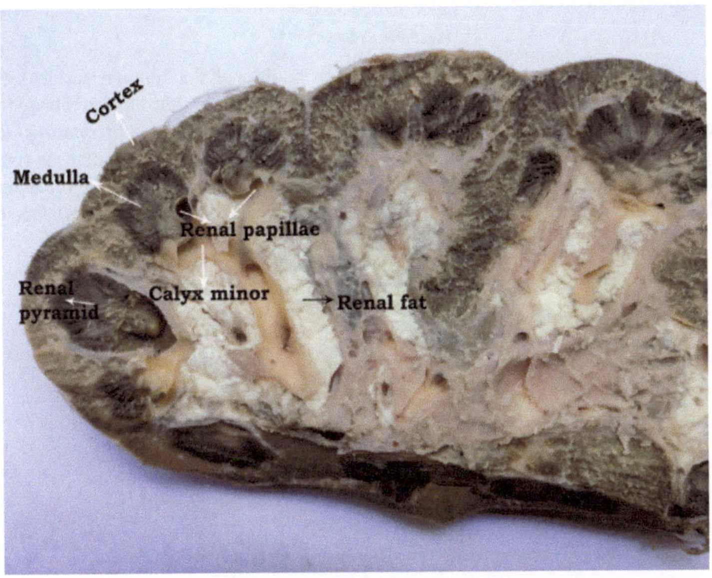

Fig. 5.59: Frontal Section of Kidney of Ox

The right kidney is an elongated elliptical or oval gland placed ventral to the **last rib and first two or three lumbar transverse processes.** It is related to liver cranially and is flattened dorsoventrally. It shows cranial and caudal extremities, dorsal and ventral surfaces, medial and lateral borders. The ***hilus is at the anterior part of ventral surface nearer to medial border*** **(Fig. 5.60).** The anterior extremity is related to liver and right adrenal. The dorsal surface is rounded, while the ventral surface is less convex. The medial border is nearly straight, while lateral border is convex **(Fig. 5.60, 5.61).**

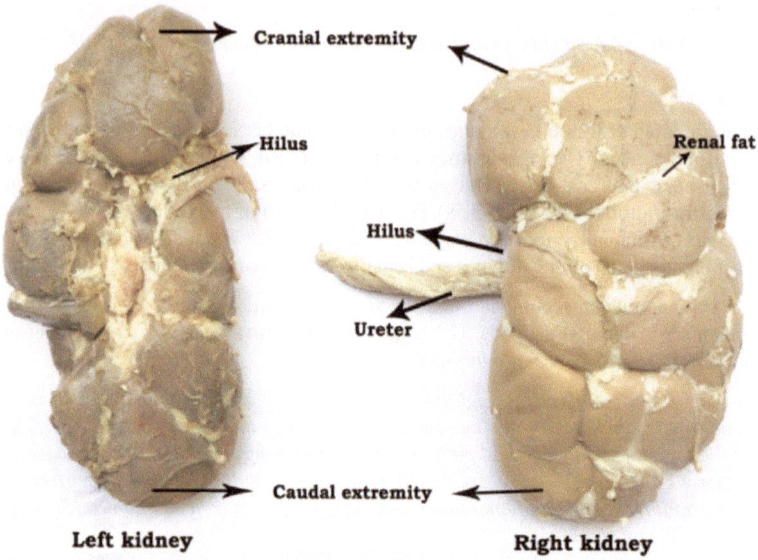

Fig. 5.60: Kidneys of Ox

The left kidney is pyramidal and presents 3 surfaces (with additional flat ruminal surface), 3 borders and 2 extremities **(Figs. 5.60, 5.61).** It extends below the bodies of **2nd or 3rd to 5th lumbar vertebrae** to the right of the median plane. The left kidney in ox can be palpated per retcum. The position is variable (***floating kidney***) because of its relation with right surface of dorsal sac of rumen and it depends on the amount of contents in rumen. The borders are medial, dorsal and ventral. The posterior extremity is large, thick and rounded, while the anterior extremity is small and pointed. The ***hilus is situated on the anterolateral aspect of the convex dorsal surface*** **(Fig. 5.60).**

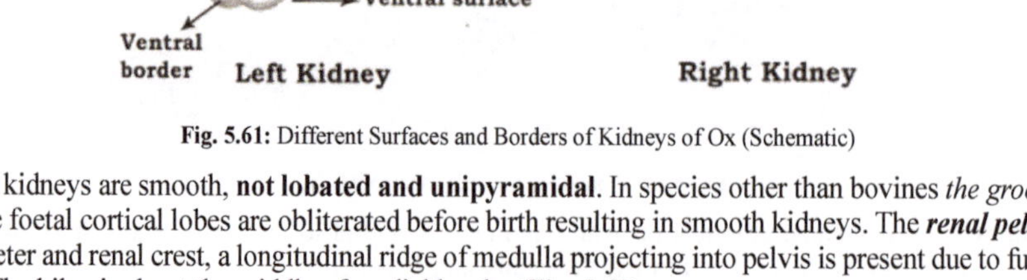

Fig. 5.61: Different Surfaces and Borders of Kidneys of Ox (Schematic)

Horse: The kidneys are smooth, **not lobated and unipyramidal.** In species other than bovines *the grooves existing* between the foetal cortical lobes are obliterated before birth resulting in smooth kidneys. The ***renal pelvis*** is dilated origin of ureter and renal crest, a longitudinal ridge of medulla projecting into pelvis is present due to fusion of renal pyramids. The hilus is about the middle of medial border **(Fig. 5.62).**

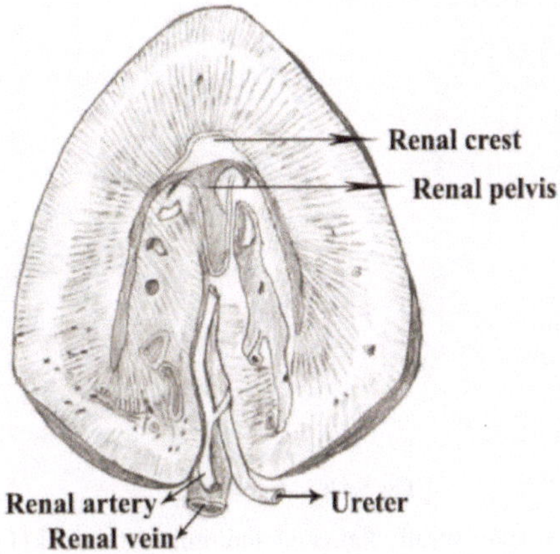

Fig. 5.62: Right Kidney of Horse (Sagittal section)

The ***right kidney*** resembles the **heart of playing cards**. It is located under the vertebral end of **last two ribs and 1st lumbar transverse process.** The anterior extremity is thicker. The ***left kidney*** is **bean shaped** and located under the last rib and first two or three lumbar transverse processes. The posterior extremity is wide and thicker **(Fig. 5.63).**

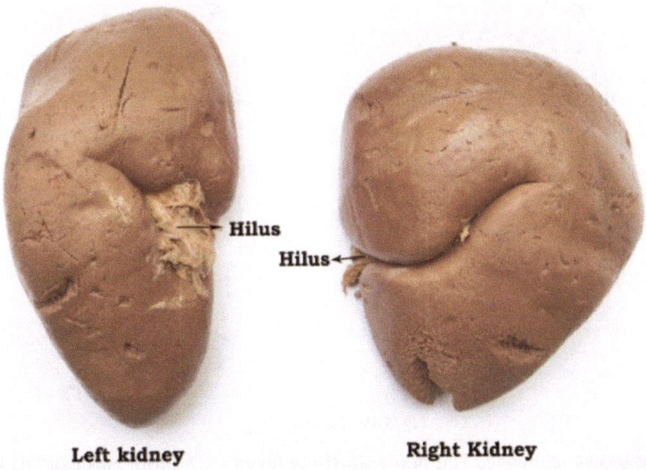

Fig. 5.63: Kidneys of Horse

Dog: The kidneys are smooth and unipyramidal and ***bean shaped*** **(Fig.5.64)**. The **renal pelvis and renal crest are present.** The hilus is about the middle of medial border. The **right kidney** is located under the bodies of the **first three lumbar vertebrae**, while the **left kidney is located under 2nd, 3rd and 4th lumbar vertebrae.**

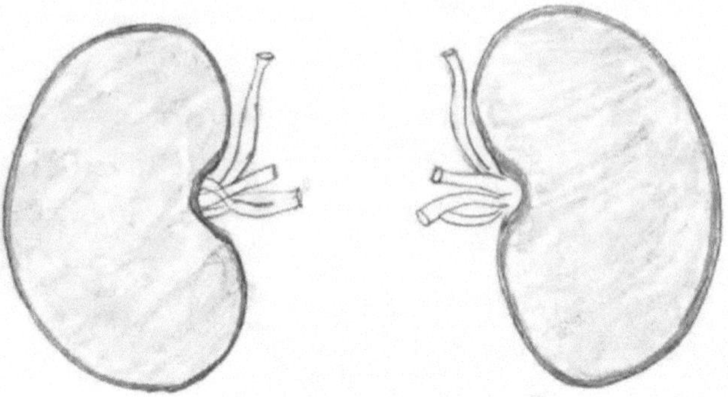

Fig. 5.64: Kidneys of Dog

Pig: The kidneys are smooth and dorsoventrally flattened and multipyramidal (**Fig.5.65**). The cranial pole of the ***right kidney*** lies ventral to the last rib and the caudal pole lies below the fourth lumbar vertebra. ***The pig is the only domestic animal in which right kidney does not contact with the liver***. The left kidney is related ventrally to the ascending colon, base of the caecum and the pancreas. The hilus is situated in the medial border. The calyx major and minor are present. The renal pelvis leads into ureter.

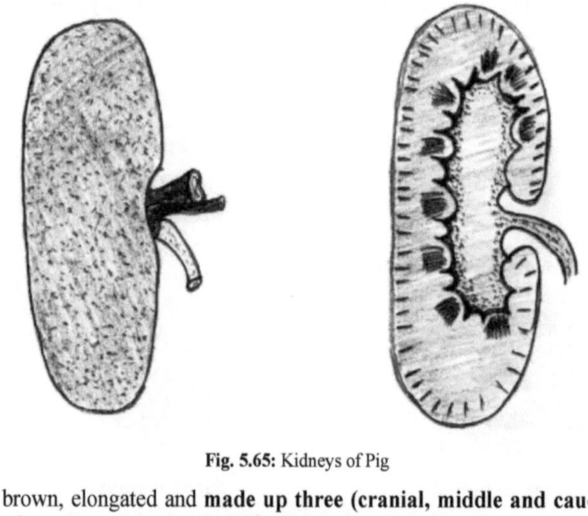

Fig. 5.65: Kidneys of Pig

Fowl: The kidneys are brown, elongated and **made up three (cranial, middle and caudal) lobes** that lie along side of vertebral column from the vertebral end of **6th rib into the iliac fossa. Cranially they are in contact with the lungs (Fig. 5.66).** The ***cranial*** **and** ***middle lobes*** are separated on their ventral surface by a transverse groove in which lies the external iliac artery and vein. The kidney is also related on its medial border to the aorta or the caudal vena cava, on its ventral surface to various loops of the intestine and to the ovary and oviduct in females, especially during the laying period and to the testes in males **(Fig. 5.66).** Between these organs and the kidney there are the abdominal air sacs. The colour of the kidney is dependent on its blood content and varies from pale pink to dark brownish-red. In the fowl it is 7-10 cm long, with an average breadth of 2 cm and a depth of 1.3-1.5 cm. It weighs 5-6g. The ***ureter*** begins at the cranial lobe of kidney and runs caudally along its ventromedial border. **In the male it crosses the ductus deferens**

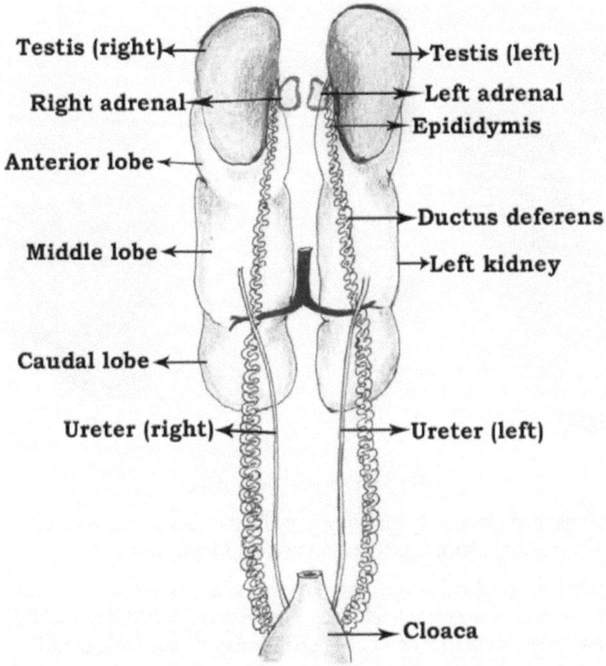

Fig. 5.66: Kidneys and Adrenal Glands of Fowl

Ureter: Each ureter consists of abdominal part (located in sublumbar region) and pelvic part. The pelvic part pierces the dorsal wall of bladder at an acute angle near the neck and opens at the base of trigonum vesicae. After penetrating muscular coat of bladder it continues for a short distance in the submucosa before opening into lumen of the bladder.

Ox: The ureter begins at the junction of calyces major and terminates at the urinary bladder. The left ureter begins on the right of median plane, then passes along right surface of its kidney and then lies ventral to right ureter for a short distance before crossing to the left.

Horse and Dog: It arises from renal pelvis.

Fowl: It arises on the anterior part of the medioventral face of the kidney and **opens into the urodeum of the cloaca,** medial to the opening of the ductus deferens or oviduct.

ADRENAL GLANDS

Adrenal Glands are **two in number** and red brown in colour. It shows an outer light coloured cortex and inner dark medulla. The cortex is yellowish and radially striated and medulla is much darker and has uniform appearance.

Ox: The ***right adrenal is V-shaped*** and located against the medial surface of anterior end of the right kidney and shows a base, an apex and three surfaces. The base is irregularly concave and is in contact with anterior end of right kidney, while the apex is pointed and lies in the angle between posterior vena cava and liver **(Figs. 5.67, 5.68).**

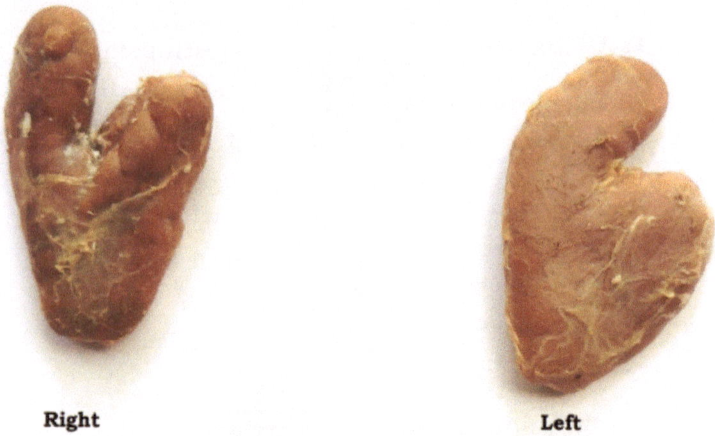

Fig. 5.67: Adrenal Glands of Ox

The medial surface is flattened and related to diaphragm, while the lateral surface is convex and lies in the renal impression of the liver. The ventral surface is grooved for posterior vena cava.

The ***left adrenal is roughly C-shaped*** and located just posterior to anterior mesenteric artery on medial surface of posterior vena cava about 5 to 8 cm anterior to left kidney. ***Hence, it is not in contact with left kidney***. It shows two (left and right) surfaces and posterior border or base which is deeply notched **(Figs. 5.67).**

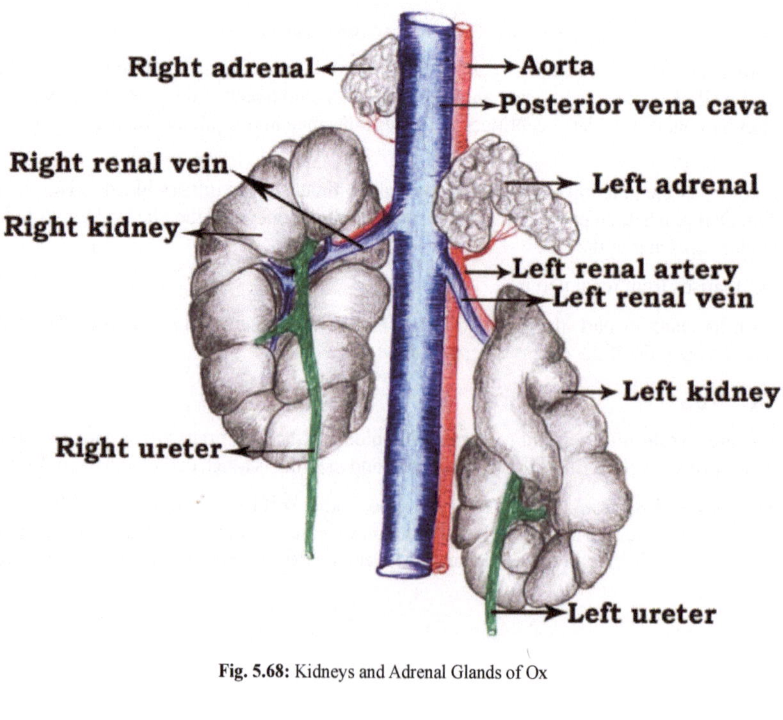

Fig. 5.68: Kidneys and Adrenal Glands of Ox

Horse: The adrenals are flattened and lie in contact with the anterior parts of medial border of the respective kidneys.

Dog: The ***right adrenal is prismatic*** and pointed at either end while the ***left adrenal is elongated*** and flattened dorsoventrally. The left adrenal is not in contact with left kidney.

Pig: They are long cylindrical organs situated on the medial surface of the kidney cranial to its hilus in the perirenal fat. The **glands are reddish brown because of poor lipid content**. The left gland is usually longer and heavier than the right.

Fowl: They are yellowish brown, **oval or triangular** and about 13 mm long and 8 mm wide. Each lies **at the cranial pole of the corresponding kidney, related ventrally to the ovary in female and epididymis in male.**

5.6 SURGICAL OPERATIONS OF THE ABDOMEN

Paralumbar fossa is a part of the ***non bony wall of abdomen (flank)*** and is clinically important. Boundaries of paralumbar fossa are superiorly longissimus dorsi muscle, anteriorly posterior border of last rib, inferiorly obliquus abdominis internus.

Palpation: Left paralumbar fossa (Hunger hollow) is an ideal space for observing the motility of rumen. Foetal movements may be observed through the abdominal wall in advanced pregnancy on either side in the mare and on the right side in the cow as right horn pregnancy is more common in ruminants.

Clinical importance of the paralumbar fossa: For rumenotomy, to record ruminal movements, to palpate rumen and laparotomy operation on left side. On right side it is a site for enterotomy and caecal biopsy.

1. Laparotomy: Means opening of the abdomen. Lateral wall of the abdominal cavity is formed by obliquus abdominis externus, intemus and transversus abdominis and floor is formed by rectus abdominis and linea alba which is formed by aponeurosis of externi, interni and transverse muscles of two sides.

Indications: (1) Gastrotomy (2) Enterotomy and Enterectomy (3) Cystotomy 4) Hysterectomy (5) Ovariotomy (6) Splenectomy and (7) Diagnostic purpose (Exploratory laparotomy)

Sites

a. **Flank site:** left side for rumenotomy and spleenctomy and right side for enterotomy. Vertical or oblique incision on the hollow of the flank (paralumbar fossa) is made.

b. **Mildline site:** Incision through the linea alba between the xiphoid cartilage of sternum and pubic symphysis for Caesarean operation. This site is preferred since it is least vascular.

c. **Paramedian site:** Parallel to the linea alba along the belly of rectus abdominis muscle for Caesarean operation.

d. **Pararectal site:** Parallel to rectus abdominis muscle along its lateral border for caesarean operation.

e. **Paracostal site:** For abomasotomy in ruminants on right side.

2. Paracentesis Abdomen: (Puncturing of abdomen)

Indications: To relieve excess gases from the rumen and for collection of rumen liquor for diagnostic purpose.

Site: Paralumbar fossa on left side in cattle.

3. Rumenocentesis (puncturing of rumen): This is preceeded by paracentesis abdominis since abdomen has to be punctured to reach rumen.

Indications: to relieve **actue tympany (bloat)** as an emergency measure and for direct medication into the rumen.

Site: Left paralumbar fossa.

4. Rumenotomy: is opening of rumen. This is preceeded by laparotomy in paralumbar fossa.

Indications: 1. Severe impaction. 2. If there are any foreign bodies in the rumen or reticulum, resulting in traumatic reticulo pericarditis.

Site: Left flank (paralumbar fossa), a vertical incision 6 to 8 inches long (laparotomy) followed by incision in ruminal wall.

Incision can be made in the direction of muscle fibers thereby avoiding sutures (**suture less laparotomy**). Then rumenotomy is done. The layers incised in wall of rumen from exterior to interior are serosa, muscularis and mucosa.

5. Abomasotomy: Abomasum is present on the right side of abdomen. Its fundus is located at xiphoid cartilage and its pyloric part extends backwards.

Indications: Obstruction due to foreign bodies and in case of abomasal ulcers.

Site: 1. On the linea alba, about two inches behind xiphoid cartilage and extending upto the umbilicus. 2. About 4 to 10 inches long paracostal incision behind the right costal arch.

6. Caesarean Operation: Caesarean operation consists of opening of abdomen and also opening of uterine cavity along greater curvature of the gravid uterine horn to extract foetus when the foetus can't be delivered normally.

Indications: When normal delivery of foetus is difficult (dystokia) or not desirable

Sites: Many sites are there for this operation. 1. Between the anterior mammary veins and the midline either on left or right side from the front of the udder forwards. 2. Parallel to milk vein. 3.Oblique flank incision downward and forward from a little below external angle of ilium on right side. 4. Vertical incision on the right paralumbar fossa.

7. Sites for Biopsy of Liver, Gall bladder and caecum:

Indications: To study histopathological changes as a part of disease diagnosis.

a. Liver Biopsy

Site: in the bovine an area at the junction of upper and middle third of 10th or 11th intercostal space on the right side as liver is located on right side of abdominal cavity.

b. Gall Bladder Biopsy:

Site: Ventral part of 11th inter costal space on right side as gall bladder projects beyond ventral border of liver.

c. Caecal Biopsy:

Site: Right side at pelvic inlet.

8. Paravertebral nerve block: The flank region is supplied by ***thirteenth thoracic and first and second lumbar spinal nerves***. Each nerve has dorsal and ventral branches. The **dorsal branch** supplies the muscles of the loin. The **ventral branch** supplies to the skin, abdominal muscles and peritoneum. In addition to this ventral cutaneous branch of 3rd lumbar spinal nerve also supplies to the flank region.

Indications: for laporotomy, rumenotomy, gastrotomy and other operations of the abdomen.

Site: The last thoracic nerve is blocked about 5 to 6 cm lateral to the mid dorsal line at a point behind the level of the last rib. The sites for blocking the first three lumbar nerves are 5 to 6 cm lateral to mid dorsal line and behind the transverse processes of first three lumbar vertebrae respectively.

5.7 SUMMARY

Fowl: The lumbar and sacral vertebrae are fused together and form lumbosacral mass (Fourteen number). This with the 7th dorsal and 1st coccygeal vertebrae, fused into a mass called synsacrum (altogether 16 in number).

ABDOMINAL MUSCLES: There are four pairs of abdominal muscles viz., 1.Obliquus abdominis externus; 2. obliquus abdominis internus; 3. Rectus abdominis and 4. Transversus abdominis muscle.

1. Obliquus abdominis externus:	1. This is the **largest and the most superficial** and extensive of all the abdominal muscles. ***2. Poupart's or inguinal ligament*** is the aponeurosis of **obliquus abdominis externus** muscle at its insertion to the prepubic tendon.
2. Obliquus abdominis internus:	1. It extends from the **lateral angle of the ilium to the last rib** 2. **Creamaster externus:** This is narrow flat band of muscle detached from the internal oblique muscle.
3. Transversus abdominis:	Arises from the transverse processes of last four lumbar vertebrae and inserts on linea alba on ventral aspect of the abdomen.
4. Rectus abdominis:	Is confined to the **floor of the abdomen** and extends from the **sternum to the pubis**.

Rumen:	1. It occupies nearly 3/4th left half of abdominal cavity from **7th or 8th intercostal** space to the pelvic inlet. ***2. Atrium ventriculi***: is the area where oesophagus enters the stomach. (i.e level of **8th and 9th ribs)**
Reticulum:	1. It extends from the level of **6th rib to 8th rib.** 2. The mucous membrane gives the **honey-comb appearance**.
Omasum:	is ellipsoidal and extends from **7th to 11th rib**.
Abomasum:	1. The most distal and true **glandular compartment** of ruminant stomach. ***2. Torus pyloricus*** is a round protuberance on the in side of lesser curvature near pylorus.

Epiploic (omental / Winslow) foramen: The lesser peritoneal sac is separated from the greater peritoneal cavity except at the epiploic (omental / Winslow) foramen, situated near the porta of the liver.

Horse: The stomach is 'U' shaped sac.

Margoplicatus: is a sinuous ridge dividing the mucous membrane into two parts, non-glandular and glandular.

Dog: The stomach is pyriform shaped and it is completely glandular.

Liver

Ox: It is situated entirely in the right half of abdominal cavity from lumbocostal angle to ventral end of 7th or 8th rib obliquely downwards and forwards.

Portal fissure: is the area where the portal vein and hepatic artery enter and bile duct leaves the liver.

Dog: The liver of dog is divided into right lateral, right medial, left medial, left lateral, quadrate and caudate lobes.

Left lateral lobe is the largest lobe of liver.

The gall bladder lies in fossa between quadrate and right medial lobe.

Pig: The liver of pig resembles that of the dog in lobation and position.

Papillary process is absent.

Fowl: The liver consists of two lobes, the right and left. The right lobe is large.

Gall Bladder

Ox: It is pear shaped present at the level of 10th or 11th intercostal space.

Horse: The gall bladder is absent.

Dog: It lies in fossa between the quadrate and right medial lobes.

Pig: It is present in fossa between the quadrate and right medial lobes.

Fowl: It lies on the visceral surface of the right lobe and is elongated.

Pancreas

Ox: is irregularly quadrilateral in shape.

Horse: is triangular in outline.

Dog: is 'U' or 'V' shaped.

In ox, left kidney has an additional flat ruminal (lateral surface) surface

Kidneys of Various Species:

Description	Ox	Horse	Pig	Dog	Sheeep & Goat
Lobes	Lobated (18-20 lobes)	Smooth & non lobated	Smooth & non lobated	Smooth	Smooth
Pyramids	Multi pyramidal	Unipyramidal	Multi pyramidal	Unipyramidal	Multi pyramidal
Renal pelvis	Absent	Present	Present	Present	Present
Renal crest	Absent	Present	Absent	Present	Present
Additional surface (Ruminal/Lateral)	Present in left kidney	Absent	Absent	Absent	Absent
Calyx major & minor	Present	Absent	Present	Absent	Absent

Renal pelvis: is a dilated origin of ureter eg: Horses, Dog and Pig

Renal crest: a longitudinal ridge of medulla projecting into pelvis due to fusion of renal pyramids eg: Horses, Dog.

The pig is the only domestic animal in which right kidney does not contact with the liver.

Location of kidneys in various species:

Species	Right Kidney	Left Kideney
Ox:	Ventral to the last rib and first two or three lumbar transverse processes.	Below the bodies of 2nd or 3rd to 5th lumbar vertebrae.
Horse	Below the vertebral end of last two ribs and 1st lumbar transverse process.	Below the last rib and first two or three lumbar transverse processes.
Dog	Below bodies of the first three lumbar vertebrae.	Below the 2nd, 3rd and 4th lumbar vertebrae.
Pig	Below L1-L4 vertebrae	Below L1-L4 vertebrae.
Fowl	Vertebral end of 6th rib into the iliac fossa.	

ADRENAL GLANDS

Species	Right Adrenal	Left Adrenal
Ox	V-shaped	C-shaped
Horse	Flattened	Flattened
Dog	Prismatic	Elongated
Pig	Cylindrical	Cylindrical
Fowl	Oval / pyramidal	Oval / pyramidal

UNIT 6
PELVIS AND HIND LIMB

6.1 BONES OF THE PELVIS AND HIND LIMB

OS COXAE

Ox: The os coxae or hip bone consists of 3 flat bones i.e ilium, ischium and pubis which fuse together to form the acetabulum.

Ilium: is largest of the 3 parts. It shows three surfaces, three borders and three angels. The **lateral (gluteal)** surface presents gluteal line parallel to cotyloid border. The **medial surface** consists of **rough medial triangular part, the sacral surface** for articulation with sacrum and a **smooth quadrilateral part, iliac surface**. The ***iliopectineal*** line separates these surfaces and bears **psoas tubercle** in its middle (**Fig. 6.1**).

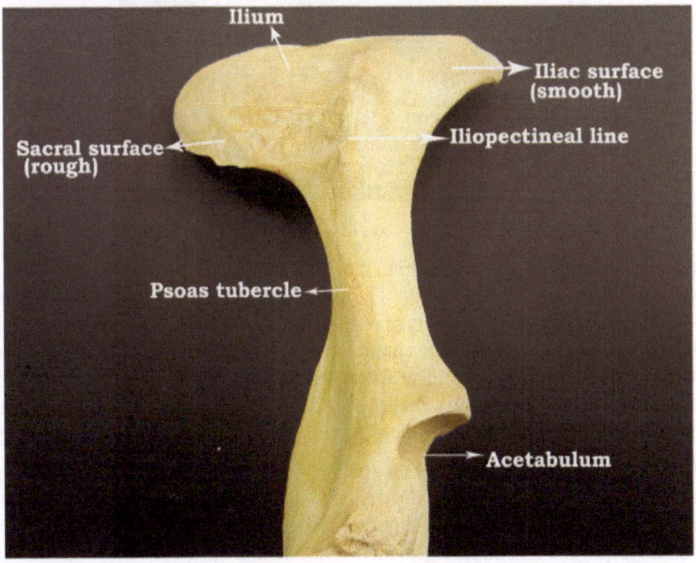

Fig. 6.1: Ilium of Ox (Medial /Pelvic view)

The **cotyloid border** leads to acetabulum and bears two depressions in front and above the acetabulum. The **ischiatic border** is concave and forms the greater sciatic notch. The **dorsal border or crest of ilium** is concave and rough. The **medial angle or tuber sacrale** is small and the **lateral angle (tuber coxae / hook bone)** is large, wide in the middle and smaller at either end. The **inferior (acetabular)** angle is thick and meets the ischium and pubis to form acetabulum (**Fig. 6.2**).

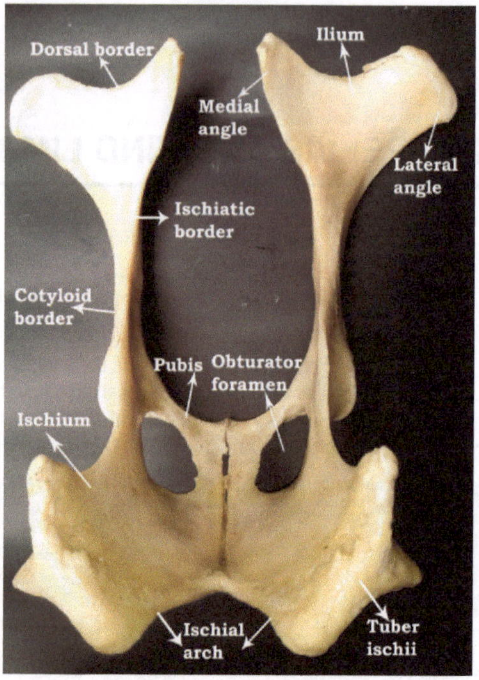

Fig. 6.2: Os coxae of Ox (Dorsal view)

Ischium: is irregularly quadrilateral and placed behind the ilium and pubis. The **dorsal surface** is slightly concave. The **ventral surface** presents a rough ridge in middle. The **anterior border** is concave and forms posterior boundary of obturator foramen. The **posterior border** meets opposite side one to form the ischial arch. The **medial border** meets the same border of its fellow to form the ischiatic symphysis which presents a ridge ventrally. The **lateral border** is concave and forms lesser sciatic notch. The **anterolateral angle** joins the ilium and pubis at the acetabulum. The **anteriomedial angle** joins pubis and forms medial boundary of obturator foramen. The **postereolateral angle (tuber ischii / pin bone)** is trifid in appearance while posterio medial angle forms symphysis (**Fig. 6.2**).

Pubis: is the smallest of the three parts. The **dorsal (pelvic) surface** forms the anterior part of the pelvic floor and the **ventral surface** is rough. The **anterior border** is thick and laterally bears illiopectineal eminence. The **posterior border** forms the anterior margin of the obturator foramen. The **medial border** meets the same border of its fellow to form pubic symphysis. The three angles medial, acetabular and posterior, form symphysis, acetabulum and inner boundary of obturator foramen respectively (**Fig. 6.2**). The **shape of the pelvic inlet is elliptical.**

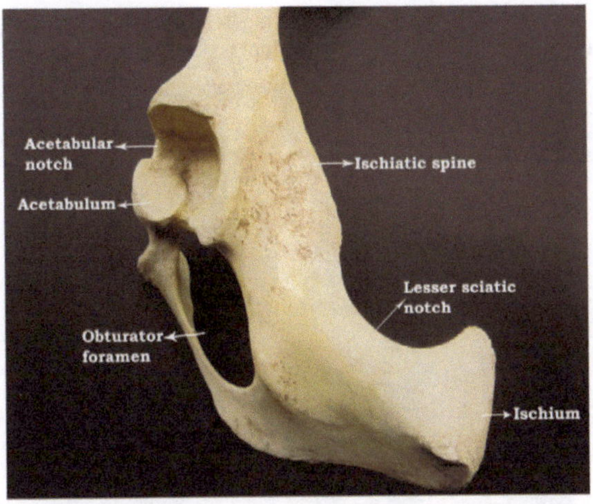

Fig. 6.3: Os coxae of Ox (Lateral view)

Acetabulum: is formed by meeting of ***three bones i.e ilium, ischium and pubis***. It consists of **articular and non articular parts.** The ***articular part*** articulates with the head of the femur. The rim of the cavity presents ***acetabuluar notch on its posteromedial aspect*** which **transmits the round ligament of the hip joint**. The **non articular part, the acetabular fossa** is situated deeply. Another **small notch may be present anteromedially**, sometimes it is **replaced by a foramen** or it is absent (**Fig. 6.3**).

Obturator foramen: is a **large, elliptical foramen** present on the floor of the pelvis and is **formed by the ischium and pubis.** It is covered in life by obturator muscles.

Sexual Differences: in female **ischial arch is wider and the pelvic outlet is larger** and the **vertical (conjugate) and transverse diameters are greater** than in the male, so that the ***cavity is more roomy in female.***

Horse: The **gluteal line is very faint**. The tuber coxae is large consisting of four tuberosities. The ischial arch is wide and shallow and there is also ventral ischiatic spine while ridge on the inferior face of ischium is absent. The **symphyseal ridge is also absent. The tuber ischii is not trifid.** The ventral face of the anterior border of pubis is crossed by pubic groove which leads to the acetabular notch which transmits the ***accessory pubio-femoral ligament*** of the hip joint to the femur (**Fig. 6.4**).The acetabular notch is medial. The shape of the pelvic inlet is nearly ***circular in mare and semi-elliptical in the stallion.***

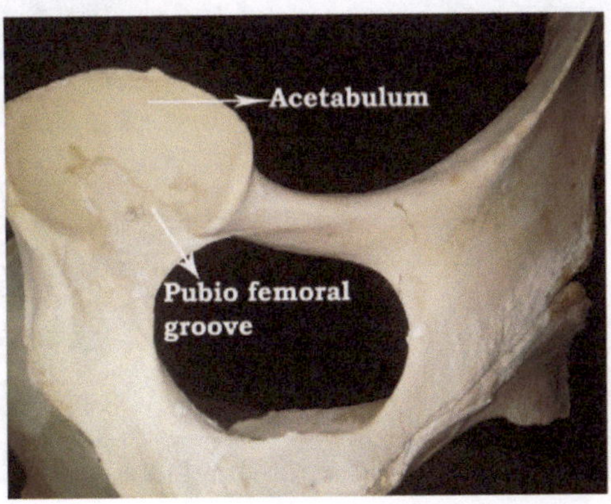

Fig. 6.4: Os coxae of Horse

Dog: The **ilium is nearly in vertical plane** and its crest is strongly convex, while the ischium has a twisted appearance. The **lesser sciatic notch is absent**. The acetabulum is deep (**Fig. 6.5**).

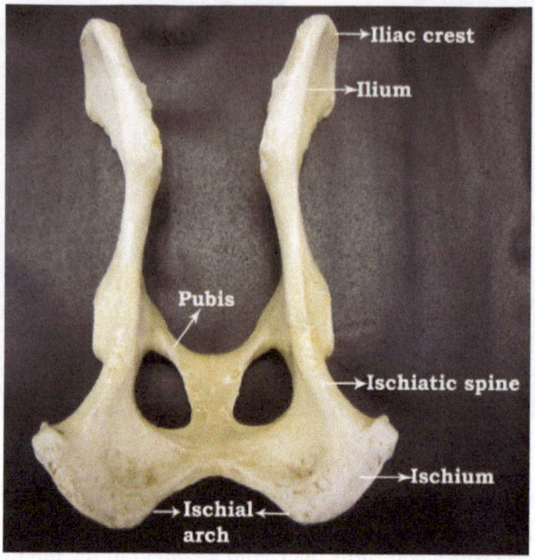

Fig. 6.5: Os coxae of Dog

Pig: The oscoxae is long and narrow. The ilium and ischium are almost in line with each other and nearly sagittal in direction. The wing of the ilium bends laterally much less than in the horse or ox. The gluteal surface is divided into two fossae by a ridge, which is continuous with the ischiatic spine caudally. The tuber coxae is everted and bears three prominences. There is a crest or tuberosity on the ventral surface. The ischiatic spine is like that of the ox but is slightly incurved and the muscular ridges on its lateral face are more pronounced. The iliopubic eminence is prominent and the psoas tubercle is well marked. The acetabulum is placed a little farther caudal than in the ox.

Fowl: The ***ilium is elongated*** and extends over the entire length of the hip bone. It is firmly fused to the transverse processes of the lumbosacral mass (**Fig. 6.6**). The pelvic face is concave (***renal fossa/ iliac fossa***) for the lodgement of **kidney** (**Fig. 6.7**).

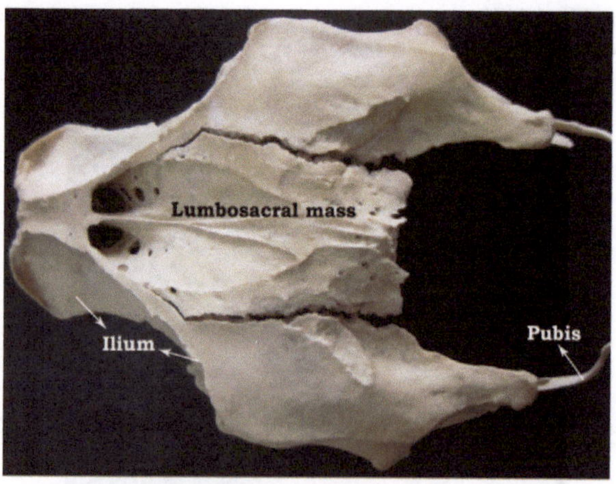

Fig. 6.6: Os coxae of Fowl with Lumbosacral mass (Dorsal view)

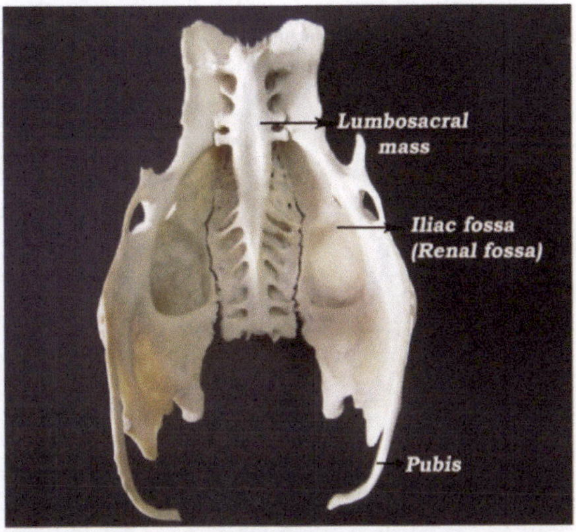

Fig.6.7: Os coxae of Fowl-Ventral view

The ***ischium*** is **smaller and triangular** and lies below and lateral to the posterior part of the ilium. The ischiatic foramen is formed between the adjacent borders of the ischium and ilium. The ventral border of the ischium forms the **obturator foramen with pubis.**

The pubis is long **slender rod like bone**, present along the ventral border of the ischium. The acetabulum is large and perforated and presents at its **superoposterior** part a process, the **antitrochanter** for articulation with the trochanter major of the femur (**Fig. 6.8**). There is **no pelvic symphysis.**

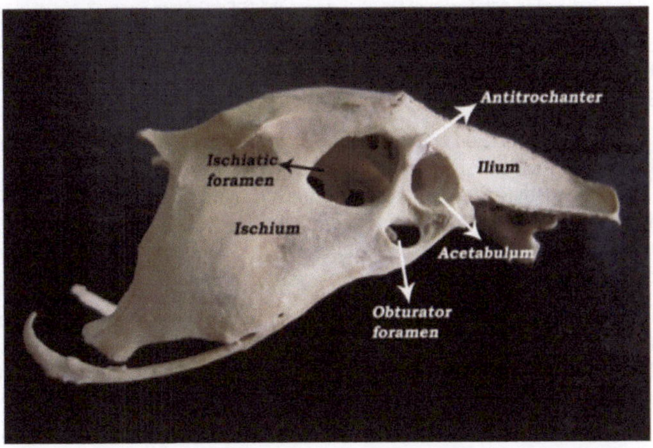

Fig. 6.8: Os coxae of Fowl (Lateral view)

FEMUR

Ox: It is a long bone and is most massive. The shaft consists of four surfaces. The **anterior, medial and lateral surfaces** are continuous and convex. The flat **posterior face** is narrow in the middle where it is rough. The upper part of medial border of this surface presents the trochanter minor. An **oblique trochanteric ridge** extends from this and joins the trochanter major forming the posterolateral boundary of the trochanetric fossa (**Fig. 6.9B**).

The **supracondyloid fossa** is present along lateral border of the distal part of posterior face which is bounded laterally by lateral supracondyloid crest. An oblique vascular groove is present below the middle of the posterior surface running downward and outward marking the course of femoral vessels (**Fig. 6.9B**).

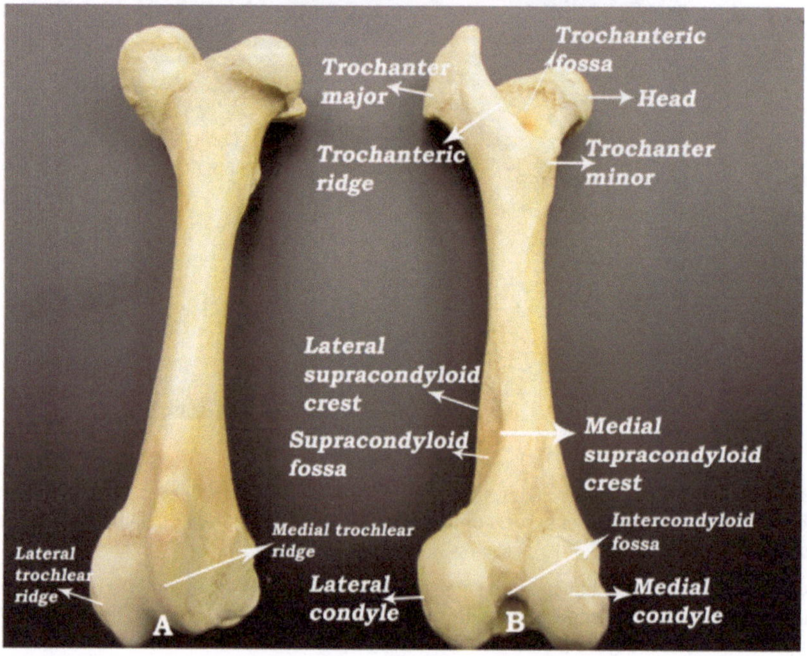

Fig. 6.9: Femur of Ox (A-Anterior and B-Posterior view)

Proximal extremity consists of **head and trochanter major**. The **head** shows a small depression on it called ***fovea capitis***. The **trochanter major** presents convex lateral face. Below its base two (upper and lower) rough tubercles are present (**Fig. 6.9B**).

The **trochlea** in front and two condyles and epicondyles behind are present in distal extremity. Two depressions on lateral condyle and an eminence on medial condyle are present. The **posterior part** of intercondyloid fossa shows one depression close to lateral condyle for attachment of **anterior cruciate ligament** and another depression close to **medial condyle** for **coronary ligament of lateral meniscus**. The medial ridge of trochlea is larger and higher (**Fig. 6.9B**). The intercondyloid fossa is present between medial and lateral condyles and ***extensor fossa*** is placed **between lateral condyle and lateral trochlear ridge**.

Horse: The trochanter minor is in the form of rough ridge and **trochanter tertius** is present at the junction of proximal and middle thirds of lateral border. The supracondyloid fossa and supracondyloid crests are well developed. The **trochanteric ridge is vertical** connecting trochanteric tertius and trochanter major. The **trochanter major is made up of convexity, summit and crest** (**Figs. 6.10, 6.11**).

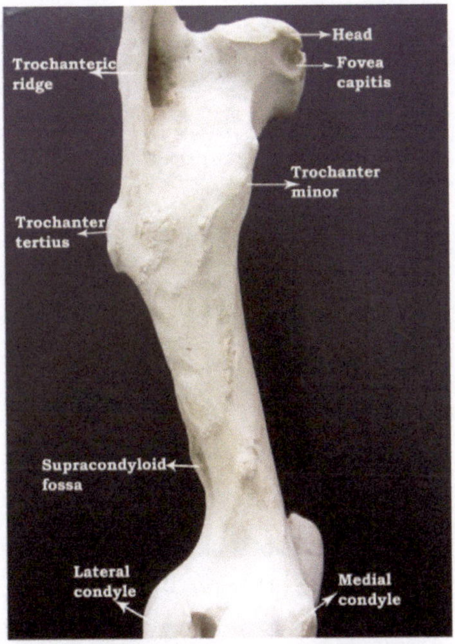

Fig. 6.10: Femur of Horse (Posterior view)

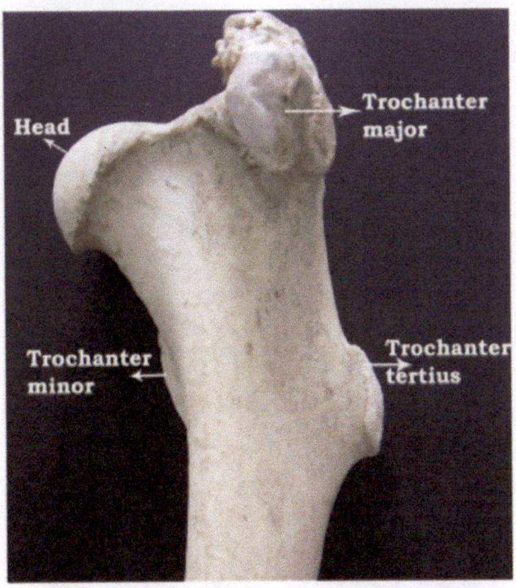

Fig. 6.11: Femur of Horse

Dog: The shaft is strongly curved and **supracondyloid fossa is absent.** The trochanteric fossa is rounded and deep. The ridges of **trochlea are sagittal and equal** and intercondyloid fossa is wide. Above the each condyle small facet is present for sesamoids, the ***fabella*** **(Fig. 6.12).**

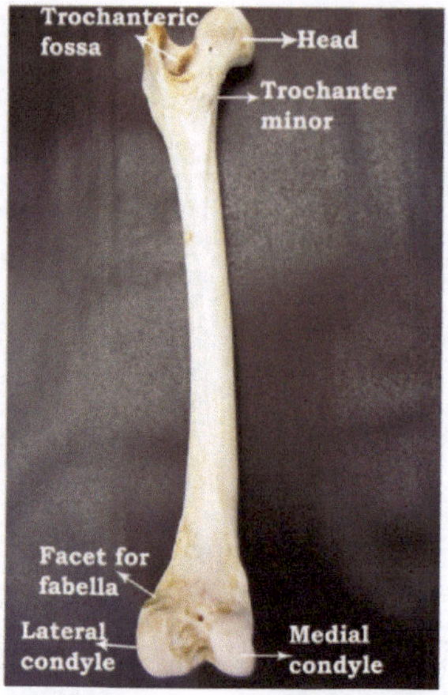

Fig. 6.12: Femur of Dog

Pig: The femur has a relatively wide and massive body. There is no supracondyloid fossa. The head is strongly curved and is marked toward the medial side. The greater trochanter, although massive, does not extend above the level of the head. The third trochanter is absent. The ridges of the trochlea are similar and almost sagittal.

Fowl: The head is prominent but smaller than the acetabulum and the articular surface extends on the trochanter. The **lateral condyle** presents on its lateral aspect a **groove for the head of the fibula (Fig. 6.13)**.

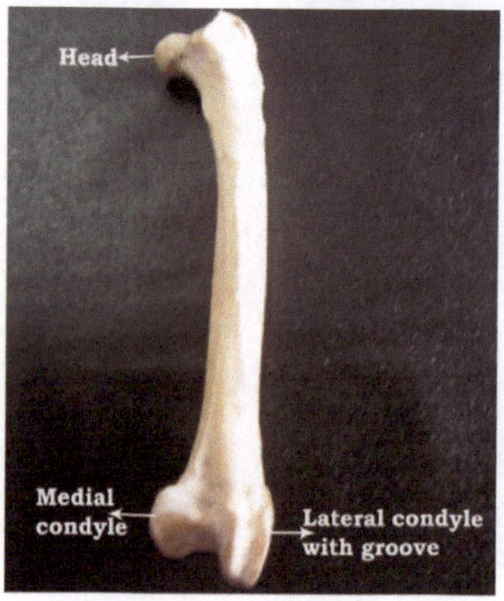

Fig. 6.13: Femur of Fowl

PATELLA

Ox: It is largest sesamoid bone and **irregularly triangular**. It consists of **two surfaces, two borders, a base and an apex**. The **anterior surface** is convex and rough. The **posterior surface** is divided by a vertical ridge into two concave areas (**Fig. 6.14**). The two borders converge at the apex below. The base faces upward and is irregular. The lateral border is convex. The medial border is concave and carries fibrocartilage in living animal.

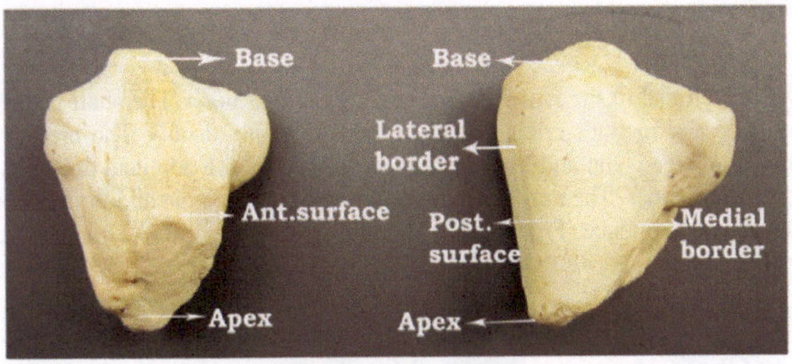

Fig. 6.14: Patella of Ox

Horse: It is quadrilateral in shape. The base is wide and large and grooved transversely (**Fig. 6.15**).

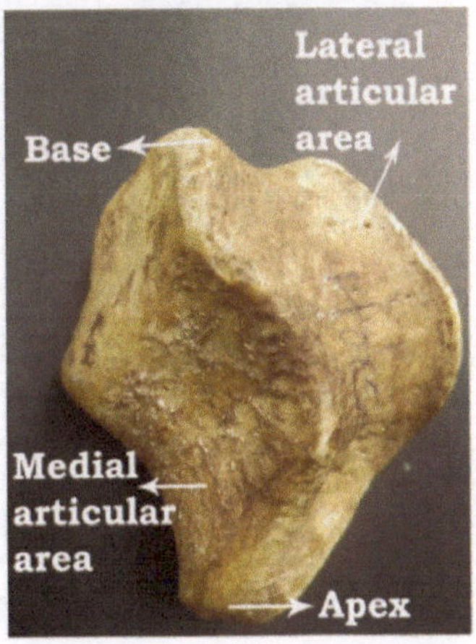

Fig. 6.15: Patella of Horse-Posterior view

Dog: It is long and narrow (**Fig. 6.16**).

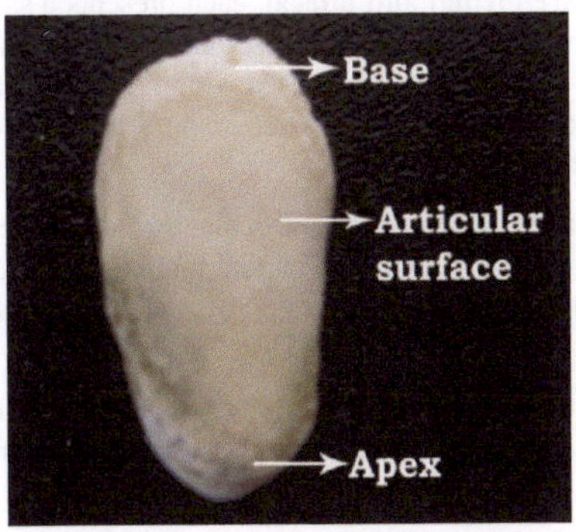

Fig. 6.16: Patella of Dog

Pig: The patella is very much compressed transversely and presents three surfaces.

Fowl: It is wide and thin.

TIBIA

Ox: It is large and well developed of the two bones of leg. It is a long bone. The shaft is curved. Its **lateral face** is wide and concave above and inclines gradually to the front of bone distally. The **medial face** is convex and subcutaneous. The **posterior face** is flat and its upper part is marked by the popliteal line (**Fig. 6.17B**). The rest of this surface is marked by rough lines. The **anterior border** of shaft is prominent and forms tibial crest which shows on its medial aspect a rough prominence (**Fig. 6.17A**). The **medial border** is thick and rounded in its upper fourth, while **lateral border** is concave.

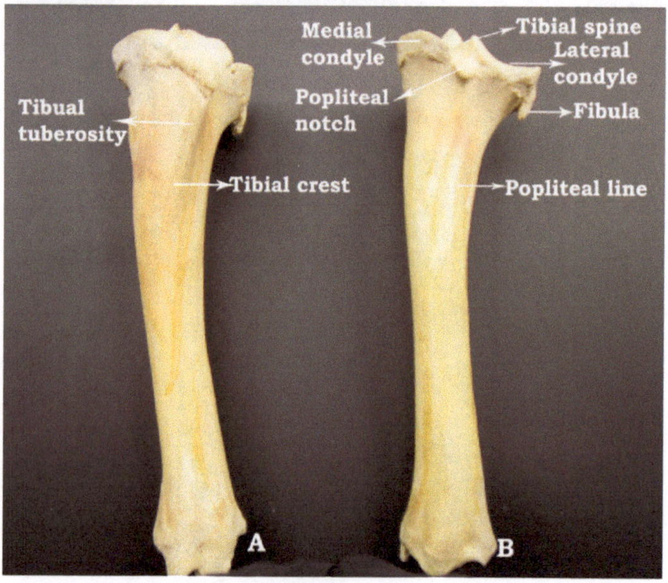

Fig. 6.17: Tibia of Ox (A-Anterior and B-Posterior view)

The proximal extremity consists of **two condyles**, a **tuberosity and spine**. The tuberosity is anterior and continued down by tibial crest. The **condyles are medial and lateral**, each presents a saddle shaped articular area. The two condyles are separated posteriorly by popliteal notch the medial aspect of which shows a tubercle (**Fig. 6.17B**). The **lateral condyle** has head of the rudimentary fibula fused with it on its lateral aspect. The **tibial spine** is placed between two condyles whose articular surfaces are continued on the spine. It is bifid at the summit. Between lateral condyle and tibial tuberosity is ***sulcus muscularis***.

The **distal extremity** is smaller than the proximal. The articular surface presents two deep sagittal grooves. The **medial groove** is bounded on the medial aspect by the medial malleolus, the anterior part of which is prolonged downward to a pointed end. The **lateral groove** is separated by a sharp ridge from an outer area which is for the **lateral malleolus** (*distal extremity of the fibula*).

Horse: The **medial border** of the shaft presents at its upper part a small tubercle. ***The popliteal line is prominent.*** The ***anterior tuberosity is grooved*** (**Fig.6.18**). Below the lateral margin of the lateral condyle is a facet for the fibula. The ***articular grooves on the distal extremity are oblique*** (**Fig.6.18**).

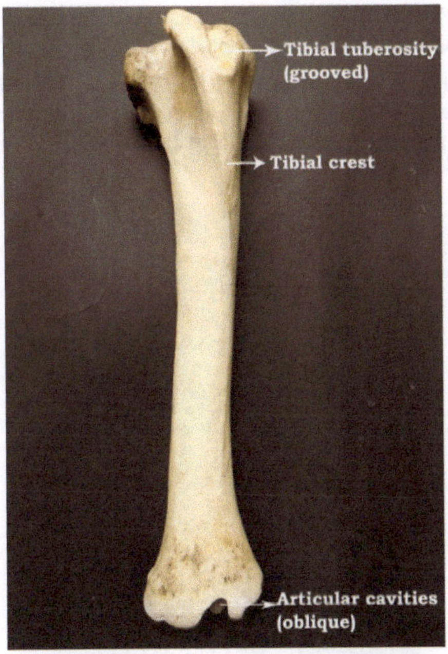

Fig. 6.18: Tibia of Horse (Anterior view)

Dog: The shaft forms double curve. The proximal part is convex medially and the distal part is convex laterally. The **tibial crest is prominent**. The facet for the fibula is on the postero- lateral aspect of the lateral condyle. The distal extremity presents laterally **a facet for the fibula (Fig. 6.19).**

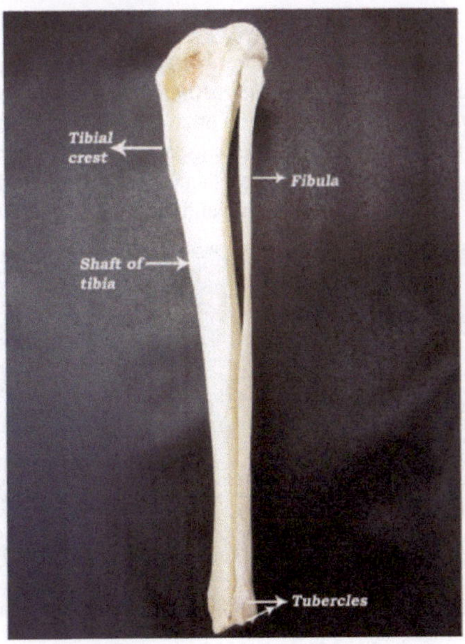

Fig. 6.19: Tibia and Fibula of Dog

Pig: The body of the tibia is slightly curved, being convex medially. The **tuberosity is grooved cranially.** The facet for the fibula is on the caudal border of the latter and is bounded medially by an eminence.

Fowl: The tibia fuses below with the upper row of tarsal bones forming the tibiotarsus. The **tibiotarsus is the longest bone** in the body. The proximal extremity is large and irregular. The distal extremity comprises of a trochlea behind and two condyles infront, representing the fused bones of the proximal row of tarsus. Distally it also shows a tendinal grove above the condyles (**Fig. 6.20**).

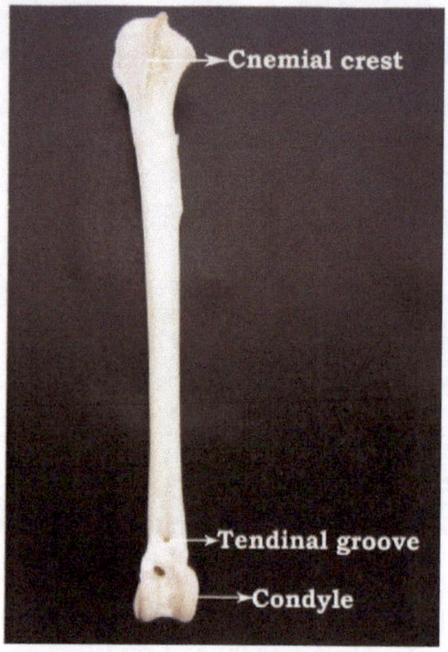

Fig. 6.20: Tibiotarsus of Fowl

FIBULA

Ox: The **fibula is rudimentary**. Its head is fused to the tibia and is continued below by a small shaft which is connected in living animal to the **distal extremity** ***(lateral malleolus)*** of the bone by fibrous cord. The **distal extremity** (**lateral malleolus**) is ***quadrilateral*** in shape. Its proximal surface is concave in front and convex behind and shows spine in the middle. It articulates with the lateral aspect of distal extremity of tibia. The **distal face** has a concave facet for the fibular tarsal. The medial face shows an articular groove which responds to the lateral ridge of the trochlea of the tibial tarsal. The **lateral face** is rough and irregular **(Fig. 6.21)**.

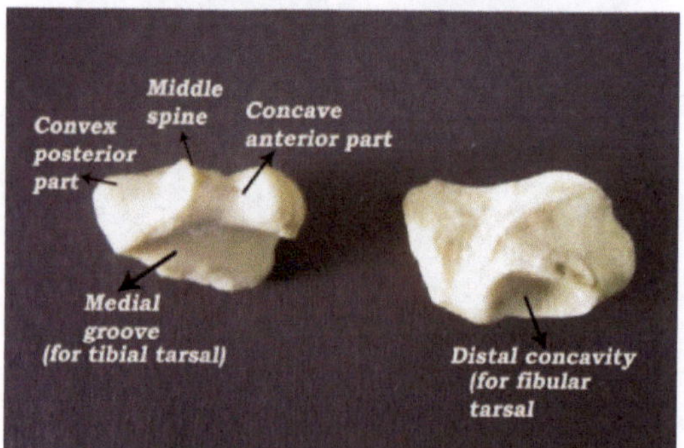

Fig. 6.21: Lateral Malleolus of Ox

Horse: The fibula is placed along the lateral border of tibia. The proximal extremity is large and flattened and bears a facet on medial face for the lateral condyle of the tibia **(Fig. 6.22)**. Its lateral face is rough. The shaft extends one half to two thirds length of tibia and ends in a pointed end. **The distal extremity (lateral malleolus) is fused to the tibia**.

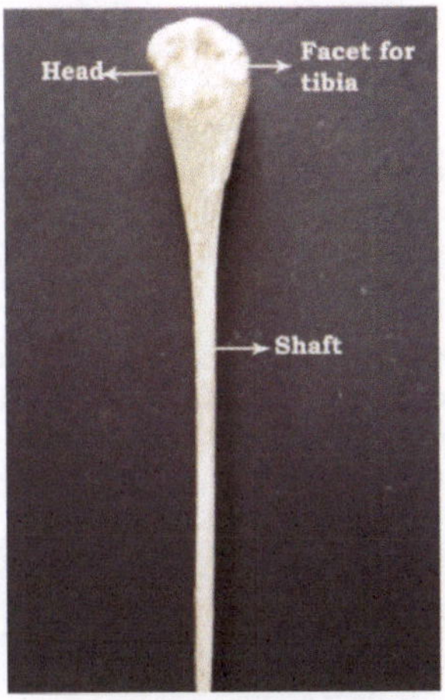

Fig. 6.22: Fibula of Horse

Dog: It is nearly as long as tibia. It is slender, somewhat twisted and enlarged at either end. The proximal and distal extremities bear facets for the tibia. The **distal extremity bears two tubercles laterally (Fig. 6.19)**.

Pig: The fibula extends the entire length of the region and is separated from the tibia by a wide interosseous space. The distal end forms the lateral malleolus. It is grooved laterally and articulates with the tibia and talus medially, and with the calcaneus distally.

Fowl: It is a thick bone reaching the lower third of the tibia. Its head is massive and articulates with lateral condyle of tibia and also above with the lateral condyle of the femur **(Fig. 6.23)**.

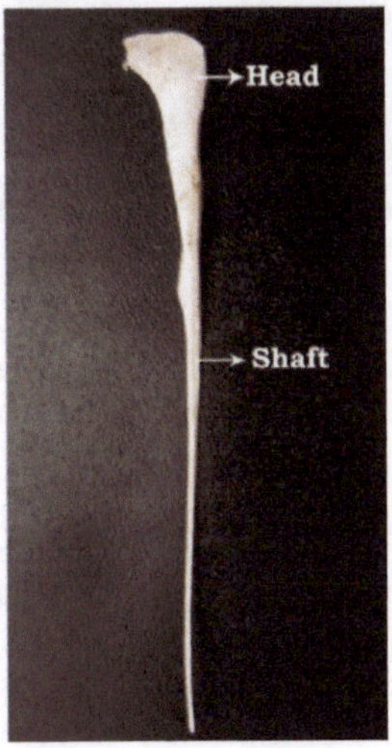

Fig. 6.23: Fibula of Fowl

TARSALS

Ox: The tarsus is composed **of five short bones** arranged in three rows **(Fig. 6.24).**

Proximal row: Tibial tarsal, fibular tarsal

Central row : Fused central and fourth

Distal row : First tarsal, fused 2nd and 3rd tarsal

Tibial tarsal (Talus): shows six surfaces. The proximal and dorsal faces are continuous and form trochlea for the tibia and lateral malleolus. The distal face articulates with fused central and 4th tarsal. Its plantar face articulates with fibular tarsal. On **posteromedial aspect** a narrow elongated area is present for articulating with ***plantar prolongation*** of fused central and 4th tarsal. The lateral face shows two facets for the fibular tarsal, while medial face is rough **(Fig. 6.24).**

Fibular tarsal (Os calcis): is ***largest tarsal*** and elongated. It is placed behind and lateral to the tibial tarsal. The **medial face of body has two facets** for the tibial tarsal, while distal face has a facet for fused central and 4th tarsal. The ***sustentaculum tali*** projects medially from body and presents a facet dorsally for tibial tarsal. The body is prolonged to form the tuber calcis which forms ***point of hock. The tuber calcis is grooved*** **(Fig. 6.24).**

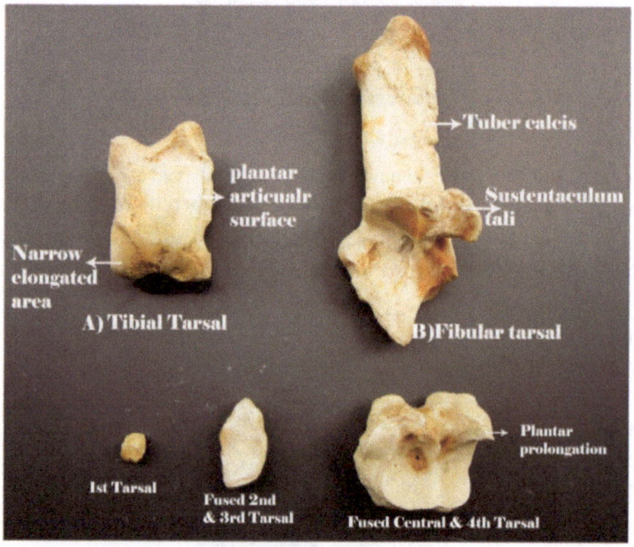

Fig. 6.24: Tarsals of Ox

Fused central and fourth tarsal: It is four sided. It shows two concave areas on ***proximal face for the tibial tarsal and a projection posteromedially*** for the narrow medial facet of the plantar face of the tibial tarsal **(Fig. 6.24).** The **distal face is uneven** and its medial half is at higher level and presents a large facet in front for fused 2 and 3rd tarsal and a small facet behind for the first tarsal. The **lateral half presents two facets** separated by a transverse groove and articulates with large metatarsal bone.

First tarsal: is a ***small quadrilateral*** piece of bone. Its proximal face articulates with the **fused central and 4th tarsal.** The distal and dorsal faces articulate with the large metatarsal and **fused 2 and 3 tarsals** respectively.

Fused 2 and 3rd tarsal: is present on medial aspect of hock. Its proximal face is concavo convex and articulates with the fused central and 4th tarsal. The distal face articulates with the large metatarsal. Its plantar face has a facet for the first tarsal. The dorsal and medial faces are continuous, convex and rough.

Horse: Tarsus consists of **six bones (Fig. 6.25).**

Proximal row : Tibial tarsal, Fibular tarsal

Central row : Central tarsal

Distal row : Fused 1st and 2nd tarsal, 3rd tarsal and 4th tarsal

Tibial tarsal: Ridges of the ***trochlea are oblique***. The lateral face has no facets for the fibular tarsal **(Fig. 6.25).**

Fibular tarsal: is short and thick. It does not articulate with lateral malleolus. The ***sustentaculum tali is larger and tuber calcis is not grooved*** **(Fig. 6.25).**

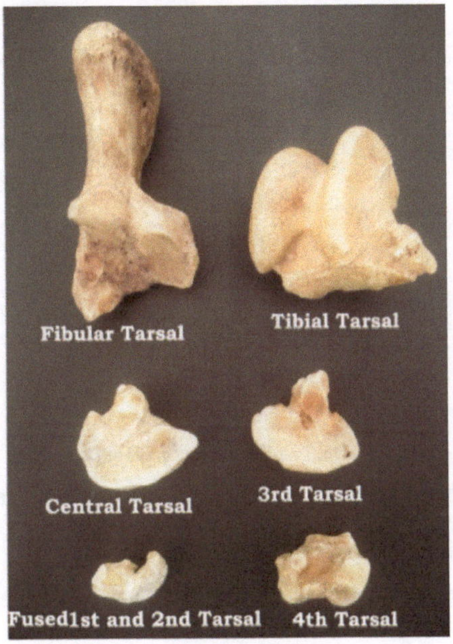

Fig. 6.25: Tarsals of Horse

Central tarsal: is flat and **irregularly quadrilateral.** Its proximal face articulates with the tibial tarsal, while distal face articulates with fused 1st and 2nd tarsal and 3rd tarsal. The lateral border presents two facets for the 4th tarsal **(Fig. 6.25).**

Fused 1st and 2nd tarsal: It is ***irregular*** in shape **(Fig. 6.25).** The medial face is convex, while lateral face is marked by a deep notch and articulates with third tarsal. The proximal face is concave and has two facets for the central tarsal, while distal face articulates with medial small metatarsal and large metatarsal. The plantar end is prolonged downwards into a nodular projection.

3rd tarsal: is triangular in outline. Its **proximal face articulates with central tarsal and distal face** articulates with **large metatarsal**. The medial border has one facet for fused ***1st and 2nd tarsal,*** while **lateral border shows two facets for the 4th tarsal.**

Fourth tarsal: is ***cuboid in shape and shows six surfaces***. The **proximal face** articulates with **tibial tarsal and fibular tarsal**. The **distal face** has two facets separated by a ridge for the **lateral small metatarsal and large metatarsal bones.** The **medial face** has facets for the **central tarsal and the 3rd tarsal (Fig. 6.25).** The dorsal, lateral and the plantar surfaces are convex and rough.

Dog: Consists of ***seven*** bones.

Proximal row : Tibial tarsal, Fibular tarsal

Central row : Central tarsal

Distal row : 1st tarsal, 2nd tarsal, 3rd tarsal, 4th tarsal

The tibial tarsal shows body, ***neck and head like in human***. The *distal row tarsal bones articulate with respective metatarsals but 4th tarsal in addition articulates with 5th metatarsal.*

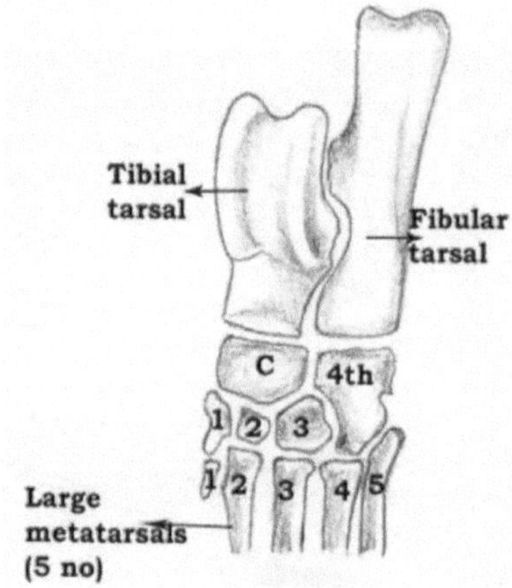

Fig. 6.26: Tarasals and Metatarsals of Dog

Pig: The tarsus comprises **seven bones**. The talus and calcaneus resemble in general those of the ox. The axis of the talus is slightly oblique (ventromedial) and its distal end bears **double trochlea** for articulation with the **central and fourth tarsals**. The **tuber calcis is deeply grooved plantarly.**

Fowl: The tarsals of proximal row fuse with the tibia, while those of the distal row fuse with the metatarsus.

METATARSUS

Ox: The metatarsus has two bones, the ***large (3rd and 4th fused)*** and ***small (second)*** metatarsal bones.The large metatarsal bone resembles the large metacarpal bone except for the following differences **(Figs. 6.27, 6.28)**.

1. It is ***longer than large metacarpal*** and shaft is four sided.
2. The ***dorsal metatarsal groove is deeper*** and plantar face presents a shallow groove. Commencing at the upper part of this groove is a ***vascular tunnel passing obliquely through proximal extremity*** and opening on its proximal surface.
3. The proximal extremity presents **laterally** a facet for the **fused central and fourth tarsal** and a large facet on the **medial aspect** for the **fused 2nd and 3rd tarsal** behind which another small facet for the **first tarsal** is present.
4. The ***posteromedial aspect of proximal extremity*** shows a small facet for the **small metatarsal bone.**
5. The dorsomedial aspect presents a tuberosity. The distal extremity resembles that of the large metacarpal.
6. The ***small metatarsal (2nd metatarsal) is a disc shaped*** structure present on ***posteromedial aspect*** of large metatarsal bone. It presents a small facet on dorsal surface for the large metatarsal bone **(Fig. 6.29)**.

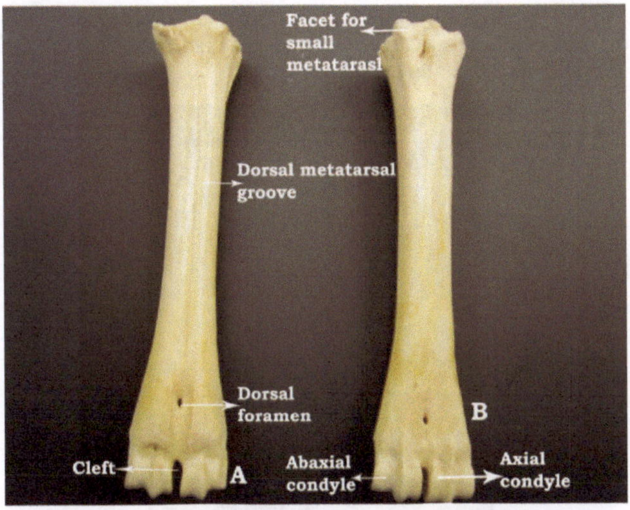

Fig. 6.27: Large Metatarsals of Ox (A-Anterior and B-Posterior view)

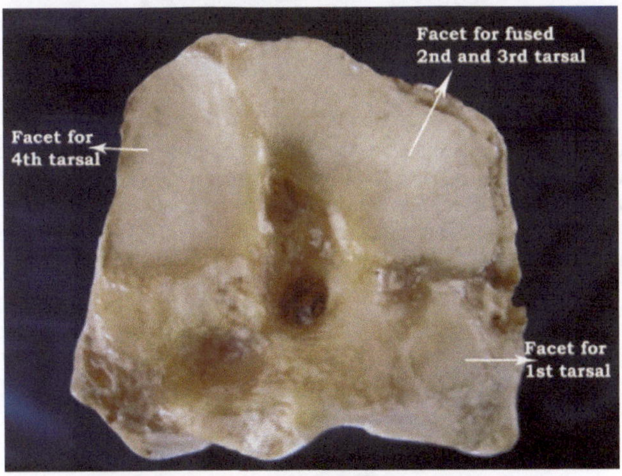

Fig. 6.28: Large Metatarsal of Ox-Proximal Extremity

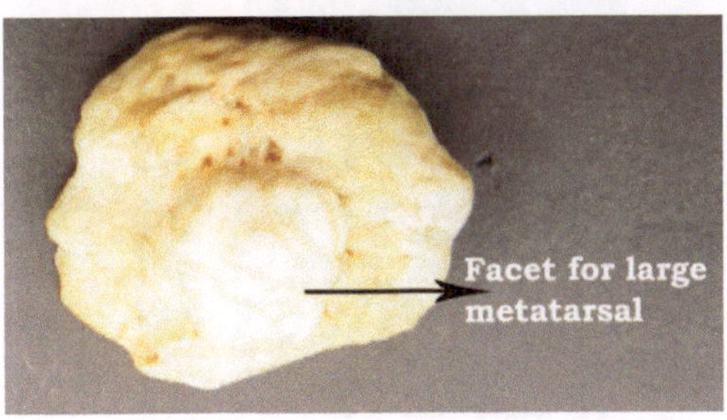

Fig. 6.29: Small Metatarsal of Ox

Horse: Has three metatarsals. One ***large (3rd) and two small (medial or second and lateral or 4th) metatarsals***. The **vertical grooves are absent** in large metatarsal and **shaft is cylindrical (Fig. 6.30)**. The proximal extremity presents facets for the **1st and 2nd tarsal, 3rd tarsal and 4th tarsal.**

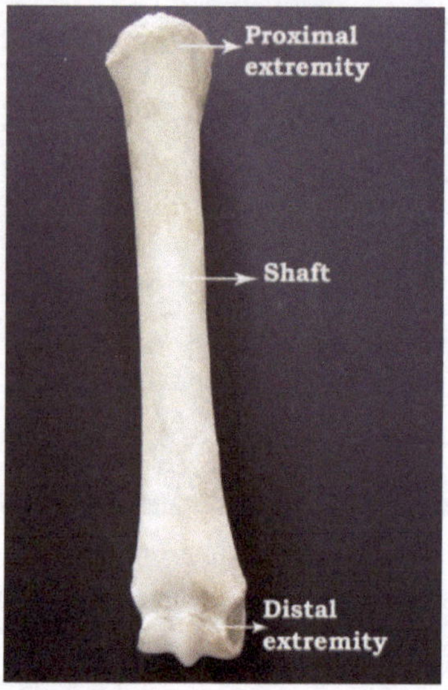

Fig. 6.30: Large Metatarsal of Horse

Both medial and lateral small metatarsals show two facets for the large metatarsal bone. The ***lateral metatarsal*** is relatively **massive especially in its upper part**. The proximal extremity is large and bears a facet for the 4th tarsal. The ***medial small metatarsal bone is more slender*** than the lateral especially in its proximal part, which bears two facets for the fused 1st and 2nd tarsal and sometimes for the 3rd tarsal **(Fig. 6.31)**. Their shafts are joined to shaft of large metatarsal by syndesmoses.

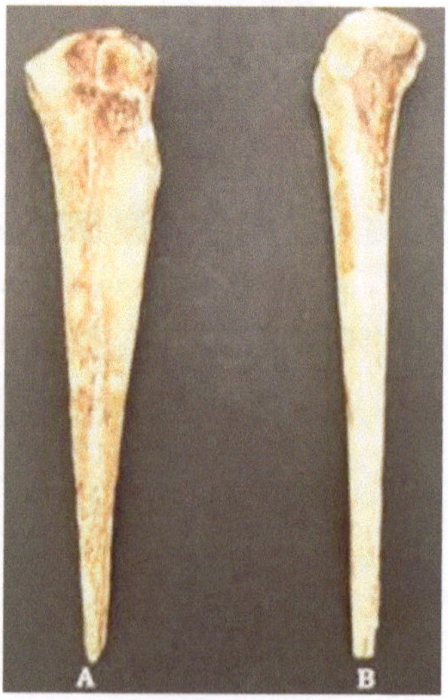

Fig. 6.31: A-Lateral and B-Medial Small metatarsals of Horse

Dog: Five metatarsals are present. The **first is small** and the other four are well developed and resemble the metacarpals **(Fig. 6.26)**. The proximal ends of the **third and fourth** show considerable plantar projections. The **second and fifth** are placed more towards the plantar aspect of 3rd and 4th than in case of forelimb.

Pig: The **four metatarsal bones** resemble the corresponding bones of the forelimb but are somewhat longer **(Fig. 6.32)**.The proximal ends or bases of the third and fourth each have a considerable plantar projection. The second and fifth are placed more toward the plantar aspect of the large bones than is the case in the forelimb.

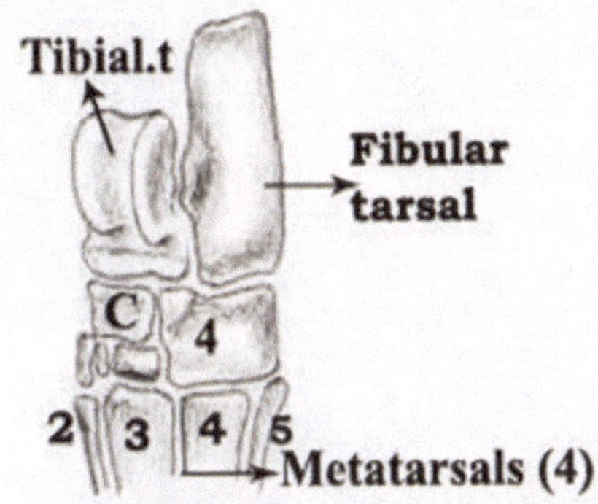

Fig. 6.32: Tarasals and Metatarsals of Pig

Fowl: The tarsometatarsus is a single bone formed by the fusion of the distal row of the tarsals with the 2nd, 3rd and 4th metatarsals. The **first metatarsal** is attached by a ligament to the **posteromedial border of lower part of the tarsometatarsus**. Above this in male is a conical projection which serves as a core for the ***horny spur or calcar*** **(Fig. 6.34)**.The ***distal extremity divides into three trochleae each representing fused 2nd, 3rd and 4th metatarsals*** **(Fig. 6.33)**. Each process is in the form of an articular convexity. The **medial one is shortest** and articulates **with the second digit**. The **middle one is the longest** and articulates **with the 3rd digit. The lateral one** articulates **with the fourth digit (Fig. 6.34)**.

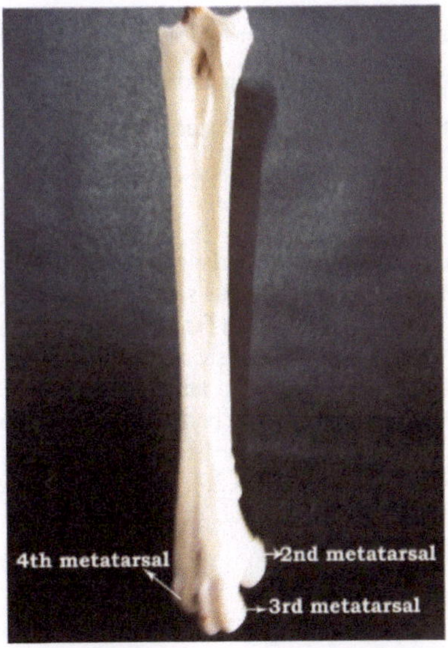

Fig. 6.33: Tarsometatarsus of Fowl

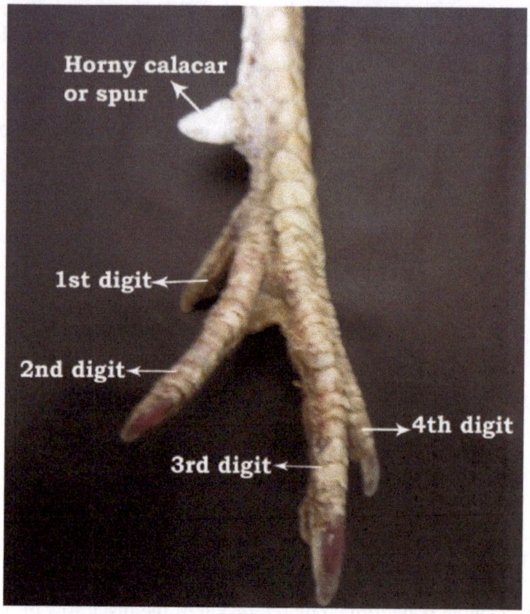

Fig. 6.34: Tarsometatarsus of Fowl with Digits

DIGITS

Ox: Resemble those of the forelimb.

Horse: compared to the phalanges of the pectoral limb the first phalanx is little short, wider above and narrow below. The proximal sesamoids are smaller and the distal sesamoids are shorter and narrower.

Dog: of the five digits the ***first is often absent***. The other four digits resemble those of the fore limb.

Pig: The proximal and middle phalanges are a little longer and narrower than those of the forelimb.

Fowl: Four digits are usually present and the number of phalanges in each digit is one more than the serial number of the respective digit.

SACRUM

Ox: It is formed by the **fusion of 5 sacral vertebrae**. It is triangular in form. It presents two surfaces, two borders, **a base and an apex**. The **dorsal surface** shows dorsal median sacral crest formed by the fusion of spinous processes of vertebrae, on either side of which the lateral sacral crest formed by the fusion of articular processes is seen. The **dorsal and ventral surfaces** show 4 dorsal and ventral sacral foramina **(Fig. 6.35)** on either side. The **ventral surface** is strongly arched and this surface is marked by a faint longitudinal groove and by transverse lines **(Fig. 6.36)**. The **base or anterior extremity** articulates with the body of the **6th lumbar vertebra** and its ventral margin projects slightly forming promontory. The lateral parts of the base are the alae or wings. **Each wing** is a **quadrilateral compressed plate** directed downward and forward **(Fig. 6.35)**. The posterior face is rough and in its lower part there is a triangular area for articulation with the ilium.

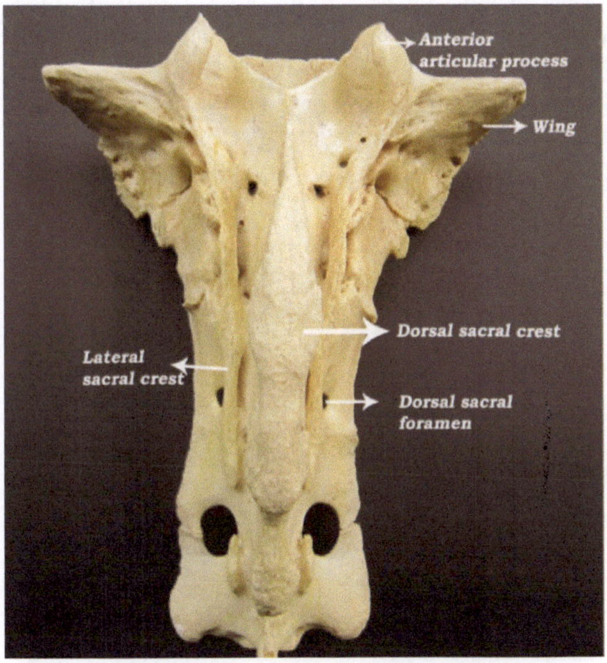

Fig. 6.35: Sacrum of Ox (Dorsal view)

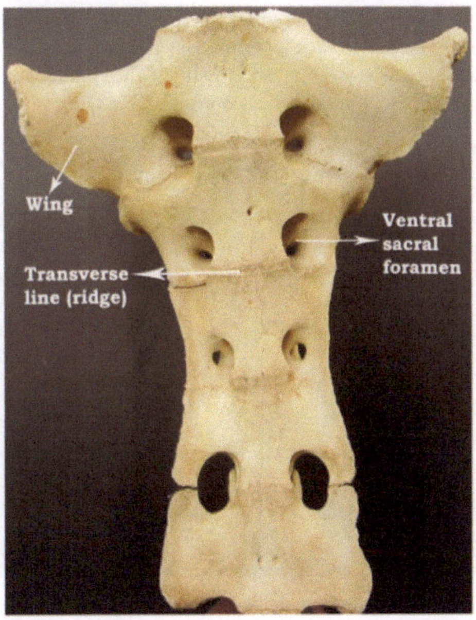

Fig. 6.36: Sacrum of Ox (Ventral view)

Horse: The sacrum presents **five dorsal spines**. The ventral surface is not so deeply arched as in the ox. The ***wings are prismatic*** with pointed ends and show **large oval facet** in front which articulates with the facet on the posterior border of the transverse process of the last lumbar vertebra **(Fig. 6.37)**.

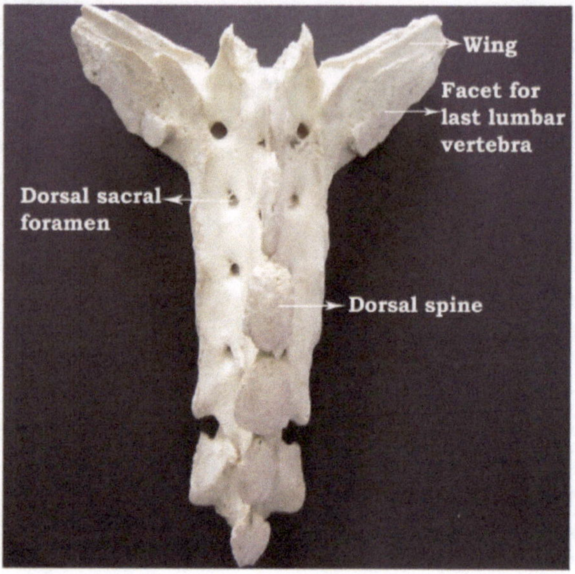

Fig. 6.37: Sacrum of Horse

Dog: It is formed by **3 bony segments**. The articular processes are vestigeal and are represented on the side of the median crest as a pair of tubercles. The **pelvic face** is deeply concave and presents **two ventral sacral foramina**. The **wings are prismatic and very high**. The promontory is distinct. The **spinal canal** is compressed dorsoventrally. The transverse processes of the last segment projects backward **(Fig. 6.38)**.

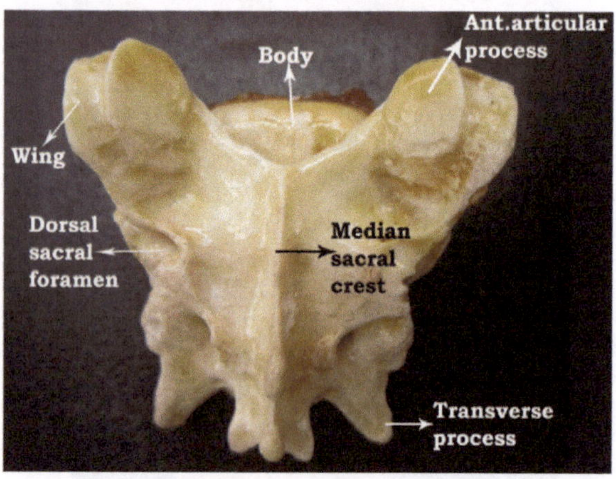

Fig. 6.38: Sacrum of Dog

Pig: consists of **four vertebrae** which fuse later. It is less curved than in the ox. The spinous processes are not well developed.

COCCYGEAL VERTEBRAE

Ox: The number varies considerably. The **first 5 or 6 are typical vertebrae** but beyond the sixth, processes and arches get gradually suppressed. The ventral surface presents a pair of processes ***called haemal processes*** between which ***sulcus vasculosus*** is present. The articular processes do not carry facets. The transverse processes are relatively large in anterior series but disappear after the 9th or 10th vertebra.

Horse: The laminae fail to meet dorsally after the fourth so that the neural arch is incomplete.

Dog: The **haemal arches** (***chevron bones***) are in the ***form of 'U' or 'Y'*** occurring ventrally at the intercentral junctions of the ***3rd, 4th and 5th*** usually. The first 3 or 4 have articular processes.

Pig: The coccygeal vertebrae are specially characterized by the presence of functional articular processes on the first four or five, beyond which these processes become non-articular and smaller.

Fowl: They are **7 in number**. First one is fused with the lumbosacral mass. The ***last is a three sided pyramid called pygostyle.*** It forms foundation for the feathers of the tail and **preen gland**. The **intermediate ones (2-6) are typical** and transverse processes are well developed and the spines are bifurcated.

6.2 JOINTS OF THE PELVIS AND HIND LIMB

SACROILIAC ARTICULATION

Articular areas: Posterior aspect of wing of sacrum and pelvic surface of ilium

Type: Simple, diarthrodial.

Ligaments

1. Tightly attached capsular ligament.
2. **Dorsal sacroiliac ligament** shows two parts i.e **a)** Short part ***(pars brevis)*** **and b)** long part ***(pars longa)*** between **sacral spines and tuber sacrale** and between **lateral border of sacrum and upper part of the ischiatic border of ilium (Fig. 6.39).**
3. **Ventral sacroiliac ligament** lies on ventral aspect of joint and extends between ilium and wing of sacrum.

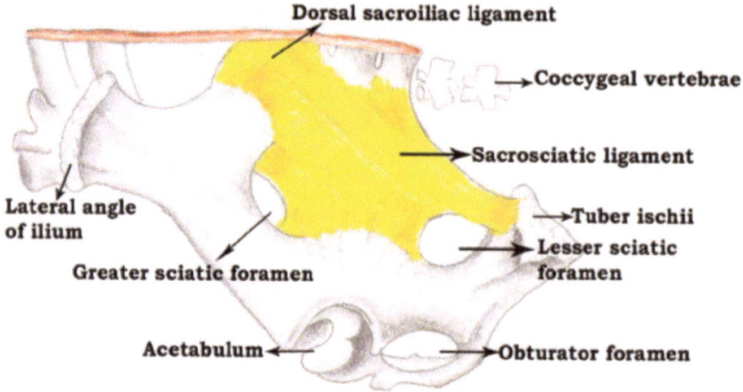

Fig. 6.39: Ligaments of Sacroiliac Articulation

4. **Broad sacrosciatic ligament** present between lateral border of sacrum and first 2 or 3 caudal vertebrae on one end and tuber ischii at other end attaching halfway below to ischiatic spine converting greater and lesser sciatic notches into greater and lesser sciatic foramina respectively. It **forms lateral wall of pelvis** and consists of two parts. The one part inserts on tuber ischii and another part inserts on ischiatic spine. The cranial border of the latter is concave and with the greater sciatic notch forms greater sciatic foramen, while the former forms lesser sciatic foarmen with lesser sciatic notch. ***In ox, the caudal border of sacrosciatic ligament is prominent under the skin resulting in ischiorectal fossa between root of tail and tuber ischii as it is not covered by ischiatic muscles unlike in horse and pig. Shortly before parturition this normally taut ligament slackens off and feels soft on palpation.***

4. **Lateral sacroiliac ligament** between lateral border of sacrum and upper part of the ischiatic border of ilium.

Movements: Inappreciable.

HIP JOINT

Articular areas: acetabulum of oscoxae and head of the femur

Type: Simple, diarthrodial (ball and socket / enarthroses)

Ligaments

1. **Capsular ligament.**
2. **Cotyloid ligament** which is nothing but a marginal (fibro) cartilage around the rim of acetabulum deepening it and converting acetabular notch into a foramen. The part of the cotyloid ligament over the notch is called **transverse acetabular** ligament **(Fig. 6.40).**
3. **Round ligment attached to fovea capitis at one end** shows three attachments at other end i.e a) Strongest from outer acetabular margin around the notch and transverse ligament b) few fibers from acetabular fossa c) others from groove on ventral surface of ischium

Movements: Extension, flexion, rotation, circumduction, abduction and adduction.

***In horse there is also an *accessory / pubio-femoral ligament which limits side kicking* (Fig. 6.40).**

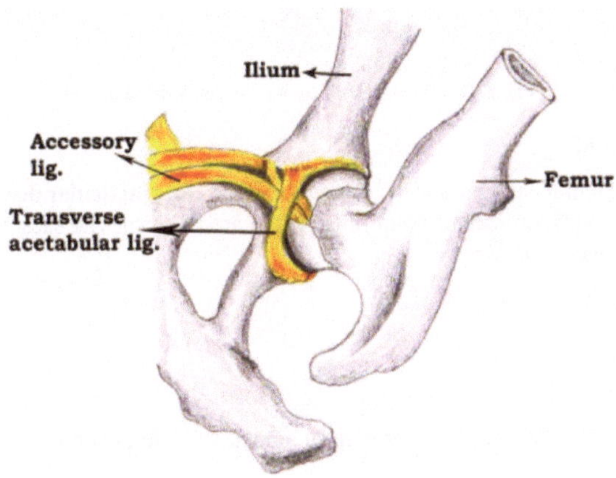

Fig. 6.40: Hip Joint of Horse

STIFLE JOINT

Stifle joint is a composite joint and consists of **femoropatellar and femorotibial** articulations.

a. Femoropatellar articulation:

Articular areas: Trochlea of femur and patella.

Type: Diarthrodial (arthrodia).

Ligaments

1. Capsular ligament,

2 & 3 The medial and lateral (collateral) femoropatellar ligaments from respective femoral condyle to respective angles of patella

4. Three (medial, middle and lateral) straight ligaments attaching base of the patella to the tibial tuberosity. They are nothing but insertions (tendons) of quadriceps femoris muscle (Fig. 6.41).

Movements: ***Gliding. Proximal fixation of patella and its fibrocartilage occurs in ox due to asymmetry of trochlear ridges of femur, which has to be relieved by sectioning medial patellar ligament.***

* **Note:** ***In dog, sheep and goat there is only one straight ligament.***

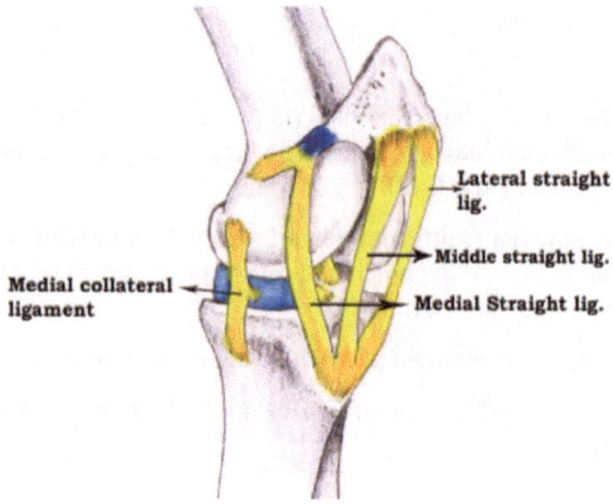

Fig. 6.41: Ligaments of Femoro-patellar Articulation

b. Femorotibial articulation:

Articular areas: condyles of femur and tibia and ***"C" shaped menisci*** (**interarticular discs**) which are fibrocartilages present between respective condyles of femur and tibia. There are two synovial sacs and each is divided into an upper and lower compartments by the meniscus.

Type: Simple, diarthrodial (hinge) joint.

Ligaments

1. Capsular ligament

2 & 3 **Medial and lateral collateral ligaments** from medial and lateral condyles of femur to medial condyle of tibia and fibula respectively.

4. **The anterior cruciate ligament** extends from summit of tibial spine passes upward and backward to posterior part of intercondyloid fossa of femur close to lateral condyle **(Fig. 6.42)**.

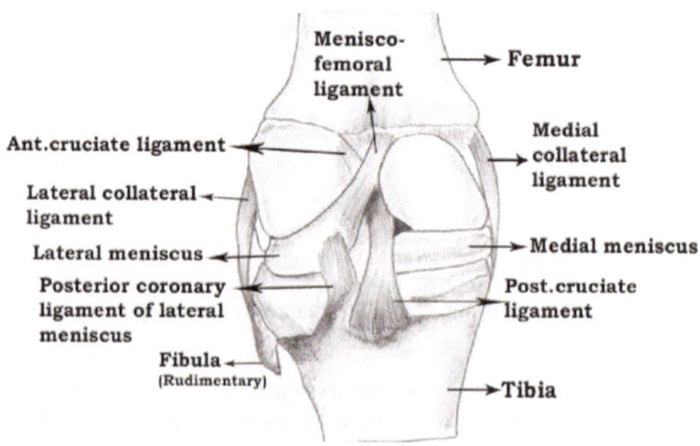

Fig. 6.42: Stifle Joint of Ox

5. **The posterior cruciate ligament** extends from a tubercle medial to popliteal notch passes upward and forward to anterior part of intercondyloid fossa **(Fig. 6.42)**. (***The cruciate ligaments are named cranial and caudal according to their attachment on tibia***)

6. **The anterior and posterior coronary** ligaments one each attach respective parts of two menisci to areas in front and behind the tibial spine. The lateral meniscus in addition shows third (***posterosuperior coronary / meniscofemoral***) ligament which attaches to posterior part of intercondyloid fossa close to the medial condyle of the femur **(Fig. 6.42)**.

7. **The strong posterior ligament** reinforces posterior aspect of the joint capsule.

Movements: Extension and Flexion.

* ***In addition in buffaloes there is an additional ligament in stifle joint that lies just lateral to the anterior cruciate ligament extending from tibial spine to the medial part of posterior part of intercondyloid fossa of femur*** **(Fig. 6.43)**.

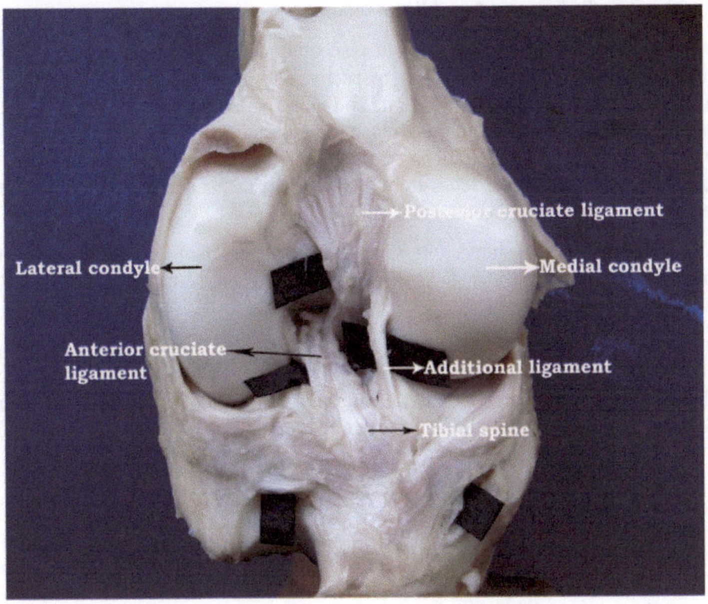

Fig. 6.43: Stifle Joint of Buffalo with an Additional Ligament

4. Tibiofibular articulations

Proximal: The head of the fibula fuses with the lateral condyle of the tibia.

Distal: distal extremity of fibula (lateral malleolus) articulates with tibia above, tibial tarsal medially and distally with fibular tarsal.

Movements: Inappreciable

HOCK JOINT

Articular areas: Tibia, **fibula *(lateral malleolus)*** tibial tarsal, fibular tarsal, fused central and 4th tarsal, 1st tarsal, fused 2 and 3rd tarsal and large metatarsal. The joint cavity is subdivided into many compartments due to presence of number of bones.

Type: Composite, diarthrodial.

It consists of **a. Tibio tarsal** (Tarso crural) articulation: Between distal extremity of tibia and fibula (lateral malleolus) and tibial tarsal and fibular tarsal. The **tuber calcis forms point of hock.**

b. **Proximal tarsal**: Between lateral and plantar aspects of tibial tarsal and fibular tarsal.

c. **Proximal intertarsal**: Between tibial tarsal and fibular tarsals above and fused central and 4th tarsal below.

d. **Distal intertarsal**: Between central and 4th tarsal above and 1st and fused 2 and 3rd tarsals below.

e. **Distal tarsal**: Between 1st and fused 2nd and 3rd tarsals of distal row.

f. **Tarsometatarsal**: Between 1st and fused 2nd and 3rd tarsal above and large metatarsal below.

Type: Diarthrodial ("a" is hinge type while b-f are arthrodia type).

Ligaments

1. **Capsular ligament** (***called plantar tarsal ligament*** on posterior aspect).
2. **Medial and lateral collateral ligaments** from respective aspects of distal extremity of tibia and fibula (**lateral malleolus and also fibular tarsal**) to respective aspects of proximal extremity of large metatarsal. The **medial collateral ligament** shows two (long and short) parts. The **superficial layer** of long part extends from medial malleolus to sustentaculum tali, plantaromedial projection of central and fourth tarsal, then to large metatarsal. The deeper layer of long part goes to tibial tarsal, fused central and fourth tarsal and finally to large metatarsal. The short part extends from medial malleolus and ends on sustentaculum tali, talus and plantaromedial projection of fused central and 4th tarsal.
3. **The lateral collateral ligament** shows long superficial part extending from lateral malleolus to calcaneus, fused central and 4th tarsal and then to large metatarsal and the short deep part extending from lateral malleolus to fibular tarsal **(Fig. 6.44)**.
4. **The calcaneometatarsal** (***long plantar***) ligament extends along posterior aspect of fibular tarsal, central and fourth tarsal to large metatarsal. The plantar annular ligament (flexor retinaculum) extends across from medial collateral ligament and large metatarsal to fused central and 4th tarsal, sustentaculum tali of fibular tarsal and long plantar ligament and forms posterior boundary of tarsal sheath/canal, (**Fig. 6.44**).

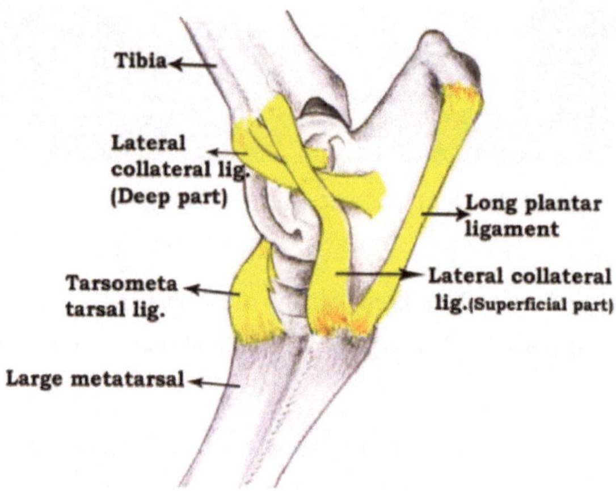

Fig. 6.44: Ligaments of Hock Joint

5. The **tarsometatarsal ligament** blends above with plantar tarsal ligament **(Fig. 6.44)**.

Movements: Extension & flexion in **Tibio tarsal** articulation & gliding in remaining joints i.e in b-d joints.

Tarsal canal: is formed in front by the **tarso-metatarsal ligament** blending with capsular ligament and **behind by the plantar annular ligament**. This canal is for passage of the tendon of **deep digital flexor, medial plantar arteries and nerves (Fig. 6.45)**.

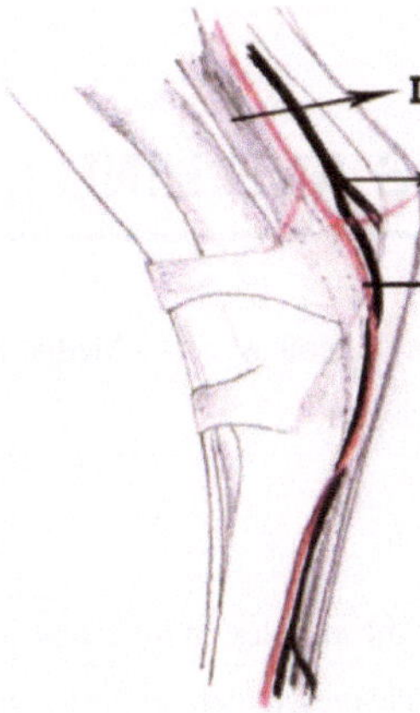

Fig. 6.45: Structures of Tarsal Canal

Intermetatarsal joint: is a simple diarthrodial joint between facet on posteromedial aspect of proximal extremity of large metatarsal and facet on discoidal small metatarsal. The movements are inappreciable.

FETLOCK, PASTERN AND COFFIN JOINTS: resemble those in forelimb.

6.3 MUSCLES OF THE PELVIS AND HIND LIMB

These are grouped into 1. Muscles of the hip and thigh a) Lateral aspect b) Medial aspect.

2. Muscles of the leg and foot a) dorsolateral b) plantar aspect.

Muscles of the Hip and Thigh

The Lateral Aspect: (Fig.6.46)

1. **Tensor fasciae latae**: This is the most anterior of the muscles on the lateral aspect of the hip and thigh.
2. **Biceps femoris:** This is a large quadrilateral muscle present behind the tensor fasciae latae.
3. **Gluteus medius (middle gluteus):** This muscle is partly covered by the preceding
4. **Gluteus profundus (Deep gluteus):** This muscle is completely under cover of the preceding.
5. **Semitendinosus:** It is a very long muscle extending from the tuber ischii to the leg, behind the biceps femoris.

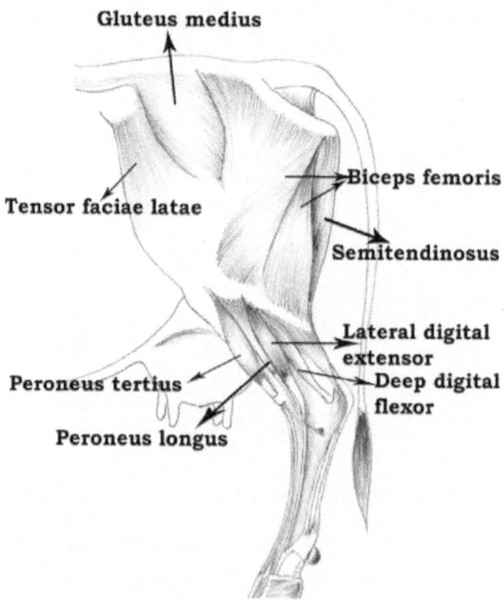

Fig. 6.46: Muscles of Hip and Thigh of Ox-Lateral Aspect

The Medial Aspect: They are arranged in three layers **(Fig.6.47).**

First layer

1. **Sartorius:** This is a long muscle and is the anterior of the two muscles of this layer.
2. **Gracilis:** This muscle is extensively united to its fellow at the origin and is the larger and wider of the two muscles of this layer.

Second layer

1. **Pectineus:** It is a small conical muscle situated under the gracillis.

   Femoral canal: is a muscular canal bounded in ***front by the Sartorius, behind by the pectineus, laterally by the ilio psoas and vastus medialis and medially by the gracilis***. The upper opeining of this canal is the femoral ring. It is bounded in front by the ***Poupart's ligament*** behind by the anterior border of the pubis and laterally by the tendon of psoas minor. It lodges the **femoral vessels, saphenous artery, vein and nerve**.The canal terminates below at the lower part of the insertion of the pectineus.

2. **Adductor:** is present on ventral surface of the pubis and ischium.

3. **Semimembranosus:** This is very large **quadrilateral muscle** situated behind the adductor and between it and the semitendinosus.

Third Layer

1. **Quadratus femoris**: It is a narrow short muscle present under cover of the origin of the adductor and semimembranosus.

2. **Obturator externus:** This muscle is made up of coarse muscular bundles situated around the obturator foramen on the ventral surface of the ischium.

3. **Obturator internus:** This muscle is extensive and is situated on the pelvic surface of the ischium.

4. **Gemellus:** This is a small muscle extending from the ventral surface of the ischium to the trochanteric fossa.

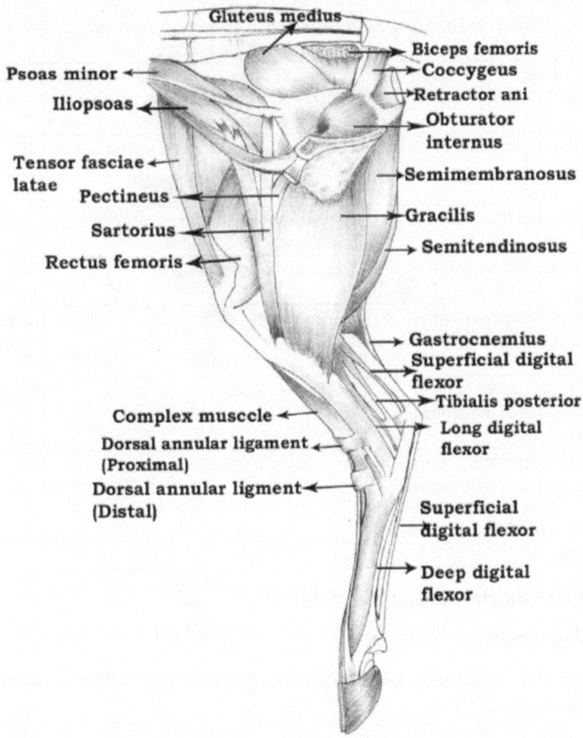

Fig. 6.47: Muscles of Thigh and Leg of Ox-Medial view

THE MUSCLES OF HIP AND THIGH (Figs: 6.46,6.47)

Name of the muscle	Origin	Insertion	Action
Lateral aspect			
Tensor fasciae latae	Lateral angle of ilium	Fascia lata and indirectly to the patella, the lateral patellar ligament and the cranial border of tibia.	Tense the fascia and flex the hip and extend the stifle.
Biceps femoris	Sacral spines, sacrosciatic ligament, tuber ischii and gluteal fascia.	The lower part of the muscle is succeded by three aponeurotic tendons which are inserted to the patella, tibial crest and fascia lata.	To extend the limb as in kicking and propulsion and to extend the stifle, hip and hock
Gluteus medius (middle gluteus)	Lateral angle of the ilium, sacrosciatic ligament, gluteal surface of the ilium and gluteal fascia.	1) By a strong tendon to the summit of the troachanter major 2) By a short tendon to the area below the trochanter major (3) By a fleshy insertion to the trochanteric ridge.	To extend the hip and abduct the limb to assist in kicking and propulsion.
Gluteus profundus (Deep gluteus)	Lateral angle of the ilium and the gluteal surface in front of the gluteal line and the lateral surface of the ischiatic spine.	A tubercle a little below the base of the trochanter major below the insertion of middle gluteus	To abduct the limb and rotate it inwards
Semitendinosus	Ventral surface of the tuber ischii	Tibial crest and fascia lata	To extend the hip and assist in kicking and propulsion
Medial aspect			
Sartorius	By two heads from iliac fascia and the tendon of psoas minor.	Medial straight ligament of patella and the fascia lata and the tuberosity of tibia.	to flex the hip and adduct the limb
Gracilis	Pelvic symphysis and prepubic tendon	Medial patellar ligament, medial surface of the tibia and fascia lata.	To adduct the limb
Pectineus	Ventral surface of the pubis and the prepubic tendon.	The middle of the medial border of the posterior surface of the femur and the medial epicondyle.	To adduct the limb, flex hip and rotate the femur inwards
Adductor	Ventral surface of the pubis and ischium	The lateral part of the posterior surface of the femur	To adduct the limb extend the hip and rotate the femur inwards.
Semimembranosus	Ventral face of the ischium and the tuber ischii.	Medial epicondyle of the femur and the medial condyle of the tibia	To extend the hip and adduct the limb
Quadratus femoris	Ventral face of the ischium	Trochanter minor of the femur	To extend the hip and adduct the thigh
Obturator externus	Ventral surface of ischium and pubis around the obturator foramen	Trochanteric fossa.	To adduct the thigh and rotate it outwards
Obturator Internus:	Pelvic surface of the ischium and pubis around the obturator foramen.	Trochanteric fossa.	To rotate the femur outwards
Gemellus	Lateral border of the ischium at the lesser sacro-sciatic foramen and from the lateral face of the posterior part of the sacro-sciatic ligament.	Trochanteric fossa	To rotate the femur outwards

The Muscles of the Thigh (Anterior Aspect, Fig.6.46)

1. Sartorius (already described)
2. **Quadriceps femoris**: This is a massive muscle composed of **total four divisions** situated around the anterior, medial and lateral faces of the femur.

a. **Rectus femoris**: is rounded.

b. Vastus lateralis: lies on the lateral surface of the femur

c. Vastus medialis: is present on the medial surface of the femur

d. Vastus intermedius: situated deeply on the anterior face of the femur covered by the preceeding divisions.

Note: The three straight ligaments of the patella are in fact the tendons of insertion of the quadriceps muscle; the patella being developed as a sesamoid bone in the tendons.

3. **Articularis genu**: This is a very small muscle situated at the lower third of the anterior surface of the femur under cover of the vastus intermedius.

Name of the muscle	Origin	Insertion	Action
Muscles of the Thigh-Anterior aspect			
1.Quadriceps femoris: a. Rectus femoris:	By two heads from the two depressions at the lower most part of the cotyloid border of the ilium, above and in front of the acetabulum.	The base and anterior surface of the patella	To extend the stifle and to flex the hip.
b. Vastus lateralis	Lateral border and surface of the femur from the great trochanter to the supracondyloid fossa.	The lateral part of the anterior surface of the patella and lateral patellar ligament.	To extend the stifle joint.
c. Vastus medialis	The medial face of the neck of the femur to the middle of the caudal surface of the femur.	Craniomedial surface of the patella and medial patellar ligament.	To extend the stifle joint.
d.Vastus intermedius	Anterior surface of the femur	Base of the patella and femoropatellar ligaments.	To extend the stifle and raise the capsule during extension of the joint.
2. Articularis genu	Lower part of anterior face of the femur	Femoro-patellar capsule	To raise the joint capsule of stifle.

THE MUSCLES OF THE LEG AND FOOT

The Dorsolateral Group: (Fig.6.47)

1. **Complex muscle**: This muscle is situated on the ***dorsolateral aspect*** of the leg. The muscular belly of this muscle divides below into three divisions i.e peroneus tertius, long digital extensor and medial digital extensor

   a. **Peroneus tertius**: is the **most superficial part**. It is succeeded by a strong flat tendon which is perforated by the tendon of the tibialis anterior. It is inserted to the tubercle at the dorsomedial aspect of the proximal extremity of the large metatarsal bone.

   b. **Long digital extensor** (extensor digitalis longus) is lateral to the preceeding. It is succeeded by a tendon which resembles the tendon of common digital extensor of the forelimb in its course and termination.

   c. **Medial digital extensor** is under cover of the preceeding two divisions. It is succeeded by a tendon which resembles that of the forelimb in its course and termination. The long and medial digital extensors have a common synovial sheath at the tarsus.

2. **Tibialis anterior:** This muscle lies under cover of the complex muscle on the lateral surface of the tibia and arises by two heads.Its tendon passes through the tendon of the peroneous tertius.

3. **Peroneus longus:** This muscle is situated between the peroneus tertius and lateral digital extensor.

4. **Lateral digital extensor:** It is situated lateral to the preceeding and is successed by a tendon which passes through synovial sheath in common with that of the preceeding muscle, crosses under that tendon and thereafter it resembles the tendon of the muscle of the fore limb in its course and termination.

5. **Extensor digitalis brevis:** It is a narrow muscle present on the dorsal surface of the metatarsus.

THE PLANTAR GROUP: (Fig.6.47)

Superficial layer

1. **Gastrocnemius:** It is a large muscle with two heads of origin. By a twist in the tendon at the lower third the tendon of superficial flexor lies behind the tendon of the gastrocnemius. The two tendons are together called as ***tendo calcaneous or hamstring or tendo achilles.***
2. **Soleus:** This is very small muscle situated along the lateral border of the lateral head of the gastrocnemius.

Deep layer

1. **Superficial digital flexor:** This muscle is very closely blended with the lateral head of the gastrocnemius. It passes over the summit of the tuber calcis, detaching two slips attached to it and passes down the metatarsal region and appears in the same way as in the fore limb.
2. **Deep digital flexor:** This muscle is situated on posterior face of the tibia and is made up of three heads. The superficial head is termed ***tibialis posterior***, the deep head is ***flexor hallucis*** and the medial head is the ***long digital flexor***. The tendons of superficial and deep heads unite above the tarsus and the common tendon passes through tarsal sheath and then descends in the metatarsal region.

THE MUSCLES OF THE LEG AND FOOT

Name of the muscle	Origin	Insertion	Action
Dorsolateral Group:			
Complex muscle	By a strong tendon from the extensor fossa of the femur	**Peroneus tertius**: Dorsomedial tubercle of proximal extremity of large metatarsal. **Long digital extensor**: Extensor process of 3rd phalanx of both digits. **Medial digital extensor**: 2nd and 3rd phalanges of medial digit.	Flex the hock. Flex the hock and extend the fetlock, pastern and coffin joints of the both the digits and approximate two digits flex the hock and extend the fetlock pastern and coffin joints of the medial digit. and abduct the medial digit
Tibialis anterior:	Tibial tuberosity and tibial crest: upper part of the lateral border of the tibia and the fibrous cord of fibula	The postero medial surface of the upper extremity of the large metatarsal and the second and third tarsal bones.	Flex the hock.
Peroneus longus	Lateral condyle of the tibia and the fibrous cord of the fibula	First tarsal and proximal end of the large metatarsal bone	Rotate the hock inwards.
Lateral digital extensor	Lateral ligament of the stifle and the lateral condyle of the tibia.	2nd and 3rd phalanges of lateral digit.	Flex the hock and extend the fetlock pastern and coffin joints of the lateral digit. and abduct the lateral digit
Extensor digitalis brevis	Depression on the dorsal surface of the metatarsus	Tendon of long digital extensor	Assist the long digital extensor in its action.
Plantar Group:			
Gastrocnemius:	The medial supracondyloid crest and the outer edge of the supracondyloid fossa.	Summit of the tubercalcis	Extend the hock.
Soleus	Lateral condyle of the tibia and proximal extremity of fibula.	Lateral head of gastrocnemius muscle	Assist the gastrocnemius in its action.
Popliteus	Lower depression on the lateral condyle of femur	Popliteal line on upper part of the posterior surface of tibia.	Flex the stifle and rotate the leg. inwards.

Superficial digital flexor	The supracondyloid fossa of femur.	Plantar aspect of 2nd phalanx of both the digits.	Extend the hock and flex the fetlock and pastren joints.
Deep digital flexor	Lateral border and posterior face of tibia, lateral condyle of the tibia and the fibrous cord of the fibula.	Plantar aspect of 3rd phalanx of both the digits.	Extend the hock and flex the fetlock, pastern and coffin joints.

THE MUSCLES OF THE TAIL

These muscles are situated around the tail enclosed in the coccygeal fascia.

1. **Coccygeus:** is included in the fold at the ventral aspect of the base of the tail.
2. **Sacro-coccygeus dorsalis:** is situated on the dorsal aspect of the tail with its fellow on either side of spines.
3. **Sacro-coccygeus lateralis:** is situated lateral to the preceding.
4. **Intertransversales caudae:** present between the transvese processes of adjacent veretebrae.
5. **Sacro-coccygeus ventralis:** is situated on the ventral aspect of the tail. It consists of two parts medial and lateral.
6. **Recto coccygeus:** It is large band of plain muscle and detached on either side from the longitudinal layer of the muscular coat of rectum to the fourth and fifth coccygeal vertebrae.

Name of the muscle	Origin	Insertion	Action
Coccygeus	Pelvic surface of the sacro-sciatic ligament, near the ischiatic spine.	The transverse processes of the second and third coccygeal vertebrae.	compress the anus, depress the tail over the perineum and flex laterally.
Sacro-coccygeus dorsalis	The last one or two sacral spines	The upper faces of the bodies of the coccygeal vertebrae, beyond third coccygeal vertebra.	elevate the tail and to incline it laterally
Sacro-coccygeus lateralis	Transverse processes of the sacral and coccygeal vertebrae.	Lateral faces of the vertebrae, except the first three	elevate the tail and flex laterally.
Intertransversales caudae	The lateral broder of the sacrum and the transverse processes of adjacent coccygeal vertebrae.	Tranverse process of the first coccygeal and the transverse process of the vertebra behind.	flex the tail laterally.
Sacro-coccygeus ventralis	Transverse process of fifth sacral vertebra.	Medial part is inserted to bodies of coccygeal vertebrae, lateral part is inserted to bodies and transverse processes of coccygeal vertebrae.	depress the tail.
Rectococcygeus	Muscular coat of rectum	4th and 5th coccygeal vertebrae	shorten the rectum and helps in evacuation of its contents.

6.4 BLOOD SUPPLY TO THE PELVIS AND HIND LIMB

The Internal Iliac Artery

It is the main arterial trunk which supplies the **pelvic wall and viscera**. Each artery passes obliquely downwards and backwards on the sacrosciatic ligament and terminates about the level of the lesser sciatic foramen by dividing into **posterior gluteal and internal pudic arteries.**

Collateral branches

1. **A large common trunk** which divides into ***umbilical and middle uterine artery in female/deferential artery in male***. The ***middle uterine artery*** in *female supplies greater part of the uterus (***Figs.6.48, 6.50, 6.51***), while* ***deferential artery*** *in male supplies vas deferens* **(Fig.6.49).**

> *The uterine artery increases in size during pregnancy. A palpable pulsation can be detected in the artery when palpated per rectum in a cow in third month of pregnancy. This pulsation is diagnostic of pregnancy and is referred to as "**whirling, thrill or fremitus**".*

The ***umbilical artery*** gives off small branch to **ureter and slender cranial vesical branch to the urinary bladder**. The **umbilical artery** is usually obliterated in the adult. In the foetus it is large and runs in the free margin of the lateral ligament of the bladder, passes through the umbilicus and ramifies in the placenta carrying impure blood for oxygenation. As this artery is no longer required after birth, it gradually gets atrophied and the lumen is obliterated. The obliterated part of the vessel forms the ***round ligament of the bladder***.

2. **A short common trunk** which divides into (a) **the sixth lumbar artery (b) lateral sacral artery** (If the middle sacral artery is absent) (c) **anterior gluteal artery** which passes out through the greater sacrosciatic foramen and supplies **middle gluteus and deep gluteus.**

3. **Vesicogenital artery** arises from the ventral face of the internal iliac artery near hip joint. It gives off *prostate artery in male / vaginal artery* in female and **caudal vesical artery** to **urinary bladder**. The ***prostatic artery*** gives off braches to seminal vesicle, urethra, prostate and Cowper's glands **(Figs.6.48, 6.49).**

The ***vaginal artery*** gives off posterior ***uterine branch supplying caudal part of body of uterus and cervix***, gives branches to urethra, vagina and ends into middle rectal and dorsal perineal artery (**Figs.6.48, 6.50, 6.51**). The latter ends in caudal rectal branches to caudal part of rectum and dorsal labial branch to labium of vulva **(Figs.6.48, 6.50)**.

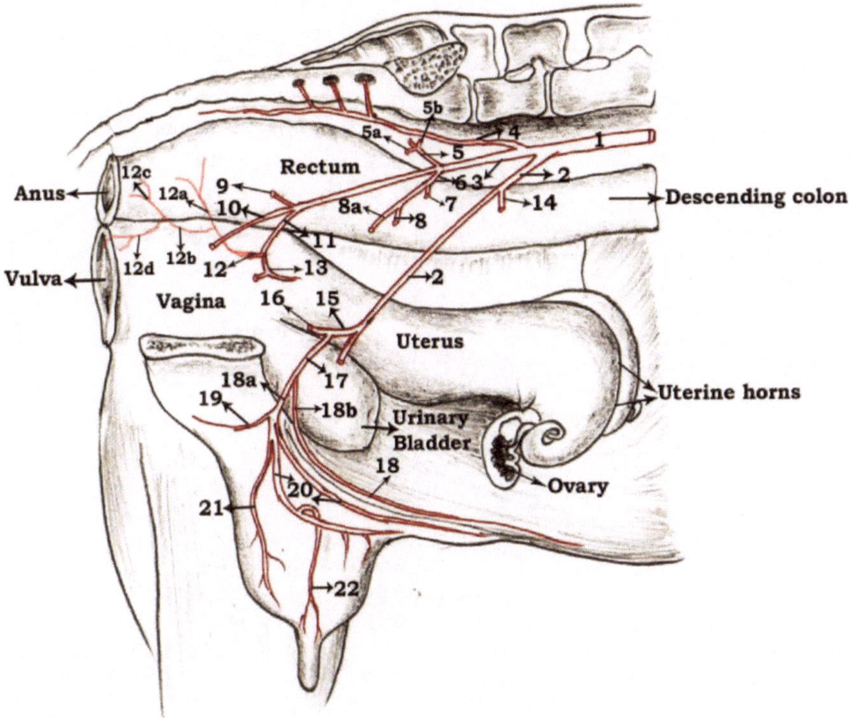

Fig. 6.48: Branches of Internal Iliac Artery in Female

1. Abdominal aorta	12a. Middle rectal artery
2. External iliac artery	12b. Dorsal perineal artery
3. Internal Iliac artery	12c. Caudal rectal artery
4. Median sacral artery	12d. Dorsal labial artery
5. Short common trunk	13. Caudal uterine artery
5a. Anterior gluteal artery	14. Circumflex iliac artery
5b. Sixth lumbar artery	15. Common trunk
6. Large common trunk	16. Deep femoral artery
7. Ureteric branch	17. Prepubic artery
8. Middle uterine artery	18a. External pudic (mammary) artery
8a. Umbilical artery	18b. Posterior abdominal artery
9. Posterior gluteal artery	19. Branch to mammary lymph node
10. Internal pudic artery	20.Cranial mammary artery
11. Vesicogenital artery	21. Caudal mammary artery
12. Vaginal artery	22. Papillary artery

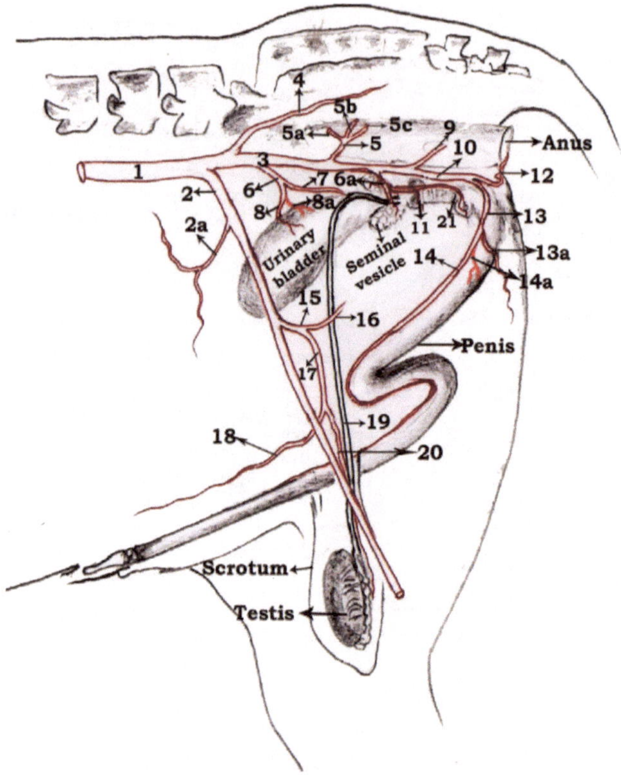

Fig. 6.49: Branches of Internal Iliac Artery in Male

1. Abdominal aorta	10. Internal pudic artery
2. External iliac artery	11. Prostate artery
2a. Circumflex iliac artery	12. Dorsal perineal artery
3. Internal Iliac artery	13. Artery of the bulb of the penis
4. Median sacral artery	13a. Ventral perineal artery
5. Short common trunk	14. Dorsal artery of the penis
5a.Anterior gluteal artery	14a. Deep artery of penis
5b. Sixth lumbar artery	15. Common trunk
6. Large common trunk	16. Deep femoral artery
6a.Vesicogenital artery	17. Prepubic artery
7. Deferential artery	18. Posterior abdominal artery
8. Umbilical artery	19. Vas deferens
8a.Cranial vesical artery	20. External pudic artery
9. Posterior gluteal artery	21. Branch to Cowper's gland from prostate artery.

After giving the above collateral branches the internal iliac artery finally terminates by dividing into posterior gluteal and internal pudic arteries.

TERMINAL BRANCHES

1. The **posterior gluteal artery** passes out of the pelvis through the lesser sacrosciatic foramen and supplies **biceps femoris and middle gluteus.**

2. The **internal pudic artery** continues the internal iliac artery and gives branches to obturator internus, retractor ani and compressor coccygeus muscles.

In **female** it gives branches to vagina, urethra and vestibule and terminates as ventral perineal artery and artery of the clitoridis. The latter divides into deep and dorsal branches to clitoris. The ventral perineal branch gives branches to labium of vulva **(Fig.6.50)**. In male **internal pudic artery** gives ***urethral artery, dorsal perineal artery, artery of the bulb of the penis*** supplying enlargement of the corpus spongiosum, then passes down the ischial arch and terminates into ventral perineal artery and artery of penis. The latter divides into ***dorsal and deep arteries of the penis***, the former passing forwards on the dorsum to the tip of the penis while the latter supplies corpus cavernosum **(Fig 6.49)**.

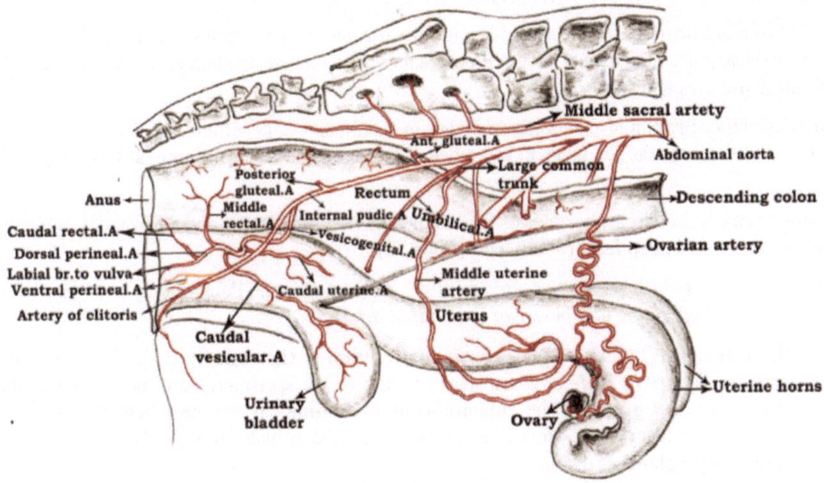

Fig. 6.50: Terminal branches of Internal Iliac Artery and Blood Vessels of Uterus

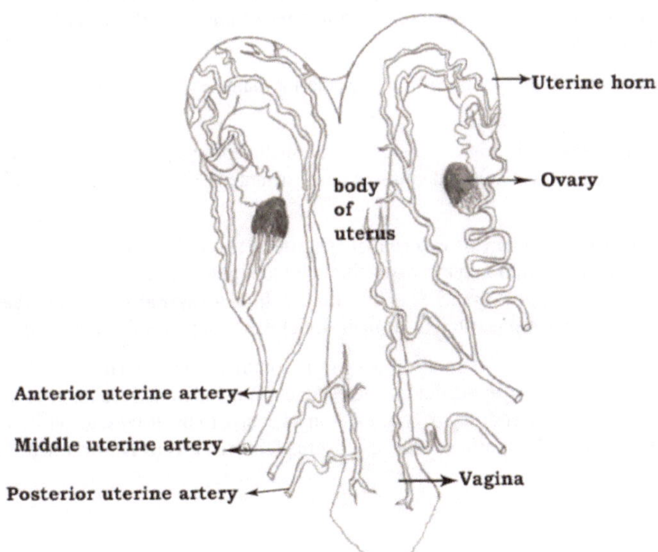

Fig. 6.51: Different Uterine Arteries of Cow

The External Iliac Artery

The ***hind limb is supplied by the external iliac artery.*** Each arises from lateral surface of aorta just in front of the internal iliac artery. It passes downward and backward along the tendon of psoas minor to the side of the pelvic inlet, crosses the tendon, reaches the anterior border of the pubis, gains the space between sartorius and pectineus and is ***continued as the femoral artery***.

Collateral Branches

1. **Circumflex iliac artery:** It is a large vessel arising from the external iliac artery close to its origin, passes outwards towards the lateral angle of the ilium supplying branches to psoas major and iliacus and divides into **superior and inferior branches (Fig.6.52).**

The superior (anterior) branch runs downwards and forwards on the transversus abdominis, then gets under the internal oblique muscle perforates it, gets under the external oblique muscle and finally reaches the skin of the flank. It supplies all these muscles and skin.

The inferior (posterior) branch also supplies branches to the iliopsoas, penetrates the abdominal wall, descends on the deep face of the tensor fasciae latae and supplies to these muscles, the **prefemoral lymph gland and skin of the thigh.**

2. **Common trunk**: arises from the anterior face of the external iliac artery and this divides into two branches i.e **the prepubic and deep femoral arteries (Fig.6.52)**.

A. Prepubic artery: This branch passes forwards from its origin crosses the Poupart's ligament and divides at the abdominal ring into ***external pudic and posterior abdominal arteries***.

i. External pudic artery: This branch supplies chiefly the **scrotum in the male**. It descends in the inguinal canal and ***exhibits a sigmoid flexure in male*** at the posterior border of the spermatic cord, passes out of the canal at the external inguinal ring and gives off the **subcutaneous abdominal artery and branches to scrotum.**The **subcutaneous abdominal artery** passes forwards on the tunica abdominalis supplies branches to **the scrotum, superficial inguinal lymph gland and skin**.

In the female, this vessel is very large and termed the **mammary artery**, which passes through the inguinal canal and divides into two branches, ***an anterior and a posterior to supply the mammary gland. In cattle, a small amount of blood comes to udder from the mammary branches of the ventral perineal artery and dorsal labial branch from the internal pudic artery.***

A small subcutaneous abdominal artery arising from the anterior mammary artery supplies the **skin in front of the mammary gland.**

ii. Posterior abdominal artery: This branch crosses the spermatic cord, supplies branches to the internal oblique muscle, runs on the deep face of the rectus abdominis and is distributed to it. Its branches anastomose with those of the anterior abdominal artery.

Artery of the cord (cremasteric artery or external spermatic artery): This is a very small vessel which arises usually from the **posterior abdominal artery** passes through the inguinal canal along the posterior border of the cremaster externus muscle and supplies branches to this **muscle, tunica vaginalis and the other structures of the cord. In the female** this branch is represented by a small vessel which supplies the mammary region.

B.Deep femoral artery: It is a large vessel usually arising from common trunk with the prepubic artery **(Fig.6.52)**. It passes under Poupart's ligament between the iliacus and pectineus muscles.It divides into two sets of vessels which supply the **biceps femoris and semitendinosus**. It supplies in its course to **pectineus, gracilis, obturator externus, obturator internus, adductor, semimembranosus, quadratus femoris, biceps femoris, semitendinosus muscles and hip joint.**

The Femoral Artery

This is the main arterial trunk of the thigh. It ***continues the external iliac artery*** below the level of the pubis, descends in the femoral canal, in company with the **femoral vein and saphenous nerve**, passes underneath the lower part of gracilis, over the vastus medialis below the insertion of the adductor. It dips in between the two heads of the gastrocnemius and ***is continued as the popliteal artery*** **(Fig.6.52)**.

> *The femoral triangle is a site used for taking pulse from the femoral artery in some animals. The sartorius muscle forms the cranial boundary and the pectineus forms the caudal boundary of the femoral canal.*

Collateral branches

1. **Anterior femoral artery:** It arises from the anterior face of the femoral artery, It gains the company of the **femoral nerve** reaches the space between the rectus femoris and vastus medialis and divides into branches to supply the **four heads of the quadriceps muscle and articularis genu**. Its muscular branches **supply pectineus, sartorius, gracilis, vastus medialis and semimembranous.**

2. **Saphenous artery:** It is given off about the middle of course of femoral artery in femoral canal. It becomes superficial by emerging between the lower parts of sartorius and gracilis, passes down in company with the saphenous vein and saphenous nerve on the medial face of the leg. **On reaching the hollow of the hock it divides into medial and lateral tarsal arteries.** It supplies branches to **sartorius and gracilis** and cutaneous branches to the skin. The **lateral tarsal artery** is smaller and it passes outwards and contributes towards the formation of the ***rete tarsi dorsale***. The **medial tarsal artery** passes down in company with the tibial nerve along the deep flexor tendon and divides into **medial and lateral plantar arteries.**

The lateral plantar artery is smaller and passes down under the deep fasica of the metatarsus in company with the lateral plantar nerve along lateral border of the deep flexor tendon runs outwards in front of the plantar ligament, gains the plantar aspect of the metatarsus, gives off a branch towards the formation of the proximal plantar arch, branches to the tendons and skin and is **continued down as the lateral plantar superficial metatarsal artery**. This furnishes a **branch to the distal plantar arch** and is continued as the **lateral (abaxial) digital artery for the lateral digit.**

The medial plantar artery is larger and it passes down the tarsal sheath along the medial border of the deep flexor tendon passes under the deep fascia of the metatarsus gives off a branch to the proximal plantar arch and is continued down as the **medial plantar superficial metatarsal artery.** At the lower part, this furnishes branches to the distal plantar arch and is continued down as the **medial (abaxial) digital artery for the medial digit.**

3. **Posterior femoral artery:** it is a large vessel which marks the lower limit of the femoral artery **(Fig.6.52)**. It divides in to **superior and inferior branches** and the former ascends between the **semimembranosus and biceps femoris** and supplies these muscles, while the latter accompanies the **lateral head of the gastrocnemius** and supplies it.

The Popliteal Artery

The vessel is very short and **continues the femoral artery** over the posterior capsular ligament of the stifle joint, detaches the posterior tibial artery and gets under cover of the popliteus muscle and is **continued as anterior tibial artery (Fig.6.52)**. It furnishes branches to the **gastrocnemius and superficial digital flexor of the digits.**

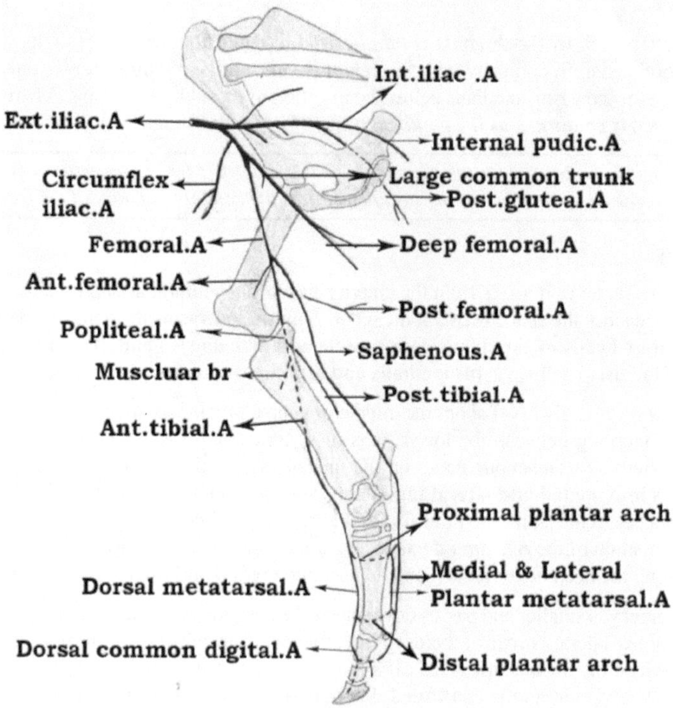

Fig. 6.52: Branches of External Iliac artery

The Posterior tibial artery: It is a slender veseel which runs down on the posterior face of the popliteus muscle and supplies **popliteus and deep digital flexor** of the digit **(Fig.6.52)**.

The Anterior tibial artery: It **continues the popliteal artery** and runs obliquely downwards and outwards under the popliteus and deep digital flexor. It passes through tibio-fibular arch and then passes successively under the origin of the **lateral digital extensor, peroneus longus** and between the muscles and bone. It here gives off a number of collateral branches to the **muscles of the dorsolateral group**. It then gains the lateral face of the tibia. It runs downwards, passes over the anterior ligament of the tarsus and **divides into perforating tarsal and dorsal metatarsal arteries (Fig.6.52).**

The perforating tarsal artery passes backwards through the **gap between central and fourth tarsal** and **fused 2nd & 3rd tarsal** and then reaches **proximal extremity of large metatarsal and passes through its vascular tunnel** and reaches the posterior face of the large metatarsal bone and unites with the branches from the **medial and lateral plantar arteries to form the proximal plantar arch** between the bone and suspensory ligament. From the ventral face of this arch a small deep plantar metatarsal artery descends on the plantar groove of the bone to the distal plantar arch.

The dorsal metatarsal artery descends in the dorsal metatarsal groove in company with the veins and the deep peroneal nerve, gives off branches to the extensor digitalis brevis, detaches at the lower third, a perforating metatarsal artery which passes through the distal foramen of large metatarsal to the posterior face of the large metatarsal bone and unites with the branches of the **medial and lateral plantar superficial metatarsal arteries** to form the **distal plantar arch (Fig.6.52).** The dorsal metatarsal artery continues downwards as the **dorsal common digital artery** which enters the interdigital space and divides into two branches. These branches unite with the like branches of the plantar common digital artery to form the two proper digital arteries for each digit.

The plantar common digital artery arises **from distal plantar arch** and divides into two branches which unite with similar branches of the dorsal common digital artery to form the proper digital ***(axial digital)*** arteries. It also anastomoses with the plantar abaxial digital arteries of medial and lateral digits.

The **axial digital arteries** are directed downward on the axial surface of the digits give branches to the axial part of the dermis/corium and then **enters axial foramina** on the extensor process of third phalanx and within the 3rd phalanx gives number of branches which emerge through the formina in the bone **to supply dermis/corium of hoof.**

Non Satellite Veins of the Hind Limb and Pelvic Cavity

Most of the veins are the satellites of the arteries and need no special description. Only such of the veins which do not follow arteries (which are not satellite) are dealt here under.

The Recurrent tarsal vein: It is a subcutaneous vein on the **lateral surface of the leg** and is **formed by the dorsal metatarsal vein and the lateral plantar metatarsal vein.** It communicates with anterior tibial and saphenous veins. It ascends at first in front of tendo achilles passes up between biceps femoris and semitendinosus and joins, the deep femoral or posterior femoral vein.

The Veins of the Udder: form a venous circle at the base of the udder, which is drained chiefly by two pairs of veins. The **paired anterior mammary or milk vein** (***subcutaneous abdominal vein***) is very large in animals of dairy breeds **(Fig.6.53).** It leaves the anterior border of the udder about 7 cm from the linea alba, runs a flexuous course forwards along the floor of the abdomen dips under the cutaneous muscle, passes through the foramen in the rectus abdominis and joins the internal thoracic vein **(Fig.6.53).**

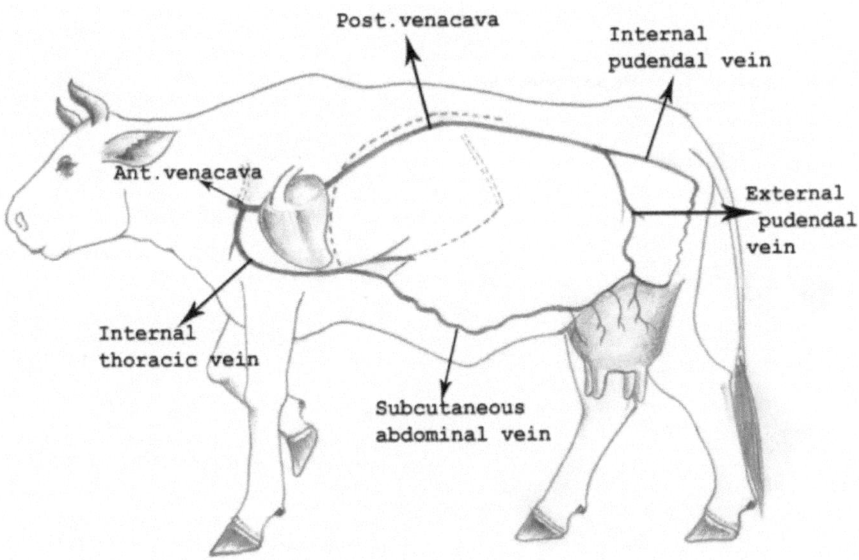

Fig. 6.53: Mammary Veins of Cow

The two **anterior mammary veins** are connected by a transverse anastomosis and each is connected with the **middle mammary vein (Fig.6.54)**. The **middle mammary vein** (***external pudic vein***) is also large and ascends in the inguinal canal as a satellite of the artery and joins the external iliac veins. Both are connected behind by a transverse branch from which a single posterior mammary vein (***perineal vein***) arises, which runs medially upwards to the perineum and joins the internal pudic vein **(Fig.6.54).**

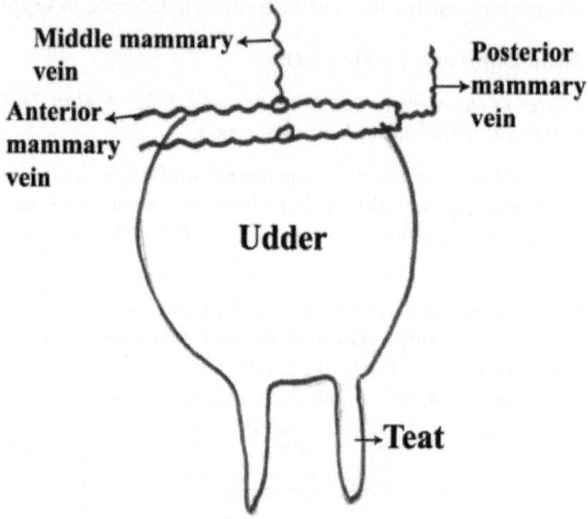

Fig. 6.54: Venous Drainage from the Udder (Schematic)

6.5 NERVE SUPPLY TO THE PELVIS AND HIND LIMB

The muscles of the hind limb are supplied by the **lumbosacral plexus**. It is formed by the convergence of the ventral primary branches of the **last three lumbar (4th, 5th and 6th) and first two or three sacral spinal nerves**. This plexus is in two parts i.e anterior and posterior parts connected by anastomotic branches.

The **anterior part is formed** by the **fourth, fifth and sixth lumbar nerves** and is situated between the psoas muscles while the **posterior part is formed** by the **sixth lumbar, first and second sacrals** and sometimes a branch of the third sacral and is on the pelvic face of the sacrosciatic ligament at the greater sciatic foramen. The nerves emerging from the anterior part of the plexus are the **iliopsoas, the femoral and the obturator nerves**. The nerves emerging from the posterior part of the plexus are the anterior gluteal, the sciatic and the posterior gluteal nerves.

1. **The iliopsoas nerve**: derives its fibres from the **fourth lumbar** and supplies **psoas minor and ilio psoas muscles.**
2. **The femoral nerve**: derives its fibers from the **fourth and fifth lumbar** spinal nerves and is the **largest nerve of the anterior part of the plexus.** It runs downward and backward between the psoas muscles, crosses the lateral face of the tendon of psoas minor gets under cover of sartorius. It detaches the **saphenous nerve** and dips in between the rectus femoris and vastus medialis to supply the **quadriceps femoris and articularis genu.**

   The saphaneous nerve is detached a little above the brim of the pelvis as the femoral nerve crosses the tendon of psoas minor, passes down at first between the sartorius and vastus medialis in **femoral canal** and then gives off a long branch which passes backward into the pectineus. The nerve gains exit with the saphenous artery and saphenous vein between the sartorius and gracilis at about the level of the stifle, divides into several branches which penetrate the deep fascia and pass subcutaneously to supply the skin on the **medial aspect of the leg.**
3. **The obturator nerve**: derives its fibres from **all the three lumbar spinal nerves**. It passes downward and backward then turns downward on the shaft of the ilium towards the obturator internus, passes through foramen, then through obturator externus supplying it and divides to supply **pectineus, adductor and gracilis muscles.**

Obturator nerve damage can occur by compression of the nerve by a large foetus during difficult parturition. The condition is characterized by a failure to adduct the limb, especially on a slippery floor.

4. **The anterior gluteal nerve:** is derived from the posterior part of the plexus and is in front of the sciatic nerve. Its fibres are derived from the **sixth lumbar and the first sacral spinal nerve**. It divides into four or five branches which leave the cavity through the greater sciatic foramen in company with the anterior gluteal vessels and then supply the **gluteus medius and gluteus profundus.** ***A long branch passes between these two muscles to supply the tensor fasciae latae.***
5. **The posterior gluteal nerve:** its fibres are derived from the **first and second sacral spinal nerves**. It divides into branches which passes backward through the greater sciatic foramen over the **gluteus medius and supply the upper part of the biceps femoris.**
6. **The sciatic nerve:** It is the ***largest nerve in the body***. It is derived from the **sixth lumbar and first and second sacral spinal nerves**. It is a wide flat band, leaves the pelvic cavity through the greater sciatic foramen, passes downward and backward between the gluteal muscles, gains the hollow between the trochanter major and tuber ischii runs over the gemellus and quadratus femoris. It dips between the **two heads of gastrocnemius** and is ***continued as the tibial nerve***.

Collateral branches of Sciatic nerve are

1. **A slender muscular branch** which passes along its posterior border through the lesser sciatic foramen to the **obturator internus.** This nerve is given off in the midway between the two sciatic foramina.
2. **A small muscular branch** from the deep face of the sciatic nerve, passes backward between the nerve and **gluteus profundus, supplies gemellus** and passes through it to supply the **quadratus femoris.**
3. **A large muscular branch** to supply the **biceps femoris, semitendinosus and semimembranosus.**
4. **The posterior cutaenous nerve of the leg** is detached from the sciatic about the middle of the thigh. It descends over the **lateral head of the gastrocnemius** under cover of biceps femoris. It runs downward in company with the recurrent tarsal vein to the lower third of the leg. It divides here into a number of branches which are distributed to the **skin on the lateral aspect of the tarsal and metatarsal regions.**
5. **The peroneal nerve** is a very large trunk detached about the middle of the thigh.It descends in front of the sciatic to the origin of the gastrocnemius, crosses over the lateral head of this muscle obliquely downward and forward, gains the level of the origin of the lateral digital extensor of the digit and ***divides into superficial and deep peroneal nerves*** **(Fig.6.55)**. It also gives off **branches to biceps femoris and the lateral cutaneous nerve of the leg**, which perforates through the biceps femoris and supplies the skin of the stifle region.

The superficial peroneal nerve: It supplies branches to the **lateral digital extensor and then passes beneath the peroneus longus.** It passes down between it and the lateral digital extensor to the lower third of the leg. Thereafter it runs down between the lateral and long digital extensors, gains the dorsolateral face of the lower part of the hock, runs down subcutaneously over the annular ligament, runs down the metatarsal region on the extensor digitalis brevis, gains the company of the dorsal superficial metatarsal vein and divides below into three branches of which the **lateral and medial branches** are continued down as the ***lateral dorsal abaxial and medial dorsal abaxial digital nerves***. The ***middle branch*** joins the dorsal branch of the ***deep peroneal to form the dorsal common digital nerve***, which divides into two **dorsal axial digital nerves (Fig.6.55).**

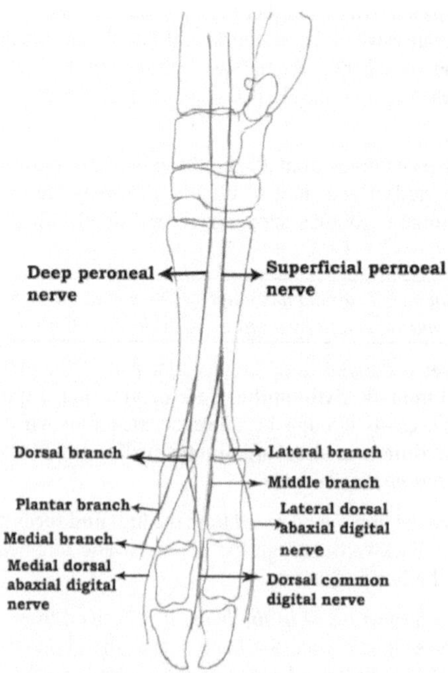

Fig. 6.55: Branches of Peroneal nerve (Schematic)

The deep peroneal nerve: It at first dips between the lateral digital extensor and peroneous longus and then between the lateral and long digital extensors. ***It gives branches to all the muscles of the dorsolateral group of the leg*** and is continued down on the lateral border of the tendon of the long digital extensor and reaches the hock, gives off cutaenous branches, passes under the annular ligament, gives off branches to extensor digitalis brevis, runs down the metatarsal groove in company with the dorsal metatarsal vessels and divides above the fetlock into **dorsal and plantar branches (Fig.6.55)**. The ***dorsal branch*** joins middle branch of the **superficial peroneal** to form the ***dorsal common digital nerve.*** The **plantar branch of deep peroneal nerve** passes through interdigital space to reach plantar aspect and joins a **lateral branch of the medial plantar nerve of tibial nerve by passing through the cleft of large metatarsal bone** to form the ***plantar common digital nerve*** which divides into **two plantar axial digital nerves (Figs.6.56 , 6.57)**.

The Tibial Nerve

It is a continuation of the sciatic nerve after it **dips between the two heads of the gastrocnemius.** It passes along the posterior border of the superficial digital flexor and becomes subcutaneous by passing under the medial head of gastrocnemius, continues in front of the tendo achilles on the medial aspect of the leg. Its collateral branches supply ***all the muscles on the posterior aspect of the leg.*** It then emerges from beneath the superficial flexor, becomes subcutaneous, descends in front of the tendoachilles on the inner face of the leg and divides on reaching the hock **into lateral and medial plantar nerves (Figs.6.56 & 6.57).**

The ***medial plantar nerve*** descends under cover of the deep fascia of the metatarsus between the tendon of superficial digital flexor and suspensory ligament, passes along the medial border of the deep digital flexor tendon and at the lower part of metatarsus divides into two branches, the medial of which supplies a few branches to the rudimentary digit and is ***continued as medial plantar abaxial digital nerve.*** The lateral branch turns round the flexor tendon, gains the inter digital space, joins the branch of the **deep peroneal to form plantar common digital nerve**, which divides into two plantar axial digital nerves **(Figs.6.56 & 6.57).**

The lateral plantar nerve descends under the metatarsal ligament, winds to the lateral aspect descends along the lateral border of the tendons under the deep fascia of metatarsus. It gives off branch to the **lateral rudimentary digit** and is ***continued as the lateral plantar abaxial digital nerve.***

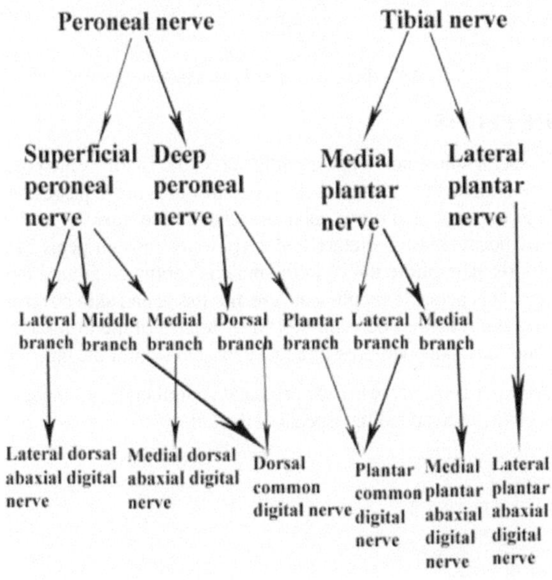

Fig. 6.56: Terminal branches of Peroneal and Tibial nerves (Schematic)

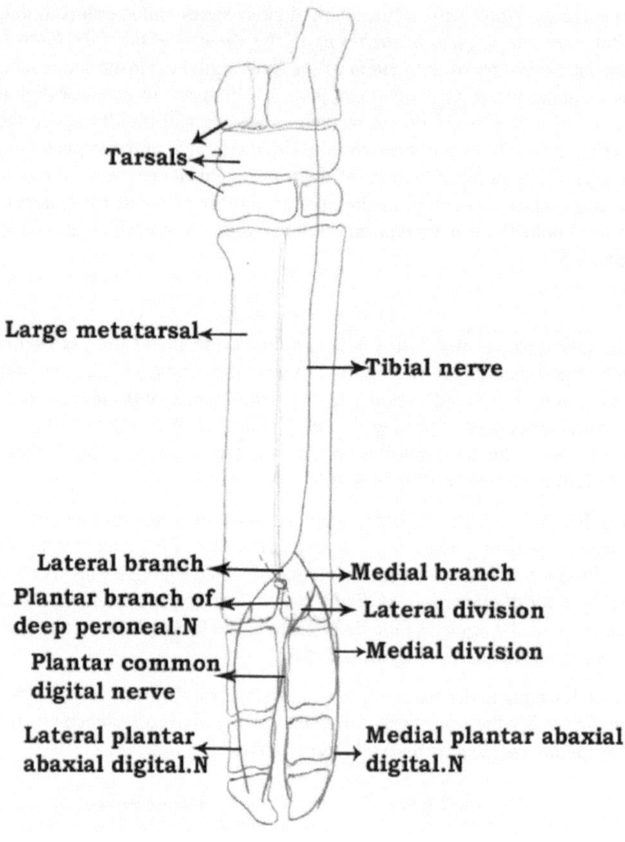

Fig. 6.57: Branches of Tibial Nerve (Schematic)

NERVE SUPPLY TO THE PELVIS

The ventral branch of the 3rd sacral spinal nerve is the pudic nerve, the fourth is the posterior haemorrhoidal nerve and the fith passes towards the sphincter ani exxternus muscle. The pudic nerve passes on the sacro sciatic ligament, gives off branches to the bladder, urethra and muscular branches to the muscles of the anus. At the ischial arch it supplies branches to the ischiocavernosus, urethra and corpus cavernosum penis in the male and vulva in the female terminating in the clitoris. The **pudic nerve** in the male is continued around the ischial arch, descends on the dorsum penis to reach the glans penis. It supplies the erectile tissue and skin covering the penis. The ***posterior haemorrhoidal nerve supplies the rectum***. The ventral primary branch of the fifth sacral spinal nerve is small and supplies the muscles of the anus and skin, compressor coccygeus and skin of the tail.

Coccygeal nerves: There are five pairs of nerves. The dorsal and ventral branches unite to form two trunks on either side and supply the muscles on the corresponding aspects of the tail.

6.6 VISCERAL ORGANS OF THE PELVIC CAVITY

The Rectum

It is a straight terminal part of alimentary canal present in pelvic cavity and extends from the pelvic inlet to anal canal.

Ox: It shows two parts i.e ***peritoneal and retro peritoneal parts***. The greater **first or peritoneal part** is suspended by mesorectum, while the **second or retro peritoneal part** is shorter and forms a flask shaped dilatation termed, ***the ampulla recti***. The rectococcygeus muscle consists of thick muscle bundles that arise dorsally from the longitudinal musculature of the rectum and are inserted on the ventral surface of the first few caudal vertebrae i.e to the first 3 coccygeal. In the cow, muscle bundles from the ventral surface of the rectum decussate in the perineal region and unite with the constrictor vulvae.

Horse: The retroperitoneal part is larger and presents a dilatation at its terminal part viz., **rectal ampulla**. The **rectococcygeus muscle** is derived from the well developed longitudinal muscle layer of of the rectum. It is a thick paired band which attaches on the ventral surface of the 4th cocygeal vertebra. **In the stallion**, the rectum is related ventrally to the bladder, pelvic urethra, deferent ducts, seminal vesicles, prostate gland and the bulbourethral glands. **In mare**, it is related to the body of the uterus, cervix, vagina and vestibule. Ventral to these are the urethra and the urinary bladder.

Pig: Ampulli recti is present.

Dog: It is short and completely covered with peritoneum and ampulla is present.

*The perineum: is the part of the body wall that closes pelvic outlet and surrounds the anal and urogenital canals.*_

The Anal Canal

Ox: The anal canal is short end portion of alimentary canal and has **anorectal and anocutaneous zones** at the junction with rectum and skin respectively. The longitudinal folds are present at anorectal zone (10 cm). The terminal opening of anal canal is ***anus.*** External and internal sphincters surround the anus and keep the opening closed.The latter is continuation of circular smooth muscle coat of rectum. The striated external anal sphincter arises from caudal vertebrae and lies superficial to internal sphincter.The levator ani originating from sacrosciatic ligament or ischiatic spine blends into external anal sphincter. The retractor penis in male / retractor clitoridis in female lies cranial to external sphincter and arises from caudal vertebrae passes on side of rectum and suspends terminal part of rectum and anal canal before reaching penis or clitoris.

Horse: The anus forms a rounded protuberance ventral to the root of tail. The mucosa is whitish and nonglandular. The anal canal proximally is continuous with the rectal mucosa at the distinct **anorectal line**, while distally at the **anocutaneous line** it is succeeded by the skin that covers the anus. The levator ani arises from sacrosciatic ligament and thus indirectly from the ischiatic spine and is inserted to lateral wall of anal canal deep to external anal sphincter. The grayish white retractor penis / clitoridis extends from ventral surface of second caudal vertebra on either side of rectum and forms a loop ventral to rectum with opposite muscle, then goes to penis in male / clitoris in female.

Dog: The mucosa is divided into three consecutive annular zones from cranial to caudal, a wider **columnar, an intermediate and a cutaneous zone**. The mucosa of columnar zone is darker than rectal mucosa and is arranged into longitudinal folds and contains anal glands. Two laterally placed anal sacs with glands in their walls are characteristic of cutaneous zone between internal and external anal sphincter muscles. The **cutaneous zone** forms transition with the skin and is bluish red and shows fine hairs and circumanal glands. The levator ani muscle is extensive and **inserts on 4th to 7th caudal vertebrae** with a few fibres attaching to external anal sphincter. It shows two parts pubocaudalis and iliocaudalis arising from pubis and ilium respectively.

Pig: It is divided as in carnivores ***i.e columnar, an intermediate and a cutaneous zone.*** The columnar zone is narrow covered with stratified squamous epithelium, light red in colour and presents longitudinal depressions (sinus anales) associated with accumulations of lymphoreticular tissue. Intermediate zone is also red covered with stratified squamous epithelium. It is separated from cutaneous zone by the anocuatneous line.

Fowl: The **cloaca** is pathway for urogenital and alimentary passages. It has three compartments.

Coprodeum: The initial expanded portion into which the ***colorectum opens.***

Urodeum: is the portion into which the ***ureter and oviduct or vas deferens open.*** The oviduct or vasdeferens opens lateral to ureter.

Proctodeum: is the last portion of cloaca and cloacal bursa (bursa of Fabricius) opens into its dorsal aspect. The bursa is a blind sac like unpaired structure found best developed in chickens about four months of age. It usually disappears at one year age. The external opening of the cloaca ***is termed, the vent.***

The Urinary Bladder

It is a musculomembranous sac located on the floor of pelvic cavity behind the pelvic inlet.

Ox: It has the shape of a long oval and has 3 parts ***i.e funds, body and neck*** **(Fig.6.58)**. The **fundus (vertex / apex)** is the flask shaped anterior blind end. It presents the vestigial connection of bladder to the urachus. ***Urachus*** is the tube that connects the **primitive urinary bladder with the allantoic sac** in the fetus.

The body is central middle and main part which presents two (dorsal and ventral) surfaces, while the neck is the constricted portion which joins the pelvic urethra. The bladder is fixed in position by three peritoneal folds i.e ***ligaments of the bladder, one middle ligament and two lateral ligaments.*** It is related ventrally to floor of pelvis and ventral abdominal wall when it is full. In males dorsally it is related to ***rectum, genital fold, vas deferens, seminal vesicles and prostate gland*** **(Fig.5.56)**. In females it is related dorsally ***to uterus and broad ligaments and neck of the bladder and urethra*** **(Fig.5.58)** ***are united with the ventral wall of vagina.***

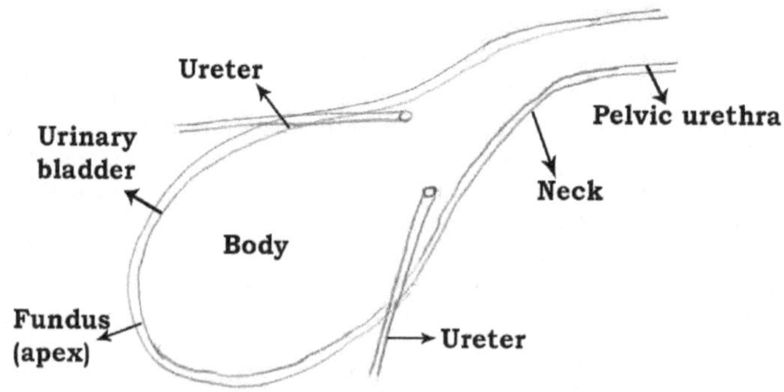

Fig. 6.58: Urinary Bladder with Ureters (Schematic)

The mucous membrane is loosely attached to submucosa and shows numerous folds in contracted state but in the superoposterior part the mucous membrane is firmly attached to submucosa without any folds over a triangular area ***called trigonum vesicae.*** This area shows the ***openings of ureters at the base and internal urethral orifice at the apex*** **(Fig.6.59)**.

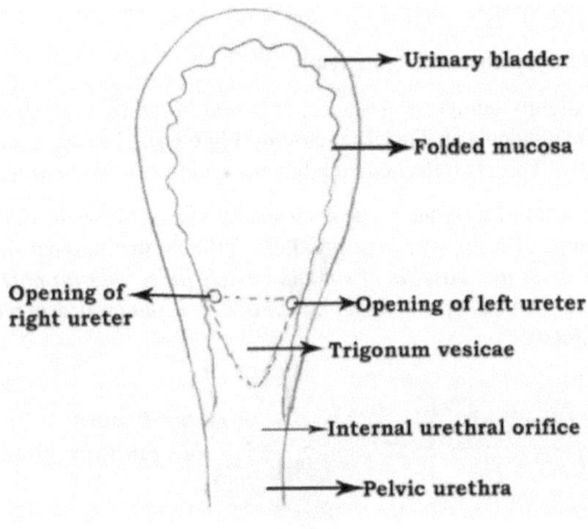

Fig. 6.59: Urinary Bladder with Trigonum Vesicae (Schematic)

Horse: It is short and wide.

Pig: The bladder is oval when empty or moderately full and spherical when full. Except neck it rests on ventral abdominal wall.

Dog: It is relatively large and whether full or empty lies on the ventral abdominal wall cranial to pubis except neck which is in pelvic cavity.

Fowl: The urinary bladder is absent and ureters open into urodeum.

THE MALE GENITAL ORGANS

The male genital system comprises of testicles with their covering (scrotum) and appendages, the ductus deferens, the accessory glands, urethra and penis with its covering, the prepuce.

The Scrotum

It is a diverticulum of the abdomen and lodges the testicles and its appendages. It contains many sweat and sebaceous glands. The ***tunica dartos* is a modified** subcutaneous tissue that lies on the deep surface of the skin and cannot be separated from it and **forms a scrotal septum**, a median partition dividing scrotum into two compartments marked externally by scrotal raphe. It contains smooth muscle bundles connected by collagen and elastic fibers. The tunica dartos contracts under the influence of cold or as a result of mechanical stimulation, wrinkling the scrotal skin. **Its contraction also helps to elevate the testes.**

Bull: It is a long and pendulous pouch present in front of inguinal region. It is oval in form and slightly compressed. It has well marked neck above the testes. The hair on the skin is sparse.

Stallion: It is in the **inguinal region** and placed high between the thighs and **globular in shape.** The skin is pigmented.

Dog: It is **behind the inguinal region** and skin is pigmented.

Boar: It lies a short distance ***ventral to the anus in perineal region*** against caudal surface of thighs and does not protrude very much from the surface of the body. The skin has few hairs. A deep groove divides scrotum into right and left halves.

Cock: Absent

The Testicles

The testes are located in scrotum together with epididymis.

Bull: Testicles are two oval slightly compressed glands, enclosed in tunica vaginalis, an evagination of parietal peritoneum passing through the inguinal canal into the scrotum **(Fig.6.60).** The ***long axis is vertical*** **(Fig.6.62)**. Each testis shows two extremities, two borders (attached / epididymal and free) and two (medial and lateral) surfaces.

The **spermatic cord** is in the form of a slender cone enclosed by visceral layer of tunica vaginalis **(Fig.6.60).** Its distal end is attached to the head of testis while the proximal end is at the inguinal ring. It ***consists of testicular artery and vein, lymphatics, nerves and bundles of smooth muscle in its anterior part and ductus deferens in its posterior part***. The testicular vein breaks up and ***forms a rich network, pampiniform plexus, which surrounds the coils of testicular artery*** **(Fig.6.60).**

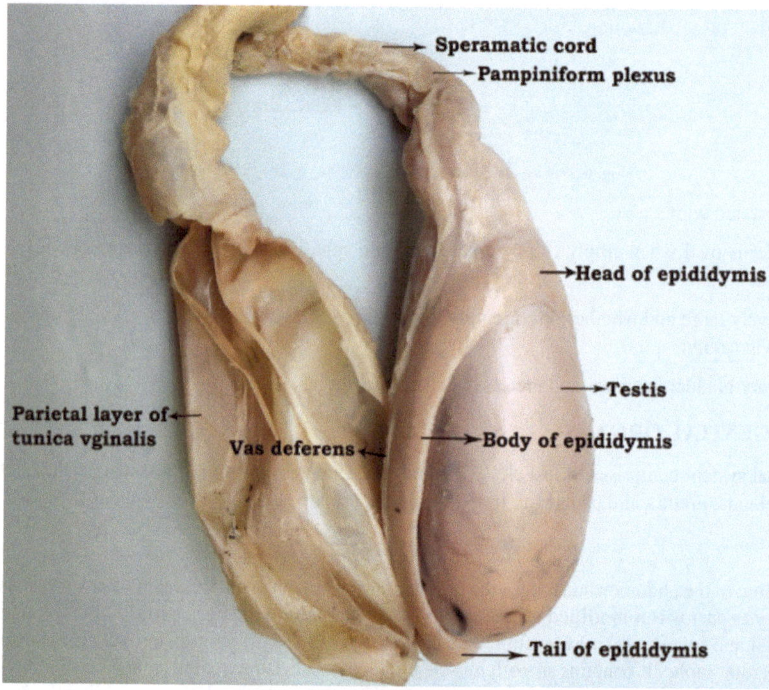

Fig. 6.60: Testis of Bull with Epididymis and Tunica Vaginalis

> *Pampiniform plexus is formed by the torturous bends of the testicular vein that wrap around the testicular artery. The pampiniform plexus is to cool the blood in testicular artery entering the testis. The temperature of the testicles* ***lowered by atleast 2-3^0 c,*** *is essential for regulation of spermatogenesis.*

The **epididymis** is an elongated structure along the posterior border of the testis. It consists of head, body and tail. The tail of epididymis is large and attached to the ventral extremity of the testis by ***proper ligament of testis*** and to the parietal layer of tunica vaginalis ***by ligament of tail of epididymis*** **(Fig.6.61)**. Both ligaments are ***remnants of the gubernaculums testis***, a gelatinous mesenchymal structure responsible for descent of testis into the scrotal sac. The ***testicular bursa*** is an elongated recess present between the body of the epididymis and the testis.

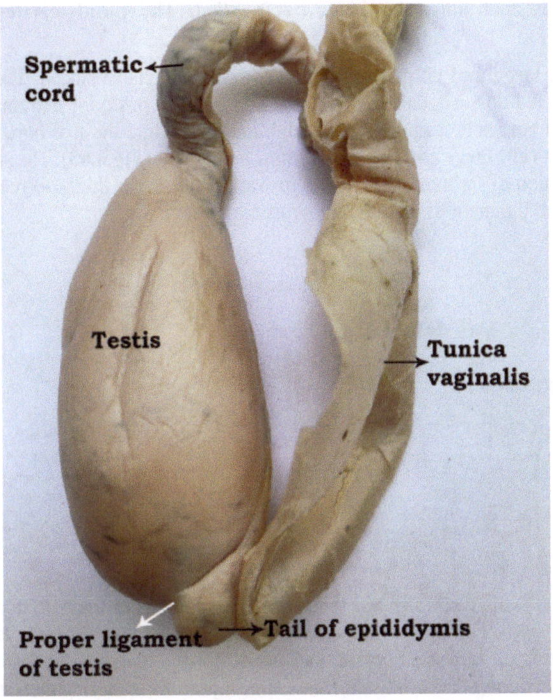

Fig. 6.61: Testis of Bull with Proper Ligament of Testis

The layer of serosal fold that suspends the ductus deferens is called mesoductus deferens. The testicular artery and vein are suspended by a similar peritoneum known as mesoorchium. The mesoductus deferens and mesoorchium are continuous with each other.

Stallion: The testes are smaller but **globular and long axis is parallel to the long axis of the body**. The epididymis lies on the dorsal border of the testis **(Fig.6.62)**.

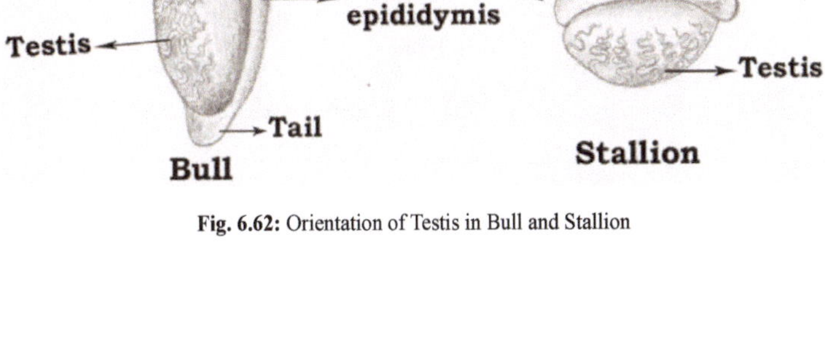

Fig. 6.62: Orientation of Testis in Bull and Stallion

Dog: The testes are relatively small and oval and ***long axis is oblique***. The **epididymis lies along the dorsal border (Fig.6.63).**

Boar: The testes are **long, large and elliptical**. The mediastinum is axially placed. The posterior extremity and tail of epididymis are directed dorsocaudally towards the anus. Hence posterior extremity lies close to anus and epididymis and epididymal border lie against caudal thigh muscles, while the free border of the testis is directed caudally. The **epididymis is very large and tail forms blunt projection (Fig.6.63)**. The spermatic cord is very long and because of caudal position of scrotum it must pass forward between the thighs to reach external inguinal ring. Proper ligament of testis and ligament of tail of epididymis are present.

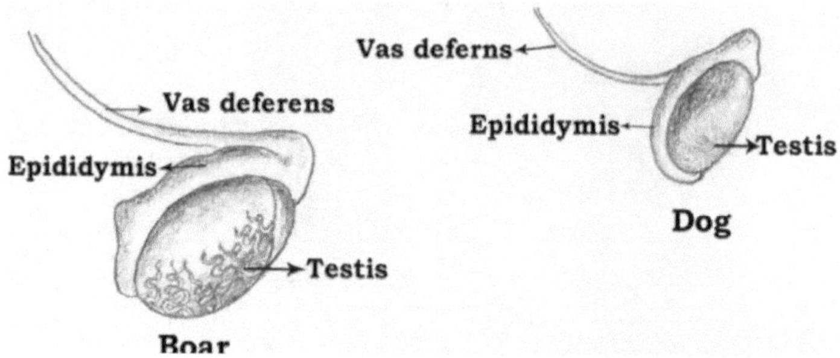

Fig. 6.63: Orientation of Testis in Boar and Dog

Cock: The two bean shaped testicles lie **ventral to the anterior lobe of kidneys** in body cavity **(Fig.6.64)**. The epididymis does not show 3 parts. During the reproductive period, the testes of the cockerel are 35-60 mm long and 25-30 mm in diameter. During the quiescent period, they are 10-19 mm long and 10-15 mm in diameter. The testis is yellowish to greyish white during the resting stage and almost pure white during the stage of activity. A cockerel can copulate or tread up to **50 times per day**. Once the sperms have been introduced into the female genital tract, they **remain fertile for 10-21 days in the fowl** and **8-10 days in the duck and goose.**

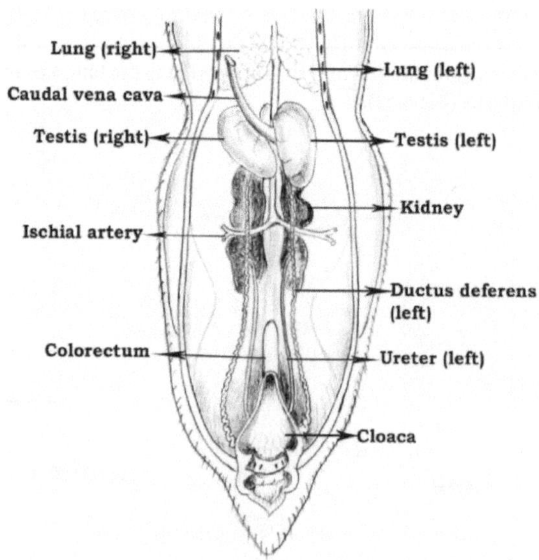

Fig. 6.64: Testes of Cock and their Relations with other Organs

The Ductus Deferens

It is the continuation of the tail of epididymis and connects the epididymis with the pelvic part of urethra. It forms the spermatic cord with testicular vessels and nerves. The mesoductus deferens is a narrow serosal fold enclosing the ductus deferens.

Bull: It has **initial coiled portion followed by straight portion** which forms the posterior part of the spermatic cord. The two ducts enter the genital fold in the cranial part of the pelvis. The terminal part shows an enlargement near the urethra ***viz., ampulla***. The ductus deferens and seminal gland open separately on colliculus seminalis.

Stallion: The **seminal glands (vesicles) and ductus deferens open on a common ejaculatory orifice.**

Dog: The ampulla is narrow. The ductus deferens passes through the substance of prostate and opens alone on indistinct colliculus seminalis.

Boar: The ductus deferens does not form ampulla and disappear ventral to extensive vesicular glands, passes through prostate and may open separately or together with duct of vesicular gland in a recess on the small colliculus seminalis.

Cock: The **ductus deferens** is extremely tortuous, arises without any clear line of differentiation from the epididymis. It accompanies the ipsilateral ureter beneath which it crosses from medial to lateral at the level of the caudal lobe of the kidney and opens into ***urodeum*** lateral to the opening of ureter. During the mating period the ductus deferens increases considerably both in length and thickness and becomes folded into numerous convolutions. It **acts as a *sperm reservoir*** and is recognisable by its white colour.

The Uterus masculinus: It is a ***remnant of the paramesonephric*** (***Mullerian***) ducts found occasionally in the genital fold between the two ductus deferens and is the homologue of the uterus and vagina.

Bull : It is vestigeal.

Stallion: It is present centrally on the dorsal surface of the neck of bladder.

Dog : It is in the form of a small compressed sac in the caudal part of genital fold.

Cock : Absent.

The Accessory Sex Glands

They are grouped around the pelvic urethra and can be palpated rectally.

Seminal Glands:

Bull: The seminal glands are **largest of the accessory genital glands**. They are two hard, compact, irregular and elongated glands (**often S-shaped**) with lobulated surface. They are present on ***posterodorsal surface of bladder*** **(Fig.6.65)**. The excretory duct, one for each gland opens on either side of the opening of the ductus deferens at the ***colliculus seminalis***.

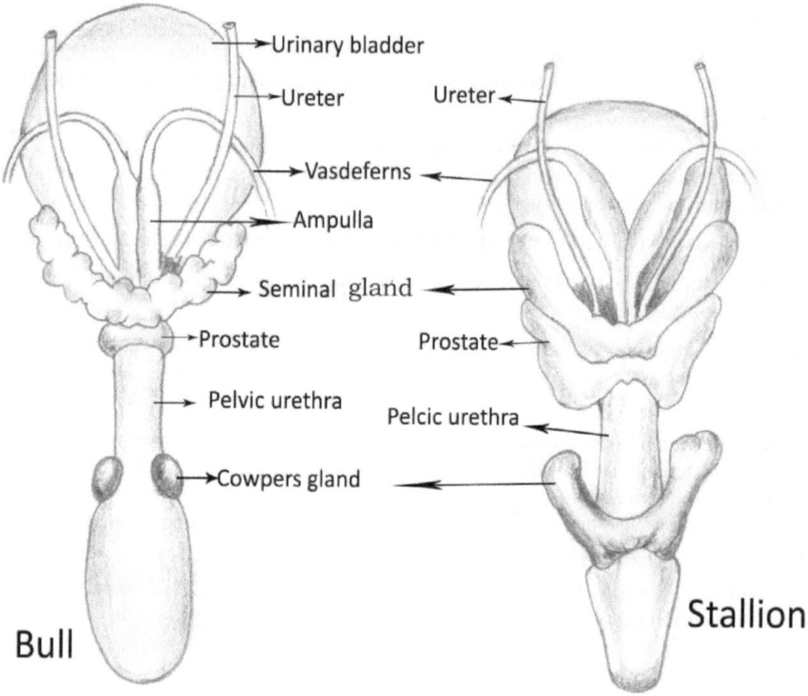

Fig. 6.65: Accessory sex glands of Bull and Stallion

Stallion: They are elongated and true sacs.They are ***pyriform shaped*** and consist of body and neck **(Fig.6.65)**. The duct opens along with ductus deferens on common ejaculatory orifice.

Dog : absent.

Boar: These glands are so large that only their caudal ends are in the pelvic cavity, the major part projects into the abdominal cavity and they are enclosed in the genital fold. The ducts of the seminal glands enter the urethra beside the ductus deferens.

The Prostate Gland

Bull: It has compact ***glandular part*, the body (corpus)** present on the dorsal face of the neck of bladder and a glandular layer in the wall of pelvic urethra (**Pars disseminata**). The ducts open into the urethra behind the colliculus seminalis in two rows on either side of mucosal folds diverging caudally from colliculus seminalis. ***In sheep and goat only pars disseminata is present.***

Stallion: It is large and consists of two lobes connected by an isthmus. There are **15 to 20 ducts** opening on either side of the opening of the ejaculatory orifice. **Pars disseminata is absent.**

Dog: It is very large and globular in shape and is divided into right and left lobes. It surrounds the neck of the bladder **(Fig.6.66A)**. Pars disseminata is less extensive and ducts are numerous and open lateral to the indistinct colliculus seminalis.

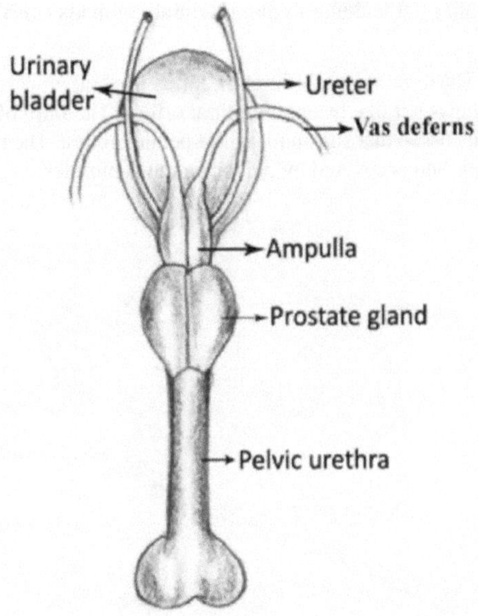

Fig. 6.66A: Prostate Gland of Dog

Boar: The bulk of the prostate is formed by disseminate part within the wall of the pelvic urethra. It has numerous small openings.

The Cowper's / Bulbourethral Glands

Ox: are two in number and present on either side of the pelvic urethra near ischial arch. Each has a single duct which opens into the dorsal wall of urethra under cover of a caudoventrally directed fold of mucous membrane (**dorsal diverticulum**).

Stallion: They are club shaped, larger and each has 6-8 ducts. The dorsal diverticulum is absent.

Dog : absent

Boar: They are very long and cranially touch the vesicular glands. They are covered dorsally by the **bulboglandularis muscles** whose contraction promotes their evacuation.

Cock : All accessory sex glands are absent.

Penis: It is a male copulatory organ.

Bull: It measures about 90 cm and is ***fibroelastic type*** and hence doesn't expand very much during erection. It consists of three parts **i.e. root, body and glans.** The root is firmly attached to the ischial arch of the pelvis by two crura. The bulbospongiosus muscle covers the bulb of the penis and ends near the junction of the crura of the penis. The body forms **'S' shaped curve (sigmoid flexure)** behind the ***scrotum*** i.e ***post scrotal (*****Fig.6.66B)**. The protrusion of penis is due to straightening of sigmoid flexure. The ***proximal curve of flexure is open caudally and distal curve is open cranially***. During erection cavernous spaces are filled with blood from deep artery of penis, ishiocavernous muscle contracts repeatedly closing off deep artery and vein at crura making the cavernosum a closed system. After erection muscle relaxes and veins resume drainage of corpus cavernosum.

The **retractor penis muscle** is attached to second bend of sigmoid flexure. The free part of the organ that lies in prepuce is twisted slightly counter clock wise. This causes urethral groove and raphe penis both ventral structures originally, to lie on the right surface of penis. The raphe penis is cranial continuation of frenulum of prepuce. ***Raphe***

penis is connected to raphe preputii by frenulum **in young animals so penis can't be protruded** but it ruptures at puberty.

The **glans is poorly developed.** The terminal part of urethra forms urethral process which is visible in a groove on the right side of tip of penis. It shows slit like external urethral orifice. The **bulb of the penis** is an enlargement of corpus spongiosum, the cavernous tissue that surrounds entire penile urethra. The bulb extends from bulbourethral glands to junction of crura of penis and is covered by bulbocavernous muscles.

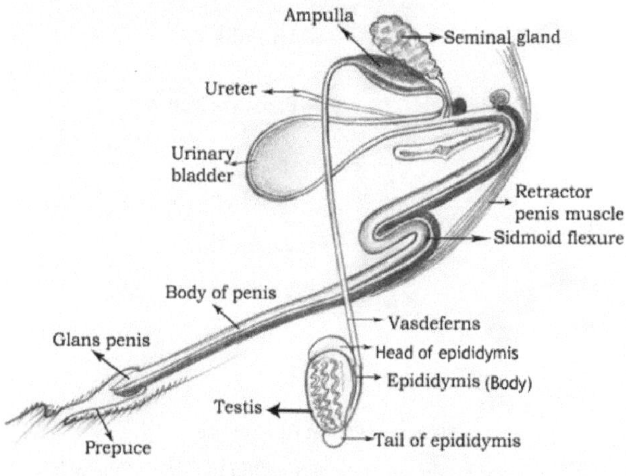

Fig. 6.66B: Genital Organs of Bull

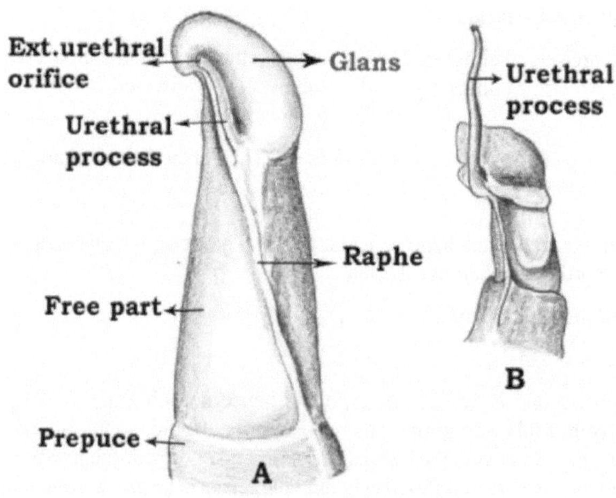

Fig. 6.67: Penis of Bull (A) and Ram (B)

In small ruminants the genital organs resemble, those of the bull. But the urethra lies in a groove on the ventral surface of the corpus cavernosum. Its terminal part projects commonly about 3-4 cm beyond the the glans penis, forming a twisted urethral process **(Fig.6.67 B)**

The sigmoid flexure is a frequent site for calculi (obstructive urolithiasis) especially in male ruminants i.e bull, buck and rams. High amounts of oxalates, calcium and legumes promote stone formation. The urethral process in small ruminants can also be a potential site for urolith obstruction. The obstructive materials are formed from mucus, proteins and minerals.

Stallion: It measures about 50 cm and undergoes 50% increase during erection. The erectile tissue is more. So ***it is vascular type***. There is no sigmoid flexure **(Fig.6.68)**. The base of the glans forms a prominent margin ***known as corona glandis*** behind which is constriction, ***collum glandis***. Its lower part presents a depression ***called fossa glandis*** **(Fig.6.69)**.

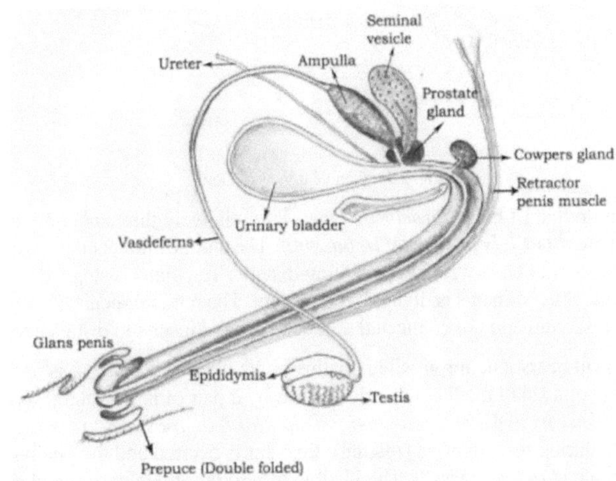

Fig. 6.68: Genital Organs of Stallion

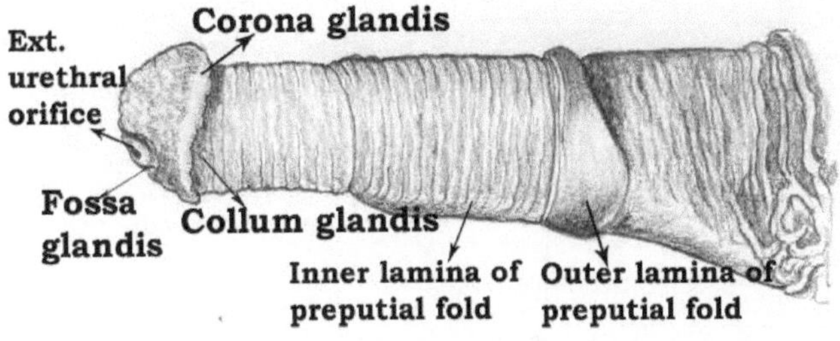

Fig. 6.69: Penis of Stallion

Dog: There is ***no sigmoid flexure***. A bone, Os penis is present in glans penis. Ventrally this bone is grooved for the lodgement of the urethra. The glans penis is very long and shows ***anterior cylindrical part, pars longa glandis*** with a pointed free end surrounding slender portion of Os penis and a posterior rounded enlarged part, bulbus glandis surrounding thick proximal portion of bone **(Fig.6.70)**. The enlargement of bulbus glandis during copulation is responsible for "***dogs stuck"***.

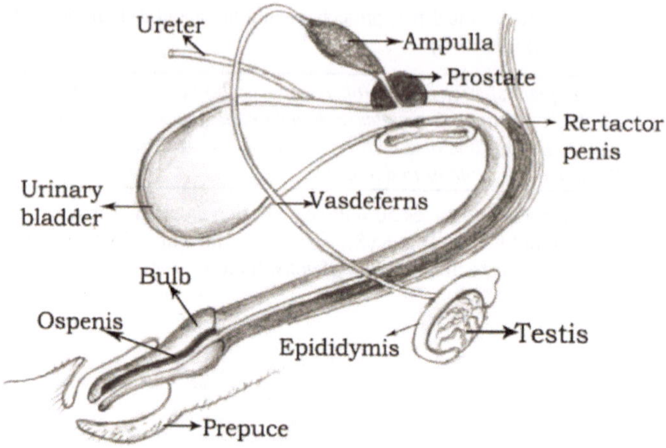

Fig. 6.70: Genital organs of Dog

Boar: The penis is similar to that of bull ***(fibroelastic type).*** It is relatively thin, about 60 cm long in flaccid state. The ***sigmoid flexure is present but it is prescrotal in position***. The shaft of the penis is twisted on its longitudinal axis by about one full turn counter clockwise when looking distally. The glans is small. The **diameter of the shaft enlarges by about 20%.** The bulb of penis is divided by a septum. The retractor penis has separate rectal and penile parts; the latter arises from sacrum and not connected to rectal part and inserts to distal curve of sigmoid flexure.

Cock: The ventral lip of vent bears a nonprotrusible phallus on its internal surface, it is in the form of **two raised folds.** The **phallus** consists of a small median tubercle flanked by a pair of larger lateral phallic bodies **(Fig.6.71).** *These protrude in the swollen and expanded state and together form a groove that receives the ejaculate from the deferens ducts* **(Fig.6.71).** During insemination (mating), the vent is everted and the phallus is pressed against the cloacal mucosa of the female (***Cloacal "Kiss"***). The phallus of **gander** (**male goose**) and the **drake** (**male duck**) have an ***intromittent*** protrusible phallus, several centimetres long and capable of intromission. It is thin cone like and exhibits a spiral groove that conveys the semen to the tip.

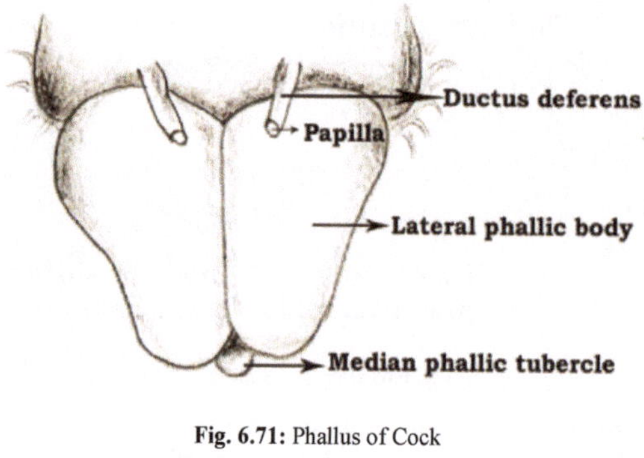

Fig. 6.71: Phallus of Cock

Day old chicks of both sexes present a minute genital protuberance at the future location of the phallus. It is rounded in males and conical in females, ***this difference enables the separation of male chicks from laying flock.***

The Prepuce

The Prepuce is a tubular structure covering the anterior part of the penis.

Bull: It consists of external and internal laminae which meet at preputial orifice. The external lamina is continuous with the skin of the abdominal wall, while internal lamina is in contact with penis and is continuous at the proximal end of preputial cavity with skin of penis. The **preputial orifice** is the opening of the prepuce. It is about 5 cm behind the umbilicus. The protractor and retractor prepuce muscles are associated with prepuce which are derivatives of cutaneous trunci.

Stallion : Prepuce is a **double invagination of the skin**.

Dog : As in bull.

Boar: The prepuce is relatively long and houses the free part of the penis. The cranial half is wider and communicates dorsally with a **preputial diverticulum,** a pouch containing a foul smelling fluid made up of cell debris soaked with urine. If the contents of the diverticulum accumulate, the cranial end of the prepuce enlarges and may mimic an **umbilical hernia** since the umbilicus is only a few centimetres cranial to the preputial orifice.

Cock : Absent.

The Male Urethra

The urethra extends from neck of urinary bladder to the external urethral orifice of glans penis.

Bull: It shows **pelvic and extra pelvic parts**. The **pelvic part** extends from urinary bladder to ischial arch. It is surrounded by thick urethralis muscle which is striated in nature. The urethralis muscle is thick ventrally and absent dorsally and continuous with the bulbospongiosus at the level of bulbourethral glands.

The **colliculus seminalis** is a rounded prominence about 5 cm behind the internal urethral orifice. This shows two slit like openings for ductus deferens and duct of seminal gland. Two mucosal folds pass caudally from colliculus seminalis and diverge. The ducts of prostate gland open in series on either side of these folds.

The penile (extra pelvic/spongy) part extends from ischial arch to external urethral orifice of glans penis. It passes between two crura of the penis and then enclosed along ventral part of penis. At the origin i.e. near ischial arch it has an enlargement, bulb of penis and then gradually diminishes in diameter. The mucosa of the spongy part of urethra forms longitudinal folds which give a rosette-like appearance on cross-section.

Stallion: The **pelvic part is 10-12 cm long**. The colliculus seminalis presents on either side a small diverticulum in which the **common ejaculatory** orifice lies into which the ducts deferens and duct of seminal gland open. The extra pelvic part is covered by bulbospongiosus muscle ventrally and laterally and continues to glans penis. It passes through the glans and projects forward about an inch in fossa glandis as a free tube, processes urethrae.

Dog: The pelvic part of the urethra is relatively long. Its first part extends from urinary bladder and is enclosed in the prostate. The **colliculus seminalis is indistinct**. The bulb of penis is well developed and divided by a median furrow and septum into two lateral lobes. The bulbospongiosus is small and extends to junction of crura of penis.

Boar: The urethralis covers ventral and lateral surfaces of pelvic urethra.The spongy part of the urethra begins at the ischial arch with an ampulliform enlargement of lumen.The bulbospongiosus muscle is divided into two halves by a septum and extends to junction of crura.

Cock: The urethra is absent.

THE FEMALE GENITAL ORGANS

The female genital system consists of two ovaries and fallopian tubes (oviduct), uterus, vagina, vestibule and vulva. The mammary glands are closely associated functionally with genital organs.

The Ovaries

Cow: The ovaries are **small, oval glands** attached to flank in front of middle of lateral margins of pelvic inlet. The ovary in the non pregnant animals lies near the lateroventral margin of the pelvic inlet. If the animal is pregnant, the ovary is drawn downward and forward. They are 3-4 cm long, 2.5 cm wide and each weighs about 15-20 gms. They are attached by anterior part of broad ligament of uterus ***called mesovarium.*** Each shows two surfaces (**medial and lateral**), two borders (**free and attached or mesovarial**) and two extremities i.e. **tubal or anterior and uterine or posterior**, (**Fig.6.73**). The proper ligament of ovary attaches uterine end of ovary to the mesometrium and ipsilateral uterine horn. The corpus luteum of pregnancy has a pronounced yellow colour and projects from surface of the ovary. The corpus luteum is partly embedded in the ovary but protrudes on the surface which canbe palpated about four days after estrus. If cow doesn't conceives it regresses. If pregnancy supervenes it is retained till parturition. Hence ovary can be evaluated per rectum for pregnancy diagnosis based on presence of corpus luteum.

Mare: The ovaries are **bean shaped, larger** and are situated in sublumbar region. They are **7-8 cm long, 3-4 cm thick** and each weighs about 70 to 80 gm. The free border of the ovary is marked by a notch which leads into a narrow depression, ***the ovulation fossa***. The corpus luteum does not project from the surface of the ovary but is embedded in the ovary.

Bitch: The ovaries are small, elongated oval in outline and flattened. They are situated a little behind (1-2 cm) the posterior pole of corresponding kidney. ***Ovarian bursa*****, a peritoneal pouch** with a slit like ventral opening is present around the ovary.

Sow: They are **cylindrical**, about 5 cm long, mobile and lie at pelvic inlet and have **tuberculate surface** because of many follicles and corpora lutea protruding from surface as they are multiparous. The **proper ligament of ovary is muscular**. The large cone shaped ovarian bursa encloses the ovary. The entrance to bursa is wide and directed ventrally.

Hen: ***Only left ovary is present.*** **The right one is rudimentary**. The left ovary is present in the dorsal part of body cavity and it weighs about 60g and ***resembles a bunch of grapes*** with **four or five large mature** and thousands of smaller immature follicles. The yellow colour of the mature follicles is due to the presence of yolk, the protein and lipids which are manufactured in the liver and travel in the blood stream to the oocyte. ***Unlike mammals there is no corpus luteum in birds.***

The Oviduct

Cow: Each is about 20-25 cm long and **less flexuous.** It has fimbriated end, the infundibulum, followed by ampulla and isthmus. The junction with uterine horn is **gradual**. It is enclosed in a **peritoneal fold, mesosalpinx derived from broad ligament**.

Mare: The oviduct is long, **more flexuous** and joins the **uterine horn abruptly**.

Bitch: The oviduct is small and **slightly flexuous**. The fimbriated end lies in ovarian bursa.

Sow: It is about 20 cm long and begins within the ovarian bursa.

Hen: The left oviduct is only developed. It is about 80 cm in length and divisible into five parts. The ***infundibulum*** has funnel shaped and tubular part. The ***magnum*** is **largest** and coiled part. The ***isthmus*** connects the magnum and uterus. The ***uterus (shell gland)*** is like a pouch. The **vagina is "S" shaped** whose walls are highly muscular. It terminates in urodeum of the cloaca by a slit like opening (**Fig.6.72**). ***The infundibulum is the site of fertilization, magnum and isthmus deposit albumen, while uterus secretes the shell.***

The egg stays in the **infundibulum for 15min**, in the **magnum for 3 hrs**, in the **isthmus for 75 minutes**, in the **uterus for 20 hours** and **in the vagina for few seconds**.

In the mature sexually active chicken the oviduct may reach size of about 65cm, but when the chicken goes out of lay, the length of the oviduct is reduced to about 15cm.

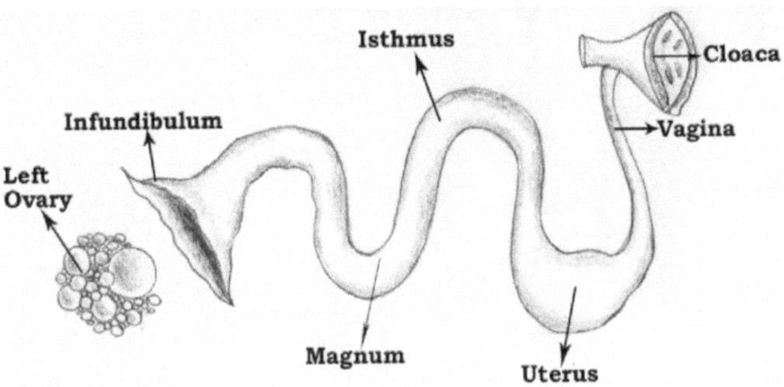

Fig. 6.72: Oviduct of Fowl

The Uterus

Cow: The uterus is a **hollow musculomembranous sac** continuous with the oviduct in front and vagina behind. It consists of ***two horns, body and a neck (cervix)***. **Most of the uterus is in the abdominal cavity, while only the cervix is in the pelvic cavity**. In pregnant state the gravid horn and body greatly increase in size and the position of the uterus varies greatly with the stage of pregnancy extending farther cranially as it enlarges with progress of gestation. It may lie directly on the right abdominal floor or it may be in the supraomental recess with the intestines. Distention of right ventral abdominal wall occurs in late pregnancy.**The junction of uterine horn with fallopian tube is not abrupt but gradual.** The mucous membrane of body and horns presents about **100 caruncles which are oval prominences (Fig.6.73)**. During pregnancy they become greatly enlarged and **pedunculated and spongy in appearance**. The intercornual ligaments at the divergence of uterine horns can be grasped per rectum to retract uterus and palpate horns.

The ***cervix is*** constricted posterior part and is **about 10 cm long** and thick walled. It is clearly marked off from body of uterus and vagina and part of it projects into cavity of vagina. It communicates with the body of uterus through **internal uterine orifice and with vagina by external uterine orifice.** The **cervical canal is spiral** as it is characterized by **three to four thick annular folds** and is ordinarily tightly closed.

The broad ligaments extend from the sublumbar region and lateral pelvic walls to the dorsal border of cornua and the lateral margins of the body of uterus. The part of broad ligament ending on the horn and body of uterus is ***mesometrium, while the other portions are mesovarium and mesosalpinx attaching to ovary and oviduct*** respectively. The round ligaments arise from lateral folds of broad ligaments and blend with parietal peritoneum over the internal inguinal ring.

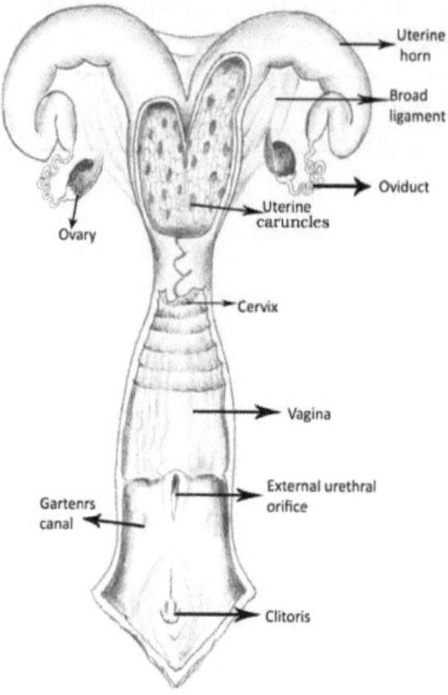

Fig. 6.73: Genitalia of Cow

Mare: The uterus has a wide lumen. The body is situated partly in the abdominal cavity and partly in pelvic cavity, while the horns lie entirely in the abdominal cavity. The body is relatively large. The mucous membrane of body and horns shows **no caruncles**. The **junction of oviduct and horns is abrupt**. The horns are slightly curved or nearly straight. The **cervical canal is straight and shows longitudinal folds (Fig.6.74)**.

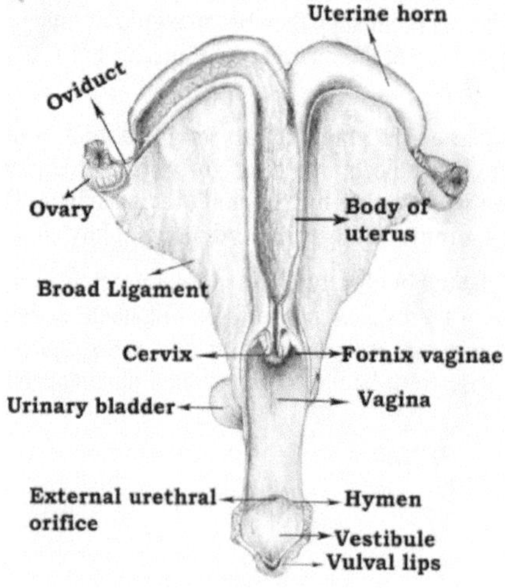

Fig. 6.74: Genitalia of Mare

Bitch: The body of uterus is short and horns are very long, slender, nearly straight and lie entirely within abdominal cavity. The horns diverge from the body in the form of a **'V' towards** kidneys. The **cervix is very short** and mucosa presents few oblique folds (**Fig.6.75**). The round ligaments of the uterus arising from lateral folds of the broad ligaments pass through inguinal canal enveloped by peritoneal pouch. The horns of **gravid uterus present dilatations, the ampullae** which contain the foetuses and are separated by constrictions.

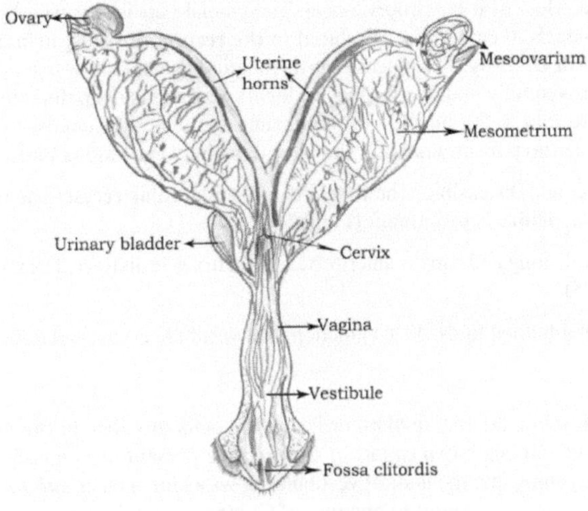

Fig. 6.75: Genitalia of Bitch

Sow: The body of the uterus is short. The horns are **very long, flexuous, thick walled, coiled and arranged like intestine coils** in non gravid state. The **cervix is very long** i.e upto 25 cm and there is no intravaginal part of cervix (**Fig.6.76**). It opens gradually into uterus and vagina without noticeable demarcation. The deeper **circular muscle** at the junction of body and horns forms ***complex sphincter*** and operates in such way that when the entrance of one horn is closed that of the other is open. This arrangement plays an ***important role at farrowing and regulates the presentation of foetuses at pelvic inlet and prevents the collision*** that otherwise might occur should both horns contract together.

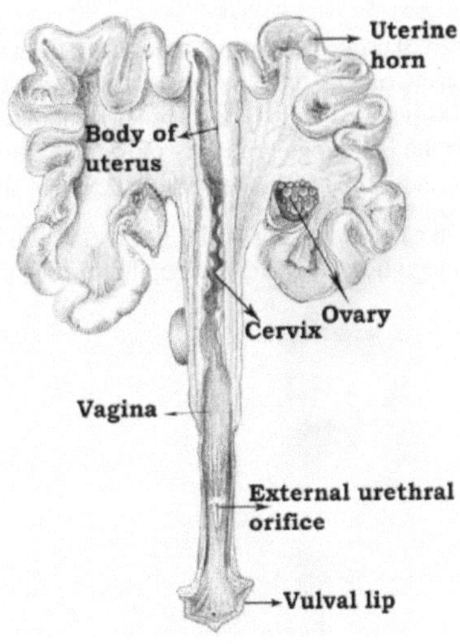

Fig. 6.76: Genitalia of Sow

The Vagina

Cow: is tubular passage **extending from neck of uterus to the vestibule**. The junction with latter is marked by external urethral orifice. Most of it is retroperitoneal. The cranial part is occupied by intravaginal part of the cervix (**Fig.6.73**). It is about 25-30 cm long. It is **related to the rectum dorsally, urinary bladder and urethra ventrally and the pelvic wall laterally**. The mucosa shows longitudinal and transverse folds. The intravaginal part of the cervix of uterus fuses ventrally with the vagina. So **fornix vaginae is deep dorsally and shallow or absent ventrally**. A low transverse fold at the junction of vagina and vestibule just cranial to external urethral orifice represents **hymen in rudimentary form, marking the boundary between vagina and vestibule.**

Mare: The vagina is shorter and distensible. The **fornix is a deep annular recess**. The **transverse fold (hymen) cranial to external urethral orifice is prominent (Fig.6.74).**

Bitch: The vagina is relatively long and narrow anteriorly. The **fornix is indistinct**. The mucosa shows longitudinal or transverse folds (**Fig.6.75**).

Sow: The mucosa shows longitudinal folds. At the junction with vestibule is an annular fold homologous to hymen.

The Vestibule

Cow: It extends from the level of external urethral orifice to the labia of vulva. In **the ventral wall of vestibule between muscular and mucosal coats two *canals of Gartner* are present** one on each side of external urethral orifice. The urethra before opening into the floor of vestibule shows a blind pouch, ***sub-urethral diverticulum***. The **major vestibular glands** are **present caudal to opening of Gartner's canals** and their ducts open on the floor of the vestibule caudal and lateral to external urethral orifice (**Fig.6.73**). Constrictor vestibuli in cow arises from fascia covering retractor ani and ends in a flat tendon which passes under the cranial end of vestibule to meet opposite one.

Mare: The mucosa is folded. **Only minor vestibular glands are present**. Their openings are arranged in two ventral and two dorsolateral rows. **There are large nodular vestibular bulbs, areas of erectile tissue in lateral wall**. The suburethral diverticulum is absent.

Bitch: The mucosa is folded. Its lateral wall shows the vestibular bulbs. On floor of the vestibule **minor vestibular glands** are arranged in two rows. The **suburethral diverticulum is absent.**

Sow: In floor of vestibule is entrance to **suburethral diverticulum**. Two rows of minor vestibular glands open onto floor of vestibule.The mucosa is **bluish red** and forms longitudinal folds.

The Vulva: The vulva is the terminal part of urogenital tract continuing in front with vestibule and opening externally at the vulval cleft below the anus. It has two thick lips, the labia vulvae which unite dorsally and ventrally to form commissures. The ventral ends of the vulval lips are pointed and show number of long hairs. The **vulval cleft is a vertical slit (Fig.6.77)**. The **clitoris** is the homologue of penis present at the ventral commissure and shows root, body and glans. The root is attached to the ischial arch, the body is flexuous and end of the **glans is pointed**.

Mare: The ventral ends of vulval **lips are rounded (Fig.6.77)**. The labial skin is pigmented. The **glans clitoridis is rounded** and covered by pigmented integument. It occupies deep fossa clitoridis.

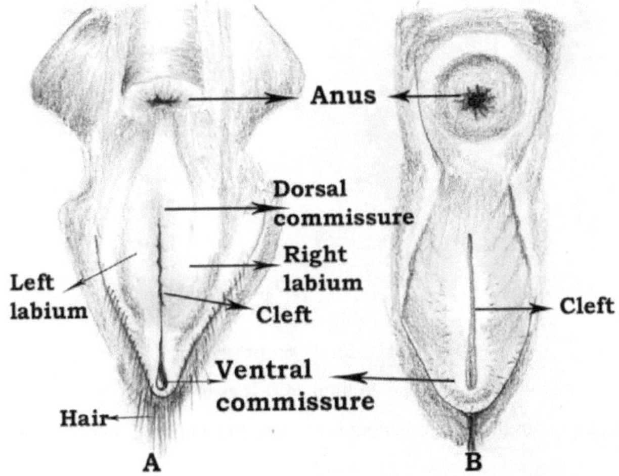

Fig. 6.77: Vulval Lips of Cow (A) and Mare (B)

Bitch: The lips are thick and ventral ends are pointed **(Fig.6.78)**. The labial skin is often pigmented. The glans clitoridis lies in fossa clitoridis.

Sow: It is somewhat ***conical and slopes so that the cleft faces dorsocaudally***. The labia are round and wrinkled and bear few hairs **(Fig.6.78)**. The ventral commissure is pointed. In some gilts the cone is upturned, making the cleft inaccessible to the boar.

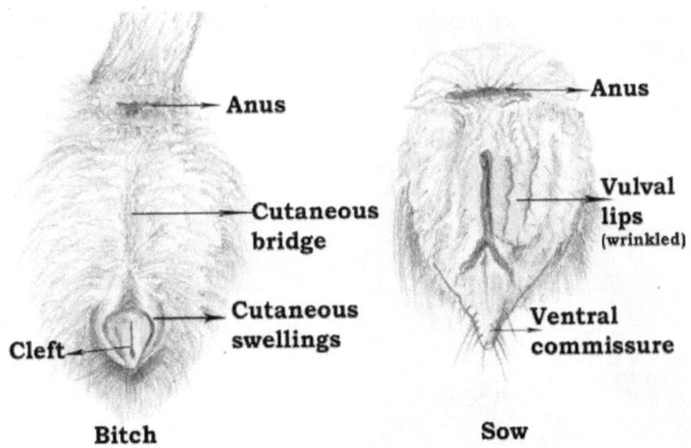

Fig. 6.78: Vulval Lips of Bitch and Sow

The Female Urethra

The female urethra has only pelvic portion which lies centrally on pelvic floor and related dorsally to the vagina.

Cow: It is short and dilatable and opens at the junction of vagina and vestibule. The urethral crest extends caudally only to the middle of the urethra. It shows a blind pouch beneath the external urethral orifice viz. ***sub-urethral diverticulum*** **(Fig.6.79)**. *Because suburethral diverticulum is ventral to urethral orifice catheter or A.I rod passed along floor of vestibule often enters diverticulum resulting in deposition of semen in improper location.*

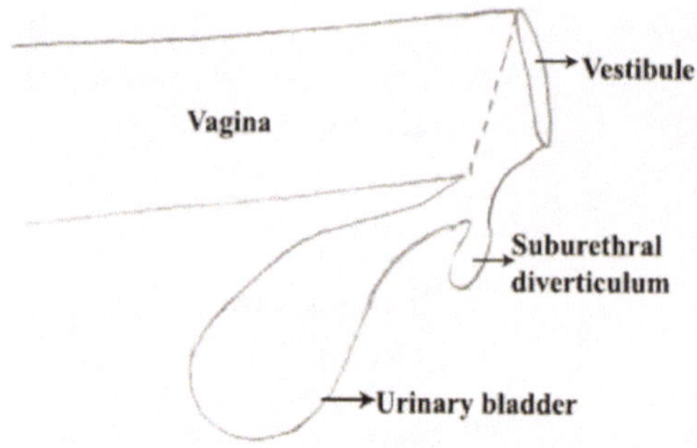

Fig. 6.79: Female Urethra (schematic)

Mare: The suburethral diverticulum is absent and urethral crest is as in cow.

Sow: The urethra is long and suburethral diverticulum is present. In addition to smooth muscle **striated urethralis muscle** is also present.

Bitch: The sub-urethral diverticulum is absent. The urethra is long. In addition to smooth muscles the striated urethralis muscle is also present.

Hen: The urethra is absent.

The Mammary Glands

The mammary glnads are characteristic of mammals and produce milk. Milk synthesis requires that a large amount of blood passes through the udder. This has been estimated as 600 litres of blood for each litre the milk produced.

Cow: The four glands are together called udder and each gland constitutes a quarter. Hence there are two fore quarters and two hind quarters. A prominent median intermammary groove marks the division of udder into right and left halves. The base of each gland is slightly concave and **attached to abdominal wall and pelvic symphysis by suspensory apparatus** consisting of four lamiane, **two of which are well developed and median in position and two are lateral laminae (Fig.6.80)**. These laminae are made up of yellow elastic tissue. Each gland consists of a ***body (glandular portion) and a cylindrical papilla (teat).***

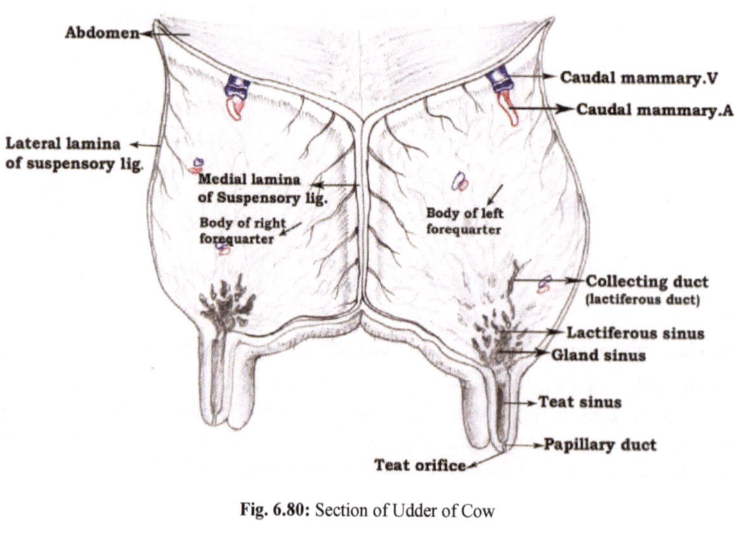

Fig. 6.80: Section of Udder of Cow

The body is ellipsoidal in form. The lateral surface of the gland is convex, while medial surface is flat. The secretory units of gland, alveoli are drained by alveolar duct into lactiferous ducts the latter opening into lactiferous sinus. The **lactiferous sinus has two parts gland sinus and teat sinus.** The latter is connected by **single** teat canal (***papillary duct***) to the exterior **(Fig.6.80)**. The annular fold and erectile venous circle (***Furstenberg's venous ring***) are present at the junction between the gland and teat sinuses. The teat canal has longitudinal folds that project into the teat sinus forming "***Furstenberg's rosette***"

> *The pudic nerve as well as first four lumbar nerves must be blocked to anaesthetise udder. The duct system of individual glands (quarters) doesn't communicate, hence drugs administered locally for treatment of mastitis must be injected into each quarter. Teat surgery can be performed with a ring block around the base of the teat.*

Mare: The **two glands** are in prepubic region on either side of mid-line and are much smaller. They are in the form of flattened cone. The ***teats have 2-4 teat canals***.

Bitch: Usually **ten glands** are present in two series from posterior part of pectoral region to inguinal region. The teats are short and ***have 6-12 teat canals***.

Sow: Most sows have **seven pairs of mammary glands** forming ventral contour of the trunk and **extending from the axilla to the stifle**. In lactating sows the caudal glands are more pendulous than the cranial ones and their teats point somewhat laterally.

Hen: Cutaneous glands (except uropygial glands) are absent in birds.

6.7 SURGICAL OPERATIONS OF THE PELVIS AND HIND LIMB

1. NERVE BLOCKS AND NEURECTOMIES OF HIND LIMB

Tibial nerve block and neurectomy: Tibial nerve supplies branches to the muscles of the plantar aspect of the leg region.

Site: On the medial aspect of the leg about a hands breadth above the point of hock and infront of the tendo achilles **(Fig.6.81)**.

Peroneal nerve block and neurectomy: The nerve gives branches to the all the dorsolateral group muscles of the leg **(Fig.6.81).**

Site: Two inches below and behind the lateral condyle of the tibia in the groove between peroneus longus and lateral digital extensor muscles.

Plantar nerve block and neurectomy:

Site: same as volar nerve block in forelimb.

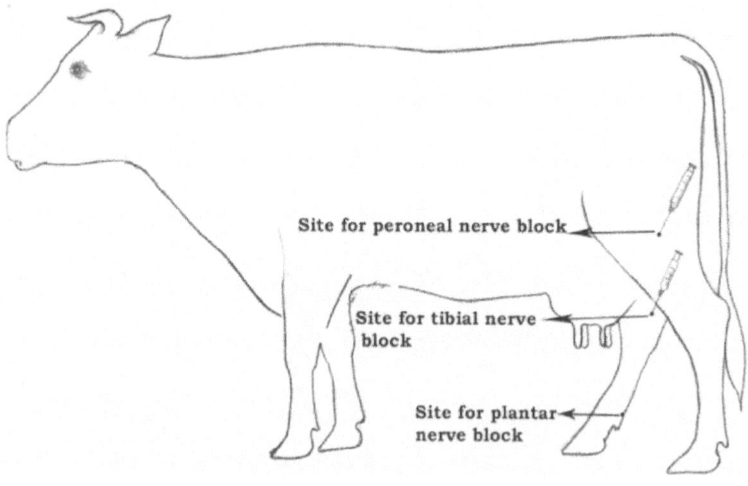

Fig. 6.81: Sites for Nerve Blocks of Hind Limb

Pudic nerve block: can be best performed by palpating per rectum the internal pudic artery and nerve on the lateroventral aspect of the pelvic cavity just cranial to the lesser sciatic foramen.

Indications: Surgical interference with the penis and prepuce.

Site: The ischiorectal fossa of either side between the anal orifice and the ischial tuberosity.

2. Patellar desmotomy

Indications: In chronic subluxation of patella, the patella gets fixed above the trochlea of femur and the medial straight ligament is tightly over stretched behind the medial trochlear ridge which prevents the downward return of the patella. This is because medial ridge of trochlea of femur is larger and higher than lateral one. So the stifle joint is in an extended state and animal drags the limb. This is more common in the emaciated animals. Two palpable dimples at the proximal end of the tibial tuberosity separate and identify three straight ligaments of patella.

The objective of the operation is to mechanically bring down the patella by cutting the tensed medial straight ligament of the patella.

Site: close to the insertion of the medial ligament to the anterior tuberosity of tibia. This is most suitable site as it is easier to locate, causes less bleeding and there is no danger of injuring the joint capsule. Bleeding if any is from geniculate artery supplying this joint which is a branch of femoral artery.

3. Intraarticular injection of stifle

The femoropatellar and medial and lateral femorotibial joint cavities communicate with each other. Injection to any one therefore spreads throughout system. Two punctures can be used, one between medial and middle patellar ligaments a short distance proximal to tibia and other in sulcus muscularis cranial to tendon of origin of complex muscle for lateral femorotibial compartment.

4. Epidural anaesthesia: Epidural space is the space between the spinal canal and the spinal duramater. This space is filled with fat and areolar tissue.

Site:1. Sacrococcygeal site: Between sacrum and first coccygeal vertebra.

Indications: Primarily for obstetrical and genital surgeries. It desensitizes inguinal region, flank, prepuce, scrotum, mammary glands and part of lumbar region. So it can be used for surgical manipulations of penis in bull and correction of prolapse of uterus and vagina in cow.

Note: In dog lumbosacral space is used for epidural anaesthesia.

Site 2: Inter coccygeal site i.e between first and second coccygeal vertebrae.

Indications: It desensitizes tail, anus, vulva, perineum, thighs and part of sacral region. This can be used for surgical manipulations of penis in bull and correction of prolapses of uterus and vagina in cow.

5. Castration of bull

A. Closed Method: The scrotum of the bull is long and pendulous with a well defined neck, located in inguinal region. The testicles are placed vertically in the scrotum along its long axis. The testicles, epididymis and the spermatic cord are enclosed by a layer of serous membrane called the tunica vaginalis. The spermatic cord consists of an anterior vascular and nervous part and a posterior part containing the vas deferens.

Indications: To prevent indiscriminate breeding and for easy management and maintenance of working cattle.

Site: Neck of the scrotum. In this method an instrument Burdizzo castrator is used to crush the spermatic cord at above mentioned site.

B. Open method: Preferable in Pigs. In this method two testicles are removed by giving a vertical incision in the scrotum.

6. Vasectomy operation: means transaction of vas deferens.As explained previously the spermatic cord consists of a **larger anterior vascular and nervous part** and a small **posterior part consisting of vas deferens**.

Indications: To prevent indiscriminate breeding and vasectomized bull can be used as a teaser to detect heat in female animals in a herd.

Site: On the neck of the scrotum.

7. Cystotomy in bovines

Indications: 1. Calculi in urinary bladder, 2. Neoplastic growth

Site: The prepubic site is chosen along linea alba starting infront of the pubic symphysis to a length of about 3 to 4 inches forward.

8. Urethrotomy in bovines: In bulls the body of the penis forms **'S' shaped (sigmoid) flexure**. It is the common seat of urethral obstruction.

Indications: Urethral obstruction.

Site: **a. Post scrotal site**: for removal of obstruction at the sigmoid flexure, it is about 3 inches behind the scrotum along the mediam line.

b. Ischial site: for removal of obstructions close to the ischial arch. It is two inches below the ischial arch downwards along the median line.

6.8 SUMMARY

Species Differences in Various Male Genital Organs

Testis

	Bull	Stallion	Dog	Boar
Location of Scrotum	Present in front of inguinal region	Present in inguinal region	Placed Behind the inguinal region	Present ventral to the anus in perineal region
Orientation of testicles	***long axis is vertical.***	long axis is ***parallel to the long axis of the body***	***long axis is oblique***	***long axis is vertical.***
Shape of testicles	Oval slightly compressed glands	Globular	Oval	Elliptical.

Accessory Sex Glands

	Bull	Stallion	Dog	Boar
Seminal glands	Paired irregular and elongated glands (often **S-shaped**)	***Pyriform sacs***	Absent	Elongated and large
Prostate Gland:	***Unpaired consists of* the body and Pars disseminata**	Consists of two lobes connected by an **isthmus.** ***Pars disseminata is absent.***	It is very large and **globular in shape** and divided into right and left lobes	The **bulk of the prostate** is formed by **disseminate part**
Cowper's or Bulbo-urethral Glands:	Two in number. **Each has a single duct**.	They are **club shaped, each has 6-8 ducts**.	Absent	Very long and cranially **touch the vesicular glands.**

Penis

	Bull	Stallion	Dog	Boar
1. Type	Fibroelastic	Vascular	Intermediate	Fibroelastic
2. Length	90 cm	50 cm	10 cm	60 cm
3. Sigmoid sigmoid flexure	**Post scrotal**	Absent	Absent	**Pre scrotal**
4.Glans penis	Poorly developed	Glans forms a prominent margin known as **corona glandis** behind which is constriction called **collum glandis**. Its lower part presents a depression called **fossa glandis.**	**Os penis is present**	
5.Prepuce	It consists of external and internal laminae	It has ***double invagination of the skin***.	as in bull	**It has a preputial diverticulum,** a pouch containing a foul smelling fluid.

Species Differences in Various Female Genital Organs

	Cow	Mare	Bitch	Sow	Hen
Ovaries	Small and oval shaped.	**Bean shaped, The *ovulation fossa is present.***	Small, elongated, oval in outline.	Ovaries are tuberculated,	Left ovary is functional, the right one is rudimentary.

Oviduct:	Less flexuous.	more flexuous and joins the uterine horn abruptly.	slightly flexuous		It is divisible into five parts. 1.Infundibulum 2. Magnum is largest 3.Isthmus 4. Uterus. (shell gland) is like a pouch, 5.Vagina is "S" shaped.
Uterus:	about 100 caruncles present .	Caruncles are absent.	The horns are 'V' like.	The horns are very long, coiled and arranged like intestine.	
Vestibule	Major vestibular glands are present.	Only minor vestibular glands are present.	Minor vestibular glands are arranged in two rows.	Two rows of minor vestibular glands are present.	
Vulva	The ventral ends of the vulval lips are pointed.	The ventral ends of vulval lips are rounded.	The lips are thick and ventral ends are pointed.	The ventral commissure is pointed.	

References

Budras K.D., Habel R.E., Wunsche A. and Buda S. 2003. Bovine Anatomy, An illustrated text: 1st Edn.Schlatersche GmbH &Co. K.G., Verlag and Drucjerei.

Dyce K.M., Sack W.O. and Wensing C.J.G. 2010. Text Book of Veterinary Anatomy. 4th Edition, Saunders Elsevier.

Konig H.E. and Liebich H.G. 2007, Veterinary Anatomy of Domestic Mammals, Textbook and Colour Atlas, Schattauer GmbH, Stuttgart, Germany.

Mansour M., Wilhite R. and Joe Rowe 2018. Guide to Ruminant Anatomy, Dissection and Clinical Aspects, 1st edn., John Wiley & Sons. Inc, U.S.A

Madras Lecture Notes prepared by Faculty of Department of Veterinary Anatomy, Madras Veterinary College, Chennai

McLeod. W.W. 1958. Bovine Anatomy, Burges Publishing Company, Minnesota

McLelland. J. 1990. A colour Atlas of Avian Anatomy: Wolfe Publishing Ltd., England.

Nickel. R, Schummer. A and Seiferle. E. 1986. The Anatomy of the Domestic Animals. The locomotor system of the domestic animals, Verlag Paul Parey, Berlin, Hamburg.

Peter Popesko.2011. Atlas of Topographical Anatomy of Domestic Animals, 4th Edition, Vydavatel'stvo Priroda, Bratislava, Slovak Republic.

Robert Getty. 1975. Sisson and Grossman's The Anatomy of the Domestic Animals, Volume I 5th Edition, W.B. Saunders Company, Philadelphia, London, Toronto.

Robert Getty. 1975. Sisson and Grossman's The Anatomy of the Domestic Animals Volume II 5th Edition, W.B. Saunders Company, Philadelphia, London, Toronto.

Schummer. A., Nickel. R and Sack. W.O.1979. The Viscera of the Domestic Mammals, 2nd Revised Edition, Verlag Paul Parey Berlin, Hamburg.

Schummer. A., Wilkens. H., Vollmerhans. B. and Habermahl. KM. 1981. The Circulatory system, the Skin and the Cutaneous organs of the Domestic Mammals. Verlag Paul Parey, Berlin.

Subject Index

D

H

I

J

K

L

M

Menisci 20, 384, 385

N

O

P

T

U

V

W

X&Z